BRAIN AND SPINE IMAGING PATTERNS

The McGraw-Hill Radiology Series
Series Editor: Robert J. Ward, MD

This innovative series offers indispensable workstation reference material for the practicing radiologist. Within this series is a full range of practical, clinically relevant works divided into three categories:

- **Patterns:** Organized by modality, these books provide a pattern-based approach to constructing practical differential diagnoses.
- **Variants:** Structured by modality as well as anatomy, these graphic volumes aid the radiologist in reducing false-positive rates.
- **Cases:** Classic case presentations with an emphasis on differential diagnoses and clinical context.

BRAIN AND SPINE IMAGING PATTERNS

Chi-Shing Zee, MD

Professor of Radiology and Neurosurgery
Keck School of Medicine
University of Southern California
Los Angeles, California

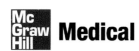 **Medical**

New York   Chicago   San Francisco   Lisbon   London   Madrid   Mexico City
Milan   New Delhi   San Juan   Seoul   Singapore   Sydney   Toronto

Brain and Spine Imaging Patterns

1 2 3 4 5 6 7 8 9 0   CTP/CTP   14 13 12 11 10

ISBN 978-0-07-146541-0
MHID 0-07-146541-3

Notice

Medicine is an ever-changing science. As new research and clinical experience broaden our knowledge, changes in treatment and drug therapy are required. The authors and the publisher of this work have checked with sources believed to be reliable in their efforts to provide information that is complete and generally in accord with the standards accepted at the time of publication. However, in view of the possibility of human error or changes in medical sciences, neither the authors nor the publisher nor any other party who has been involved in the preparation or publication of this work warrants that the information contained herein is in every respect accurate or complete, and they disclaim all responsibility for any errors or omissions or for the results obtained from use of the information contained in this work. Readers are encouraged to confirm the information contained herein with other sources. For example and in particular, readers are advised to check the product information sheet included in the package of each drug they plan to administer to be certain that the information contained in this work is accurate and that changes have not been made in the recommended dose or in the contraindications for administration. This recommendation is of particular importance in connection with new or infrequently used drugs.

This book was set in TradeGothic Light by Aptara®, Inc.
The editors were Michael Weitz and Robert Pancotti.
The production supervisor was Catherine Saggese.
Project management was provided by Samir Roy, Aptara®, Inc.
The text designer was Eve Siegel; the cover designer was The Gazillion Group.
China Translation & Printing Services, Ltd. was printer and binder.

This book is printed on acid-free paper.

Library of Congress Cataloging-in-Publication Data

Zee, Chi S. (Chi Shing)
   Brain and spine imaging patterns / Chi-Shing Zee.
       p. ; cm.
   Includes index
   ISBN-13: 978-0-07-146541-0 (alk. paper)
   ISBN-10: 0-07-146541-3 (alk. paper)
1. Brain—Imaging—Handbooks, manuals, etc. 2. Spine—Imaging--Handbooks, manuals, etc. I. Title.
   [DNLM: 1. Brain Diseases—diagnosis—Handbooks. 2. Diagnostic Techniques, Neurological—Handbooks.
3. Magnetic Resonance Imaging—methods—Handbooks. 4. Spinal Diseases—diagnosis—Handbooks.
5. Tomography, X-Ray Computed—methods—Handbooks. WL 39 Z43b 2010]
   RC473.B7Z44 2010
   616.8′04754—dc22   2009047847

To my wife, Rosa Zee

Each Pattern Highlights Findings, Differential Diagnoses, and Comments

Icons are used to create a grading system

The innovative grading system for the images provides the relative frequency of each diagnosis within the differential, ranging from "common" (five circles) to "unusual" (one circle). The aim of this grading system is to give the reader a sense of appropriateness regarding the practical use of alternate diagnostic considerations.

IMAGE KEY

Common

●●●●●
●●●●
●●●
●●
●

Rare

CONTENTS

CONTRIBUTORS

Jamshid Ahmadi, MD
Professor of Radiology, Keck School of Medicine,
University of Southern California, Los Angeles, California

Kemin Chen, MD
Professor and Chairman of Radiology, Ruijin Hospital,
Jiao Tong University, China

Jingliang Cheng, MD
Professor and Director of Radiology, Henan University
Medical School, China

Xiaoyuan Feng, MD
Professor and Dean, Fudan University
Medical School, China

Daoying Geng, MD
Professor and Vice-Chairman, Huashan Hospital, Fudan
University, China

John L. Go, MD
Assistant Professor of Radiology, Keck School of
Medicine, University of Southern California, Los Angeles,
California

John Grimm, MD
Assistant Professor of Radiology, Department of
Radiology, Children's Hospital of Los Angeles, Keck
School of Medicine, University of Southern California,
Los Angeles, California

Paul E. Kim, MD
Assistant Professor of Radiology, Keck School of
Medicine, University of Southern California, Los Angeles,
California

Ming Law, MD
Professor of Radiology and Neurosurgery, Director of
Neuroradiology, Keck School of Medicine, University
of Southern California, Los Angeles, California

Alex Lerner, MD
Assistant Professor of Radiology, Keck School of
Medicine, University of Southern California, Los Angeles,
California

Ying-Hsuan Li, MD
Medical Staff of Imaging Department, Changhua Christian
Hospital, Taiwan

William Lo, MD
Professor of Radiology, Keck School of Medicine,
University of Southern California, Los Angeles, California

Guangming Lu, MD
Professor and Chairman of Radiology, Nanjing
Jinling Hospital Medical College, Nanjing University,
China

Yong Lu, MD
Associate Professor of Radiology, Ruijin Hospital, Jiao
Tong University, China

C. Mark Mehringer, MD
Professor and Chair of Radiology, Chief of Neuroradiology,
Harbor-UCLA School of Medicine, Torrance, California

Monique Morgensen, MD
Assistant Professor of Radiology, Keck School of
Medicine, University of Southern California, Los Angeles,
California

Maven Nelson, MD
Professor and Chairman, Department of Radiology,
Children's Hospital of Los Angeles, Keck School of
Medicine, University of Southern California, Los Angeles,
California

Steven Rothman, MD
Professor of Radiology, Keck School of Medicine,
University of Southern California, Los Angeles,
California

Hervey D. Segall, MD
Professor of Radiology, Keck School of Medicine,
University of Southern California, Los Angeles,
California

Mark Shiroishi, MD
Assistant Professor of Radiology, Keck School of
Medicine, University of Southern California, Los Angeles,
California

Zhenwei Yao, MD
Huashan Hospital, Fudan University, China

Chi-Shing Zee, MD
Professor of Radiology and Neurosurgery, Keck School of
Medicine, University of Southern California, Los Angeles,
California

FOREWORD

It is with substantial anticipation and excitement that I introduce *Brain and Spine Imaging Patterns*. Chi-Shing Zee, MD, is a recognized expert in neuroimaging and has labored to bring forth an astounding breadth and depth of case material that encompasses the essential patterns of brain and spine imaging.

The Patterns series is meant to assist radiologists at the workstation in the synthesis of practical differential diagnoses. With the material in each book organized by image appearance rather than pathology, the Patterns series carefully guides the reader toward a group of potential diagnoses. We hope that this unique approach will aid the radiologist with comprehensive, intuitive decision support.

Many patterns in this book include a colored box of "Related Patterns" images. These images serve as cross-references to alternate differential schemes in an attempt to efficiently direct the reader to the pertinent information.

The innovative grading system for the images provides the relative frequency of each diagnosis within the differential, ranging from "common" (five circles) to "unusual" (one circle). The aim of this grading system is to give the reader a sense of appropriateness regarding the practical use of alternate diagnostic considerations.

Our ultimate aim for the Patterns series is to create a practical resource for radiologists at the workstation, to which they can refer on a regular basis. Please look forward to future books in the Patterns series, as well as the corresponding volumes *Brain and Spine Imaging Cases,* which will feature a library of cases, and *Brain and Spine Imaging Variants*, with its exhaustive cross-modality lists of pitfalls and variants.

Congratulations to Dr. Zee! He has done an exemplary job in creating a practical and comprehensive work.

Robert J. Ward, MD, CCD
Chief, Division of Musculoskeletal Radiology
Department of Radiology
Tufts Medical Center
Director, Medical Student Education
Assistant Professor of Radiology and Orthopaedics
Tufts University School of Medicine
Boston, Massachusetts

Consultant
Sullivan's Island Imaging, LLC
Sullivan's Island, South Carolina

PREFACE

Since the introduction of computed tomography (CT) in 1974, there has been a tremendous change in the medical management of patients. Literally thousands of patients have been saved or their quality of life improved as a result of an accurate diagnosis provided by CT. Although the improvement in diagnosis and management has occurred in all medical specialties, it has been most impressive in the neurologic diseases. As the evolution and refinement of CT equipment have been remarkable in the development of patient diagnosis, the development of magnetic resonance imaging (MRI) since the early 80s has been just as impressive. An imaging modality has evolved into something well beyond anyone's imagination. A repeat of the CT revolution has occurred with MRI. This time, MRI gradually has taken over CT as the imaging modality of choice for neurologic disorders. Recently, more sophisticated imaging techniques using MRI have evolved into tools of molecular imaging, including diffusion tensor imaging, proton spectroscopy, and perfusion imaging. However, these new techniques are beyond the scope of this book.

This book uses an approach that is quite different from that of the usual radiology textbooks. It is based on various patterns seen on CT or MRI; an exemplary disease illustrating the pattern is presented, followed by a list of differential diagnoses. The book is divided into chapters according to anatomic locations of intracranial pathology. Chapters that cover lesions of the brain and lesions of the spine are grouped into separate sections within each part of the book. MRI findings for lesions with various imaging patterns involv-ing the skull are included in Chapter 1, and so on. CT and MRI findings of disease entities are separated into two different parts because of the logistics of this book. The book includes only one chapter on plain radiography of the skull because this modality is now seldom used to evaluate neurologic diseases. CT patterns and MRI patterns are vastly different. Almost all of the CT scans currently performed to evaluate neurologic diseases are without intravenous contrast injection. Therefore, the usefulness of CT in neuroimaging is limited to the evaluation of density of lesions and the presence or absence of calcification. Hence, more attention is paid to evaluate various patterns recognized on MRI, including contrast-enhanced MRI.

The aim of this book is to make the process of differential diagnosis easier based on patterns seen on imaging studies. The book is designed as a handy reference for radiology and neuroscience residents, fellows, clinicians, and radiologists in their daily practice. The book is not intended as an all-inclusive neuroradiology reference. Disease processes without specific imaging patterns on CT or MRI are not included in this book. For more in-depth treatment of given topics, the reader is encouraged to refer to the current literature or to recently published neuroradiology textbooks.

In summary, this pattern-based teaching file is intended to be integrated, practical, and efficient. I hope that the goals of this book have been reached and that readers will find it useful in their daily practice.

Chi-Shing Zee, MD

ACKNOWLEDGMENTS

Most of the CT and MRI studies in this book were performed at the hospitals of Keck School of Medicine, University of Southern California by an outstanding group of technologists. Special thanks go to Samuel Valencerina for his extraordinary skill and leadership in the supervision of daily performance of MRI studies.

I thank all of my colleagues in the Division of Neuroradiology at Keck School of Medicine, University of Southern California for their support and contribution of their collection of best cases. My sincere appreciation also goes to Dr. Lijun Qian at Renji Hospital and Dr. Yuxin Li at Huashan Hospital, Shanghai, China, and Alan Chia Yi Lin at Midwestern University for their excellent work in organizing a large volume of imaging cases for this book. I also thank Michael Weitz, Acquisitions Editor, and Robert Pancotti, Senior Project Development Editor, of the Medical Publishing Division at McGraw-Hill for their support and pursuit of perfection. I thank Yvonne Klausmeier and Susana Fung for their assistance.

PART I

MAGNETIC RESONANCE IMAGING

SECTION I

BRAIN

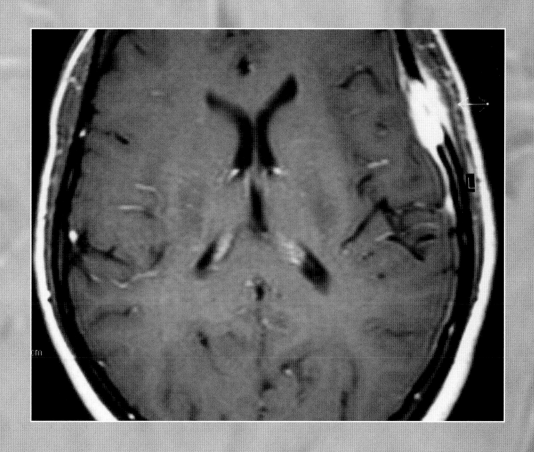

Chapter 1

Skull Defects and Lesions

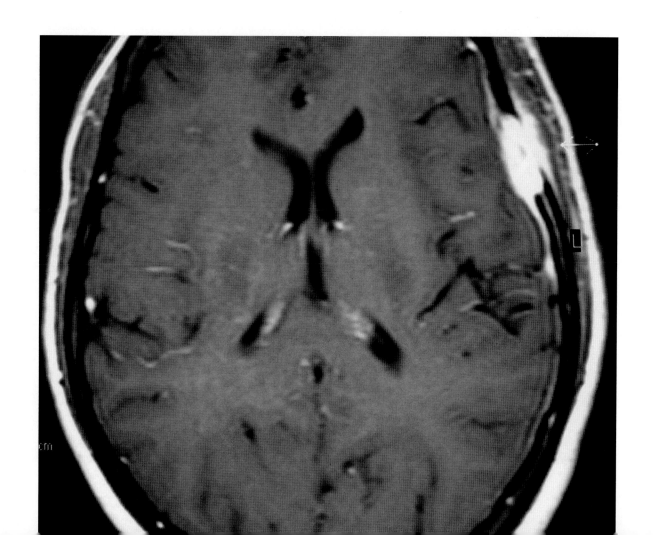

LANGERHANS CELL GRANULOMATOSIS

The skull defect has a characteristic beveled edge, which could be seen on skull X-ray, CT, and MR. **Langerhans cell granulomatosis (Eosinophilic granulomas)** arise from the diploic space, most commonly in the parietal and temporal bones. It is a disease of children and young adults, predominantly in males.

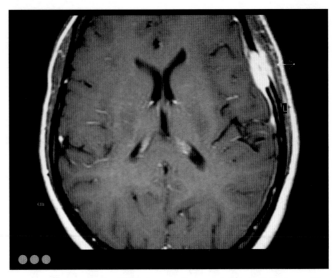

A. A contrast-enhanced MR image shows a lytic skull lesion with an enhancing mass. Adjacent dural enhancement and scalp soft tissue enhancement are also seen.

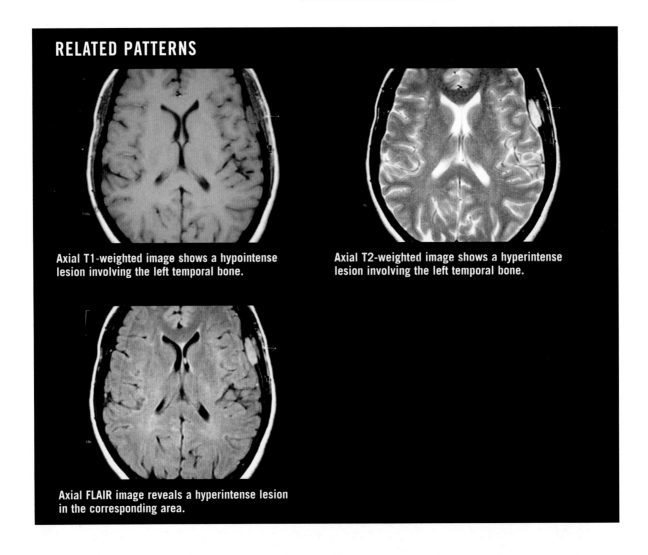

RELATED PATTERNS

Axial T1-weighted image shows a hypointense lesion involving the left temporal bone.

Axial T2-weighted image shows a hyperintense lesion involving the left temporal bone.

Axial FLAIR image reveals a hyperintense lesion in the corresponding area.

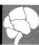

DIFFERENTIAL DIAGNOSIS

At a Glance:

- *Aneurysm Bone Cyst*
- *Arachnoid Granulation*
- *Epidermoid*
- *Hamangioma*
- *Hemangiopericytoma*
- *Lymphoma*
- *Meningioma*

- *Meningoencephalocele*
- *Metastatic Disease (Breast Carcinoma)*
- *Metastatic Disease (Melanoma)*
- *Osteoblastoma*
- *Plasmacytoma*
- *Ostemyelitis* (not pictured)
- *Paget's Disease* (not pictured)
- *Radiation Necrosis* (not pictured)
- *Venous Lake (Normal Structure)* (not pictured)

ANEURYSM BONE CYST

An **aneurysm bone cyst** is an expansile, osteolytic lesion with a thin wall containing blood-filled cystic cavities. A common presentation includes pain of relatively acute onset that rapidly increases in severity over 6–12 weeks. Trauma is considered an initiating factor in the pathogenesis of some cysts in well-documented cases involving acute fracture. Local hemodynamic alterations related to venous obstruction or arteriovenous fistulae after an injury are important in the pathogenesis of an aneurysm bone cyst. Sometimes, the lesion is a component of, or arises within, a preexisting bone tumor, this finding further substantiates the fact that aneurysm bone cysts occur in an abnormal bone as a result of associated hemodynamic changes. An aneurysm bone cyst can arise from a preexisting chondroblastoma, a chondromyxoid fibroma, an osteoblastoma, a giant cell tumor, or fibrous dysplasia.

On MR imaging, mixed signal intensity is seen on both T1-weighted and T2-weighted images depending on the presence of blood by-product with or without fluid levels. A rim of low signal intensity with internal septa may produce a multicystic appearance.

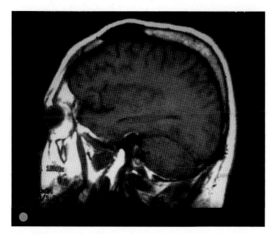

B1. Sagittal T1-weighted image demonstrates an expansile hypointense lesion involving the left frontal bone.

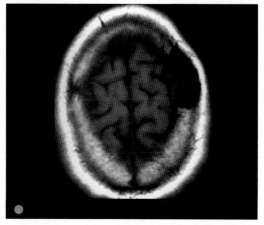

B2. Axial T1-weighted image demonstrates an expansile hypointense lesion involving the left frontal bone.

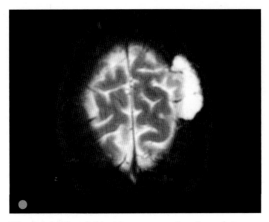

B3. Axial T2-weighted image reveals a hyperintense cystic lesion in the left frontal bone. Sometimes, a fluid–blood level may be seen in these small cysts.

ARACHNOID GRANULATION

Arachnoid granulations are growths of arachnoid membrane into the dural sinuses, through which the cerebrospinal fluid (CSF) is absorbed into the venous system from the subarachnoid space. Arachnoid granulations increase in numbers and enlarge with age in response to increased CSF pressure from the subarachnoid space and are usually quite apparent by 4 years of age. They usually measure a few millimeters in size but may grow to expand the inner table of the skull, most commonly around midline in the posterior frontal or anterior parietal area. Occasionally, they even expand into the diploic space and eventually involve the outer table, mimicking osteolytic lesions.

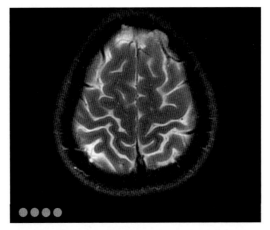

C1. Axial T2-weighted images show a hyperintense structure with remodeling of the inner table of the skull in the parasagittal region.

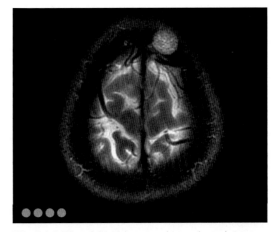

C2. Axial T2-weighted images show a hyperintense structure with remodeling of the inner table of the skull in the parasagittal region.

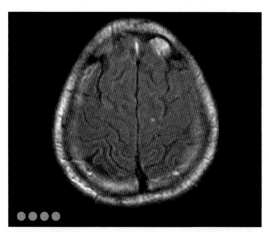

C3. Axial FLAIR images reveal a hyperintense structure in the parasagittal region.

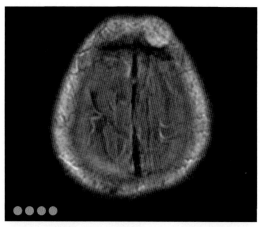

C4. Axial FLAIR images reveal a hyperintense structure in the parasagittal region.

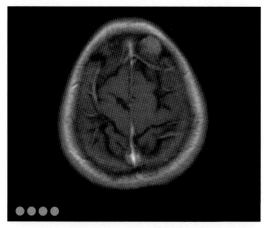

C5. Axial post-contrast T1-weighted image shows an enhancing structure in the parasagittal region.

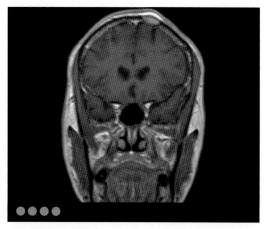

C6. Coronal post-contrast T1-weighted image shows an enhancing structure in the parasagittal region.

ARACHNOID GRANULATION (CASE TWO)

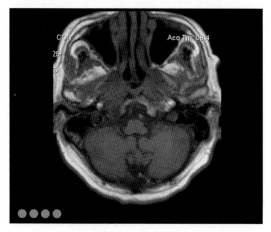

D1. Axial T1-weighted image shows a hypointense lesion involving the inner table and diploic space of the skull in the region of transverse sinus.

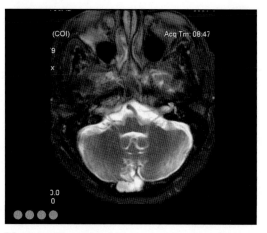

D2. Axial T2-weighted image reveals a hyperintense lesion involving the inner table of the skull and diploic space in the region of transverse sinus.

9

EPIDERMOID

Epidermoids consist of an epithelial capsule filled by desquamated epithelial cells and keratin. Epidermoid are derived from epithelial cell rests ectopically included in the bone during development. They are commonly seen in or near the midline in the vertex, the frontal or occipital regions or in the temporal bone. They originate in the diploe and enlarge in both directions expanding and thinning both tables of the skull. Sclerotic change may be seen at the edge of the lesion. The lesion may break through the thin tables and expand under the scalp or extradurally. The swelling under the scalp is firm, rubbery and non-tender. Giant intradiploic epidermoids tend to get infected resulting in osteomyelitis.

Epidermoids usually exhibit hypointensity on T1-weighted images and hyperintensity on T2-weighted images, similar to CSF. Occasionally, they can show hyperintensity on both T1- and T2-weighted images due to saponification of its content or hemorrhage. Diffusion-weighted imaging of epidermoids exhibits restricted diffusion, thus differentiating them from arachnoid cysts.

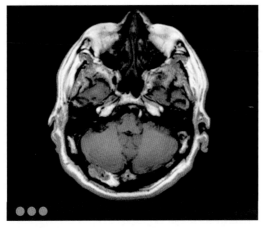

E1. Axial T1-weighted image shows a predominantly hyperintense lesion within the occipital bone on the right side.

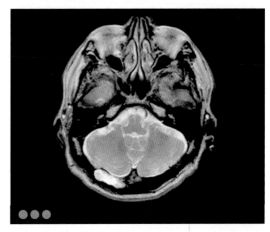

E2. Axial T2-weighted image shows a predominantly hyperintense lesion within the occipital bone on the right side.

EPIDERMOID (CASE TWO)

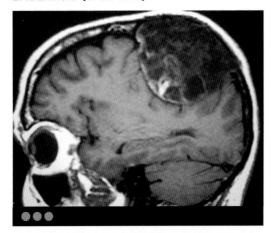

F1. Axial T2-weighted image shows a large, predominantly hyperintense mass involving the skull and epidural space.

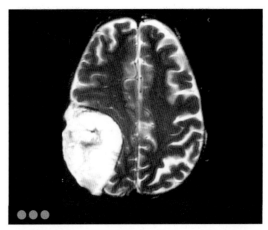

F2. Axial post-contrast T1-weighted image reveals a heterogeneously hypointense mass involving the skull and epidural space. Some marginal dural enhancement is seen.

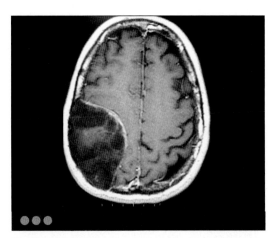

F3. Axial T1-weighted image reveals a heterogeneously hypointense mass involving the skull and epidural space. Some marginal dural enhancement is seen.

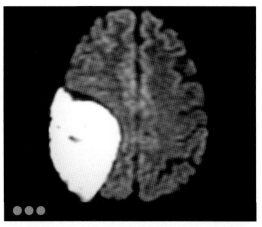

F4. Diffusion-weighted image shows restricted diffusion in the mass.

HEMANGIOMA

Hemangiomas arise from the diploic space and expand the outer table. Magnetic resonance imaging may show evidence of previous hemorrhage. There are four types of hemangioma, namely, capillary, cavernous, arteriovenous and venous types. Bone hemangiomas are predominantly of the capillary and cavernous types. Skull hemangiomas are usually of the cavernous variety.

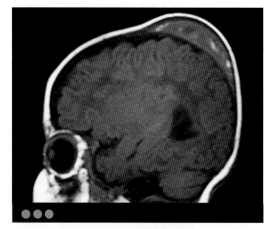

G1. Sagittal and axial T1-weighted images show a predominantly isointense lesion with small areas of hyperintensity (probably due to hemorrhage) involving the calvarium.

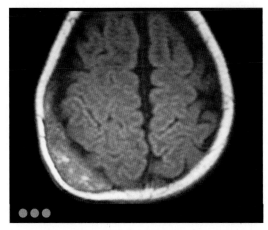

G2. Sagittal and axial T1-weighted images show a predominantly isointense lesion with small areas of hyperintensity involving the calvarium.

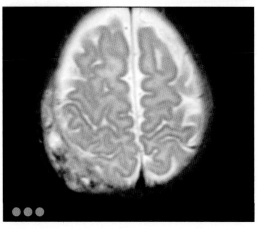

G3. Axial T2-weighted image shows a heterogeneously hyperintense lesion involving the calvarium.

11

HEMANGIOPERICYTOMA

Hemangiopericytoma of the meninges is an aggressive, highly vascular neoplasm. It arises from vascular pericytes and is therefore a distinct entity. On imaging studies, it is a heterogeneous mass with cystic, necrotic areas, and prominent vascular channels. Associated bony destruction is frequently seen.

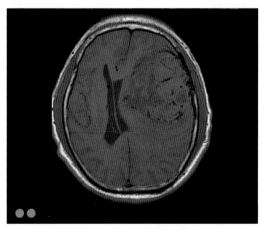

H1. Axial T1-weighted image shows a slightly hypointense mass with cuvilinear signal voids and cystic, necrotic changes in the left frontal convexity with associated bony destruction.

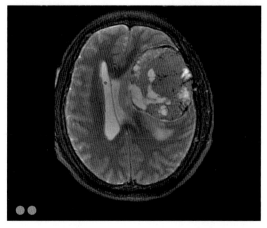

H2. Axial T2-weighted image reveals a hyperintense mass with cuvilinear signal voids and cystic, necrotic changes in the left frontal convexity with associated bony destruction.

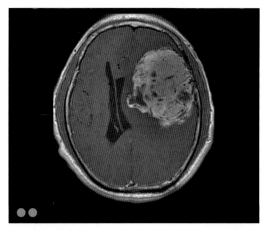

H3. Axial and coronal, post-contrast T1-weighted images show a heterogeneously enhancing mass in the left frontal convexity.

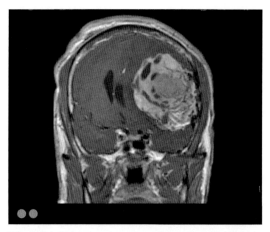

H4. Axial and coronal, post-contrast T1-weighted images show a heterogeneously enhancing mass in the left frontal convexity.

LYMPHOMA

About 10% of the patients with systemic **lymphoma** develop CNS involvement in clinical series, and secondary CNS lymphoma may be found in up to 26% of the cases in autopsy series. Primary CNS lymphomas are more common than secondary CNS lymphoma. Approximately 20 to 40% of lesions are multiple. Some 31% of patients with primary lymphoma develop leptomeningeal disease. They can present as scalp lesions, skull lesions, and epidural lesions in addition to parenchymal, leptomeningeal, and subependymal disease.

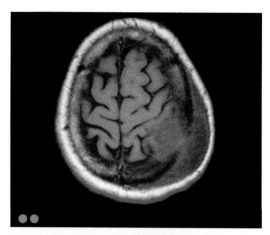

I1. Axial T1-weighted image shows a lytic, hypointense lesion involving the calvarium with a large extracranial component and a small epidural component.

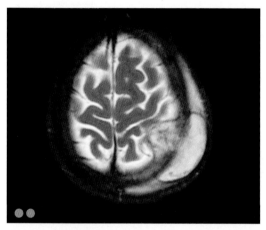

I2. Axial T2-weighted image reveals a hyperintense lesion involving the skull, epidural space, and extracranial scalp.

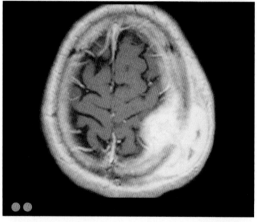

I3. Axial T1-weighted, post-contrast image shows a large enhancing mass involving the bony calvarium, epidural space, and extracranial scalp.

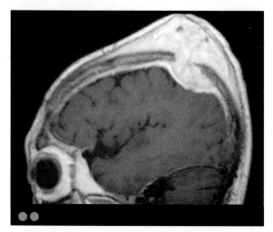

I4. Sagittal T1-weighted, post-contrast image shows a large enhancing mass involving the bony calvarium, epidural space, and extracranial scalp.

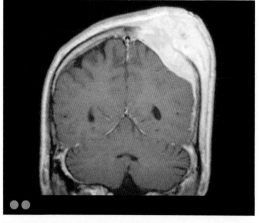

I5. Coronal T1-weighted, post-contrast image shows a large enhancing mass involving the bony calvarium, epidural space, and extracranial scalp.

MENINGIOMA

Meningiomas usually cause bony hyperostosis of the adjacent skull, but occasionally they can produce lytic changes of the skull and even extend extracranially. On MRI, they usually show isointensity on both T1 weighted and T2 weighted images. Contrast enhancement is usually homogeneous. Cystic and necrotic changes may occasionally be seen. Tumor calcification is better demonstrated by CT.

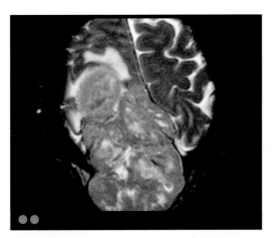

J1. Axial T2-weighted image shows a mixed hyperintense mass involving the skull, epidural space, and extracranial scalp. Several small cystic areas are seen within the mass.

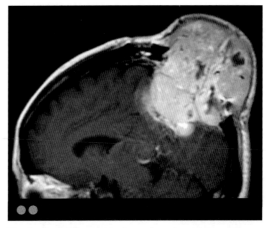

J2. Sagittal T1-weighted, post-contrast image shows a large enhancing epidural mass with bony destruction and extracranial extension. Small cystic areas are seen within the enhancing mass.

MENINGOENCEPHALOCELE

A **meningoencephalocele** is the result of failure of the surface ectoderm to separate from neuroectoderm. A skull and dural defect occurs, which allows the herniation of CSF, brain tissue and meninges. Encephaloceles located in the occipital region are more commonly seen in Europe and North America whereas those involving the forehead and nose are more commonly seen in Southeast Asia.

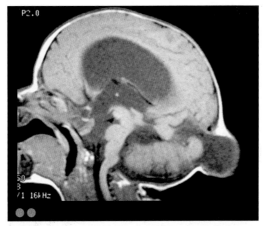

K1. Sagittal and axial T1-weighted images show a skull defect in the occipital region with herniation of the meninges, cerebral spinal fluid, and dysplastic neuronal tissue through the defect.

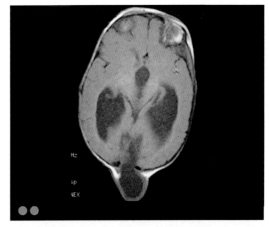

K2. Sagittal and axial T1-weighted images show a skull defect in the occipital region with herniation of the meninges, cerebral spinal fluid, and dysplastic neuronal tissue through the defect.

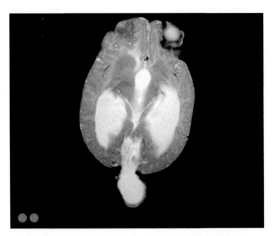

K3. Axial T2-weighted image demonstrates herniation of the meninges containing CSF and dysplastic tissue.

METASTATIC DISEASE

Primary sites are usually breast, lung, prostate, kidney, thyroid, and melanoma. Diploic space is involved before the inner or outer table of the skull. Because of its rich blood supply, the calvarium is more commonly involved than the skull base. Bone metastases are usually due to hematogenous spread of tumor cells and typically multiple although direct tumor extension and retrograde venous flow may also occur. About 70% of the bone metastases occur in the ribs, spine including sacrum, and skull (sites with residual red marrow).

METASTATIC DISEASE (BREAST CARCINOMA)

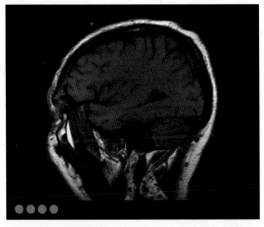

L1. Sagittal and axial T1-weighted images show a lytic, isointense skull lesion in the right parietal, parasagittal region with a small epidural and scalp components.

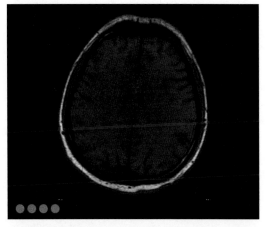

L2. Sagittal and axial T1-weighted images show a lytic, isointense skull lesion in the right parietal, parasagittal region with a small epidural and scalp components.

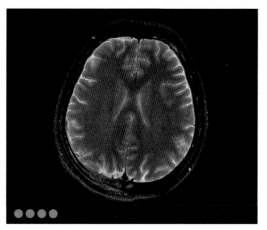

L3. Axial T2-weighted image shows a slightly hyper-intense lesion involving the skull, epidural space, and scalp.

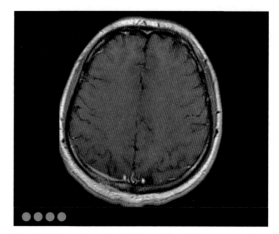

L4. Axial, post-contrast T1-weighted image reveals an enhancing mass involving the calvarium, epidural space, and scalp.

METASTATIC DISEASE (MELANOMA)

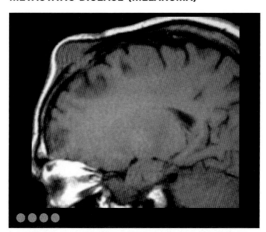

M1. Sagittal and axial T1-weighted images show an isointense lesion involving the frontal bone with extracranial extension into the scalp.

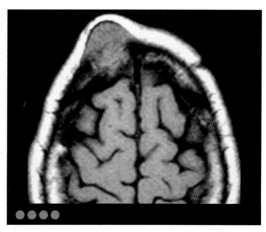

M2. Sagittal and axial T1-weighted images show an isointense lesion involving the frontal bone with extracranial extension into the scalp.

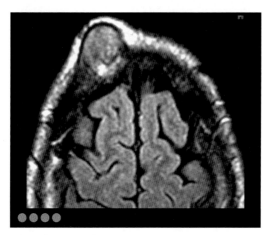

M3. Axial FLAIR imaging shows a mixed hyperintense lesion involving the skull and scalp.

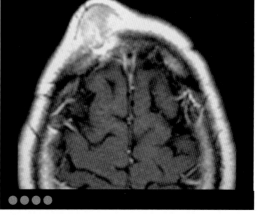

M4. Axial and coronal T1-weighted, post-contrast images show an enhancing mass involving the frontal bone and scalp.

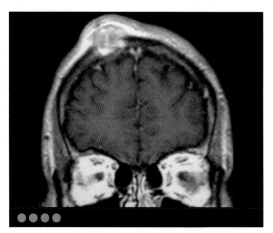

M5. Axial and coronal T1-weighted, post-contrast images show an enhancing mass involving the frontal bone and scalp.

OSTEOBLASTOMA

Benign **osteoblastomas** are rare tumors and their etiology is unknown. Histologically, osteoblastomas are similar to osteoid osteomas, producing both osteoid and primitive woven bone amidst fibrovascular connective tissue. The average age of occurrence is 17 years. They are commonly seen involving the vertebra, femur, mandible, and tibia, skull lesions are extremely rare.

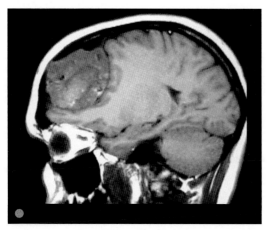

N1. Sagittal T1-weighted image shows a right frontal inner table skull defect associated with a large, extra-axial, mixed signal intensity soft tissue mass.

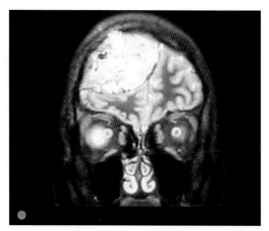

N2. Coronal T2-weighted image reveals a large, extra-axial, hyperintense mass in the right frontal region associated with a skull defect involving inner table.

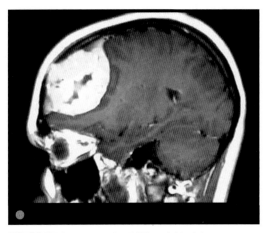

N3. Sagittal, post-contrast T1-weighted image shows marked enhancement of the mass lesion.

PLASMACYTOMA

Solitary **plasmacytomas** of the skull are lesions that, by definition, arise from the skull or dura, are not the result of extension from extracranial skeletal sites of myeloma, and are not associated with plasmacytosis within bone marrow or extracranial myeloma. Urine test for Bence Jones protein (monoclonal light chain) is negative.

Solitary craniocerebral plasmacytoma is a relatively benign entity that is potentially curable, whereas multiple myeloma generally has a poor prognosis. The most common sites of solitary plasmacytomas arising from the skull are the parietal bone and the bones of the skull base. Solitary plasmacytoma of bone may progress to multiple myeloma even as long as 7–23 years after presentation.

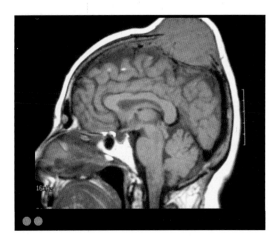

01. Sagittal and coronal T1-weighted images demonstrate an isointense mass involving the skull, epidural space, and extracranial scalp.

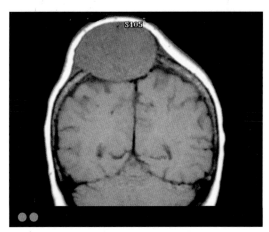

02. Sagittal and coronal T1-weighted images demonstrate an isointense mass involving the skull, epidural space, and extracranial scalp.

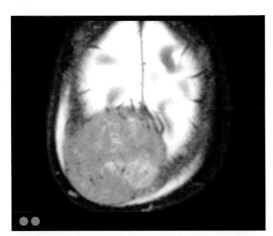

03. Axial T2-weighted image shows a large slightly hypointense mass involving the calvarium, epidural space with extracranial extension. Plasmacytoma tends to exhibit hypointensity on T2-weighted images due to its high cellularity and high nucleus to cytoplasma ratio.

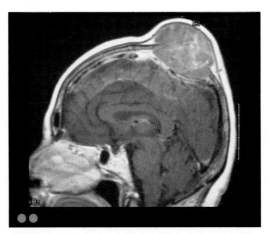

04. Sagittal, coronal, and axial T1-weighted, post-contrast images show a large enhancing mass involving the calvarium with epidural and extracranial extension.

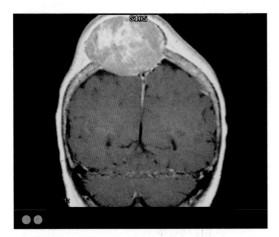

05. Sagittal, coronal, and axial T1-weighted, post-contrast images show a large enhancing mass involving the calvarium with epidural and extracranial extension.

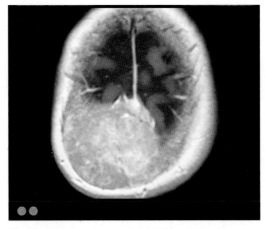

06. Sagittal, coronal, and axial T1-weighted, post-contrast images show a large enhancing mass involving the calvarium with epidural and extracranial extension.

MULTIPLE MYELOMA

Multiple myeloma manifests as an osteolytic process similar to metastatic disease. The skull is the third most frequently affected structure after the vertebral column and ribs. Classically, multiple myeloma appears as multiple rounded, well-circumscribed lesions a few millimeters in diameter, without reactive sclerosis. Mandibular involvement is seen in a third of the cases and may help to differentiate myeloma from metastatic disease.

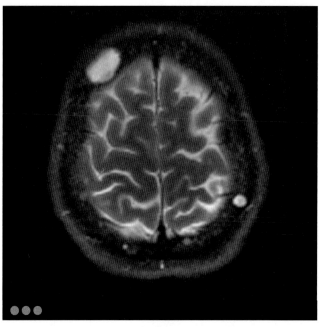

A1. Serial axial T2-weighted images show multiple hyperintense skull lesions due to multiple myeloma.

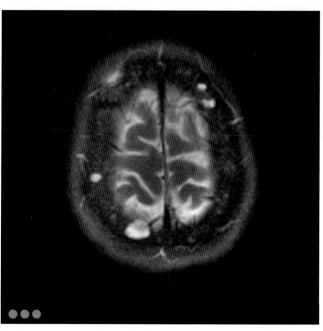

A2. Serial axial T2-weighted images show multiple hyperintense skull lesions due to multiple myeloma.

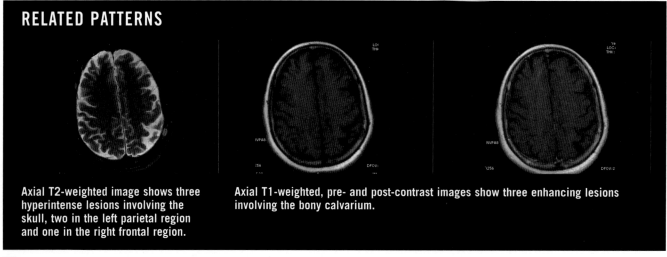

RELATED PATTERNS

Axial T2-weighted image shows three hyperintense lesions involving the skull, two in the left parietal region and one in the right frontal region.

Axial T1-weighted, pre- and post-contrast images show three enhancing lesions involving the bony calvarium.

DIFFERENTIAL DIAGNOSIS

At a Glance:

- *Lymphoma*
- *Metastatic Lesions*
- *Histiocytosis*
- *Hyperparathyroidism*
- *Osteomyelitis*
- *Pacchionian Granulation* (not pictured)
- *Parietal Foramina* (not pictured)
- *Radiation Necrosis* (not pictured)
- *Venous Lake* (not pictured)

LYMPHOMA

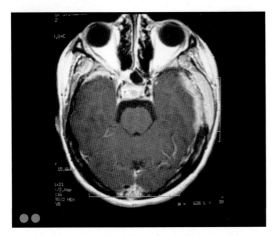

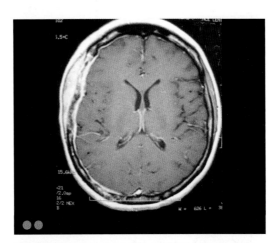

B1. Aixal, post-contrast T1-weighted images show multiple skull lesions associated with epidural enhancing masses in both temporal regions, right frontal and parietal regions.

B2. Aixal, post-contrast T1-weighted images show multiple skull lesions associated with epidural enhancing masses in both temporal regions, right frontal and parietal regions.

METASTATIC LESIONS

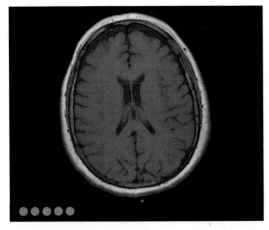

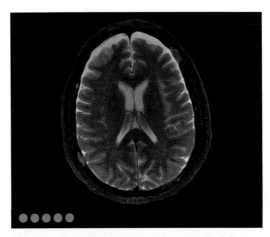

C1. Axial T1-weighted image shows left frontal and right parietal isointense lesions.

C2. Axial T2-weighted images demonstrate left frontal and right parietal hyperintense lesions.

21

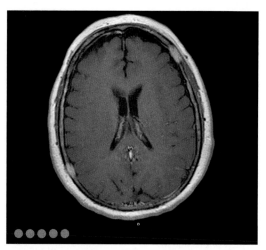

C3. Axial and coronal, post-contrast T1-weighted images reveal enhancing lesions in the left frontal and right parietal region.

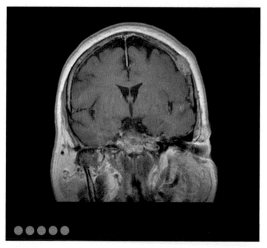

C4. Axial and coronal, post-contrast T1-weighted images reveal enhancing lesions in the left frontal and right parietal region.

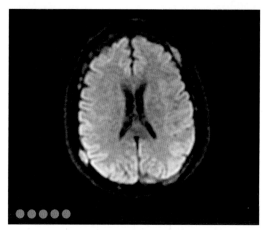

C5. Diffusion-weighted image shows restricted diffusion of these lesions.

INTRAOSSEOUS MENINGIOMA

Intraosseous meningiomas are likely the rarest manifestation of meningioma.

An enhancing dural component may or may not be present. There is usually blastic expansion of both the inner and outer table of the skull.

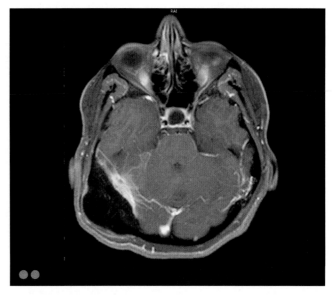

A. Axial T1-weighted, fat-suppressed, post-contrast image shows an enhancing, thin epidural lesion with marked focal thickening of the adjacent occipital bone.

RELATED PATTERNS

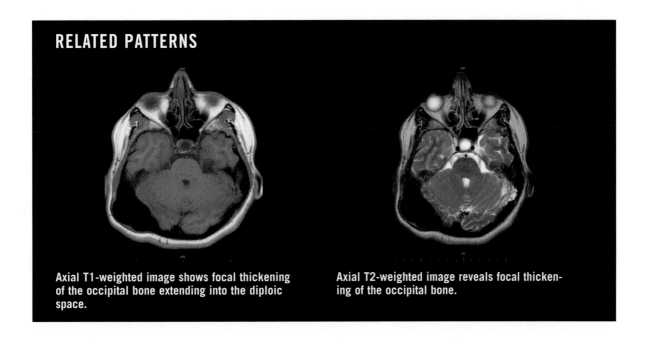

Axial T1-weighted image shows focal thickening of the occipital bone extending into the diploic space.

Axial T2-weighted image reveals focal thickening of the occipital bone.

FIBROUS DYSPLASIA

Fibrous dysplasia is a skeletal developmental anomaly. The medullary bone is replaced by fibrous tissue. Malignant degeneration, although uncommon, may occur in fibrous dysplasia. On plain X-ray, it has a classic "ground glass" appearance. MRI shows predominantly hypointensity on both T1 and T2 weighted images. Contrast enhancement is seen on post-contrast images.

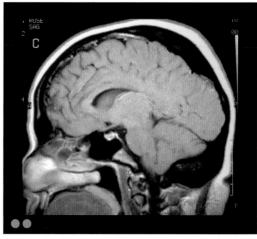

B. Sagittal T1-weighted image shows focal expansion of the calvarium in the parietal and occipital region with replacement of the fatty marrow in the diploic space.

MENINGIOMA

MENINGIOMA (CASE ONE)

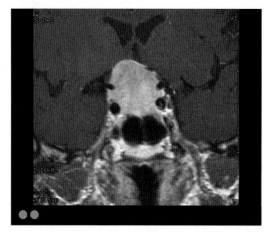

C1. Sagittal and coronal, post-contrast T1-weighted images demonstrate a planum sphenoidal meningioma with suprasellar extension. Note the focal hyperostosis seen in the planum sphenoidale.

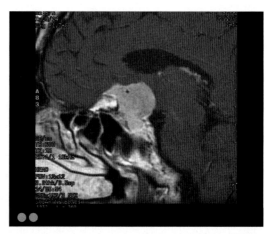

C2. Sagittal and coronal, post-contrast T1-weighted images demonstrate a planum sphenoidal meningioma with suprasellar extension. Note the focal hyperostosis seen in the planum sphenoidale.

MENINGIOMA (CASE TWO)

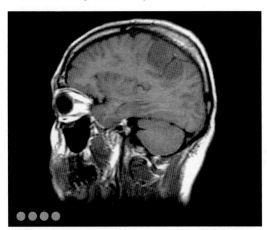

D1. Sagittal and axial T1-weighted images show a hypointense mass with adjacent calvarial hyperostosis in the left parietal region.

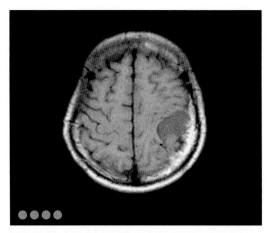

D2. Sagittal and axial T1-weighted images show a hypointense mass with adjacent calvarial hyperostosis in the left parietal region.

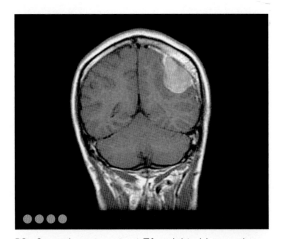

D3. Coronal, post-contrast T1-weighted image shows an enhancing extra-axial mass with adjacent skull hyperostosis in the left parietal region.

OSTEOMA

Osteomas are the most common primary tumors of the bony calvaria, affecting approximately 0.4% of the general population. They are most commonly seen in the paranasal sinuses, especially the frontal sinus, followed by maxilla and mandible. Multiple osteomas of the skull, sinus, and mandible associated with soft tissue tumors of skin and colon polyps are seen in Gardner's syndrome. They are benign mesenchymal osteoblastic tumors composed of well differentiated mature bone tissue with a predominantly laminar structure with slow growth.

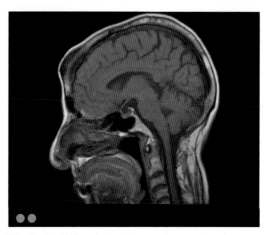

E1. Sagittal T1-weighted image shows a hypointense lesion involving both the inner and outer table of the skull with sparing of the diploic space.

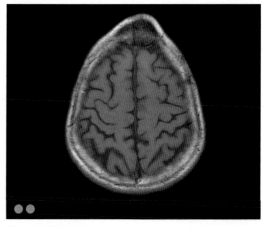

E2. Axial T1-weighted image shows a hypointense lesion involving both the inner and outer table of the skull with sparing of the diploic space.

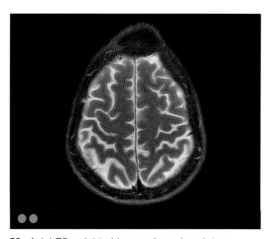

E3. Axial T2-weighted image shows hypointense lesion.

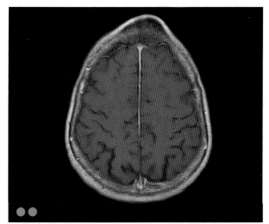

E4. Axial T1-weighted, post-contrast image with fat-suppression reveals a hypointense lesion without any contrast enhancement.

OSTEOMYELITIS

Osteomyelitis is an infection of the bony cortex and bone marrow. It may be divided into acute, subacute and chronic stages. Chronic osteomyelitis may be the initial presentation. Chronic osteomyelitis is uncommon in the United States, but may be seen in developing nations.

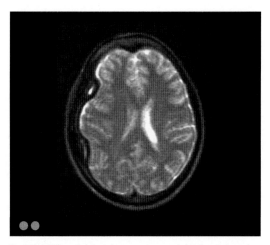

F. Axial T2-weighted image shows right frontal and parietal focal calvarial thickening containing some hyperintense tissue.

PAGET'S DISEASE

Paget's disease is usually diagnosed in people over 40 years of age and becomes more common as people get older. The disease tends to run in families. In the Unites States, it is found more frequently in the northern states, with up to 3% of all people over 55 years of age are affected with the disease. In the skull, lytic phase is termed "osteoporosis circumscripta". This is followed by osteogenesis. Frontal and/or occipital regions are more frequently involved. The disease may progress to involve the entire skull. Basilar invagination secondary to bone softening may be seen. Facial bone involvement is less frequently seen than in fibrous dysplasia.

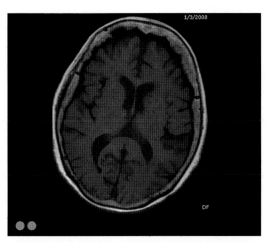

G1. Axial T1-weighted image shows focal thickening of the skull in the frontal region due to Paget's disease.

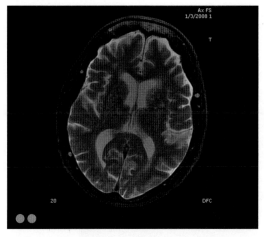

G2. Axial T2-weighted image shows focal thickening of the skull in the frontal region due to Paget's disease. Note the presence of abnormal signal in the frontal bone on T2-weighted image.

PAGET'S DISEASE

The lytic phase of **Paget's disease** is followed by evidence of osteogenesis. Areas of osteolysis and osteosclerosis merge imperceptibly with each other. The trabecular pattern is thickened and disorganized and the tables of the skull become thickened. The third stage of Paget's disease is the inactive or healing phase. The lesions become more sclerotic and thickening of the tables of the skull is more obvious.

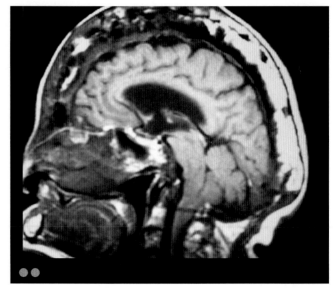

A. Sagittal T1-weighted image shows diffuse calvarial thickening with mixed hyper- and hypointensity seen within the diploic space.

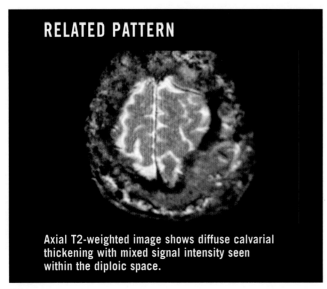

RELATED PATTERN

Axial T2-weighted image shows diffuse calvarial thickening with mixed signal intensity seen within the diploic space.

DIFFERENTIAL DIAGNOSIS

At a Glance:

- *Acromegaly*
- *Sickle Cell Anemia*
- *Thalassemia*
- *Fibrous Dysplasia* (not pictured)
- *Fluorosis* (not pictured)
- *Mucolipidosis* (not pictured)
- *Myelofibrosis* (not pictured)
- *Osteomyelitis* (not pictured)
- *Osteopetrosis* (not pictured)
- *Phenytoin* (not pictured)
- *Shunted Hydrocephalus* (not pictured)

ACROMEGALY

Acromegaly is an endocrine disorder due to increased secretion of growth hormone and characterized by enlargement of many skeletal parts. Endochondral bone formation is reactivated and periosteal bone formation is stimulated.

There is also overgrowth of soft tissue. Such excessive growth is prominent particularly in the hands, feet and skull, especially lower jaw. The skull demonstrates an enlarged sella turcica, increased thickness of the cranial vault, and prominent sinuses and supraorbital ridges.

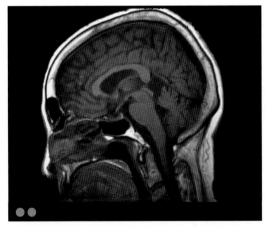

B1. Sagittal T1-weighted image shows diffuse calvarial thickening in a patient with acromegaly.

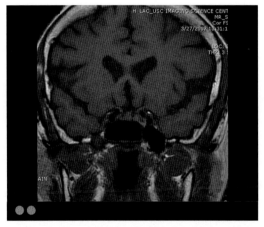

B2. Coronal T1-weighted image shows diffuse calvarial thickening in a patient with acromegaly.

SICKLE CELL ANEMIA

Sickle cell disease denotes all genotypes that contain at least 1 sickle gene in which HbS makes up at least half the hemoglobin present. Sickle cell anemia is the most severe and most common form. Repeated cycles of deoxygena- tion and morphologic sickling irreversibly damage red cell membranes and result in hemolysis. Bone marrow in- creases red blood cell production but is insufficient to compensate for the rate of hemolysis. Increased skull thickness results from expansion of the diploic space, which contains red marrow.

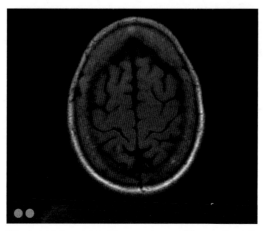

C1. Axial T1-weighted image shows diffuse calvarial thickening in a patient with sickle cell anemia.

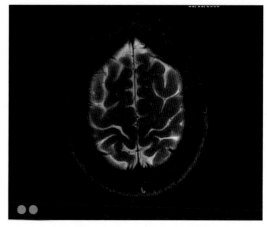

C2. Axial T2-weighted image shows diffuse calvarial thickening in a patient with sickle cell anemia.

THALASSEMIA

Thalassemia is an inherited autosomal recessive disorder. In thalassemia, the genetic defect results in reduced rate of synthesis of one of the globin chains that make up hemoglobin resulting in the formation of abnormal hemoglobin molecules. There are two major types of thalassemia.

Alpha thalassemia occurs predominantly in people from Southeast Asia, Middle East, China and Africa whereas Beta thalassemia is seen in people from Mediterranean region. The skull shows increased thickness due to hyperplasia of the red marrow in an attempt to compensate for the anemia. Widening of the diploic space and thinning of the outer table of the skull are seen.

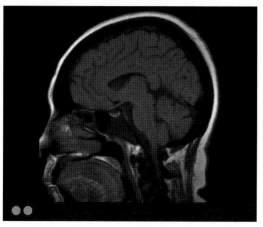

D1. Sagittal T1-weighted image shows diffuse calvarial thickening in a patient with thalassemia. Fatty marrow (hyperintense) in the diploic space and clivus is replaced by cellular marrow (hypointense).

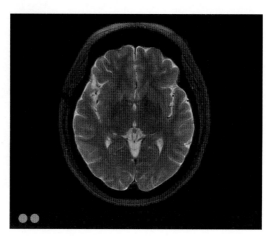

D2. Axial T2-weighted and FLAIR images show skull thickening.

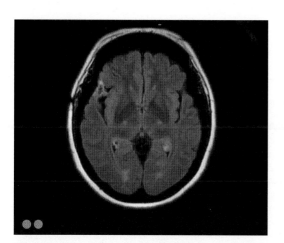

D3. Axial T2-weighted and FLAIR images show skull thickening.

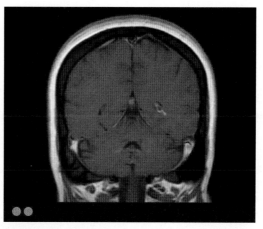

D4. Coronal, post-contrast T1-weighted image reveals no abnormal enhancement in the marrow.

UNILATERAL MEGALENCEPHALY

Unilateral megalencephaly is a rare neurological condition in which one side of the brain or part of the one side is abnormally larger than the other. The enlarged side is usually associated with abnormal neuronal migration. As a consequence, the abnormal and enlarged brain tissue causes frequent seizures, usually followed with mental retardation. Unilateral megalencephaly may occur as an isolated finding in an infant or it may be associated with other syndromes.

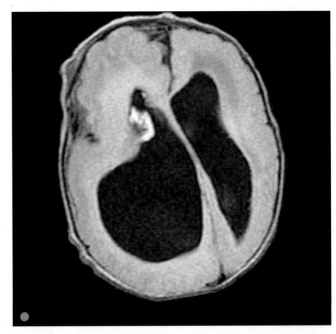

A. Axial T2-weighted FLAIR image shows enlargement of the right hemisphere, right lateral ventricle. There is poor differentiation of the gray and white matter and poor development of sulcation of the right hemisphere. The hyperintensity in the frontal horn of the right lateral ventricle is due to hemorrhage. Although there is no distinct calvarial change, the skull on the side with smaller cerebral hemisphere may appear to be slightly thickened.

RELATED PATTERNS

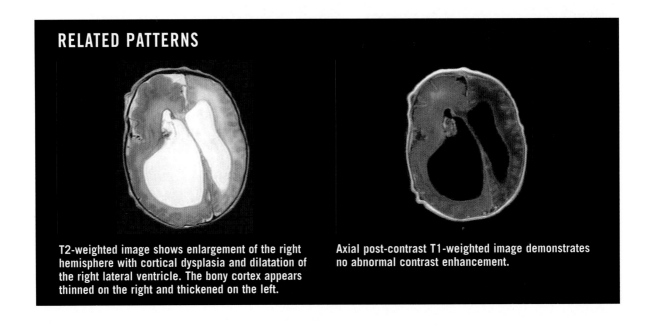

T2-weighted image shows enlargement of the right hemisphere with cortical dysplasia and dilatation of the right lateral ventricle. The bony cortex appears thinned on the right and thickened on the left.

Axial post-contrast T1-weighted image demonstrates no abnormal contrast enhancement.

DIFFERENTIAL DIAGNOSIS

At a Glance:

- *Dyke–Davidoff–Mason Syndrome*
- *Sturge–Weber Syndrome*

DYKE–DAVIDOFF–MASON SYNDROME

The characteristic findings of **Dyke–Davidoff–Mason syndrome** consist of unilateral calvarial thickening (especially of the diploic space), expansion of the ipsilateral ethmoid, frontal sinuses and mastoid, and asymmetry of the planum sphenoidale, anterior clinoid processes.

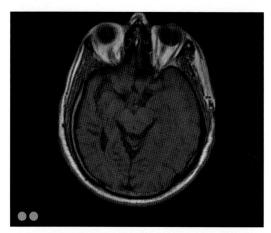

B1. Axial T1- and T2-weighted images show right-sided cerebral hemiatrophy with thickening of the calvarium and dilatation of the ipsilateral lateral ventricle.

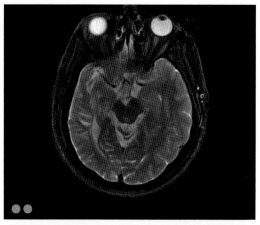

B2. Axial T1- and T2-weighted images show right-sided cerebral hemiatrophy with thickening of the calvarium and dilatation of the ipsilateral lateral ventricle.

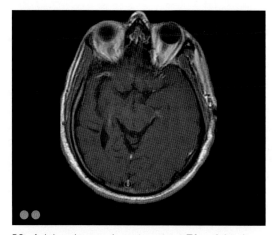

B3. Axial and coronal, post-contrast T1-weighted images demonstrate right-sided cerebral hemiatrophy with dilatation of the right lateral ventricle and thickening of the calvarium on the right side.

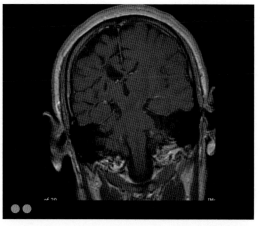

B4. Axial and coronal, post-contrast T1-weighted images demonstrate right-sided cerebral hemiatrophy with dilatation of the right lateral ventricle and thickening of the calvarium on the right side.

STURGE–WEBER SYNDROME

Sturge–Weber syndrome, also known as encephalotrigeminal angiomatosis, is a congenital vascular disorder of the brain, meninges, and the face in the trigeminal distribution, often involving the eye. The intracranial lesion is an ipsilateral leptomeningeal vascular malformation between the pia and arachnoid membranes. Abnormal cerebral venous drainage is the primary abnormality, with resultant venous hypertension leading to gradual cell death, progressive atrophy, and calcification of the cortex. A parietal, occipital location is most common. Angiomas may involve the choroid plexus and eye.

Noncontrast CT shows the typical "tram track" calcification. MRI shows the leptomeningeal, gyral, and choroid enhancement. Abnormal deep draining veins and veins with the diploic space may be seen. Cerebral hemiatrophy is present.

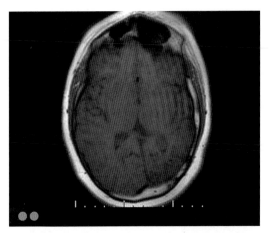

C1. Axial T1-weighted image demonstrates unilateral calvarial thickening on the left with enlarged left frontal sinus. There is volume loss in the left hemisphere and abnormal curvilinear hypointensity in the left parietooccipital region due to calcification caused by angiomatosis.

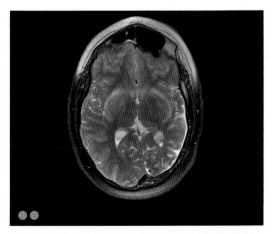

C2. Axial T2-weighted image demonstrates unilateral calvarial thickening on the left with enlarged left frontal sinus. There is volume loss in the left hemisphere and abnormal curvilinear hypointensity in the left parietooccipital region due to calcification caused by angiomatosis.

Chapter 2

Meningeal and Sulcal Diseases

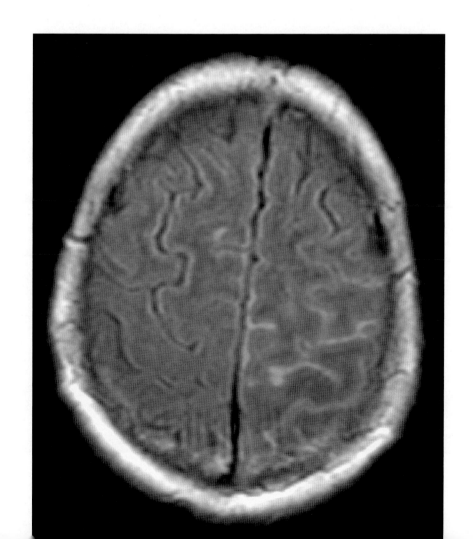

MENINGITIS

Meningitis is an inflammation of the leptomeninges and subarachnoid space. It can be caused by a number of factors, including bacterial, fungal, and viruses. MR on T2-weighted FLAIR sequence may demonstrate sulcal hyperintensity of the subarachnoid spaces. Subcortical hypointensity has been reported in some cases on T2 weighted images. Leptomeningeal enhancement is seen following intravenous injection of contrast material due to breakdown of the blood-brain barrier.

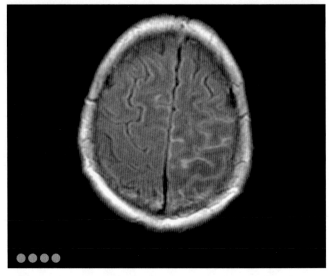

A. Axial T2-weighted FLAIR image demonstrates sulcal hyperintensity due to meningitis.

RELATED PATTERNS

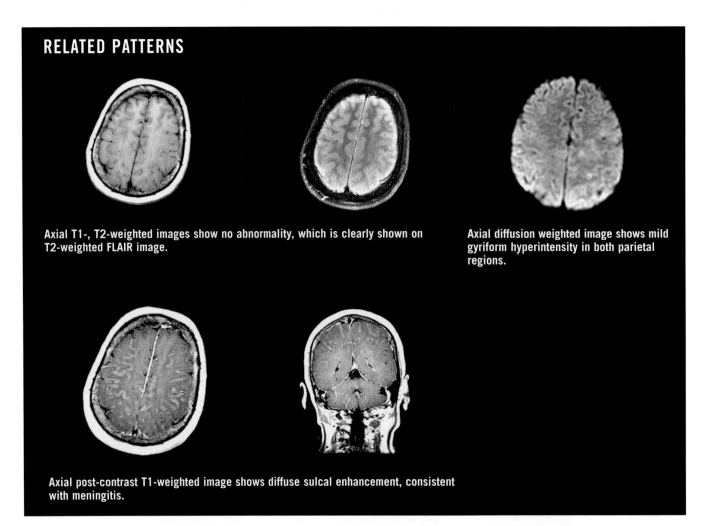

Axial T1-, T2-weighted images show no abnormality, which is clearly shown on T2-weighted FLAIR image.

Axial diffusion weighted image shows mild gyriform hyperintensity in both parietal regions.

Axial post-contrast T1-weighted image shows diffuse sulcal enhancement, consistent with meningitis.

DIFFERENTIAL DIAGNOSIS

At a Glance:

- *Tuberculous Meningitis*
- *Carcinomatous Meningitis*
- *Moyamoya Disease*
- *Hyperoxygenation*
- *Propofol*
- *Subarachnoid Hemorrhage*

TUBERCULOUS MENINGITIS

Tuberculous meningitis occurs as a result from the hematogenous spread of tuberculous bacilli from a primary lesion in the chest or genitourinary tract or from direct extension from an intracerebral focus. Primarily, the very young and very old persons as well as the immunocompromised patients are affected. The presence of thick exudate in the subarachnoid space causes sulcal hyperintensity on T2 weighted FLAIR sequence.

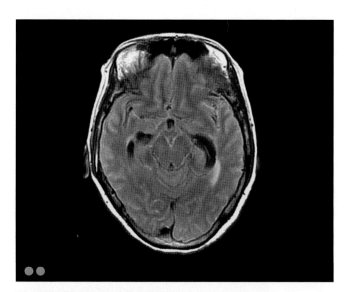

A1. Axial T2-weighted FLAIR image shows diffuse sulcal hyperintensity with dilated temporal horns.

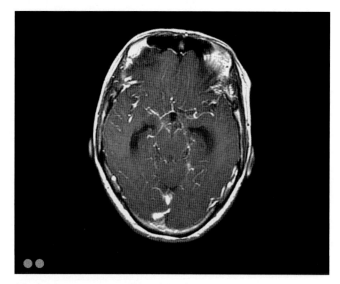

A2. Axial, post-contrast T1-weighted image shows diffuse leptomeningeal enhancement.

CARCINOMATOUS MENINGITIS

Carcinomatous meningitis occurs when neoplastic cells gain entry into the cerebrospinal fluid. It is recognized clinically in 4–7% of all cancer patients with solid tumors. In affected patients, meningeal involvement is the presenting manifes-tation of illness in 5–11%. The majority of the patients are asymptomatic at the time of presentation. Carcinomatous meningitis is seen in 20% of cancer patients at the time of autopsy. Carcinomatous meningitis is seen more frequently in certain cancers, particularly lymphoma and leukemia, melanoma, breast, and gastrointestinal cancers.

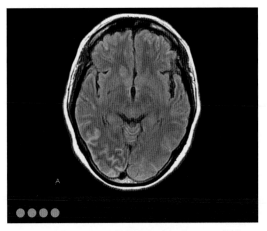

B1. Axial T2-weighted FLAIR image shows sulcal hyperintensity in the right temporal, parietooccipital region.

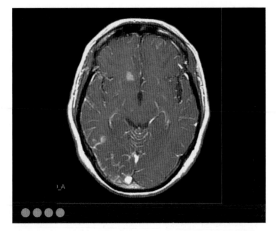

B2. Axial, post-contrast T1-weighted image shows diffuse leptomeningeal enhancement, most prominent in the right parietooccipital region.

MOYAMOYA DISEASE

Sulcal hyperintensity on T2-weighted FLAIR images in **moy-amoya disease** may be due to engorged pial vasculature from leptomeningeal anastomoses. The alteration of the underlying hemodynamics in the involved sulcal space may play a role in the failure of nulling the normal CSF signal causing sulcal hyperintensity.

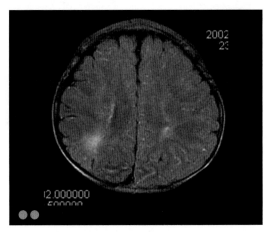

C1. Axial T2-weighted FLAIR image shows bilateral parietal sulcal hyperintensity. In addition, hyper-intense areas are seen in the deep white matter.

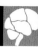

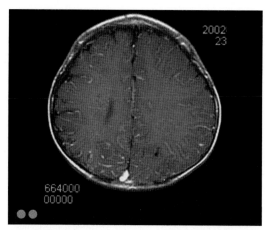

C2. Axial, post-contrast T1-weighted image demonstrates diffuse leptomeningeal enhancement.

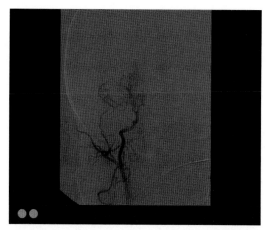

C3. AP view of DSA reveals occlusion of the right supraclinoid internal carotid artery with dilated lenticulostriate arteries in a "moya moya" type of appearance.

HYPEROXYGENATION

Evidence from numerous studies conducted in vivo and in vitro confirms the occurrence of sulcal hyperintensity on T2-weighted FLAIR images and high concentration of oxygen.

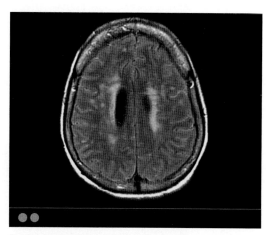

D. Axial T2-weighted FLAIR image shows diffuse sulcal hyperintensity in a patient receiving high concentration of oxygen. White matter hyperintensity is probably due to ischemic changes.

PROPOFOL

Sulcal hyperintensity on T2-weighted FLAIR images is caused by shortening of the T1 relaxation time associated with increased protein content in the CSF. There are different views in the literature whether the sulcal hyperintensity is caused by propofol or high concentration of oxygen. In our case, the patient received oxygen in both the initial study and follow-up study, whereas propofol was given to the patient only on the initial study.

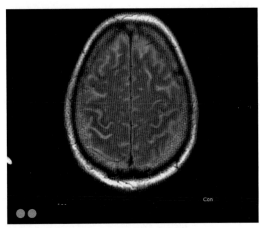

E1. Axial T2-weighted FLAIR images demonstrate diffuse sulcal hyperintensity in a patient anesthetized by propofol for the MR study because the patient was uncooperative and agitated. Diffuse periventricular white matter ischemic change is seen.

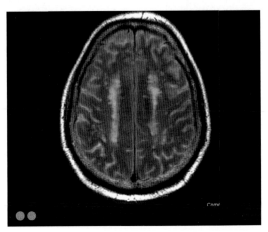

E2. Axial T2-weighted FLAIR images demonstrate diffuse sulcal hyperintensity in a patient anesthetized by propofol for the MR study because the patient was uncooperative and agitated. Diffuse periventricular white matter ischemic change is seen.

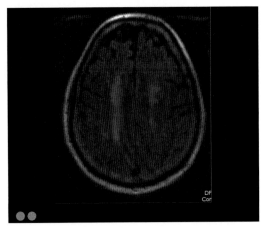

E3. Axial T2-weighted FLAIR image on the follow-up study shows no evidence of sulcal hyperintensity. Diffuse periventricular white matter ischemic change is seen. (Patient's condition improved and no sedation was required this time.)

SUBARACHNOID HEMORRHAGE

Subarachnoid hemorrhage (SAH) is bleeding into the sub-arachnoid space around the brain and spinal cord. Three layers of meninges surround the brain and spinal cord: the pia mater, the arachnoid, and the dura mater. The subarachnoid space is the space between the pia mater and the arachnoid. This space is normally filled with clear, colorless cerebrospinal fluid (CSF). Common causes of subarachnoid hemorrhage include: (1) head trauma, (2) intracranial aneurysms, (3) benign perimesencephalic hemorrhage.

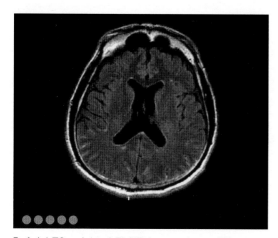

F. Axial T2-weighted FLAIR image shows diffuse sulcal hyperintensity as well as hyperintensity in the occipital horns of the lateral ventricles, consistent with subarachnoid hemorrhage and intraventricular hemorrhage.

SUBARACHNOID HEMORRHAGE

Acute hemorrhage in the stage of deoxyhemoglobin or chronic hemorrhage in the stage of hemosiderin may present as hypointensity on T2-weighted and particularly, T2*-weighted images.

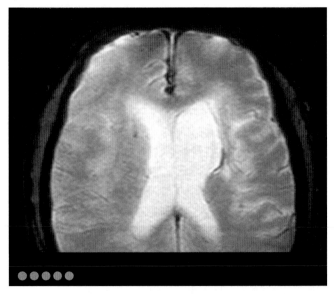

A. Axial gradient-echo sequence shows hypointensity in the frontal interhemispheric fissure and sulci, consistent with subarachnoid hemorrhage.

DIFFERENTIAL DIAGNOSIS

At a Glance:

- *Superficial Siderosis*

SUPERFICIAL SIDEROSIS

Superficial siderosis is a condition in which hemosiderin (a byproduct of the breakdown of hemoglobin) is deposited in the subpial layer of the brain and spine, which typically leads to irreversible and progressive neurological dysfunction. They usually occur secondary to previous subarachnoid hemorrhage, which may be idiopathic or result due to various etiology.

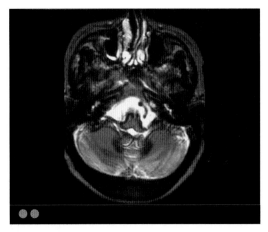

B1. Axial T2-weighted images show diffuse hypointensity on the surface of the brain parenchyma on T2-weighted images.

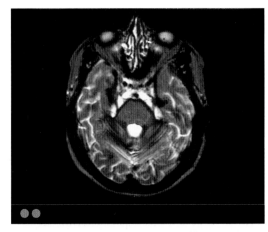

B2. Axial T2-weighted images show diffuse hypointensity on the surface of the brain parenchyma on T2-weighted images.

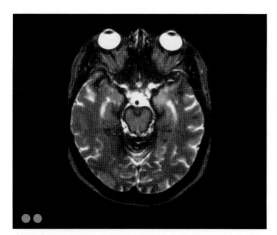

B3. Axial T2-weighted images show diffuse hypointensity on the surface of the brain parenchyma on T2-weighted images.

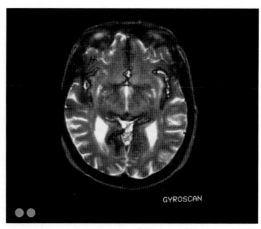

B4. Axial T2-weighted images show diffuse hypointensity on the surface of the brain parenchyma on T2-weighted images.

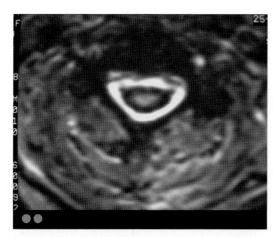

B5. Axial T2-weighted image of the cervical spine shows hypointensity surrounding the cervical cord.

MENINGITIS

The primary mechanism of leptomeningeal enhancement in **meningitis** is breakdown of the blood–brain barrier without angiogenesis. Bacterial and viral meningitis typically show thin and linear enhancement pattern. Fungal meningitis may produce thicker, lumpy, or nodular enhancement in the subarachnoid space.

Aspergillus fumigatus infection is seen predominantly in immunocompromised patients. CNS **aspergillosis** is more commonly caused by hematogenous spread of pulmonary disease and less commonly caused by direct extension of disease in the nasal cavity and paranasal sinuses. Pathologically, diffuse vascular invasion with thrombosis of cerebral vessels occurs. Necrotizing arteritis of small vascular channels is also seen.

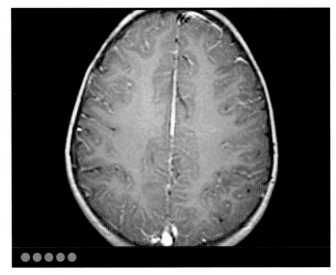

A. Axial post-contrast, T1-weighted images show diffuse sulcal enhancement, consistent with meningitis.

RELATED PATTERNS
MENINGITIS

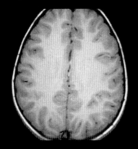

Axial T1-weighted image shows no abnormality.

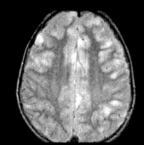

Axial T2 FLAIR image demonstrates gyriform hyperintnesity, suggesting early cerebritis.

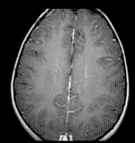

Axial post-contrast T1-weighted image shows sulcal and interhemispheric enhancement.

ASPERGILLOSIS

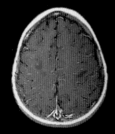
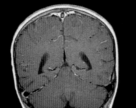

Axial and coronal post-contrast T1-weighted image shows sulcal enhancement due to cerebral aspergillosis.

COCCIDIOMYCOSIS

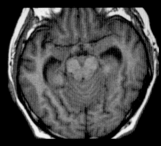

Axial T1-weighted image shows isointense material in the region of interpeduncular cistern. Dilatation of the temporal horns is seen due to hydrocephalus.

Coccidioidomycosis is caused by the airborne fungus *Coccidioides immitis*. This fungus is endemic in the southwestern United States as well as in portions of Mexico, Central and South America.

Pathologically, coccidioidomycosis is characterized by thickened, congested leptomeninges and multiple granulomas in the basal cisterns. Meningitis is most intense at the base of the brain. Hydrocephalus is seen as a result of granulomatous meningitis. Meningeal involvement is the most common manifestation of CNS disease, occurring in up to 50% of the patients with disseminated systemic disease. Males are affected five to seven times more commonly than females. Adult nonwhites often have acute, rapidly fatal meningitis, whereas children and adult whites usually have subacute or chronic meningitis.

Cryptococcosis is a systemic infection that has a worldwide distribution. Despite the high prevalence of cryptococci in the environment, cryptococcal infection is uncommon but commonly occurs in immunocompromised patients. A selective impaired lymphocyte response to cryptococci in otherwise healthy patients has been demonstrated. Cryptococcosis is the most common fungal infection in patients with AIDS. CNS infection is usually secondary to pulmonary infection. CNS cryptococcosis may present as meningitis, meningoencephalitis, or cryptococcal mass. Meningitis is the most common presentation. Hydrocephalus is seen as a result of the meningitis. Meningeal infection may extend from the basal cistern via dilated Virchow–Robin spaces into the basal ganglia and thalami.

COCCIDIOMYCOSIS (continued)

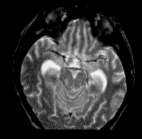

Axial T2-weighted image shows hyperintense material in the region of interpeduncular fossa, indistinguishable from CSF.

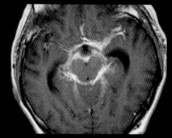

Axial post-contrast T1-weighted image shows intense enhancement in the basal cisterns.

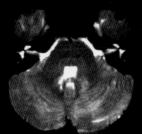

Axial T2-weighted image reveals linear hyperintensity along the cerebellum.

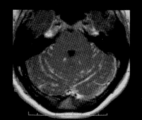

Axial and coronal T1-weighted, post-contrast images demonstrate diffuse leptomeningeal enhancement in the posterior fossa.

CRYPTOCOCCUS

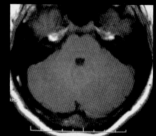

Axial T1-weighted image is unremarkable.

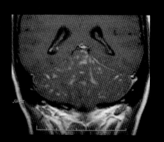

Tuberculous meningitis results from the hematogenous spread of bacilli from a primary lesion in the chest or genitourinary tract or from direct extension from an intracerebral focus. Primarily, this affects very young and very old persons, with the highest incidence in the first 3 years of life. Tuberculosis is also seen in immunocompromised patients. In the patient with tuberculous meningitis, the exudate, which is commonly seen in the basal cisterns, tends to be thick and adhesive. Communicating hydrocephalus may result from obstruction at the level of the basal cisterns. Vascular involvement of the arteries at the base of the brain or sylvian fissures may result from vasculitis and surrounding meningeal inflammation.

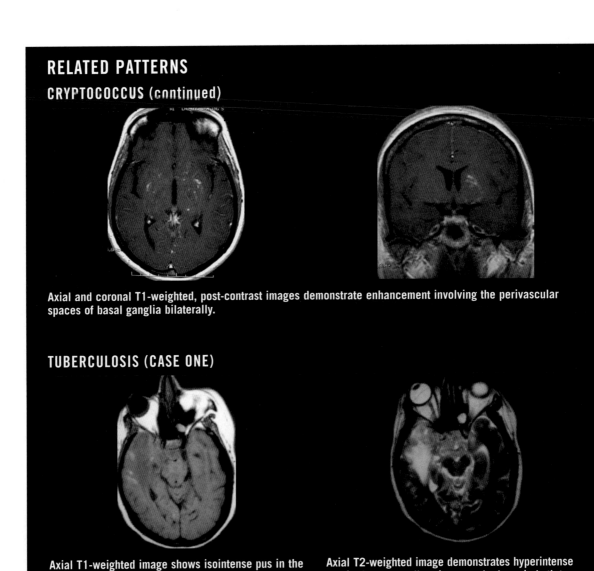

RELATED PATTERNS
CRYPTOCOCCUS (continued)

Axial and coronal T1-weighted, post-contrast images demonstrate enhancement involving the perivascular spaces of basal ganglia bilaterally.

TUBERCULOSIS (CASE ONE)

Axial T1-weighted image shows isointense pus in the suprasellar cistern and edema in the right temporal lobe.

Axial T2-weighted image demonstrates hyperintense pus in the suprasellar cistern and edema in both temporal lobes.

DIFFERENTIAL DIAGNOSIS

At a Glance:

- *Contusion*
- *Cysticercosis*
- *Infarct*
- *Leptomeningeal Metastasis*
- *Sarcoid*
- *Sturge Weber Syndrome*
- *Syphilis*

TUBERCULOSIS (CASE ONE) (continued)

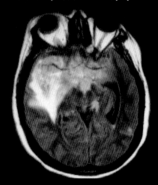

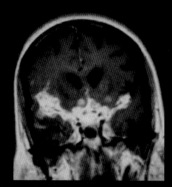

Axial T2-weighted image demonstrates hyperintense pus in the suprasellar cistern and edema in both temporal lobes.

Coronal, post-contrast T1-weighted image shows extensive enhancement in the suprasellar cistern, sylvian cistern bilaterally.

TUBERCULOSIS (CASE TWO)

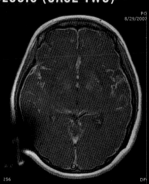

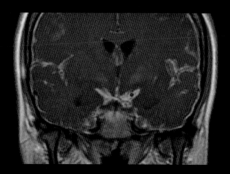

Axial and coronal, post-contrast T1-weighted images show diffuse leptomeningeal enhancement as well as pachymeningeal enhancement.

CONTUSION

A contusion is a type of traumatic brain injury that causes bruising of the brain tissue. A contusion may result from a blunt trauma on the head that causes damage to the brain.

The most common cause of traumatic brain injury is motor vehicle accidents. Sports or physical activity is the second most common cause, and assaults are third. Leptomeningeal enhancement results from breakdown of the blood–brain barrier.

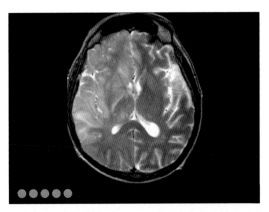

B1. Axial T2-weighted image reveals abnormal signal intensity in the region of right temporal lobe with effacement of the cortical sulci due to cerebral contusion.

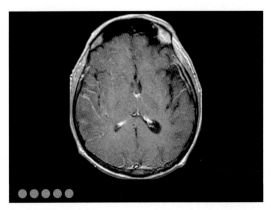

B2. Axial post-contrast, T1-weighted image demonstrates abnormal sulcal enhancement in the right temporal lobe.

CYSTICERCOSIS

Intracranial cysticercosis has four types, namely, intraparenchymal, cisternal, ventricular, and mixed. When cisternal cysts degenerate in the subarachnoid space, they can cause leptomeningeal enhancement.

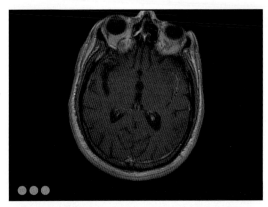

C1. Axial and coronal, post-contrast T1-weighted images show leptomeningeal enhancement in the region of left sylvian fissure.

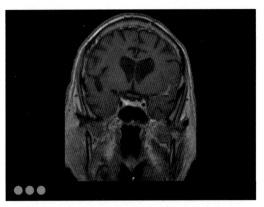

C2. Axial and coronal, post-contrast T1-weighted images show leptomeningeal enhancement in the region of left sylvian fissure.

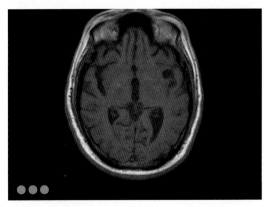

C3. Axial T1-weighted image of the same patient obtained 3 years earlier show cysticercosis cyst in the region of left sylvian fissure.

INFARCT

Detection of very early infarcts is better with MR imaging than with CT because of its superior contrast resolution. MR can detect ischemic infarcts in 96% of the cases with conventional MR scanning techniques in the first 24 hours. MR imaging may demonstrate the absence of flow void in a major vessel, loss of gray–white differentiation, focal edema, and leptomeningeal enhancement. MR diffusion imaging and MR perfusion imaging are now regarded as the imaging techniques of choice because they permit accurate, reliable diagnosis and characterization of ischemic strokes within the critical first 6-hour time period needed to initiate thrombolytic therapy.

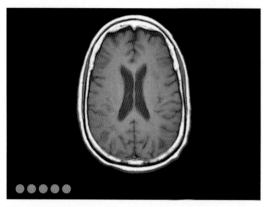

D1. Axial T1-weighted image shows mild effacement of the cortical sulci in the right parietal region.

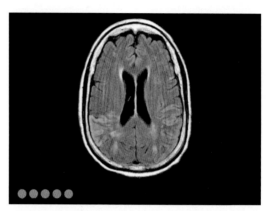

D2. Axial FLAIR image demonstrates gyriform hyper-intensity in both parietal lobes.

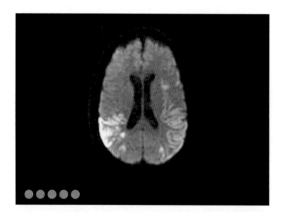

D3. Axial diffusion-weighted image shows restricted diffusion in both parietal lobes with extension into the left temporal lobe.

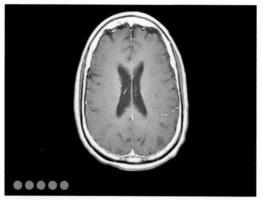

D4. Axial post-contrast T1-weighted image demon-strates subtle sulcal enhancement in the parietal lobes bilaterally.

LEPTOMENINGEAL METASTASIS

The enhancement due to leptomeningeal carcinomatosis can appear as multiple nodules, diffuse leptomeningeal enhancement, ependymal or subependymal enhancement, dural enhancement, or a combination of the above. In the nodular form, pial enhancement is difficult to distinguish from intraparenchymal enhancement, although recognizing that the nodules follow the course of sulci assists in the diagnosis. High resolution MRI with contrast enhancement and fat-suppression technique in axial and coronal planes can assist in the detection of cranial nerve involvement by the metastatic disease.

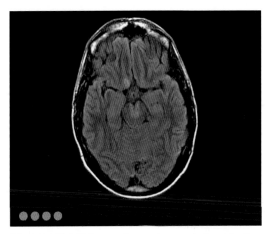

E1. Axial FLAIR image shows abnormal signal in the interpeduncular fossa and right posterior frontal lobe.

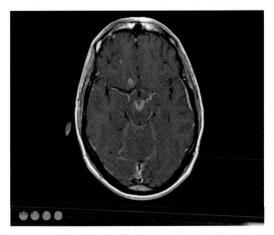

E2. Axial post-contrast T1-weighted image demonstrates enhancement in the interpeduncular fossa and right posterior frontal lobe.

LEPTOMENINGEAL METASTASIS (CASE TWO)

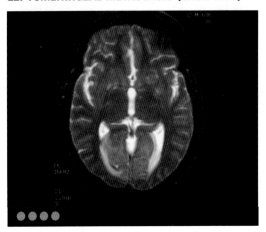

F1. Axial T2-weighted image shows hyperintensity in both parietooccipital regions.

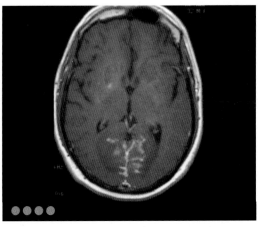

F2. Axial, post-contrast T1-weighted images demonstrate sulcal enhancement in parietooccipital region bilaterally.

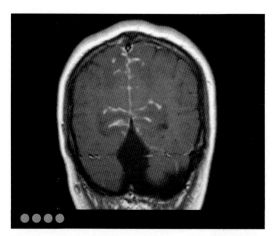

F3. Coronal, post-contrast T1-weighted images demonstrate sulcal enhancement in parietooccipital region bilaterally.

SARCOID

The intracranial compartment is involved in 15% of patients with known **sarcoidosis**. On rare occasions, CNS involvement may be the sole manifestation of sarcoidosis. Sarcoid is more prevalent in the 3rd and 4th decades of life. It may present as leptomeningitis or intracerebral granulomas. A third form of sarcoidosis, **meningoencephalitis**, is occasionally seen. Granulomatous meningitis often involves the basal cisterns in the region of the optic chiasm and hypothalamic-pituitary axis. Hydrocephalus may occur as a result of obstruction at the aqueduct, fourth ventricle, or leptomeninges.

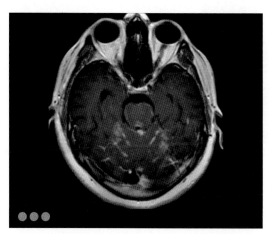

G1. Axial and coronal, post-contrast T1-weighted image shows diffuse leptomeningeal enhancement in the cerebellum.

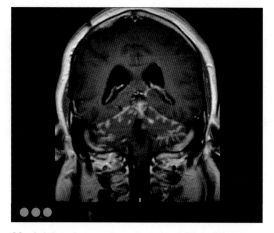

G2. Axial and coronal, post-contrast T1-weighted image shows diffuse leptomeningeal enhancement in the cerebellum.

STURGE WEBER SYNDROME

Leptomeningeal enhancement in patients with **Sturge Weber syndrome** is probably caused due to enhance-ment of the leptomeningeal angiomatosis and may allow early diagnosis of Sturge Weber syndrome. Enhance-ment of an enlarged ipsilateral choroid plexus may be seen.

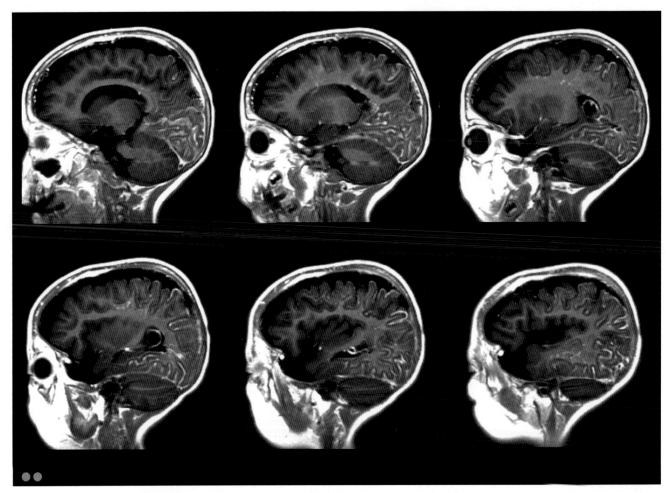

H. Sagittal, post-contrast T1-weighted images show extensive leptomeningeal enhancement. Note the enhancement of a large, cystic choroid plexus.

SYPHILIS

Pathologically, **meningovascular syphilis** is manifested by widespread thickening of the meninges, with lym-phocytic infiltration involving the meninges and around the small vessels. Contrast-enhanced MRI shows curvi-linear, nonhomogeneous enhancement of the leptome-ninges.

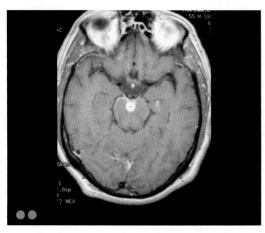

I1. Axial, post-contrast T1-weighted images show slightly thick leptomeningeal enhancement. Nodular enhancement is seen at the interpeduncular fossa and along the falx.

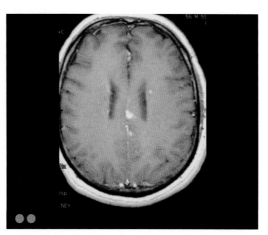

I2. Axial, post-contrast T1-weighted images show slightly thick leptomeningeal enhancement. Nodular enhancement is seen at the interpeduncular fossa and along the falx.

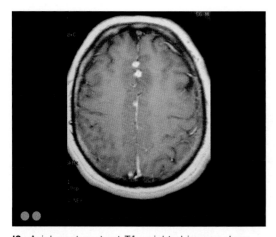

I3. Axial, post-contrast T1-weighted images show slightly thick leptomeningeal enhancement. Nodular enhancement is seen at the interpeduncular fossa and along the falx.

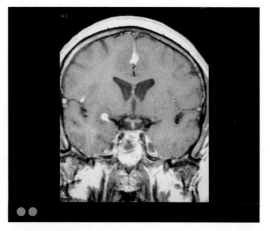

I4. Coronal, post-contrast T1-weighted image shows thick leptomeningeal enhancement along the inter-hemispheric fissure and right sylvian fissure.

POST-SHUNT

Pachymeningeal enhancement is seen in postoperative patients. Pia-arachnoid enhancement is not typical of benign intracranial hypotension, but may be seen in post-operative patients.

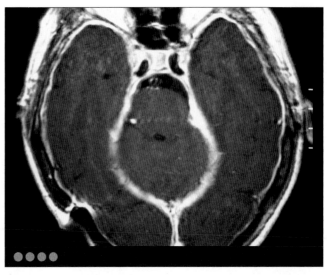

A. Axial post-contrast T1-weighted image reveals smooth enhancement along the tentorial edge in a patient with previous shunt placement.

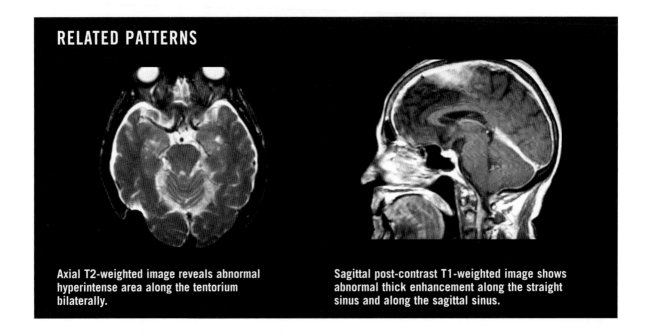

RELATED PATTERNS

Axial T2-weighted image reveals abnormal hyperintense area along the tentorium bilaterally.

Sagittal post-contrast T1-weighted image shows abnormal thick enhancement along the straight sinus and along the sagittal sinus.

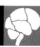

DIFFERENTIAL DIAGNOSIS

At a Glance:

- *Dural Sinus Thrombosis*
- *Wegner's Granulomatosis*
- *Granulomatous Disease*
- *Intracranial Hypotension*
- *Lymphoma*
- *Meningeal Carcinomatosis*

DURAL SINUS THROMBOSIS

Dural sinus thrombosis may be related to a number of predisposing factors including infection, tumor, trauma, dehydration, pregnancy, oral contraceptives, and hypercoagulable states. Imaging findings include detection of thrombus in the venous sinus, venous collateral flow, and venous infarction. **Pachymeningeal enhancement** along the tentorium and falx is seen as evidence of collateral flow.

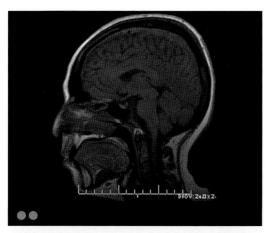

B1. Sagittal T1-weighted image demonstrates abnormal hyperintensity in the region of superior sagittal sinus instead of the usual flow void.

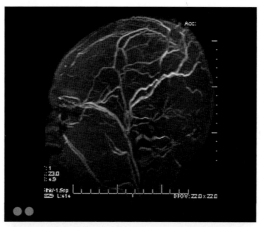

B2. Sagittal venogram reveals thrombosis of the superior sagittal sinus.

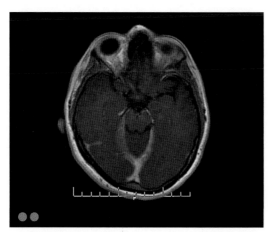

B3. Axial and coronal post-contrast T1-weighted images show enhancement along the tentorium and falx.

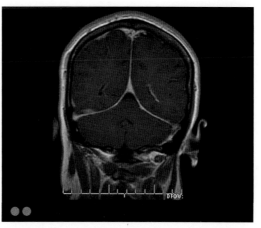

B4. Axial and coronal post-contrast T1-weighted images show enhancement along the tentorium and falx.

WEGNER'S GRANULOMATOSIS

Wegener granulomatosis is a multisystem disease characterized by necrotizing granuloma of the upper and lower respiratory tracts, disseminated vasculitis, and glomerulonephritis. Central nervous disease occurs in 20% of patients, with mononeuritis multiplex the most common manifestation. Central nervous system involvement can be in the form of cranial nerve dysfunction, diffuse cerebral vasculitis, or hypothalamic granulomas with diabetes insipidus. Rarely granulomatous meningitis can occur. It is now widely presumed that the antineutrophil cytoplasmic antibodies (ANCAs) are responsible for the inflammation in Wegener's. The typical ANCAs in Wegener's are those that react with proteinase, an enzyme prevalent in neutrophil granulocytes. ANCAs activate neutrophils, increase their adherence to endothelium, and lead to their degranulation. This causes extensive damage to the vessel wall, particularly of arterioles.

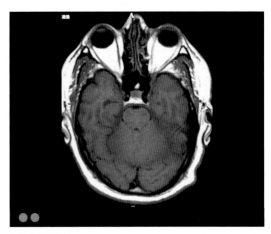

C1. Axial T1-weighted image shows isointense thickening of the tentorium with effacement of cerebellar sulci.

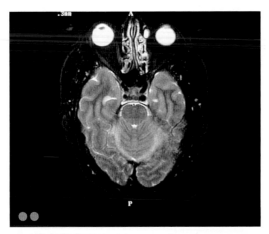

C2. Axial T2-weighted and FLAIR images demonstrate hyperintense thickening of the tentorium.

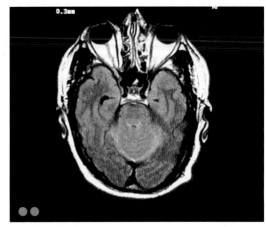

C3. Axial T2-weighted and FLAIR images demonstrate hyperintense thickening of the tentorium.

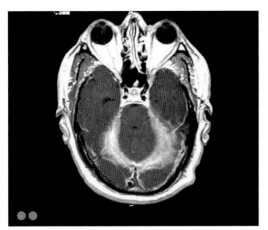

C4. Axial and coronal, post-contrast T1-weighted images demonstrate diffuse pachymeningeal enhancement along the tentorium.

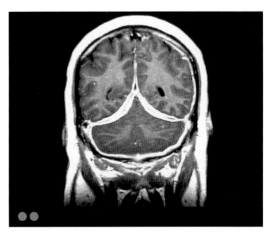

C5. Axial and coronal, post-contrast T1-weighted images demonstrate diffuse pachymeningeal enhancement along the tentorium.

GRANULOMATOUS DISEASE

Granulomatous disease usually involves the basilar meninges rather than the meninges in the convexity.

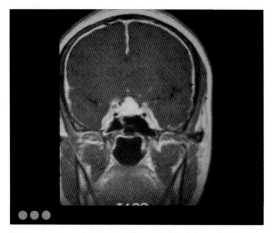

D. Coronal, post-contrast T1-weighted image shows diffuse pachymeningeal thickening and lesion in the sellar, suprasellar region as well as in both cavernous sinuses.

INTRACRANIAL HYPOTENSION

Intracranial hypotension is a benign cause of pachymeningeal enhancement that may be localized or diffuse and can be seen on MR images in patients after surgery or with idiopathic loss cerebrospinal fluid pressure. When the cerebrospinal fluid pressure drops, there may be secondary fluid shifts that increase the volume of capacitance veins in the subarachnoid space. Prolonged intracranial hypotension may lead to vasocongestion and interstitial edema, findings similar to those seen in the dural tail of a meningioma.

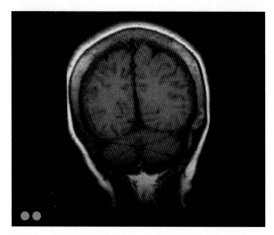

E1. Coronal T1- and axial T2-weighted images show increased thickness of hypointensity in the extracerebral space on T1-weighted image and of hyperintensity on T2-weighted image.

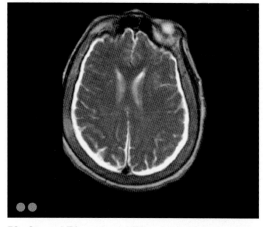

E2. Coronal T1- and axial T2-weighted images show increased thickness of hypointensity in the extracerebral space on T1-weighted image and of hyperintensity on T2-weighted image.

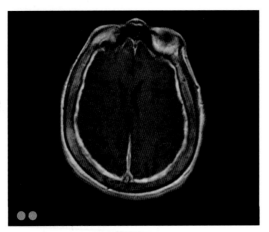

E3. Axial and coronal, post-contrast T1-weighted images demonstrate diffuse pachymeningeal enhancement. Intracranial hypotension is a benign cause of pachymeningeal enhancement that may be localized or diffuse and can be seen on MR images in patients after surgery or with idiopathic loss cerebrospinal fluid pressure. Prolonged intracranial hypotension may lead to vasocongestion and interstitial edema, findings similar to those seen in the dural tail of a meningioma.

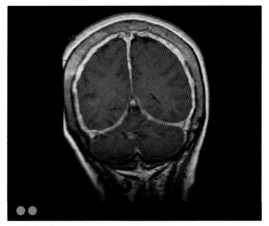

E4. Axial and coronal, post-contrast T1-weighted images demonstrate diffuse pachymeningeal enhancement. Intracranial hypotension is a benign cause of pachymeningeal enhancement that may be localized or diffuse and can be seen on MR images in patients after surgery or with idiopathic loss cerebrospinal fluid pressure. Prolonged intracranial hypotension may lead to vasocongestion and interstitial edema, findings similar to those seen in the dural tail of a meningioma.

LYMPHOMA

Secondary central nervous system **lymphoma** is usually extraaxial in location and may be epidural, dural, subdural, and subarachnoid.

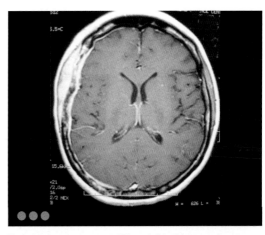

F. Axial, post-contrast, T1-weighted image shows pachymeningeal enhancement involving the right frontal and parietal region with adjacent skull and scalp involvement.

MENINGEAL CARCINOMATOSIS

Meningeal carcinomatosis most often arises from the breast carcinoma in female and prostate carcinoma in male. They can also be seen in melanoma, lymphoma or leukemia. Patients usually present with headache, cranial nerve palsies. Intracranial metastasis can involve the brain, leptomeninges, dura, and skull. Dural involvement is not common. They are usually thick and nodular in contour.

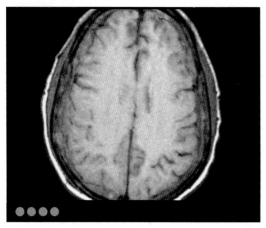

G1. Axial T1-weighted image shows abnormal hypo- to isointensity along the convexity bilaterally.

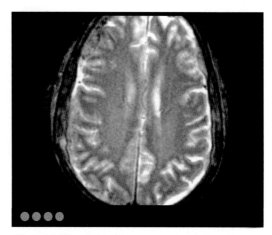

G2. Axial T2-weighted image reveals abnormal mixed signal intensity along the convexity bilaterally.

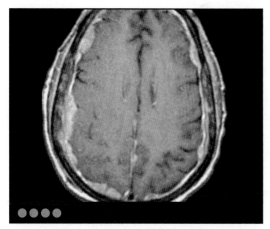

G3. Axial post-contrast T1-weighted image shows irregular pachymeningeal enhancement along the convexity bilaterally in a patient with prostate carcinoma.

SUBDURAL EMPYEMA

Subdural empyema is a crescentic collection of pus bet-ween the meningeal dura and arachnoid mater. Subdural empyema can occur secondary to direct extension of infec-tion from adjacent sinusitis or mastoiditis or through the hematogenous route. Subdural empyema usually exhibits restricted diffusion on diffusion-weighted sequence.

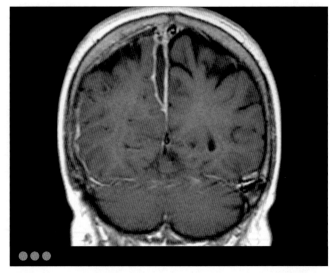

A. Coronal post-contrast T1-weighted image shows a large fluid collection along the falx with enhancing membrane. Subdural empyema shows restricted diffusion on diffusion-weighted images (not shown here).

RELATED PATTERNS

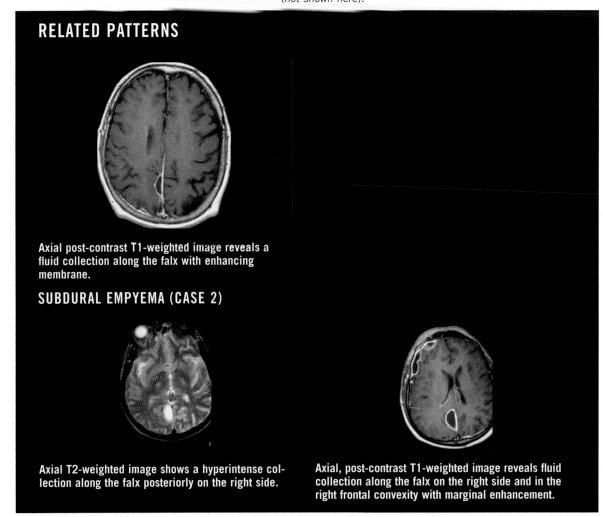

Axial post-contrast T1-weighted image reveals a fluid collection along the falx with enhancing membrane.

SUBDURAL EMPYEMA (CASE 2)

Axial T2-weighted image shows a hyperintense col-lection along the falx posteriorly on the right side.

Axial, post-contrast T1-weighted image reveals fluid collection along the falx on the right side and in the right frontal convexity with marginal enhancement.

DIFFERENTIAL DIAGNOSIS

At a Glance:

- *Arachnoid Cyst*
- *Epidural Empyema*
- *Epidural Hematoma*
- *Subdural Hematoma*

ARACHNOID CYST

Arachnoid cysts are sacs that are filled with cerebrospinal fluid and form in the surface region of the brain around the base of the skull, or on the arachnoid membrane. The majority of arachnoid cysts are developmental anomalies. A small number of them are acquired, such as those in association with neoplasms or those that are due to adhesions following leptomeningitis, hemorrhage, or surgery. They constitute approximately 1% of intracranial masses, with 50–60% occurring in the middle cranial fossa. Cysts in the middle cranial fossa are found more frequently in males and on the left side.

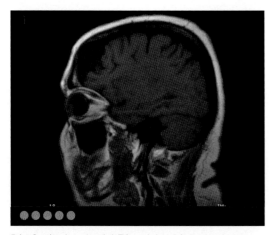

B1. Sagittal and axial T1-weighted images show a hypointense, extra-axial lesion in the left frontal region.

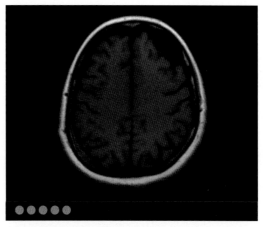

B2. Sagittal and axial T1-weighted images show a hypointense, extra-axial lesion in the left frontal region.

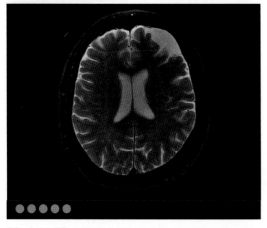

B3. Axial T2-weighted image demonstrates a hyperintense, extra-axial lesion in the left frontal region.

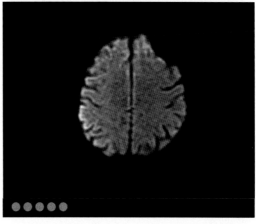

B4. Diffusion-weighted image shows no evidence of restricted diffusion.

61

EPIDURAL EMPYEMA

Epidural empyema is a collection of pus between the skull and underlying dura. It can result from spread of infection of the paranasal sinuses, middle ear, or mastoids. Routes of spread include direct spread from osteomyelitis, septic thrombus entering emissary veins, and hematogenous spread. Intracranial epidural empyema may rarely occur as a result of metastatic hematogenous seeding.

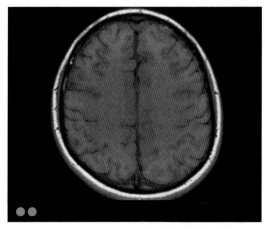

C1. Axial T1-weighted image shows two isointense collections in the frontal region.

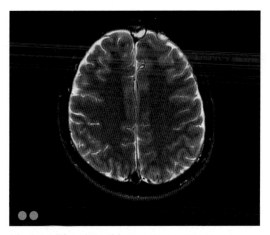

C2. Axial T2-weighted image demonstrates two hyperintense collections in the frontal region.

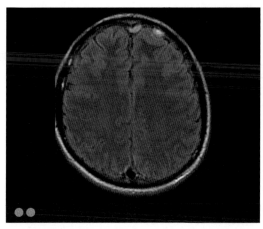

C3. Axial T2-weighted FLAIR image demonstrates two hyperintense collections in the frontal region.

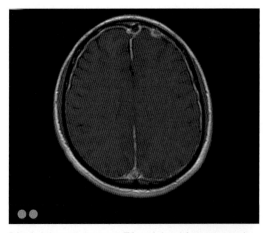

D1. Axial, post-contrast T1-weighted image reveals marginal enhancement of the two small epidural collections.

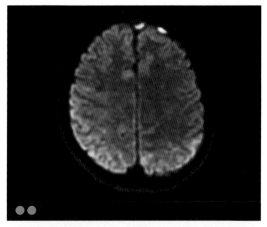

D2. Diffusion-weighted image clearly shows restricted diffusion in these two small collections.

EPIDURAL HEMATOMA

An **epidural hematoma (EDH)** is a biconves collection of blood, which lies beneath the calvarium, external to the periosteal dura. It rarely extends beyond the suture margin due to the firm attachment of periosteal dura to the suture margin. An EDH most frequently occurs over the convexity from a lacerated meningeal or periosteal artery at the frac-

tured bone edges. An EDH may also occur from the venous bleeding due to a dural sinus injury. An EDH is almost always the result of a coup injury at the site of impact. Conversely, an SDH is often the results of a contracoup injury away from the impact site. An EDH may cross the midline by displacing the interhemispheric fissure and falx away from the inner table of the skull.

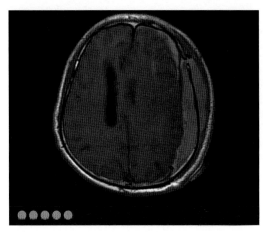 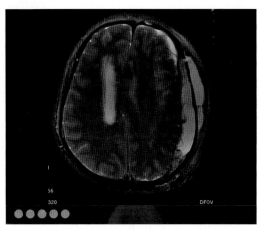

E1. Axial T1- and T2-weighted images demonstrate a large frontoparietal epidural hematoma (hyperintense on both T1- and T2-weighted images corresponding to the presence of methemoglobin) associated with frontal skull fracture and extracranial hematoma. Note there is a small left frontal subdural hematoma present as well.

E2. Axial T1- and T2-weighted images demonstrate a large frontoparietal epidural hematoma (hyperintense on both T1- and T2-weighted images corresponding to the presence of methemoglobin) associated with frontal skull fracture and extracranial hematoma. Note there is a small left frontal subdural hematoma present as well.

SUBDURAL HEMATOMA

Subdural hematoma (SDH) is an accumulation of blood between the meningeal dura and arachnoid mater. An SDH may occur from the rupture of bridging cortical veins, the bending of vessels from deceleration, or by direct injury to pial veins, great veins, or pacchionian granulation. An SDH

tends to extend along the meningeal dura and the underlying arachnoid, forming a crescentic hematoma with a long tail. An SDH may extend from the convexity to the interhemispheric fissure and the tentorial edge. An SDH is not confined by the suture line, but it cannot cross the midline due to the presence of dural folding in the midline.

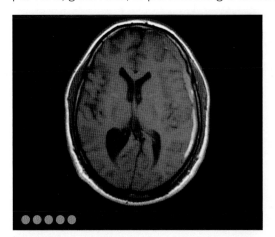 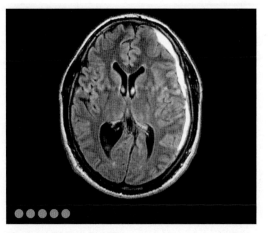

F1. Axial T1 and FLAIR images show a hyperintense subdural fluid collection on the left side, consistent with subdural hematoma.

F2. Axial T1 and FLAIR images show a hyperintense subdural fluid collection on the left side, consistent with subdural hematoma.

ARACHNOID CYST

Posterior fossa arachnoid cyst is a retrocerebellar cyst with no communication with the subarachnoid space. The vermis, cerebellum and fourth ventricle are normal, but may be displaced by a large arachnoid cyst. The posterior fossa may be enlarged. Hypoplastic changes of the adjacent vermis and cerebellar hemisphere may be seen. When the cyst is small, it may be difficult to differentiate from a giant cisterna magna. Phase-contrast cine MRI may be used to evaluate the arachnoid cysts and detect their communication with subarachnoid space.

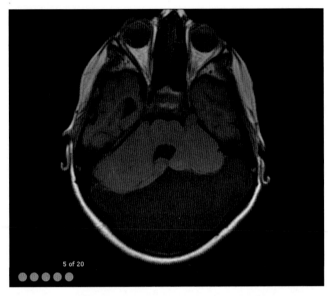

A. Axial T1-weighted image shows a large, retrocerebellar hypointense cystic lesion. Note the vermis is present between the fourth ventricle and the cyst.

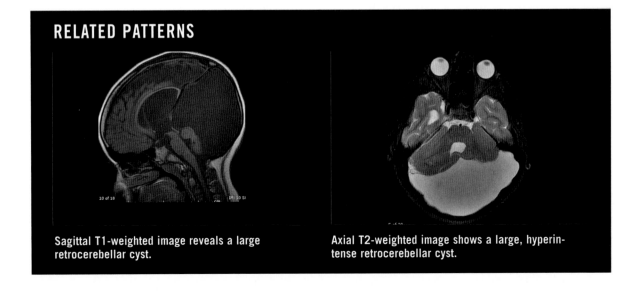

RELATED PATTERNS

Sagittal T1-weighted image reveals a large retrocerebellar cyst.

Axial T2-weighted image shows a large, hyperintense retrocerebellar cyst.

> **DIFFERENTIAL DIAGNOSIS**
>
> At a Glance:
>
> • *Dandy–Walker Malformation*
>
> • *Giant Cisterna Magna*

DANDY–WALKER MALFORMATION

Dandy–Walker malformation consists of cystic dilatation of fourth ventricle, vermian hypoplasia or agenesis, and large posterior fossa with high position of torcular. About 70–90% of patients have hydrocephalus, which often develops postnatally.

It may be associated with callosal agenesis (20–25%), colpocephaly, lipoma of the corpus callosum, holoprocen-

cephaly (20%), gray matter heterotopias (5–10%), polymicrogyria, malformation of the cerebellar folia, and etc. Dandy–Walker variant consists of varying degree of cerebellar hypoplasia, especially involving the inferior vermis. The fourth ventricle may be enlarged. The posterior fossa volume is normal.

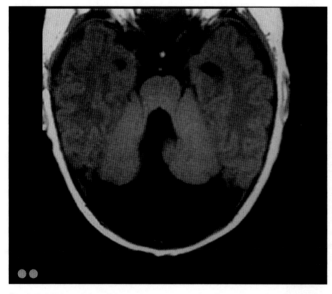

B. Axial T1-weighted image shows cystic dilatation of the fourth ventricle with agenesis of the vermis.

GIANT CISTERNA MAGNA

The **cisterna magna** is one of three principal openings in the subarachnoid space between the arachnoid and pia mater layers of the meninges surrounding the brain. The cisterna magna is located between the cerebellum and the posterior aspect of the medulla oblongata. Cerebrospinal fluid produced in the fourth ventricle drains into the cisterna magna via the lateral recess and median recess. A large cisterna magna is usually asymptomatic and a normal variation.

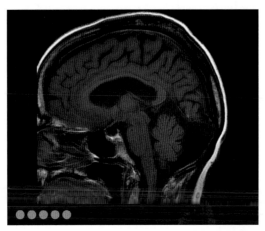

C1. Sagittal T1-weighted image shows a large, retro-cerebellar cystic lesion, cosistent with giant cisterna magna.

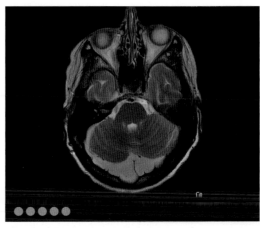

C2. Axial T2-weighted and FLAIR images show a large retrocerebellar cystic area. The signal intensity of the cyst fluid is the same as CSF.

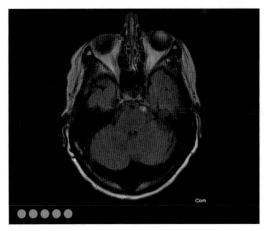

C3. Axial T2-weighted and FLAIR images show a large retrocerebellar cystic area. The signal intensity of the cyst fluid is the same as CSF.

Chapter 3

Extracerebral Masses

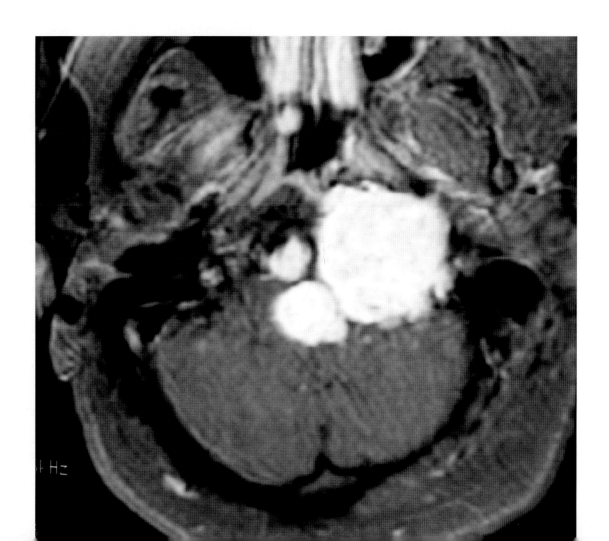

SCHWANNOMAS (NINTH CN)

The right jugular foramen is larger than the left in 68%, equal in 12% and smaller than the left in 20%, possibly due to the difference in the size of the sigmoid sinus and the jugular bulb. The jugular foramen is traditionally divided into a large posterolateral compartment (pars venosa) and a smaller anteromedial compartment (pars nervosa). The ninth cranial nerve goes through the pars nervosa, whereas the tenth and eleventh cranial nerve go through the pars venosa along with jugular vein.

Schwannomas of the cranial nerve IX, X, XI, when arising from jugular foramen, enhance homogeneously or contain cystic components on MRI. They show only mild to moderate vascularity on angiography with small scattered "puddles" of contrast in midarterial, capillary, and venous phases, and no early draining veins. Schwannomas of the jugular foramen are rare and tend to extend superomedially toward the medulla along the course of the cranial nerve from which they arise.

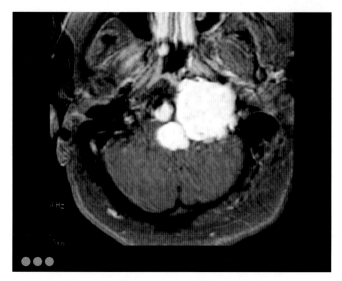

A. Axial post-contrast, fat-suppressed, T1-weighted image shows a lobulated enhancing mass in the region of the left jugular foramen. This is an exceedingly rare case of schwannoma of the ninth cranial nerve.

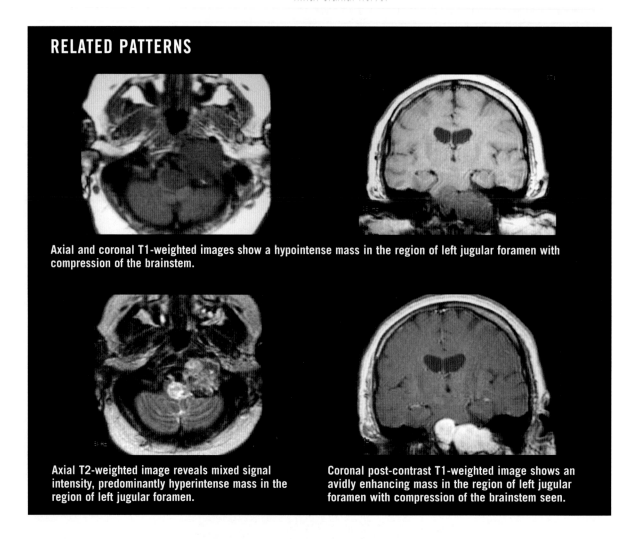

RELATED PATTERNS

Axial and coronal T1-weighted images show a hypointense mass in the region of left jugular foramen with compression of the brainstem.

Axial T2-weighted image reveals mixed signal intensity, predominantly hyperintense mass in the region of left jugular foramen.

Coronal post-contrast T1-weighted image shows an avidly enhancing mass in the region of left jugular foramen with compression of the brainstem seen.

DIFFERENTIAL DIAGNOSIS

At a Glance:

- *Eleventh Nerve Schwannoma*
- *Twelfth Nerve Schwannoma*
- *Chondrosarcoma*
- *Glomus Jugulare Tumor*
- *High Jugular Bulb*
- *Meningiomas*
- *Metastasis*
- *Cholesteatoma* (not pictured)
- *Histiocytosis* (not pictured)
- *Lymphoma* (not pictured)
- *Plasmacytoma* (not pictured)

ELEVENTH NERVE SCHWANNOMA

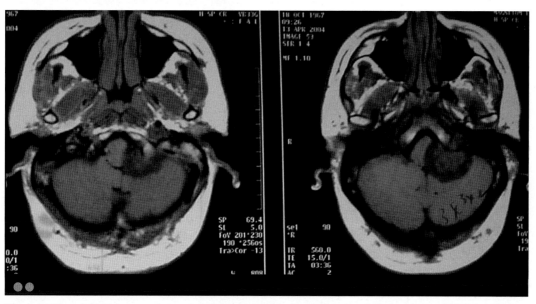

B1. Axial T1-weighted images show a hypointense mass in the left perimedullary cistern and left jugular foramen.

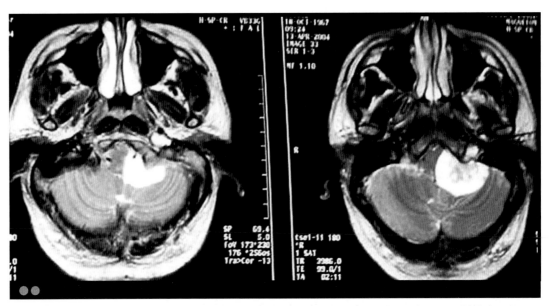

B2. Axial T2-weighted images reveal a hyperintense mass in the left perimedullary cistern and left jugular foramen.

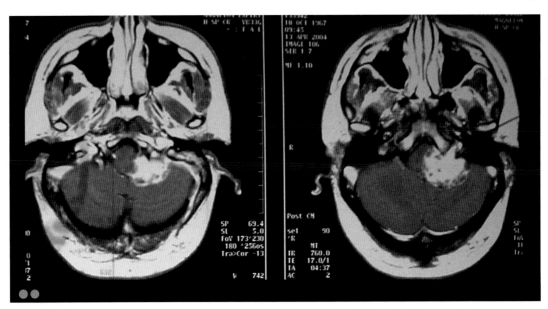

B3. Axial and coronal, post-contrast T1-weighted images demonstrate avidly enhancing mass in the left perimedullary cistern and jugular foramen.

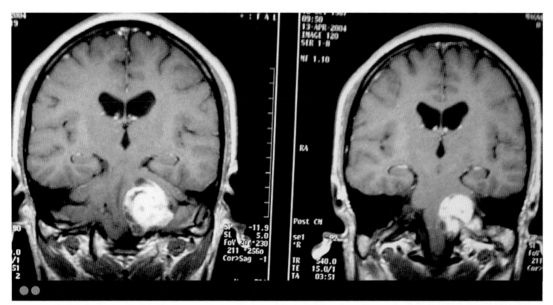

B4. Axial and coronal, post-contrast T1-weighted images demonstrate avidly enhancing mass in the left per-imedullary cistern and jugular foramen.

TWELFTH NERVE SCHWANNOMA

Schwannoma of the hypoglossal nerve is rare. The twelfth cranial nerve supplies all the intrinsic muscle of the tongue and three of the four extrinsic muscles including genioglossus, styloglossus and hyoglossus. Although the twelfth cranial nerve passes through the hypoglossal canal, not the jugular foramen, schwannoma of the twelfth nerve may present as mass lesion in the region of jugular foramen.

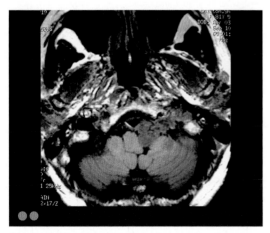

C1. Axial T1-weighted image shows a hypointense mass involving the hypoglossal canal and in the region of left jugular foramen.

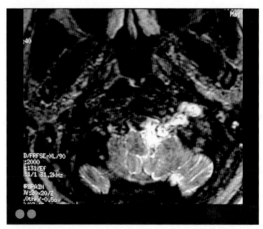

C2. Axial T2-weighted image shows a slightly heterogeneous, hyperintense mass involving the hypoglossal canal and in the region of left jugular foramen.

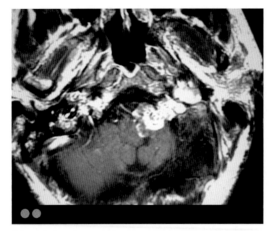

C3. Axial and coronal, post-contrast T1-weighted images demonstrate a lobulated, heterogeneously enhancing mass in the region of left hypoglossal canal.

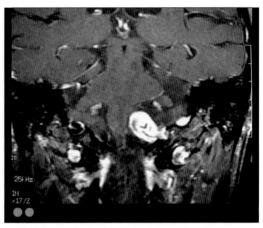

C4. Axial and coronal, post-contrast T1-weighted images demonstrate a lobulated, heterogeneously enhancing mass in the region of left hypoglossal canal.

CHONDROSARCOMA

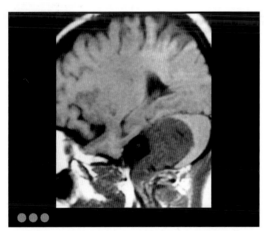

D1. Sagittal T1-weighted image shows a hypo-intense mass in the left posterior fossa with extension into the jugular foramen.

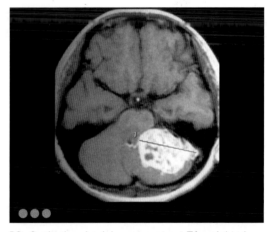

D2. Sagittal and axial, post-contrast T1-weighted images demonstrate an enhancing mass in the left posterior fossa with extension into the jugular foramen.

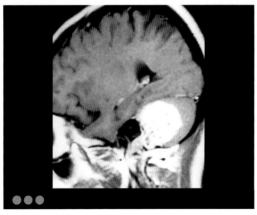

D3. Sagittal and axial, post-contrast T1-weighted images demonstrate an enhancing mass in the left posterior fossa with extension into the jugular foramen.

GLOMUS JUGULARE TUMOR

Paraganglioma is the second most common tumor in the temporal bone after vestibular schwannoma. Paraganglioma consists of glomus jugulare, glomus tympanicum and glomus vagale. These tumors are three times more common in females and are often multiple. MRI shows "salt-and-pepper" inhomogeneity and arborizing flow voids in tumors larger than 2 cm. They tend to extend from the jugular foramen into the hypotympanum superolaterally.

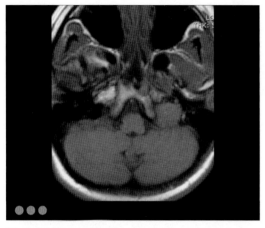

E1. Axial T1 weighted image shows an isointense mass in the region of left jugular foramen.

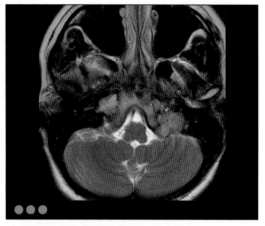

E2. Axial T2 weighted image reveals a slightly hyperintense mass with some internal flow voids in the region of left jugular foramen.

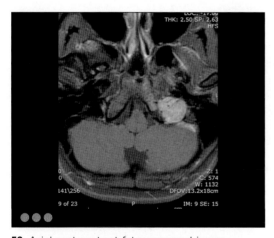

E3. Axial post contrast fat-suppressed image shows an avidly enhancing mass.

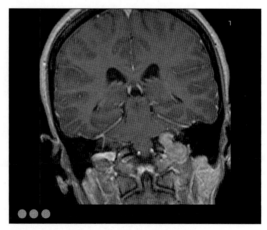

E4. Coronal post contrast T1 weighted image reveals an enhancing mass.

GLOMUS VAGALE TUMOR

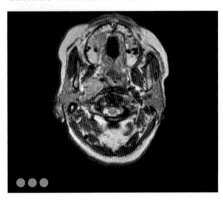

F1. Axial T2-weighted and fat-suppressed images show a hyperintense mass in the region of right jugular foramen.

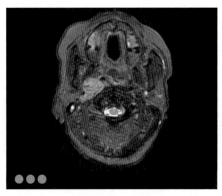

F2. Axial T2-weighted and fat-suppressed images show a hyperintense mass with curvilinear signal voids in the region of right jugular foramen.

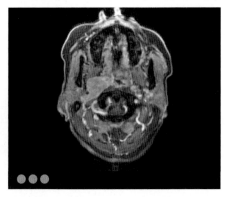

F3. Axial, post-contrast, fat-suppressed image shows an avidly enhancing mass in the region of right jugular foramen.

GLOMUS TYMPANICUM

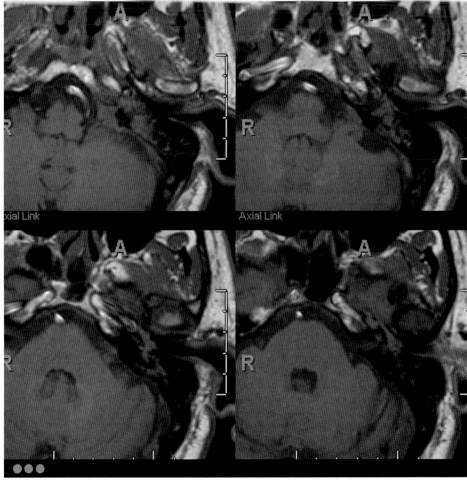

G1. Axial T1-weighted images show an isointense, heterogeneous mass with irregular margin in the left temporal bone.

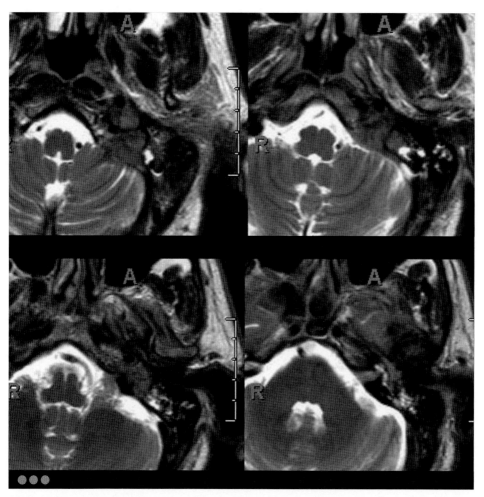

G2. Axial T2-weighted images reveal a slightly heterogeneous, hypointense mass with irregular margin in the left temporal bone.

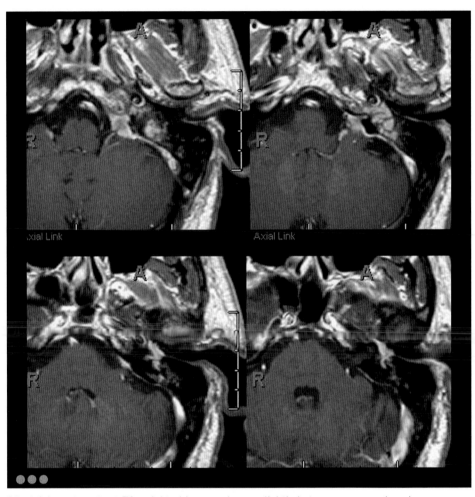

G3. Axial, post-contrast T1-weighted images show a slightly heterogeneous, enhancing mass with irregular margin in the left temporal bone.

HIGH JUGULAR BULB

The jugular bulb is the dilated portion of the upper portion of jugular vein, at its junction with the sigmoid sinus. A high jugular bulb extends into the middle ear, above the level of the bony annulus of temporal bone. A protruding jugular bulb on CT is seen as a dehiscence of the bony floor of the hypotympanum with a soft tissue mass in the middle ear. A dehiscent high jugular bulb is visible at otoscopy as a smooth, convex, bluish mass, different from the pulsating reddish mass of a glomus tumor.

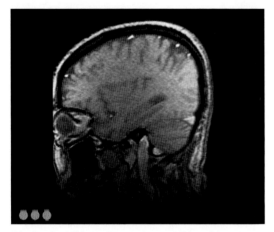

H1. Sagittal T2 gradient echo and T1-weighted images show a high riding right jugular bulb.

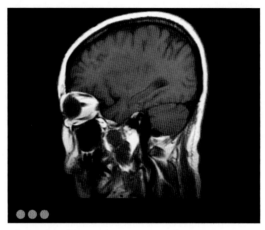

H2. Sagittal T2 gradient echo and T1-weighted images show a high riding right jugular bulb.

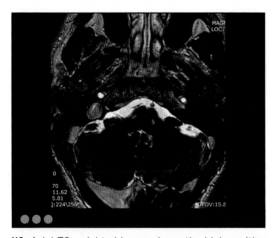

H3. Axial T2-weighted image shows the high position of right jugular bulb.

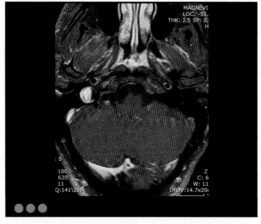

H4. Axial, post-contrast T1-weighted image shows enhancement in the high riding jugular bulb, mimicking an enhancing lesion.

MENINGIOMAS

Meningiomas arising from the jugular foramen are characterized by diffuse, centrifugal skull base infiltration. They may involve the foramen itself as well as the hypotempanum, the posterior fossa, the jugular tubercle, occipital condyle, clivus, and extracranial carotid space of the suprahyoid neck. On MRI, they exhibit isointensity on both T1-weighted and T2-weighted images and are homogeneous with moderate enhancement.

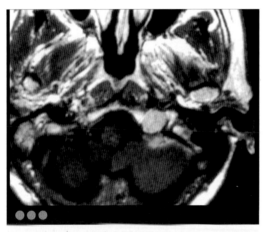

I1. Axial and coronal, post-contrast T1-weighted images demonstrate a moderately enhancing mass in the left jugular foramen.

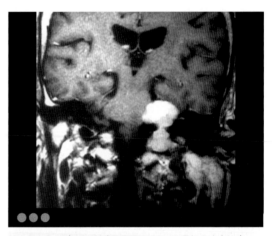

I2. Axial and coronal, post-contrast T1-weighted images demonstrate a moderately enhancing mass in the left jugular foramen.

METASTASIS

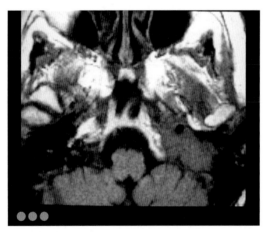

J1. Axial T1-weighted image shows a large mass in the region of left jugular foramen with adjacent bone destruction.

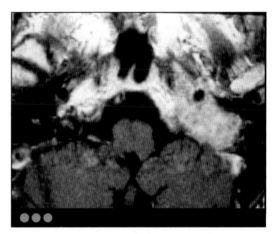

J2. Axial, post-contrast T1-weighted image reveals an enhancing mass in the region of left jugular foramen.

CHORDOMA

Approximately 35% of chordoma arise from clivus, which is the second most common site. Chordoma arise from the remnants of primitive notochord, which extends from Rathke's pouch to the clivus, continuing caudally to the vertebral bodies. Typical features of clival chordoma include a mid-line partially calcified tumor, with bony destruction of the clivus and causing a soft tissue mass in the sphenoid sinus or nasopharynx. There is a high incidence of unilateral bone erosion, erosion of the tip of the clivus and odontoid peg and sometimes sclerotic bone reaction to the tumor. Chordomas tend to displace the dura before transgressing it so that the subarachnoid space is usually patent adjacent to quite large tumors.

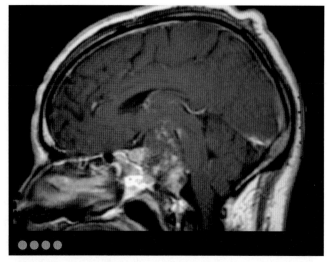

A. Sagittal, post-contrast T1-weighted image shows a patchy heterogeneously enhancing mass in the region of clivus with bony destruction, extending into the prepontine cistern and displacing the brainstem posteriorly.

RELATED PATTERNS
CHORDOMA (CASE TWO)

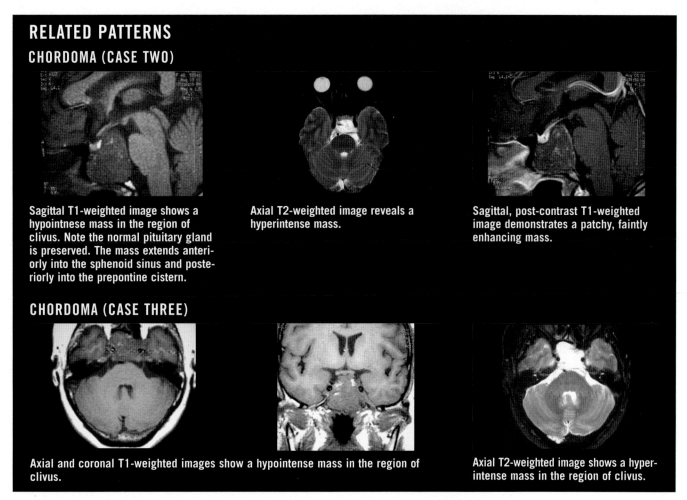

Sagittal T1-weighted image shows a hypointnese mass in the region of clivus. Note the normal pituitary gland is preserved. The mass extends anteriorly into the sphenoid sinus and posteriorly into the prepontine cistern.

Axial T2-weighted image reveals a hyperintense mass.

Sagittal, post-contrast T1-weighted image demonstrates a patchy, faintly enhancing mass.

CHORDOMA (CASE THREE)

Axial and coronal T1-weighted images show a hypointense mass in the region of clivus.

Axial T2-weighted image shows a hyperintense mass in the region of clivus.

RELATED PATTERNS (continued)

CHORDOMA (CASE THREE) (continued)

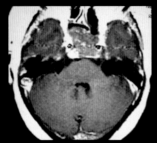 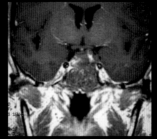

Axial and coronal, post-contrast T1-weighted images demonstrate a faintly, patchy enhancing mass in the region of clivus.

CHORDOMA (CASE FOUR)

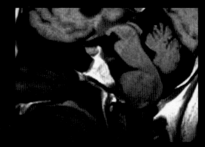

Sagittal T1-weighted image shows a large, round, isointense extra-axial mass with a small attachment to the inferior aspect of clivus.

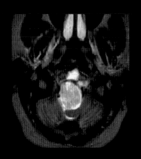 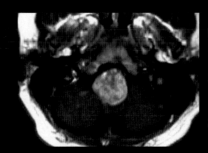

Axial T2-weighted image shows a hyper-intense mass.

Axial, post-contrast T1-weighted image shows a round enhancing mass.

DIFFERENTIAL DIAGNOSIS

At a Glance:

- Adenoid Cystic Carcinoma
- Chondrosarcoma
- Ecchordosis Physaliphora
- Lymphoma
- Meningioma
- Metastasis (Renal Cell Carcinoma)
- Nasopharyngeal Carcinoma
- Pituitary Adenoma
- Cholesteatoma (Atypical Location) (not pictured)
- Plasmacytoma (not pictured)

ADENOID CYSTIC CARCINOMA

Adenoid cystic carcinoma represents less than 10% of all salivary gland neoplasms, but is about 40% of all malignancies of major and minor salivary glands. The characteristics of this tumor include slow growth, multiple recurrences, pro-longed clinical course, and late metastasis. Adenoid cystic carcinoma occurs most frequently in the fifth decade of life. There is no sex predilection. It is the most common malignancy in the submandibular gland and the minor salivary glands. Adenoid cystic carcinoma has the tendency for perineural invasion, which is seen in about 80% of all patients.

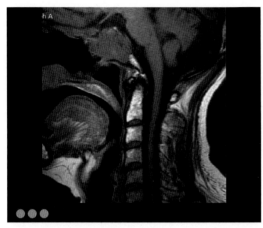

B1. Sagittal T1-weighted image shows a soft tissue mass involving the bony clivus.

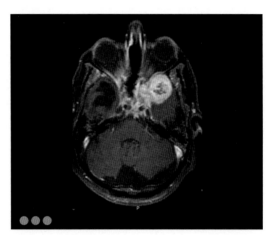

B2. Axial and coronal, post-contrast, fat-suppressed T1-weighted images show an enhancing mass involving the clivus as well as the left cavernous sinus, left temporal fossa.

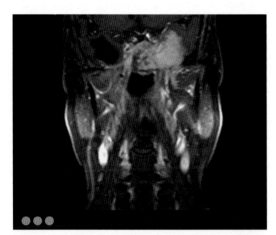

B3. Axial and coronal, post-contrast, fat-suppressed T1-weighted images show an enhancing mass involving the clivus as well as the left cavernous sinus, left temporal fossa.

CHONDROSARCOMA

Chondrosarcomas usually arise from different locations associated with sutures. In the clival region, they arise from the petrooccipital suture. Most craniofacial chondrosarcomas are low grade. They are rare, slow growing, and locally invasive tumors. On T1 weighted images, they typically show low to intermediate signal intensity, and on T2 weighted images show hyperintense signal. Signal may be heterogeneous due to calcifications or hemorrhage. Significant contrast enhancement is usually seen. Amorphous, snowflake calcifications may be seen in high grade tumors, better demonstrated with CT.

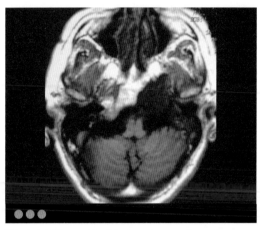

C1. Axial T1-weighted image shows a large hypointense mass involving the left petrous apex and left side of the clivus.

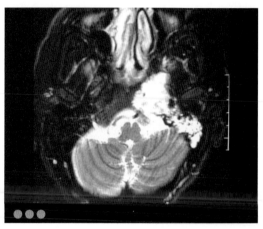

C2. Axial T2-weighted image reveals a large hyperintense mass involving the left petrous bone and left side of the clivus with extension into the skull base and associated mastoid disease.

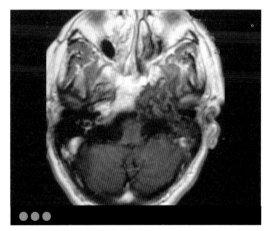

C3. Axial and coronal, post-contrast T1-weighted images demonstrate a patchy enhancing mass involving the left petrous bone, clivus, and skull base.

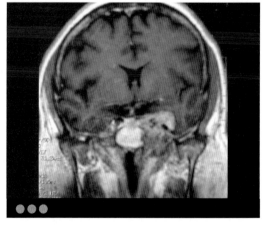

C4. Axial and coronal, post-contrast T1-weighted images demonstrate a patchy enhancing mass involving the left petrous bone, clivus, and skull base.

ECCHORDOSIS PHYSALIPHORA

Ecchordosis physaliphora (EP) is a small, gelatinous tissue that is considered an ectopic notochordal remnant. Intracranial EP is typically found intradurally in the prepontine cistern, where it is attached to the dorsal wall of the clivus via a small pedicle. Ecchordoses in this region are usually asymptomatic and found in about 2% of autopsies.

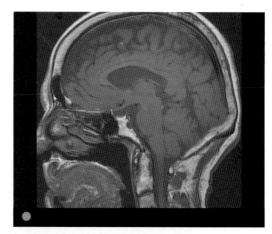

D1. Sagittal and axial T1-weighted image shows a hypointense lesion in the upper clivus in contrast to the hyperintense fatty marrow in the clivus.

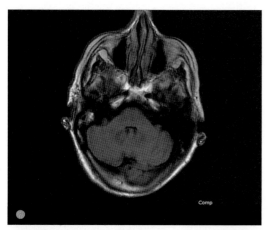

D2. Sagittal and axial T1-weighted image shows a hypointense lesion in the upper clivus in contrast to the hyperintense fatty marrow in the clivus.

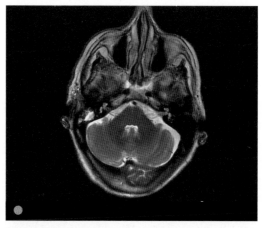

D3. Axial T2-weighted image reveals a bilobular hypointense lesion in the upper clivus.

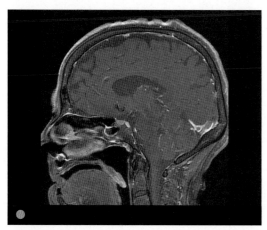

D4. Sagittal, post-contrast T1-weighted, fat-suppressed images demonstrate a nonenhancing mass in the upper clivus with disruption of the enhancing dura seen.

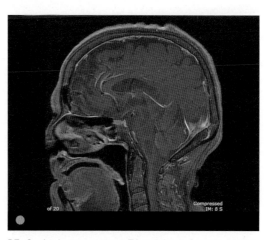

D5. Sagittal, post-contrast T1-weighted, fat-suppressed images demonstrate a nonenhancing mass in the upper clivus with disruption of the enhancing dura seen.

LYMPHOMA

Lymphoma involving the clivus may or may not demonstrate bone destruction. MR is superior to CT in the evaluation of lymphoma. Lymphomatous infiltration of the clivus with replacement of the normal fatty marrow may be seen on T1-weighted images without discrete bone destruction. Lymphoma may involve the cavernous sinus without narrowing of the carotid artery lumen whereas meningioma usually cause encasement of the carotid with luminal narrowing.

Perineural spread is a well-known property of head and neck lymphoma that invade the skull base. Tumor can selectively infiltrate a nerve or the sheath of a nerve to reach and ultimately pass through a foramen of the skull base. Occasionally, the presence of a long dural tail may be seen.

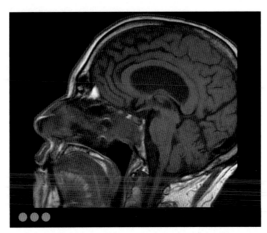

E1. Sagittal and coronal T1-weighted images show a slightly hypointense mass in the region of clivus with bony destruction and extension into the sphenoid sinus.

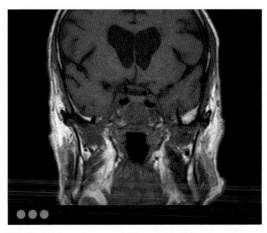

E2. Sagittal and coronal T1-weighted images show a slightly hypointense mass in the region of clivus with bony destruction and extension into the sphenoid sinus.

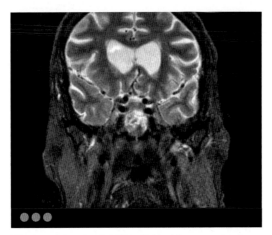

E3. Coronal and axial T2-weighted images reveal a hyperintense mass in the region of clivus.

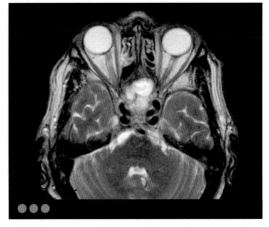

E4. Coronal and axial T2-weighted images reveal a hyperintense mass in the region of clivus.

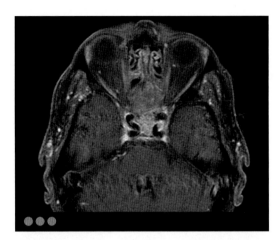

E5. Axial and coronal, post-contrast T1-weighted images demonstrate enhancement of the mass lesion.

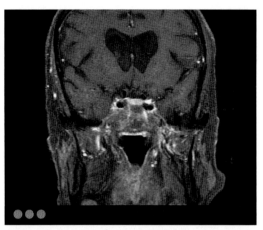

E6. Axial and coronal, post-contrast T1-weighted images demonstrate enhancement of the mass lesion.

MENINGIOMA

Meningioma of the clivus is usually associated with bony hyperostosis and calcification, bone destruction is unusual. Meningioma is a benign, slow-growing tumor of the meninges, probably arising from the arachnoid cap cells. Meningioma is the most common extraaxial tumor in adults and represents approximately 15% of all intracranial tumors in adults. Common locations for meningiomas include parasagittal (50%), sphenoid wing (20%), floor of the anterior cranial fossa (10%), parasellar region (10%), tentorium, and cerebellopontine angle cistern region. Clival meningiomas are uncommon lesions. Clival meningioma is a posterior fossa meningioma located over the middle or rostral part of the clivus. On MRI, they usually show isointensity on both T1 weighted and T2 weighted images, but may also be variable. Meningiomas enhance intensely and homogeneously following intravenous injection of gadolinium. The edema may be more apparent on MRI than on CT scan. An enhancing "dural-tail" involving the dura adjacent to the meningioma may be apparent on contrast enhanced MRI. On proton MR spectroscopy, meningiomas may show markedly increased choline peak, decreased or no NAA, and presence of alanine (at 1.5ppm).

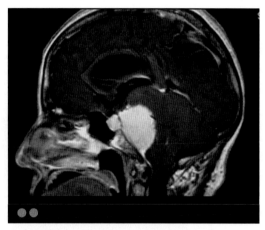

F. Sagittal, post-contrast T1-weighted image demonstrates an avidly enhancing mass along the clivus. Note the clivus and pituitary gland are intact.

METASTASIS (RENAL CELL CARCINOMA)

Metastatic disease to the clivus is not uncommon. Bone destruction is associated with replacement of normal fatty marrow within the clivus.

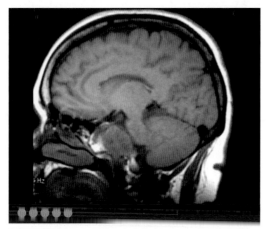

G1. Sagittal T1-weighted image reveals an isointense mass in the region of clivus with bony destruction.

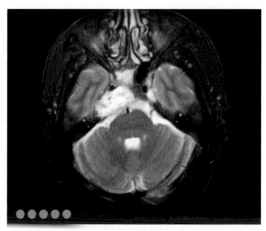

G2. Axial T2 weighted image shows a hyperintense mass on the right side of the clivus.

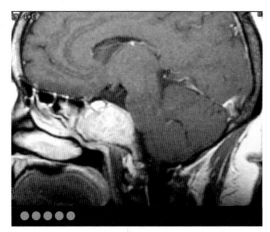

G3. Sagittal, post-contrast T1-weighted image demonstrates a mass lesion involving the clivus with intense contrast enhancement.

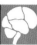

NASOPHARYNGEAL CARCINOMA

Nasopharyngeal carcinoma is a squamous cell carcinoma (SCC) that occurs in the epithelial lining of the nasopharynx. It is rare in the United States; however, it is endemic in southern China where incidence rates as high as 25 to 50 per 100,000 per year have been reported. The fossa of Rosenmuller (lateral nasopharyngeal recess) is the most common location for nasopharyngeal carcinoma.

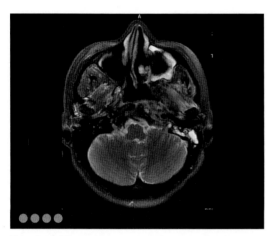

H1. Axial T2-weighted image shows a left nasopharyngeal mass invading the clivus on the left side.

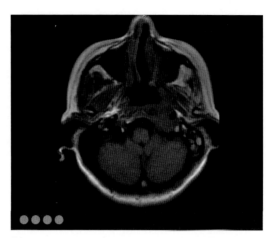

H2. Axial, pre- and post-contrast T1-weighted images show an enhancing mass at the left nasopharynx with invasion of the clivus on the left side.

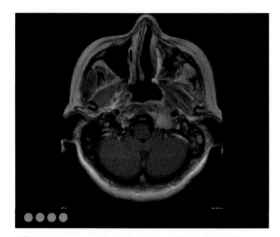

H3. Axial, pre- and post-contrast T1-weighted images show an enhancing mass at the left nasopharynx with invasion of the clivus on the left side.

PITUITARY ADENOMA

Invasive **pituitary adenoma** can grow aggressively with bone erosion and destruction.

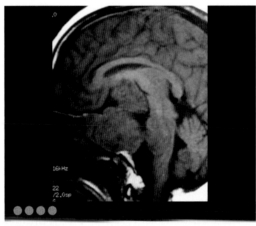

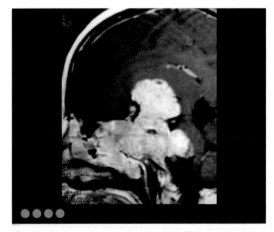

I1, Sagittal, pre- and post-contrast T1-weighted images show a large pituitary tumor eroding the clivus with extension of the tumor into the sphenoid sinus, prepontine cistern and suprasellar cistern.

I2. Sagittal, pre- and post-contrast T1-weighted images show a large pituitary tumor eroding the clivus with extension of the tumor into the sphenoid sinus, prepontine cistern and suprasellar cistern.

MENINGIOMA

Meningiomas are the most common nonglial primary neoplasm of the central nervous system. Extension of meningioma enhancement into adjacent dura may be seen in 60% of the cases. This "dural-tail" sign does not necessarily mean tumor infiltration into the adjacent dura, but it may represent a reactive change of the adjacent dura, which is due to vasocongestion and accumulation of interstitial fluid.

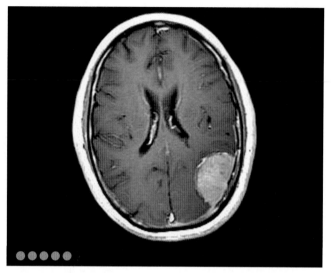

A. Axial, post-contrast T1-weighted image shows an enhancing mass in the left temporal, parietal region with broad-based dural attachment.

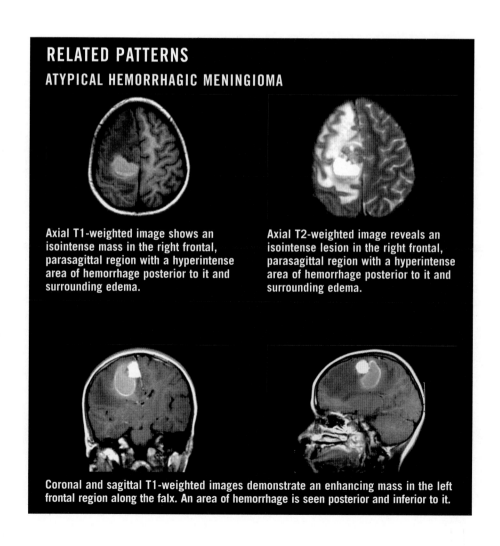

RELATED PATTERNS
ATYPICAL HEMORRHAGIC MENINGIOMA

Axial T1-weighted image shows an isointense mass in the right frontal, parasagittal region with a hyperintense area of hemorrhage posterior to it and surrounding edema.

Axial T2-weighted image reveals an isointense lesion in the right frontal, parasagittal region with a hyperintense area of hemorrhage posterior to it and surrounding edema.

Coronal and sagittal T1-weighted images demonstrate an enhancing mass in the left frontal region along the falx. An area of hemorrhage is seen posterior and inferior to it.

RELATED PATTERNS (continued)
CONVEXITY MENINGIOMA

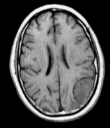 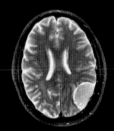 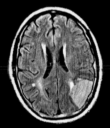

Axial T1-weighted image shows an extra-axial, hypointense lesion in the left temporal, parietal region.

Axial T2-weighted and FLAIR images reveal a hyperintense mass.

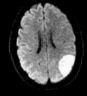 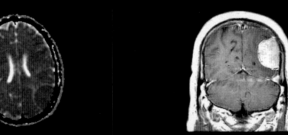

Axial diffusion-weighted image and ADC map image demonstrate a mass with restricted diffusion. Restricted diffusion is seen in atypical or malignant meningiomas. This is a case of atypical meningioma.

Coronal, post-contrast T1-weighted image shows a large, broad-based, enhancing mass lesion along the convexity in the temporal, parietal region.

INTRAOSSEOUS MENINGIOMA

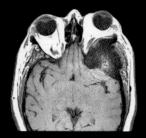

Axial T1-weighted image demonstrates focal hyperostosis of the left sphenoid bone with expansion into the left orbit. The hyperostotic bone is hypointnese with a small central component of isointnesity seen extending toward the temporal fossa.

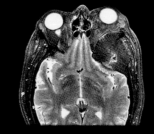

Axial T2-weighted image reveals focal hyperostosis of the left sphenoid bone with a central area of hyperintensity.

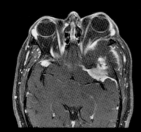

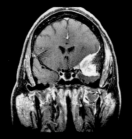

Axial and coronal, post-contrast T1-weighted, fat-suppressed images demonstrate contrast enhancement of the meningeal surface of the mass with extension of the enhancement into the central portion of hyperostosis.

DIFFERENTIAL DIAGNOSIS

At a Glance:

- *Chondrosarcoma of the Falx*
- *Hemangiopericytoma*
- *Lymphoma*
- *Meningeal Melanocytoma*
- *Metastatic Carcinoma of Prostate*
- *Metastatic Disease (Melanoma)*
- *Metastatic Melanoma (Case Two)*
- *Plasmacytoma*
- *Sarcoid*
- *Solitary Fibrous Tumor of the Meninges*

CHONDROSARCOMA OF THE FALX

Extraskeletal mesenchymal **chondrosarcoma** is a rare neoplasm. The tumor occur most often in the second and third decades. There is a moderate tendency to local recurrence.

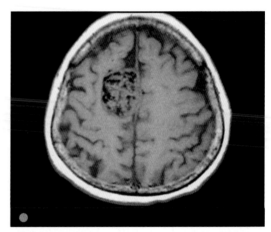

B1. Axial T1-weighted image shows an isointense mass with multiple small hypointense areas in the right frontal region along the falx. The small hypointense areas are consistent with calcification.

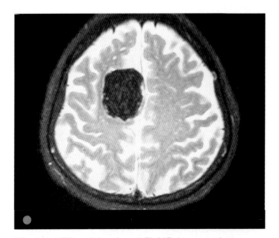

B2. Axial T2-weighted and FLAIR images show a predominantly hypointense mass along the flax in the right frontal region.

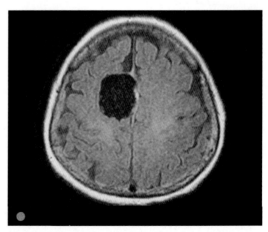

B3. Axial T2-weighted and FLAIR images show a predominantly hypointense mass along the flax in the right frontal region.

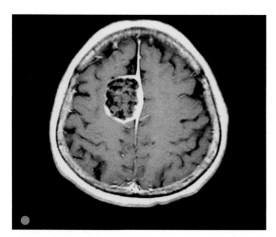

B4. Axial and coronal, post-contrast T1-weighted images show a peripheral rim of enhancement extending into the falx.

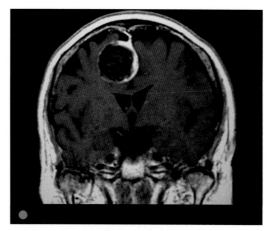

B5. Axial and coronal, post-contrast T1-weighted images show a peripheral rim of enhancement extending into the falx.

HEMANGIOPERICYTOMA

Hemangiopericytoma of the meninges is an aggressive, highly vascular neoplasm. It arises from vascular pericytes and is therefore a distinct entity. On imaging studies, it is a heterogeneous mass with cystic, necrotic areas and prominent vascular channels.

HEMANGIOPERICYTOMA (CASE ONE)

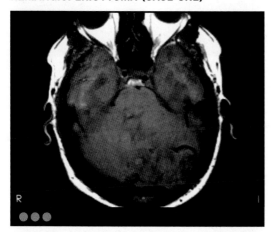

C1. Axial T1-weighted image shows an isointense mass in the left posterior fossa extraaxial mass with multiple curvilinear signal void areas within it. Note a small round area of hyperintensity is seen on the right side of the mass due to focal hemorrhage. Bony erosion is seen adjacent to the mass.

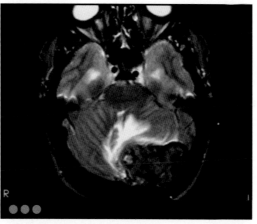

C2. Axial T2-weighted image shows a mixed signal intensity mass with a focal hemorrhage seen on the right side and surrounding edema.

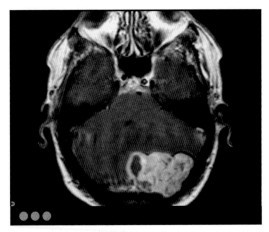

C3. Axial and coronal, post-contrast T1-weighted images show an extraaxial, heterogeneously enhancing mass in the left posterior fossa.

C4. Axial and coronal, post-contrast T1-weighted images show an extraaxial, heterogeneously enhancing mass in the left posterior fossa.

HEMANGIOPERICYTOMA (CASE TWO)

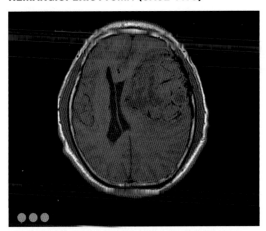

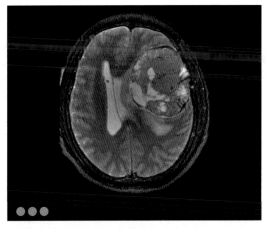

C5. Axial T1-weighted image shows a slightly hypointense mass with cuvilinear signal voids and cystic, necrotic changes in the left frontal convexity with associated bony destruction.

C6. Axial T2-weighted image reveals a hyperintense mass with cuvilinear signal voids and cystic, necrotic changes in the left frontal convexity with associated bony destruction.

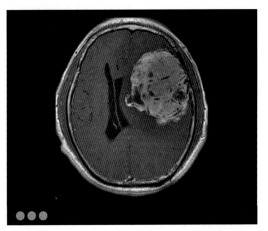

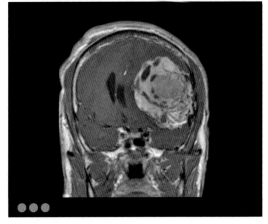

C7. Axial and coronal, post-contrast T1-weighted images show a heterogeneously enhancing mass in the left frontal convexity.

C8. Axial and coronal, post-contrast T1-weighted images show a heterogeneously enhancing mass in the left frontal convexity.

LYMPHOMA

LYMPHOMA (CASE ONE)

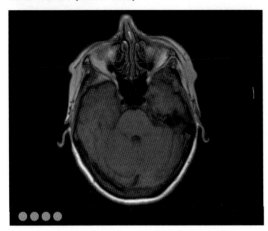

D1. Axial T1-weighted image shows an isointense lesion in the occipital region on the left side.

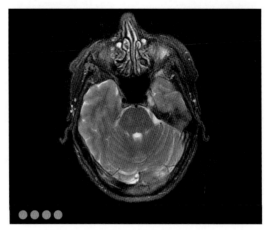

D2. Axial T2-weighted and FLAIR images demonstrate a hypointense lesion in the left occipital region with abnormal signal seen in the adjacent skull and a minimal amount of surrounding edema.

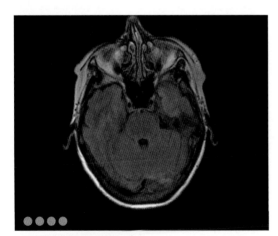

D3. Axial T2-weighted and FLAIR images demonstrate a hypointense lesion in the left occipital region with abnormal signal seen in the adjacent skull and a minimal amount of surrounding edema.

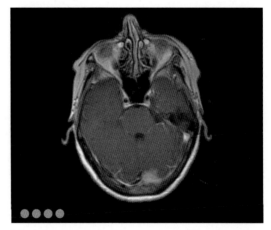

D4. Axial and coronal, post-contrast T1-weighted images reveal an avidly enhancing extradural mass in the left occipital region.

LYMPHOMA (CASE TWO)

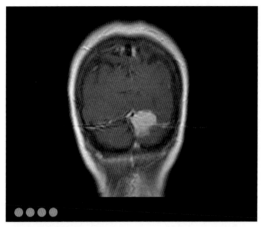

D5. Axial and coronal, post-contrast T1-weighted images reveal an avidly enhancing extradural mass in the left occipital region.

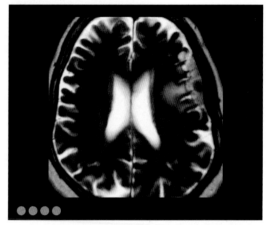

E1. Axial T2-weighted and FLAIR images show a hyperintense, extra-axial lesion in the left frontal region. Some adjacent parenchymal edema is seen.

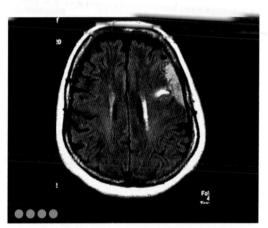

E2. Axial T2-weighted and FLAIR images show a hyperintense, extra-axial lesion in the left frontal region. Some adjacent parenchymal edema is seen.

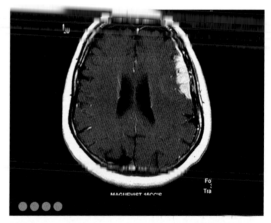

E3. Axial, post-contrast T1-weighted image shows an enhancing extra-axial mass in the left frontal region.

MENINGEAL MELANOCYTOMA

These tumors are very rare and arise in the particular distribution of normally existing melanocytes in the central nervous system. Mean age of patients is the fifth decade. Most frequent location is foramen magnum, followed by cerebellopontine angle and Meckel's cave. The MR appearance varies depending on the degree of melanization and accompanying intratumoral hemorrhage. Usually, iso- to hypointense on T1 images and low in signal on T2 images. Intense homogeneous contrast following administration of contrast.

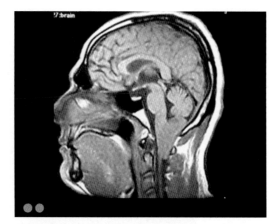

F1. Sagittal T1-weighted image shows an isointense, extra-axial mass at the craniovertebral junction posteriorly.

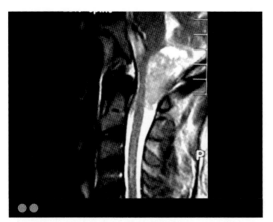

F2. Sagittal T2-weighted image shows a heterogeneously hyperintense mass at the craniovertebral junction posteriorly.

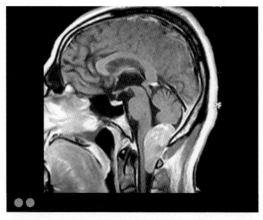

F3. Sagittal, post-contrast T1-weighted image shows a homogeneously enhancing mass.

METASTATIC CARCINOMA OF PROSTATE

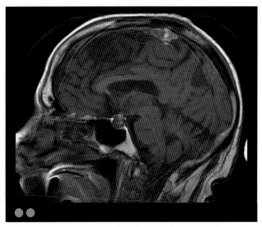

G1. Sagittal T1-weighted image shows extra-axial, hyperintense, and isointense lesions in the fronto-parietal region (the pituittary gland is enlarged due to metastatic disease to the pituitary).

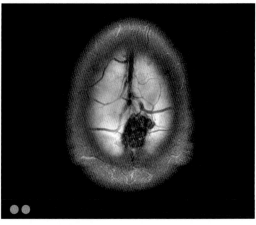

G2. Axial T2-weighted image reveals a hypointnese mass near the vertex.

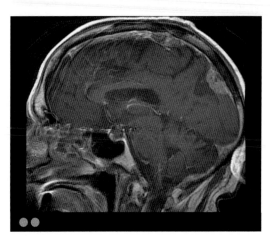

G3. Sagittal, post-contrast T1-weighted image demonstrates enhancing extra-axial masses.

METASTATIC DISEASE (MELANOMA)

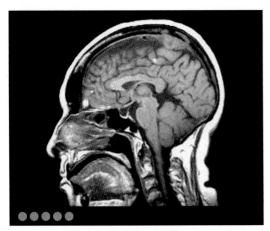

H1. Sagittal T1-weighted image shows an extraaxial mass with bony destruction of the calvarium in the parietal region.

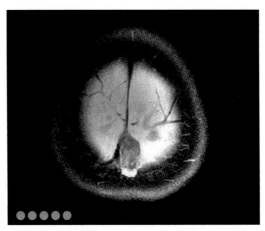

H2. Axial T2-weighted image shows a hypointense mass along the falx on the left side.

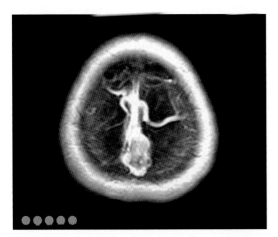

H3. Axial and coronal, post-contrast T1-weighted images demonstrate an enhancing mass along the falx with adjacent bony destruction and invasion of the superior sagittal sinus.

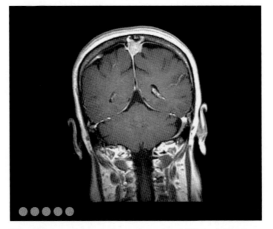

H4. Axial and coronal, post-contrast T1-weighted images demonstrate an enhancing mass along the falx with adjacent bony destruction and invasion of the superior sagittal sinus.

METASTATIC MELANOMA (CASE TWO)

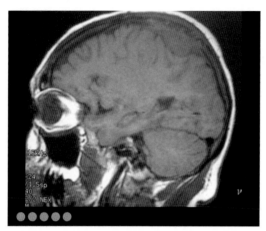

I1. Sagittal and axial T1-weighted images show a slightly hypointense, extra-axial mass with evidence of bony destruction involving the skull and extracranial extension.

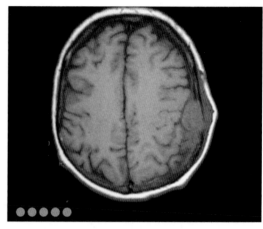

I2. Sagittal and axial T1-weighted images show a slightly hypointense, extra-axial mass with evidence of bony destruction involving the skull and extracranial extension.

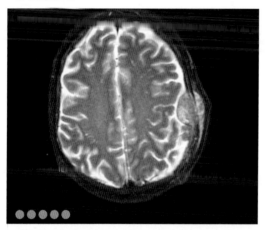

I3. Axial T2-weighted image reveals a hyperintense, extra-axial mass with bone destruction and extracranial extension.

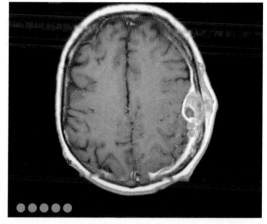

I4. Axial, coronal and sagittal, post-contrast T1-weighted images demonstrate a heterogeneously enhancing mass with dural tail and extracranial extension.

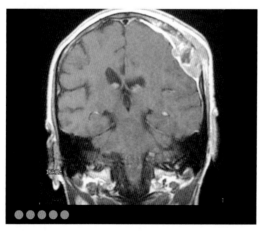

I5. Axial, coronal and sagittal, post-contrast T1-weighted images demonstrate a heterogeneously enhancing mass with dural tail and extracranial extension.

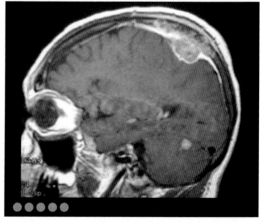

I6. Axial, coronal and sagittal, post-contrast T1-weighted images demonstrate a heterogeneously enhancing mass with dural tail and extracranial extension.

PLASMACYTOMA

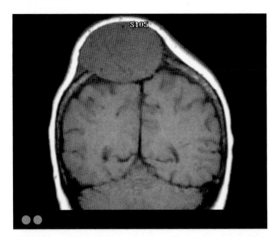

J1. Coronal T1-weighted image shows an extra-axial, slightly hypointense mass with bony destruction of the skull and extracranial extension.

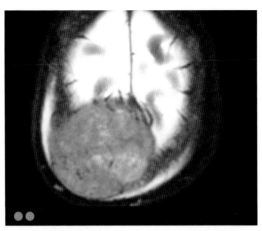

J2. Axial T2-weighted image shows a large slightly hypointense mass involving the calvarium, epidural space with extracranial extension. Plasmacytomas tend to exhibit hypointnesity on T2-weighted images due to its high cellularity and high nucleus to cytoplasma ratio.

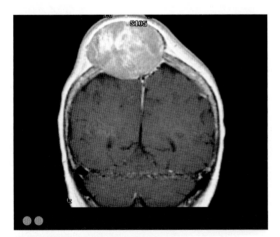

J3. Coronal, post-contrast T1-weighted image reveals an avidly enhancing mass.

SARCOID

Granulomatous disease usually involves the basilar meninges rather than the meninges in the convexity, but occasionally this can occur. Sarcoidosis can involve the meninges (cranial nerve palsies, pituitary, and hypothalamic effects), peripheral nerves (symmetric polyneuropathy, multifocal neuropathy), and brain or spinal cord. Solitary sarcoid mass lesion of the CNS, mimicking tumors are rare. They may either arise from the dura or be located entirely within the brain parenchyma, with imaging appearances which resemble meningioma and glioma respectively.

SARCOID (CASE ONE)

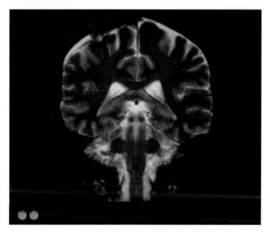

K1. Axial T2-weighted image shows a right focal dural-based hypointense lesion.

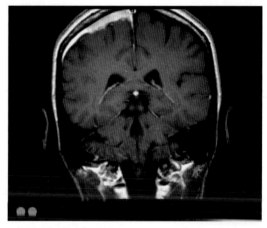

K2. Axial post-contrast T1-weighted image shows a dural-based enhancing lesion in the right parietal region.

SARCOID (CASE TWO)

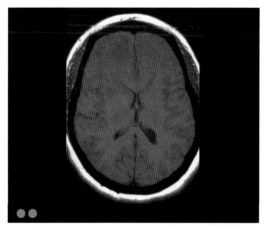

L1. Axial T1-weighted image shows hypointensity in both frontal lobes.

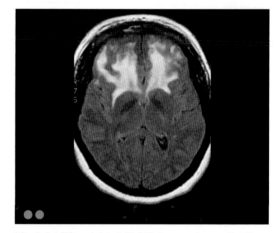

L2. Axial T2-weighted FLAIR image shows slightly hypointense lesion along the falx anteriorly with hyperintense edema seen in both frontal lobes.

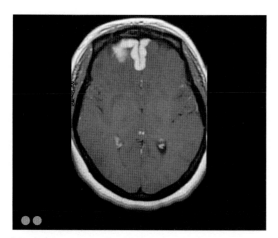

L3. Axial, post-contrast T1-weighted image shows an enhancing mass along the falx. There is an area of enhancement in the right frontal lobe, suggesting involvement of the parenchyma in the right frontal lobe.

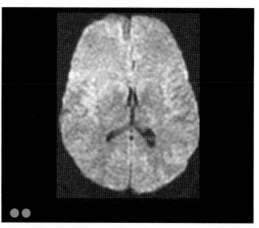

L4. Diffusion-weighted image shows no evidence of restricted diffusion.

SOLITARY FIBROUS TUMOR OF THE MENINGES

Solitary fibrous tumor occurs most frequently within the pleura, they are rarely seen intracranially. Most of these tumors are benign, but malignant cases have been reported. The solitary fibrous tumor is now recognized as a dural-based neoplasm distinct from fibrous meningioma. Histological examination showed a mixture of spindle-shaped and round cells arranged in a collagen matrix. Immunohistochemical staining of the tumor demonstrated diffuse positive staining for CD34 and vimentin. Ultrastructural studies support attributing a mesenchymal, rather than meningothelial, nature to the tumor.

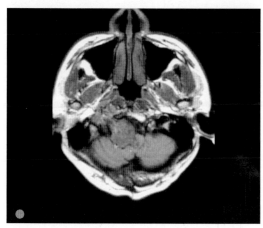

M1. Axial T1-weighted image shows an isointense mass in the region of right perimedullary cistern with extension into the skull base through hypoglossal canal.

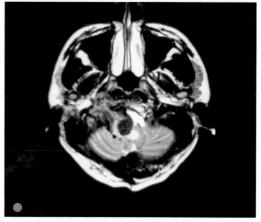

M2. Axial T2-weighted and FLAIR images demonstrate the mass to be hypointense in the center and hyperintense in the periphery.

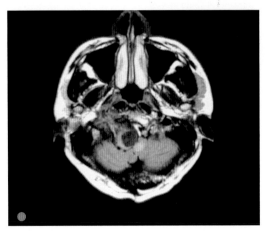

M3. Axial T2 weighted and FLAIR images demonstrate the mass to be hypointense in the center and hyperintense in the periphery.

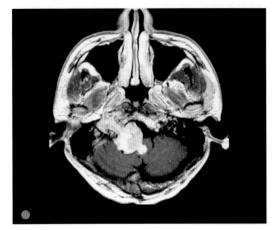

M4. Axial and coronal, post-contrast T1-weighted images show a lobulated, enhacning mass with extension into the skull base.

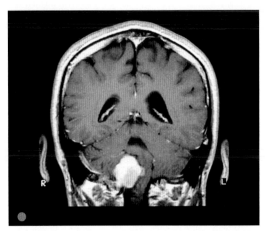

M5. Axial and coronal, post-contrast T1-weighted images show a lobulated, enhacning mass with extension into the skull base.

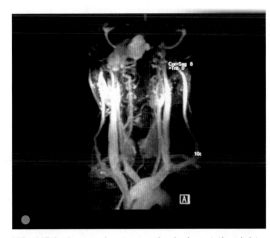

M6. MRA shows a hypervascular lesion at the right skull base.

VESTIBULAR SCHWANNOMA

Vestibular schwannoma is the most common neoplasm of the cerebellopontine angle. It arises from the Schwann cells that envelop the eighth cranial nerve, particularly the superior vestibular division. The presence of cystic or necrotic changes favors the diagnosis of a vestibular schwannoma.

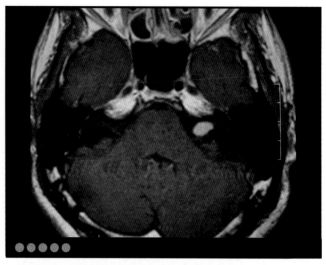

A. Axial, post-contrast T1-weighted image shows an enhancing mass in the left internal auditory canal.

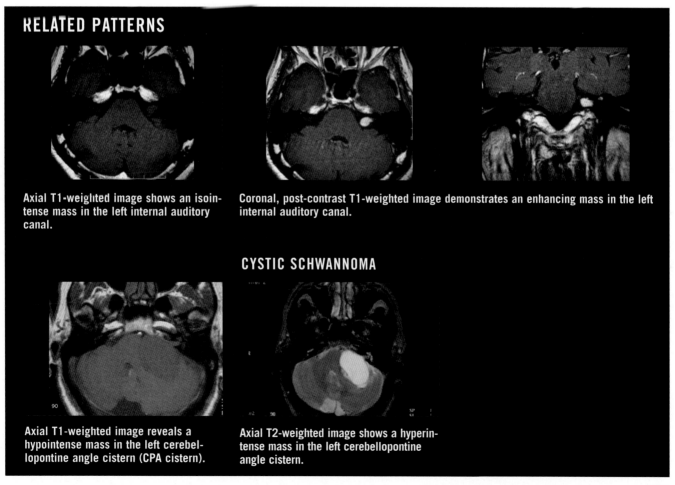

RELATED PATTERNS

Axial T1-weighted image shows an isointense mass in the left internal auditory canal.

Coronal, post-contrast T1-weighted image demonstrates an enhancing mass in the left internal auditory canal.

CYSTIC SCHWANNOMA

Axial T1-weighted image reveals a hypointense mass in the left cerebellopontine angle cistern (CPA cistern).

Axial T2-weighted image shows a hyperintense mass in the left cerebellopontine angle cistern.

RELATED PATTERNS (continued)
CYSTIC SCHWANNOMA (continued)

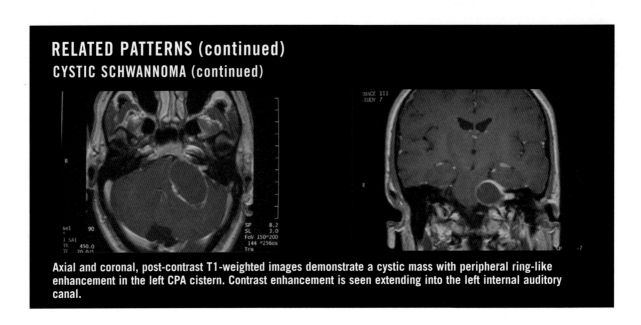

Axial and coronal, post-contrast T1-weighted images demonstrate a cystic mass with peripheral ring-like enhancement in the left CPA cistern. Contrast enhancement is seen extending into the left internal auditory canal.

DIFFERENTIAL DIAGNOSIS

At a Glance:

- BIlateral Vestibular Schwannoma
- Chondrosarcoma
- Endolymphatic Sac Tumor
- Facial Nerve Schwannoma
- Fifth Nerve Schwannoma
- Glomus Tumor
- Lymphoma
- Meningioma
- Metastasis
- Neurofibromatosis Type II

BILATERAL VESTIBULAR SCHWANNOMA

Bilateral Vestibular schwannoma are diagnostic of neurofibromatosis type II.

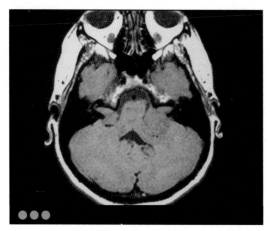

B1. Axial T1-weighted image reveals bilateral mass lesions in the CPA cisterns with extension of the mass into the internal auditory canal. Bilateral vestibular schwannomas are seen in patients with neurofibromatosis type II.

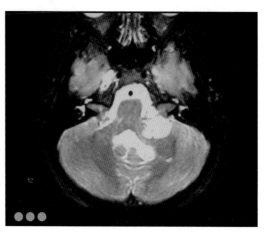

B2. T2-weighted image shows bilateral hyperintense masses in the CPA cisterns.

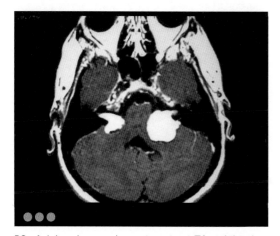

B3. Axial and coronal , post-contrast T1-weighted images demonstrate enhancing masses bilaterally.

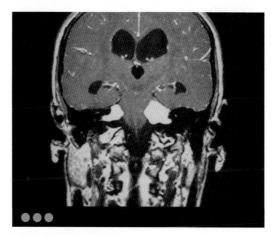

B4. Axial and coronal , post-contrast T1-weighted images demonstrate enhancing masses bilaterally.

CHONDROSARCOMA

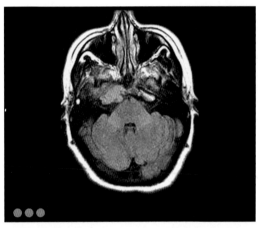

C1. Axial FLAIR image shows an isointense mass on the right side of clivus at the cerebellopontine angle.

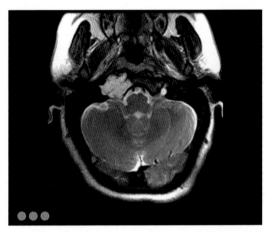

C2. Axial T2-weighted image reveals a hyperintense mass on the right side of clivus.

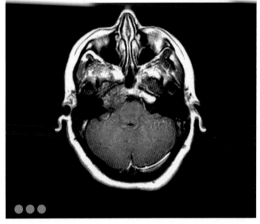

C3. Axial, post-contrast T1-weighted images show a patchy enhancing mass. Chondrosarcomas generally show more contrast enhancement than chordoma.

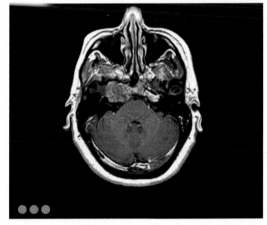

C4. Axial, post-contrast T1-weighted images show a patchy enhancing mass. Chondrosarcomas generally show more contrast enhancement than chordoma.

ENDOLYMPHATIC SAC TUMOR

The tumor is a very rare neuroectodermal tumor of the petrous temporal bone and contains areas of hemorrhage, hemosiderin, and cholesterol clefts with scattered inflammatory giant cell reactions. These aggressive papillary tumors are actually low-grade papillary adenocarcinomas of the temporal bone and demonstrate glandular features that suggest they originate in the endolymphatic sac. Most endolymphatic sac tumors occur sporadically. Patients with Von Hippel Lindau disease have a high incidence of endolymphatic sac tumors.

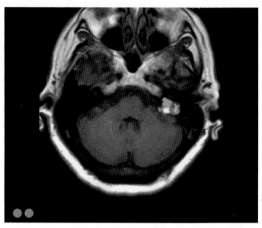

D1. Axial T1-weighted image shows a hyperintense mass at the left CPA cistern with irregular contour.

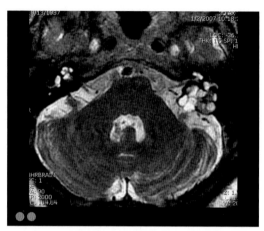

D2. Axial T2-weighted image shows a hyperintense mass at the left CPA cistern, just posterior to the seventh and eighth nerve complex.

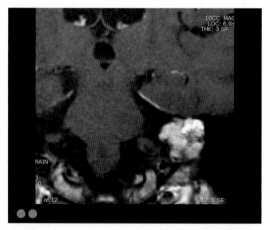

D3. Coronal, post-contrast T1-weighted image demonstrates enhancement of the mass lesion.

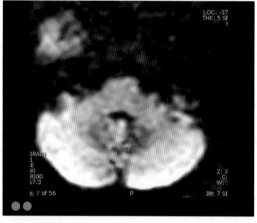

D4. Diffusion-weighted image shows no evidence of restricted diffusion.

FACIAL NERVE SCHWANNOMA

Schwannomas of the facial nerve can occur along any segment of the facial nerve, but they frequently involve the geniculate ganglion and extend proximally or distally from there. When facial nerve schwannoma cross the petrous bone to involve the posterior and middle fossa, they cross the midportion of the petrous bone, whereas trigeminal schwannomas cross near the petrous apex.

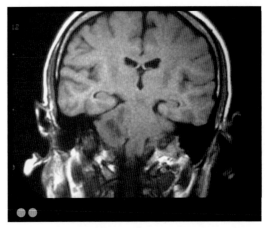

E1. Coronal T1-weighted image shows a mixed signal intensity mass at the right CPA cistern.

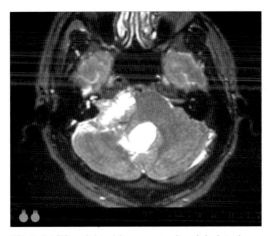

E2. Axial T2-weighted image reveals a lobulated hyperintense mass.

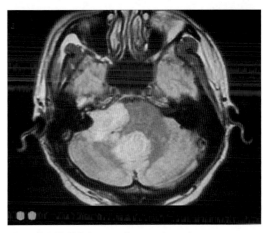

E3. Axial FLAIR image shows a hyperintense mass.

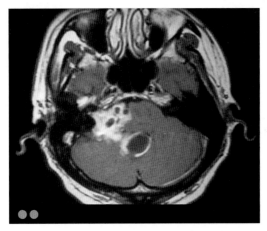

E4. Axial and coronal, post-contrast T1-weighted image demonstrate a multilobulated enhancing mass with cystic areas.

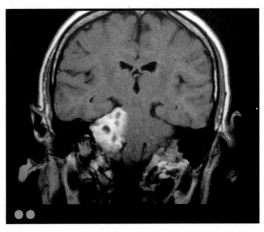

E5. Axial and coronal, post-contrast T1-weighted image demonstrate a multi-lobulated enhancing mass with cystic areas.

FIFTH NERVE SCHWANNOMA

Trigeminal schwannoma occur along the course of the fifth nerve. Tumor may extend from the ambient cistern into the Meckel's cave and cavernous sinus along the course of the fifth nerve. Bony destruction of the petrous apex is seen.

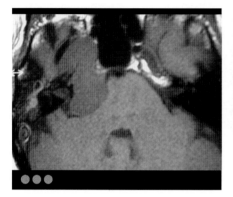

F1. Axial T1-weighted image shows a hypointense mass extending from CPA cistern into the medial aspect of the middle cranial fossa.

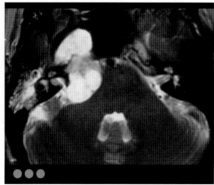

F2. Axial T2-weighted image shows a predominantly hyperintense mass.

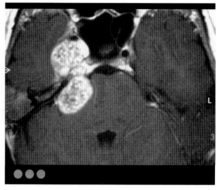

F3. Axial, post-contrast T1-weighted image shows a heterogeneously enhancing mass.

GLOMUS TUMOR

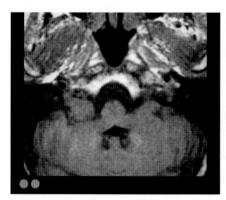

G1. Axial T1-weighted image shows a hypointense mass in the region of right CPA cistern.

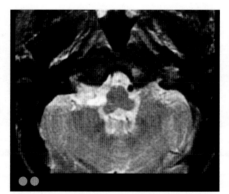

G2. Axial T2-weighted image demonstrates a slightly heterogeneous, hyperintense mass in the region of right CPA cistern.

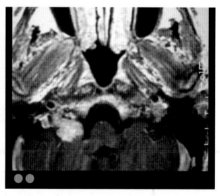

G3. Axial post-contrast T1-weighted image reveals an enhancing mass with slightly lobulated margin.

LYMPHOMA

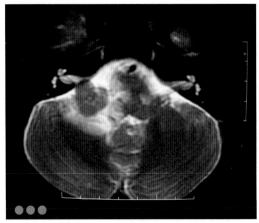

H1. Axial T2-weighted and FLAIR images demonstrate an isointense, intra-axial mass at the cerebellopontine angle cistern region with surrounding edema.

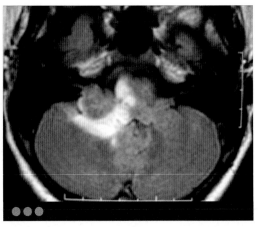

H2. Axial T2-weighted and FLAIR images demonstrate an isointense, intra-axial mass at the cerebellopontine angle cistern region with surrounding edema.

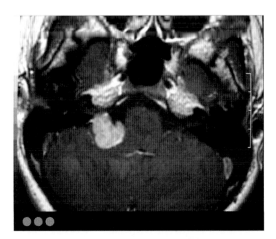

H3. Axial and coronal, post-contrast T1-weighted images show avid enhancement of the mass with irregular margin.

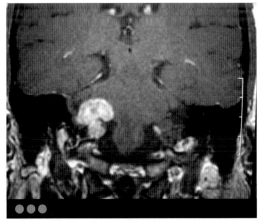

H4. Axial and coronal, post-contrast T1-weighted images show avid enhancement of the mass with irregular margin.

MENINGIOMA

Meningioma is the second most common diagnosis of a primary CPA lesion. Meningioma can arise within the CPA, extend from the middle fossa to the CPA. The presence of calcification and "dural tail" favors the diagnosis of meningioma. However, a number of other lesions may exhibit dural tail.

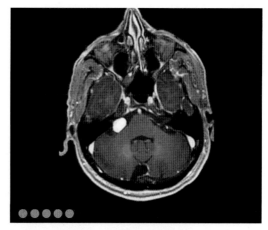

I. Axial, post-contrast T1-weighted image shows an enhancing mass in the right CPA cistern. Note there is no dural tail seen in this case.

METASTASIS

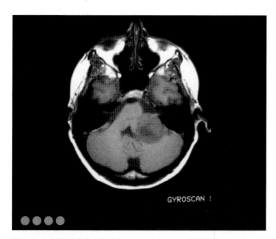

J1. Axial T1-weighted image shows a heterogeneously hypointense mass in the left brachium pontis and cerebellum at the cerebellopontine angle cistern.

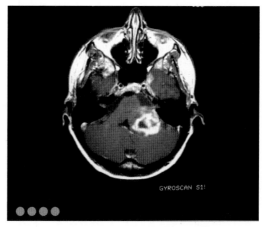

J2. Axial and coronal, post-contrast T1-weighted images demonstrate a heterogeneously enhancing mass.

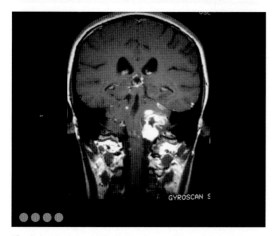

J3. Axial and coronal, post-contrast T1-weighted images demonstrate a heterogeneously enhancing mass.

113

NEUROFIBROMATOSIS TYPE II

In approximately 90% of the patients with **neurofibromatosis type II**, bilateral vestibular schwannomas are detected on MR imaging. Meningiomas, other cranial nerve schwannomas or spinal lesions are seen in about 50% of the patients. In the spine, both intramedullary tumors, such as astrocytomas or ependymomas, and extramedullary intradural tumors, such as meningiomas and schwannomas, may be detected on MR imaging studies. The gene for Neurofibromatosis type II is on band 22q11.

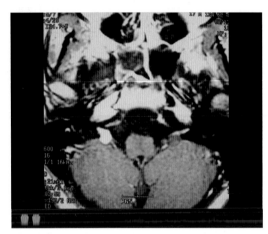

K1. Axial and coronal, post-contrast T1-weighted images show a hypothalamic astrocytoma, bilateral fifth and ninth nerve schwannomas. (Bilateral vestibular schwannomas are not shown here.)

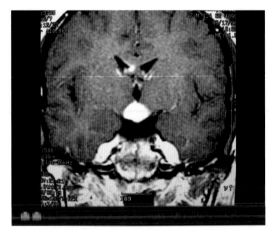

K2. Axial and coronal, post-contrast T1-weighted images show a hypothalamic astrocytoma, bilateral fifth and ninth nerve schwannomas. (Bilateral vestibular schwannomas are not shown here.)

EPIDERMOID

Epidermoids are congenital masses, but their clinical presentation usually in the third or fourth decade. They are predominantly located in basal cisterns and are usually paramedian in location as opposed to the midline location of dermoids. Epidermoids are the third most common masses of CPA. Epidermoids have similar signal intensity features to those of CSF on both T1-weighted and T2-weighted images. Sometimes, an internal stranded appearance can be seen, giving a "dirty-CSF" appearance. FLAIR imaging may show a slightly hyperintense lesion as compared to CSF. Diffusion-weighted images can be useful in differentiating epidermoids from arachnoid cysts. Epidermoids show restricted diffusion whereas arachnoid cysts do not show restricted diffusion.

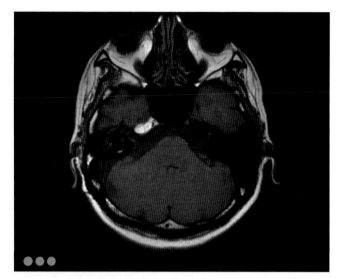

A. Axial T1-weighted image shows slight expansion of the right CPA cistern.

RELATED PATTERNS

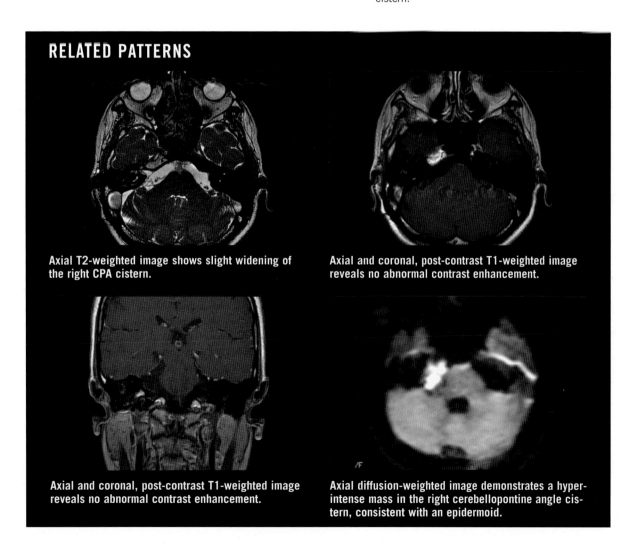

Axial T2-weighted image shows slight widening of the right CPA cistern.

Axial and coronal, post-contrast T1-weighted image reveals no abnormal contrast enhancement.

Axial and coronal, post-contrast T1-weighted image reveals no abnormal contrast enhancement.

Axial diffusion-weighted image demonstrates a hyperintense mass in the right cerebellopontine angle cistern, consistent with an epidermoid.

RELATED PATTERNS (continued)

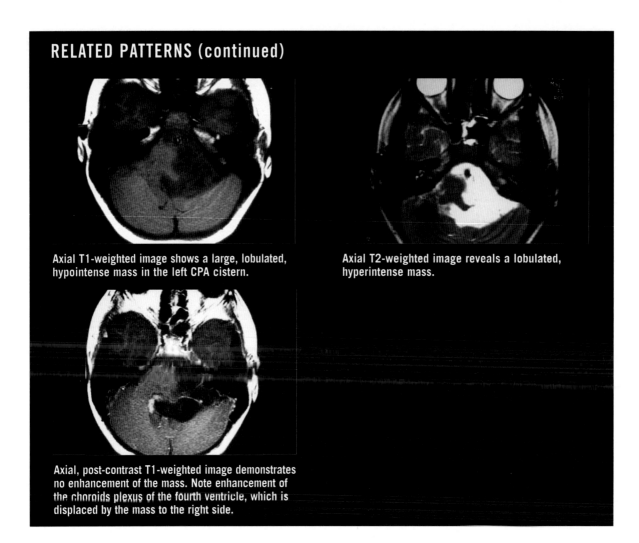

Axial T1-weighted image shows a large, lobulated, hypointense mass in the left CPA cistern.

Axial T2-weighted image reveals a lobulated, hyperintense mass.

Axial, post-contrast T1-weighted image demonstrates no enhancement of the mass. Note enhancement of the choroids plexus of the fourth ventricle, which is displaced by the mass to the right side.

DIFFERENTIAL DIAGNOSIS

At a Glance:

- *Arachnoid Cyst*
- *Cholesterol Granuloma*
- *Cysticercosis Cyst*

ARACHNOID CYST (CASE ONE)

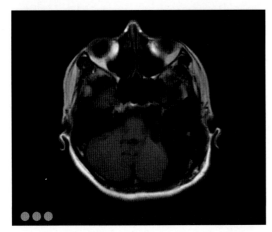

B1. Axial T1-weighted image shows a cerebrospinal fluid signal intensity lesion in the left cerebellopontine angle cistern.

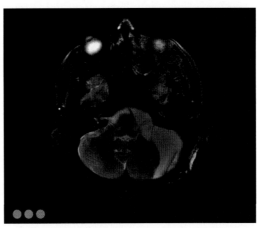

B2. Axial T2-weighted image reveals a hyperintense lesion at the left cerebellopontine angle cistern.

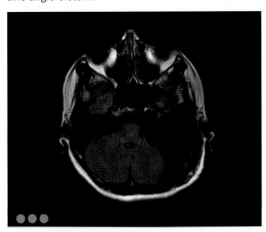

B3. FLAIR image shows the lesion to be of cerebrospinal fluid signal intensity.

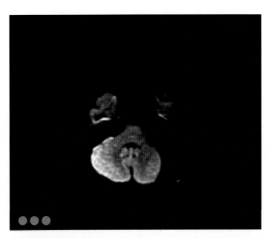

B4. Diffusion-weighted image shows no evidence of restricted diffusion.

ARACHNOID CYST (CASE TWO)

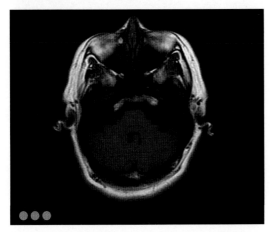

C1. Axial T1-weighted image shows a hypointense lesion in the left cerebellopontine angle cistern.

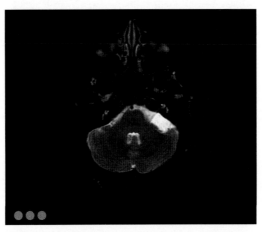

C2. Axial T2-weighted and FLAIR images demonstrate a hyperintense lesion in the left cerebellopontine angle cistern.

117

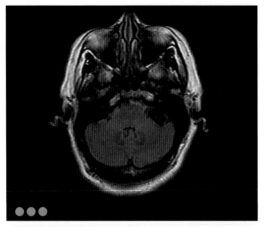

C3. Axial T2-weighted and FLAIR images demonstrate a hyperintense lesion in the left cerebellopontine angle cistern.

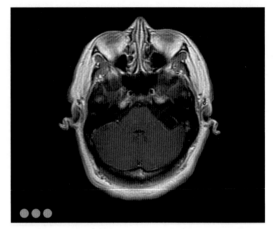

C4. Axial, post-contrast T1-weighted image reveals no abnormal enhancement.

CHOLESTEROL GRANULOMA

Cholesterol granuloma usually involves the petrous apex. Recurrent hemorrhage into the obstructed air cell at petrous apex with secondary inflammatory changes is thought to be the cause for cholesterol granuloma. Products of blood degradation, cholesterol crystals form a slowly expansile, fluid filled lesion at the petrous apex.

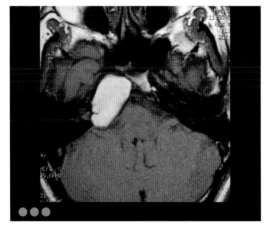

D1. Axial T1-weighted image shows an ovoid, hyperintense mass at the right petrous apex.

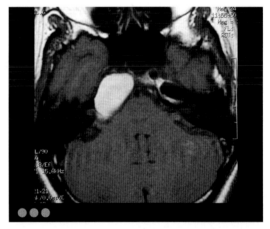

D2. Axial, post-contrast T1-weighted image reveals no enhancement of the hyperintense mass.

CYSTICERCOSIS CYST

Cysticercosis cysts in the basal cisterns usually take the racemose form and they do not contain the scolex. Since they are cysts of CSF signal intensity, they are difficult to differentiate from arachnoid cysts or epidermoids. Sometimes, contrast enhancement may be seen adjacent to the cysticercosis cysts due to the presence of inflammatory reaction adjacent to these cysts. They are similar to arachnoid cysts and do not exhibit restricted diffusion.

CYSTICERCOSIS (CASE ONE)

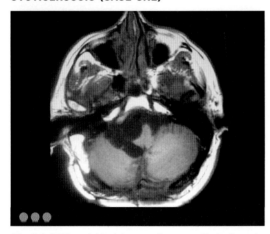

E1. Axial T1 weighted image shows cystic lesion at the right CPA cistern, prepontine cistern and left CPA cistern.

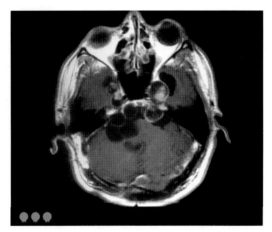

E2. Axial, post-contrast T1 weighted image demonstrate no enhancement of the cysts in the right CPA cistern, but ring enhancement is seen in a cyst in the left CPA cistern. Additional cysts with and without enhancement are seen in the middle cranial fossa.

CYSTICERCOSIS (CASE TWO)

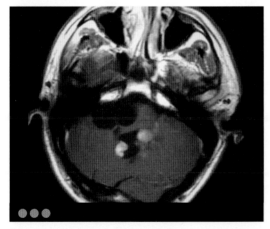

E3. Axial, post-contrast T1 weighted image shows cystic lesions in the right cerebellopontine angle cistern. In addition, two enhancing scoleces are seen in fourth ventricular cysts.

119

ESTHESIONEUROBLASTOMA

Esthesioneuroblastoma is a rare malignant neoplasm of the nasal vault, probably arising from the olfactory epithelium. Imaging is important in staging the neoplasm to detect the involvement of the skull base, its foramina, orbits and intracranial compartment.

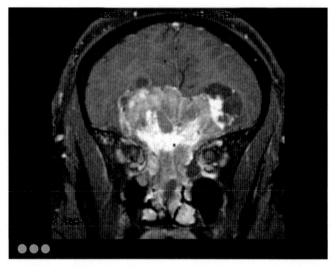

A. Coronal, post-contrast T1 weighted, fat-suppressed image shows a large enhancing mass extending from nasal cavity, ethmoid sinus through the cribriform plate into the frontal fossa.

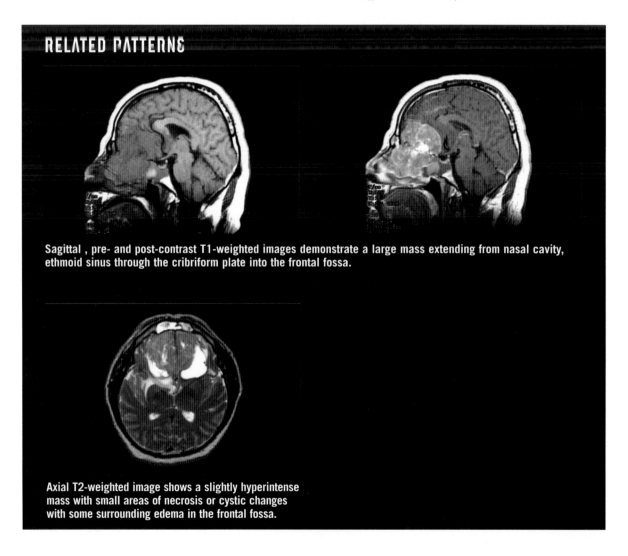

RELATED PATTERNS

Sagittal, pre- and post-contrast T1-weighted images demonstrate a large mass extending from nasal cavity, ethmoid sinus through the cribriform plate into the frontal fossa.

Axial T2-weighted image shows a slightly hyperintense mass with small areas of necrosis or cystic changes with some surrounding edema in the frontal fossa.

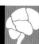

DIFFERENTIAL DIAGNOSIS

At a Glance:

- *Adenoid Cystic Carcinoma*
- *Chondrosarcoma*
- *Juvenile Angiofibroma*

- *Meningioma*
- *Neuroendocrine Tumor*
- *Rabdomyosarcoma*
- *Encephalocele* (not pictured)
- *Metastasis* (not pictured)

ADENOID CYSTIC CARCINOMA

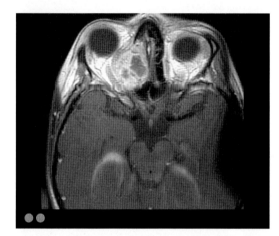

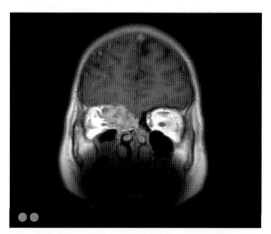

B1. Axial and coronal, post-contrast T1-weighted image shows an enhancing mass invading the right orbit and through the orbital roof as well as the cribriform plate.

B2. Axial and coronal, post-contrast T1-weighted image shows an enhancing mass invading the right orbit and through the orbital roof as well as the cribriform plate.

CHONDROSARCOMA

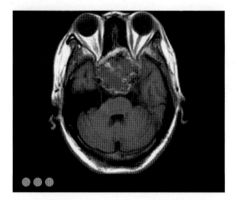

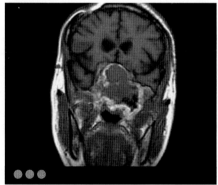

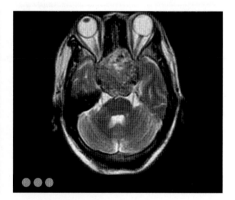

C1. Axial and coronal T1-weighted images show heterogeneous signal intensity mass with central isointensity and peripheral hyperintensity involving the clivus, sphenoid sinus, ethmoid sinus with parasellar extension and involvement of the cribriform plate.

C2. Axial and coronal T1-weighted images show heterogeneous signal intensity mass with central isointensity and peripheral hyperintensity involving the clivus, sphenoid sinus, ethmoid sinus with parasellar extension and involvement of the cribriform plate.

C3. Axial T2-weighted image reveals a predominantly hypointense mass with some hyperintense areas involving the clivus, parasellar region.

121

JUVENILE ANGIOFIBROMA

Juvenile angiofibroma occurs adjacent to the sphenopalatine foramen in the nasal cavity. Large tumors are frequently bilobed or dumbbell-shaped, with one portion of the tumor filling the nasopharynx and the other portion extending to the pterygopalatine fossa. Lateral spread of the tumor is directed toward the pterygopalatine fossa, bowing the posterior wall of the maxillary sinus. The infratemporal fossa is subsequently involved. Occasionally, the greater wing of the sphenoid may be eroded, exposing the middle fossa dura. Involvement of the cribriform plate is unusual.

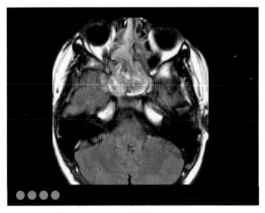

D1. Axial T2-weighted FLAIR image shows a hyperintense mass in the sphenoid and ethmoid sinuses with bone erosion.

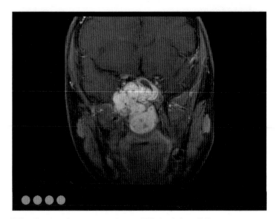

D2. Coronal, post contrast T1 weighted fat suppressed image reveals an enhancing mass extending into the right temporal fossa and in the region of cribriform plate.

MENINGIOMA

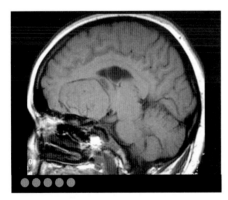

E1. Sagittal T1-weighted image shows an isointense mass in the subfrontal region on the cribriform plate.

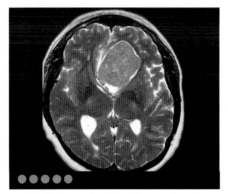

E2. Axial T2-weighted image reveals the mass to be isointense to gray matter.

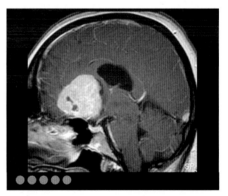

E3. Sagittal, post-contrast T1-weighted image shows intense enhancement of the mass.

NEUROENDOCRINE TUMOR

Neuroendocrine tumors arise from distinct cells in the body that are ubiquitous in the human body. They most commonly arise from the GI tract, but can also arise from the pituitary gland, the thyroid, the adrenals, the pancreas, and the lungs. neuroendocrine tumors can be quite diverse in terms of their malignant potential. Some can be benign in nature while others can be malignant. Neuroendocrine tumors of the ethmoid sinus are rare.

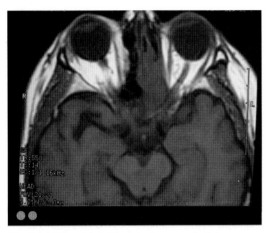

F1. Axial T1-weighted image shows an isointense mass in the region of left ethmoid sinus.

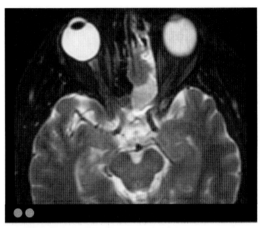

F2. Axial T2-weighted image shows an isointense mass in the region of left ethmoid sinus. Note the hyperintense area surrounding the mass is due to sinus mucosal disease.

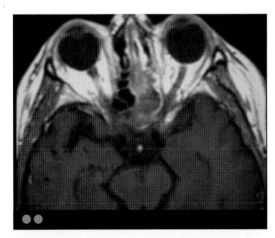

F3. Axial and coronal, post-contrast T1-weighted images show an enhancing mass in the left ethmoid sinus extending through the cribriform plate at the inferior frontal fossa.

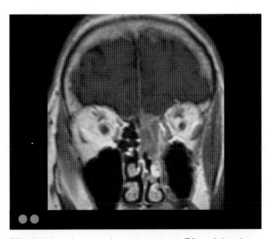

F4. Axial and coronal, post-contrast T1-weighted images show an enhancing mass in the left ethmoid sinus extending through the cribriform plate at the inferior frontal fossa.

RABDOMYOSARCOMA

Rabdomyosarcoma is the most frequent sinonasal malignancy in children, although it has been reported in adults. Rhabdomyosarcoma (RMS) is the most common soft tissue sarcoma in children. Since skeletal muscle is present throughout the body, RMS can be seen at numerous locations in the body. However, the common sites in decreasing order are the head and neck (approximately 35–40%), particularly around the eyes, the genitourinary tract (20%), the extremities (15–20%), and the trunk (chest and lungs)

(10–15%). RMSs account for 5–8% of childhood cancers and 70% of all rhabdomyosarcoma cases are diagnosed in the first ten years of life. RMS rarely affects adults, no obvious race predilection exists and overall, RMS occurs slightly more frequently in males than females. There are two main types of RMS that occur in children: (1) Embryonal type, this is the most common type and it tends to occur in the head and neck area, bladder, vagina, and in or around the prostate and testes. (2) Alveolar type, this type occurs more often in large muscles of the trunk, arms, and legs and typically affects older children or teenagers.

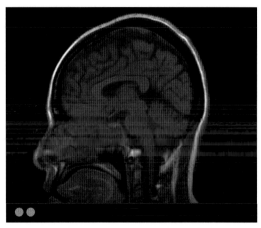

G1. Sagittal T1-weighted image shows a mass lesion extending from nasal cavity into the ethmoid sinus and through the cribriform plate. Note the sphenoid sinus contains mucous material, which has different signal intensity compared to the tumor mass.

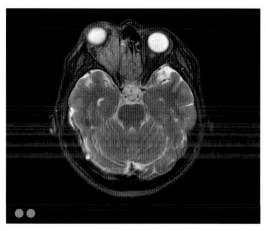

G2. Axial T2-weighted image shows an isointense mass involving the ethmoid sinus with extension into the right orbit.

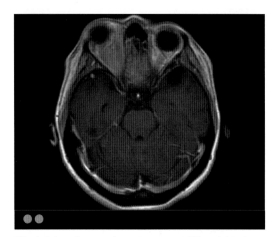

G3. Axial and coronal, post-contrast T1-weighted images show an enhancing mass in the nasal cavity, ethmoid sinus with extension into the frontal fossa. Dural enhancement just above the cribriform plate is seen due to tumor invasion.

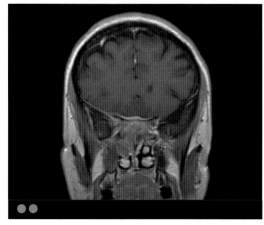

G4. Axial and coronal, post-contrast T1-weighted images show an enhancing mass in the nasal cavity, ethmoid sinus with extension into the frontal fossa. Dural enhancement just above the cribriform plate is seen due to tumor invasion.

ARACHNOID CYST

Arachnoid cysts constitute 1% of all intracranial masses. There is a male predominance with 3:1 ratio. Arachnoid cysts can be seen in any age group, but mostly in children. Common locations include middle cranial fossa, suprasellar cistern, and convexity. Focal bony erosion may be seen on imaging studies. They are of similar signal intensity to CSF on both T1-weighted and T2-weighted images.

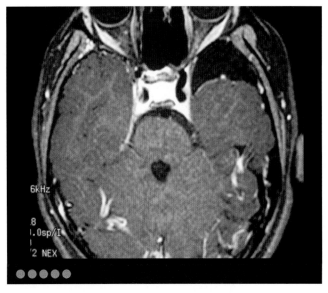

A. Axial, post-contrast T1-weighted image shows a hypointense, extraaxial, cystic mass in the left anterior temporal fossa.

RELATED PATTERNS

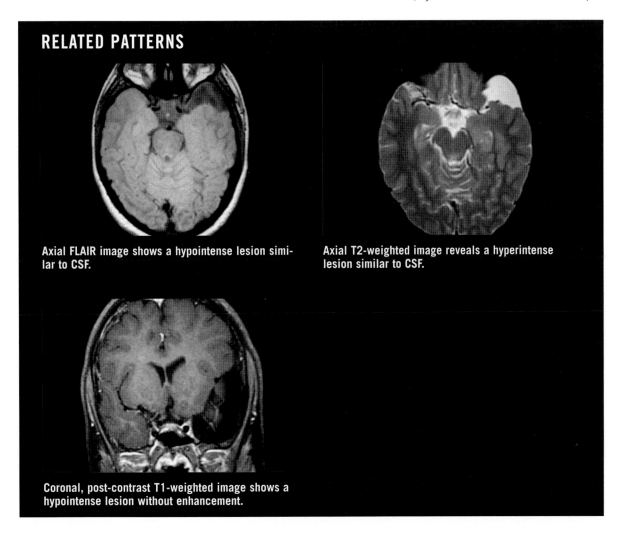

Axial FLAIR image shows a hypointense lesion similar to CSF.

Axial T2-weighted image reveals a hyperintense lesion similar to CSF.

Coronal, post-contrast T1-weighted image shows a hypointense lesion without enhancement.

DIFFERENTIAL DIAGNOSIS

At a Glance:

- *Cysticercosis*
- *Cysticercosis (Interhemispheric)*
- *Epidermoid*
- *Epidermoid (Suprasellar)*

CYSTICERCOSIS

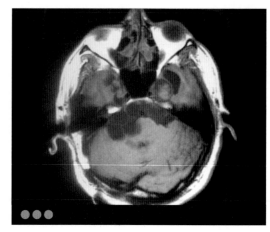

B. Axial T1-weighted image shows cysticercosis lesions in the prepontine cistern, right CPA cistern and cavernous sinuses bilaterally.

CYSTICERCOSIS (INTERHEMISPHERIC)

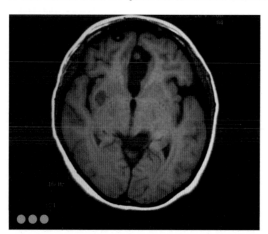

C1. Axial T1-weighted image shows a cyst in the interhemispheric fissure. In addition, there are several parenchymal cysts seen.

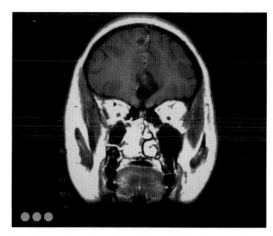

C2. Coronal, post-contrast T1-weighted image shows an interhmispheric cyst with enhancing vasculature seen adjacent to it. In addition, a ring-like enhancing cyst is seen in the right frontal lobe.

EPIDERMOID

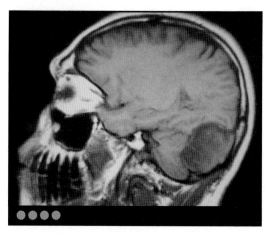

D1. Sagittal T1-weighted image reveals a hypointense, extraaxial mass in the posterior fossa.

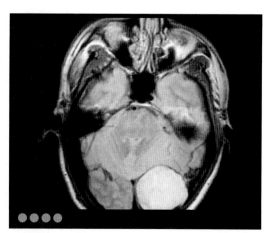

D2. Axial FLAIR image shows a hyperintense mass in the left posterior fossa. CSF is hypointense on FLAIR sequence, but epidermoid is hyperintense. On T1- and T2-weighted images, epidermoid is similar to CSF in signal intensity and sometimes called "dirty CSF" due slight internal signal inhomogeity.

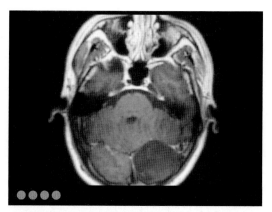

D3. Axial and sagittal, post-contrast T1-weighted images reveals no enhancement.

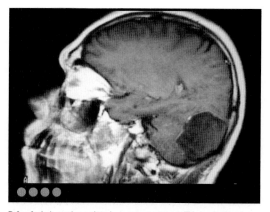

D4. Axial and sagittal, post-contrast T1-weighted images reveals no enhancement.

EPIDERMOID (SUPRASELLAR)

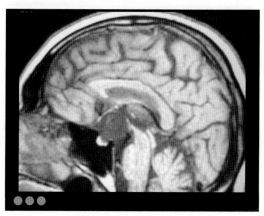

E1. Sagittal and axial T1-weighted images show a hypointense mass in the suprasellar cistern.

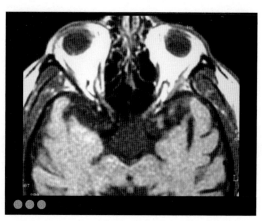

E2. Sagittal and axial T1-weighted images show a hypointense mass in the suprasellar cistern.

127

DERMOID WITH SEEDING

Dermoid tumors arise from incomplete separation of epithelial ectoderm from neuroectoderm at the region of the anterior neuropore; usually during the fourth week of gestation. The cyst wall often includes hair follicles, sweat glands, and sebaceous glands. The cyst grows slowly and gradually becomes filled by desquamated epithelium, sweat, and sebaceous materials. Aseptic meningitis can occur when a dermoid cyst ruptures. Intracranial dermoid cyst is a rare entity accounting for 0.1–0.7% of all intracranial tumors. The most common location is in the posterior fossa, at or near the midline. It may be extradural, vermian, or intraventricular. A dermal sinus may be connected to the mass and may be detected clinically or by MRI. Dermoids are usually seen in children whereas epidermoids are usually seen in adults.

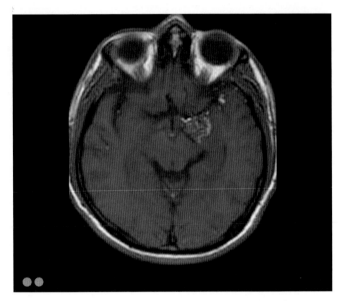

A. Axial T1-weighted image demonstrates a mixed hyperintense and isointense mass in the left medial temporal fossa. Note a small speckle of hyperintensity in the left sylvian fissure due to rupture of the dermoid.

RELATED PATTERNS

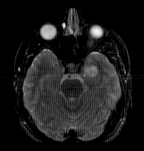

Axial T2-weighted image shows the mass to be predominantly hyperintense.

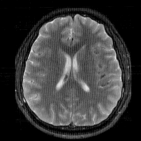

Axial T2-weighted image shows the seeding of fatty component to be hypointense.

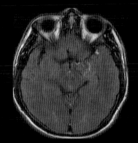

Axial FLAIR image shows the mass to be mixed signal intensity and seeding in the left sylvian fissure to be hyperintense.

DERMOID (CASE TWO)

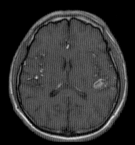

Axial T1-weighted image demonstrates seeding of the dermoid to be hyperintense, consistent with fat signal intensity.

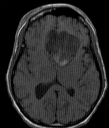

Axial and sagittal T1-weighted image shows a hypointense mass with some hyperintensity seen at the posterior aspect of the mass.

DERMOID (CASE TWO) (continued)

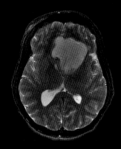

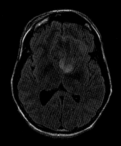

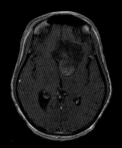

Axial T2-weighted image reveals a predominantly hyperintense mass.

Axial T2-weighted FLAIR image shows a hypointense mass with a hyperintense compoent seen posteriorly.

Axial, post-contrast T1-weighted image demonstrates no abnormal enhancement.

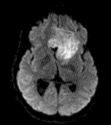

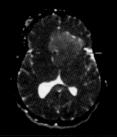

Diffusion-weighted image and ADC map shows some degree of restricted diffusion involving the mass.

RELATED PATTERNS (continued)

DERMOID (CASE THREE)

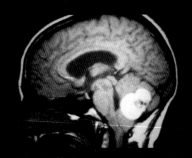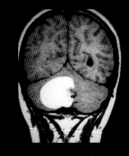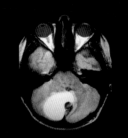

Sagittal and coronal T1-weighted images show a hyperintense lesion in the posterior fossa.

Axial T2-weighted FLAIR image shows a hyperintense lesion in the posterior fossa.

DIFFERENTIAL DIAGNOSIS

At a Glance:

- *Cholesterol Granuloma*
- *Epidermoid*
- *Lipoma*

CHOLESTEROL GRANULOMA

Cholesterol granulomas can occur in any obstructed air cells. They usually arise from the petrous apex and may expand in the posterior fossa causing cranial disturbances. Cholesterol granulomas are believed to be secondary to chronic otitis media. They are rare, benign expanding cysts that contain fluids, lipids, and cholesterol crystals surrounded by a fibrous lining. Cholesterol granulomas can form when the air cells in the petrous apex are obstructed due to infection. The obstruction creates a vacuum that causes blood to be drawn into the air cells. As red blood cells break down, cholesterol in the hemoglobin is released. The immune system reacts to the cholesterol as a foreign body, producing an inflammatory response. Associated small blood vessels rupture as a result of the inflammation. Recurrent hemorrhaging causes further expansion of the mass.

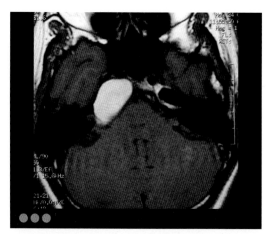

B. Axial, post-contrast, T1-weighted image shows pachymeningeal enhancement involving the right frontal and parietal region with adjacent skull and scalp involvement. Axial T1-weighted image shows a hyperintense lesion at the right petrous apex with evidence of bone erosion. A hypointense rim is seen surrounding the mass, representing expanded cortical bone.

EPIDERMOID

Epidermoids are composed of ectodermal elements and are lined with stratified squamous epithelium containing epithelial keratinaceous debris and cholesterol crystals. On MRI, they are usually hypointense on T1-weighted images and hyerintense on T2-weighted images, similar to CSF, but occasionally they can exhibit hyperintensity on T1-weighted images.

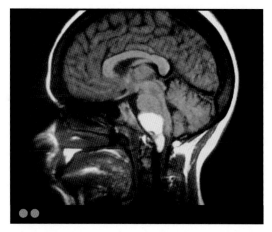

C1. Sagittal and axial T1-weighted images show a hyperintense lesion in the prepontine cistern and perimedullary cistern.

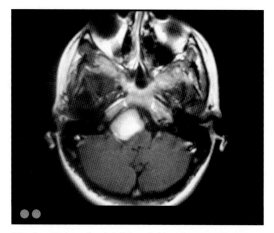

C2. Sagittal and axial T1-weighted images show a hyperintense lesion in the prepontine cistern and perimedullary cistern.

LIPOMA

Lipomas are believed to result from the maldifferentiation of the meninx primitive during the formation of the subarachnoid cistern and are associated with dysgenesis of the adjacent cerebral tissue in 55% of the cases. Their common locations include dorsal pericallosal, quadrigeminal cistern, superior vermian cistern, suprasellar cistern, and cerebellopontine angle cistern and sylvian fissure. On MRI, they are usually hyperintense lesions on T1-weighted images. MRI is useful in demonstrating associated anomalies, such as dysgenesis of corpus callosum.

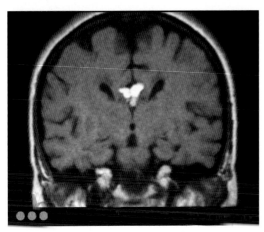

D1. Sagittal and coronal T1-weighted images show a hyperintense lesion in the region of corpus callosum that exhibits agenesis.

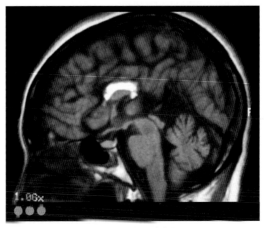

D2. Sagittal and coronal T1-weighted images show a hyperintense lesion in the region of corpus callosum that exhibits agenesis.

Chapter 4

Intracerebral Masses

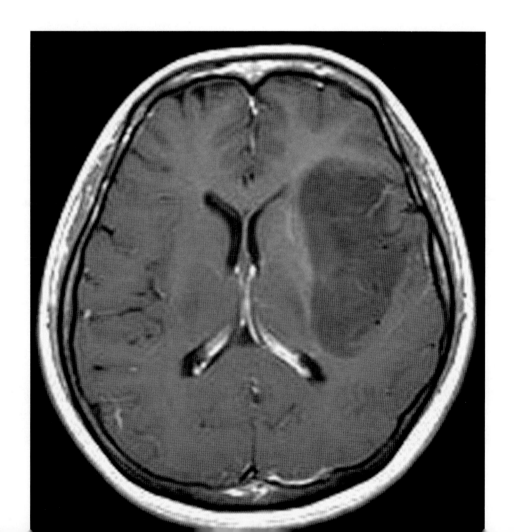

OLIGODENDROGLIOMA

Oligodendrogliomas constitute 5% of all cerebral gliomas. They are seen in young and middle aged adults. There is a male predominance of 2:1. These tumors typically involve the cerebral cortex and the subcortical white matter in the frontal and frontotemporal region. Oligodendroglioma is a hypointense mass on T1-weighted images. On T2-weighted images, they exhibit hyperintensity. Foci of calcification or hemorrhage may be seen within the tumor, thus causing heterogeneous signal intensity on both T1-weighted and T2-weighted images. About half of the tumor will show contrast enhancement and the other half will not enhance. Cystic changes are frequently seen. Peritumoral edema is mild or absent.

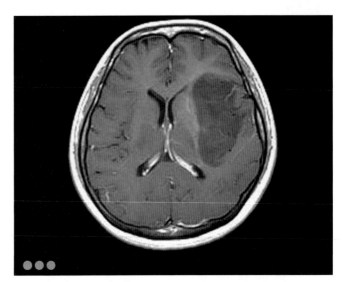

A. Axial, post-contrast T1-weighted image shows a nonenhancing, hypointense mass in the region of left insular cortex, and frontotemporal operculum.

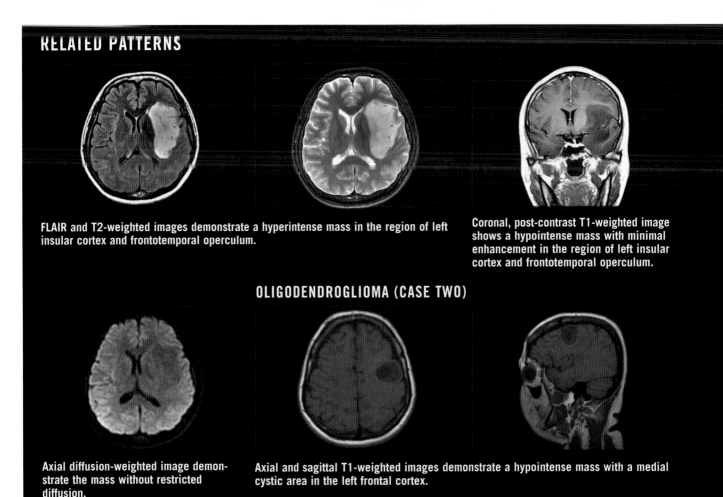

RELATED PATTERNS

FLAIR and T2-weighted images demonstrate a hyperintense mass in the region of left insular cortex and frontotemporal operculum.

Coronal, post-contrast T1-weighted image shows a hypointense mass with minimal enhancement in the region of left insular cortex and frontotemporal operculum.

OLIGODENDROGLIOMA (CASE TWO)

Axial diffusion-weighted image demonstrate the mass without restricted diffusion.

Axial and sagittal T1-weighted images demonstrate a hypointense mass with a medial cystic area in the left frontal cortex.

OLIGODENDROGLIOMA (CASE TWO) (continued)

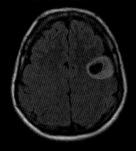 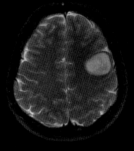

Axial T2 FLAIR and T2-weighted images show a hyperintense mass with a medial cystic component in the left frontal cortex.

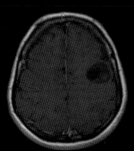 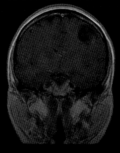

Axial and coronal, post-contrast T1-weighted image show a left frontal cortical, minimally enhancing mass with a cystic component medially.

DIFFERENTIAL DIAGNOSIS

At a Glance:

- *Dysembryoplastic Neuroepithelial Tumor*
- *Gangliogioma*
- *Low-Grade Astrocytoma*
- *Lymphoma*

DYSEMBRYOPLASTIC NEUROEPITHELIAL TUMOR

Dysembryoplastic neuroepithelial tumors (DNETs) are most commonly seen in the temporal and frontal lobes. They are neuroepithelial tumors that present in patients with seizures in their second or third decades.

They are superficially located and cortically based masses, often associated with underlying skull remodeling. The mass is hypointense on T1-weighted images and hyperintense on T2-weighted images on MRI and grows very slowly. Focal cystic changes may be seen. There is usually no surrounding edema. Focal cortical dysplasia can be associated with DNET in approximately 50% of the cases.

DYSEMBRYOPLASTIC NEUROEPITHELIAL TUMOR (DNET) (CASE ONE)

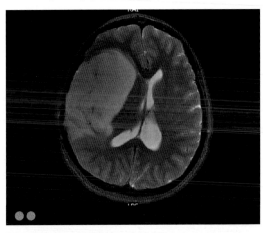

B1. Axial T2-weighted and FLAIR images demonstrate a large hyperintense mass in the right frontotemporal region.

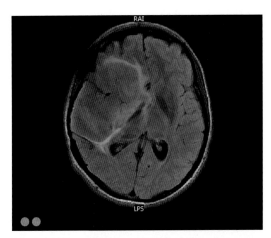

B2. Axial T2-weighted and FLAIR images demonstrate a large hyperintense mass in the right frontotemporal region.

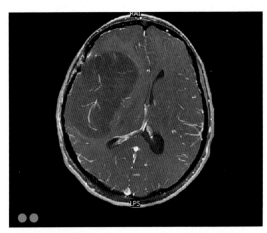

B3. Axial and coronal, post-contrast T1-weighted images show no enhancement of this hypointense mass.

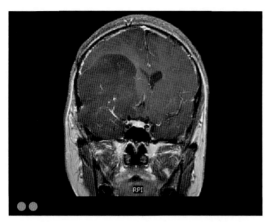

B4. Axial and coronal, post-contrast T1-weighted images show no enhancement of this hypointense mass.

B5. Diffusion tensor imaging and tractography demonstrate the benign nature of this mass. The adjacent white matter tracts are displaced by the tumor mass without evidence of destruction.

DYSEMBRYOPLASTIC NEUROEPITHELIAL TUMOR (DNET) (CASE TWO)

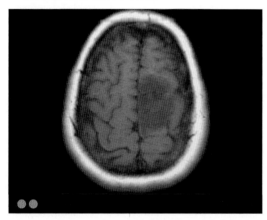

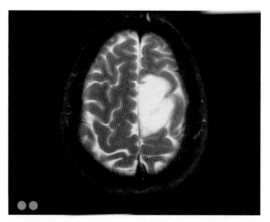

C1. Axial T1-weighted image shows a hypointense mass in the left frontal, parasagittal region.

C2. Axial T2-weighted image shows a hyperintense mass in the left frontal parasagittal region.

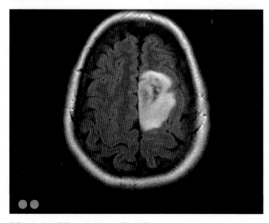

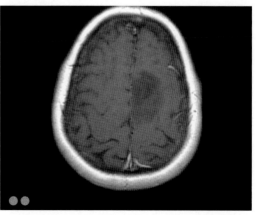

C3. Axial T2-weighted FLAIR image shows a predominantly hyperintense mass with small irregular foci of hypointensity, consistent with cystic changes.

C4. Axial and coronal, post-contrast T1-weighted images demonstrate no definite enhancement of the mass lesion. Small cystic changes are seen.

137

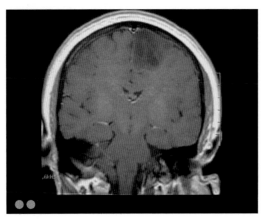

C5. Axial and coronal, post-contrast T1-weighted images demonstrate no definite enhancement of the mass lesion. Small cystic changes are seen.

GANGLIOGIOMA

Gangliogliomas are predominantly seen in children and young adults. They are the most common mixed glioneural tumors. They are typically hypointense on T1-weighted images and hyperintense on T2-weighted images and appear cystic in up to 50% of the cases. Calcification is seen in 30% of the cases and faint contrast enhancement is seen in 50% of the cases. A proton MR spectroscopy signal from *N*-acetylaspartate is an endogenous marker for functioning neurons. The choline-to-creatine ratio is lower and the *N*-acetylaspartate-to-creatine ratio is higher in gangliogliomas than in gliomas. A high *N*-acetylaspartate-to-creatine ratio may be due to a neoplastic neuronal component.

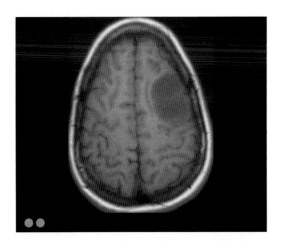

D1. Axial T1-weighted image shows a hypointense, cortical-based mass in the left frontal lobe.

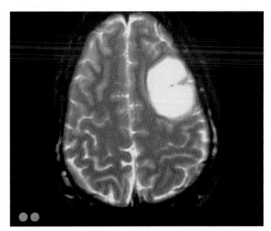

D2. Axial T2-weighted and FLAIR images reveal a hyperintense, cortical-based mass in the left frontal lobe.

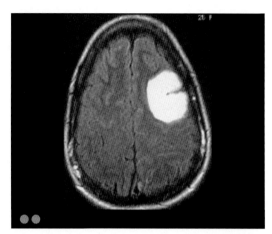

D3. Axial T2-weighted and FLAIR images reveal a hyperintense, cortical-based mass in the left frontal lobe.

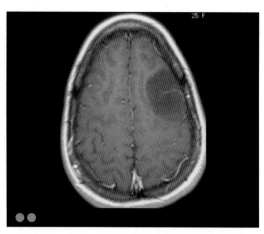

D4. Axial and coronal, post-contrast T1-weighted images show no enhancement of the hypointense mass.

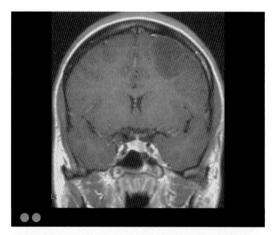

D5. Axial and coronal, post-contrast T1-weighted images show no enhancement of the hypointense mass.

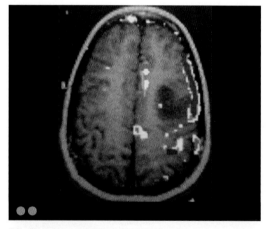

D6. Functional MRI demonstrates the motor cortex just posterior to the mass lesion.

LOW-GRADE ASTROCYTOMA

Low-grade astrocytomas constitute about 25% of all cerebral gliomas. Peak incidence of low-grade astrocytoma is between the ages of 20 and 40 years and is generally 10 years below that for glioblastoma. Astrocytomas may show hypointensity on T1-weighted images and hyperintensity on T2-weighted images. Peritumoral edema is absent or minimal. Tumor calcification is detected in 20% of astrocytomas, but better seen on CT. The pattern of contrast enhancement is quite variable with 40% of low-grade astrocytomas exhibiting some degree of contrast enhancement.

LOW-GRADE ASTROCYTOMA (CASE ONE)

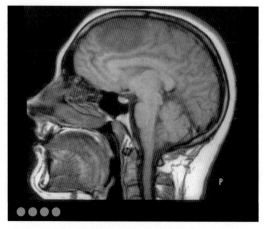

E1. Sagittal and coronal T1-weighted images show a hypointense, cortical-based mass in the left frontal lobe.

139

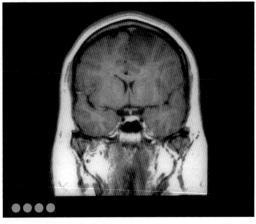

E2. Sagittal and coronal T1-weighted images show a hypointense, cortical-based mass in the left frontal lobe.

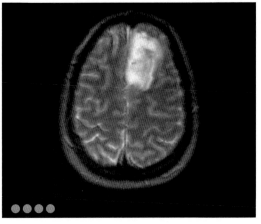

E3. Axial T2-weighted image shows a hyperintense, cortical-based mass in the left frontal lobe.

LOW-GRADE ASTROCYTOMA (CASE TWO)

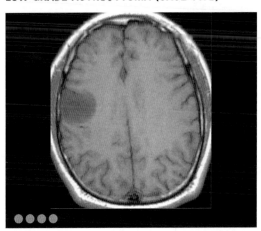

F1. Axial T1-weighted image shows a hypointense, cortical-based mass in the right frontal lobe.

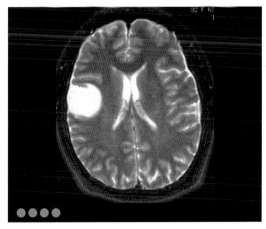

F2. Axial T2-weighted image reveals a hyperintense, cortical-based mass in the right frontal lobe.

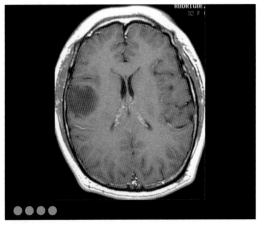

F3. Axial, post-contrast T1-weighted image shows no enhancement of the right frontal hypointense mass.

LYMPHOMA

Primary central nervous system (CNS) lymphoma is a non-Hodgkin lymphoma, usually B-cell origin, which represents 1–2% of all primary CNS tumors. It occurs with increased frequency in immunocompromised patients and patients with AIDS, but may occur in immunocompetent patients as well. Although the tumors are radiosensitive, the overall prognosis is poor, with a median survival after diagnosis +/− of 13.5 months, with chemotherapy and radiation treatment. Although the origin of PCNSL is determined as a B cell lymphoma, how these neoplastic cells come to proliferate within the central nervous system is not well understood and why they are so frequently multifocal at presentation add to the interesting nature of the tumor. The CNS has neither lymphatic circulation nor physiological accumulations of lymphoid tissue, which has led to different theories regarding the origin of the neoplastic lymphoid cells in the CNS.

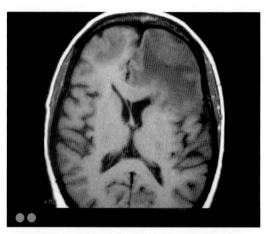

G1. Axial T1-weighted image shows a slightly hypointense mass in the left frontal region with surrounding edema. Note a small hypointense area in the right frontal region.

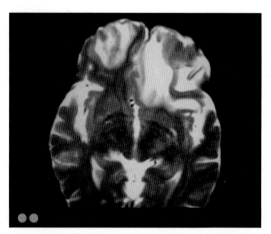

G2. Axial T2-weighted and FLAIR images show a slightly hyperintense mass in the left frontal region with surrounding edema. Note a small hyperintense area in the right frontal region.

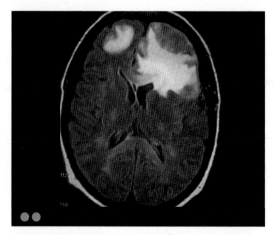

G3. Axial T2-weighted and FLAIR images show a slightly hyperintense mass in the left frontal region with surrounding edema. Note a small hyperintense area in the right frontal region.

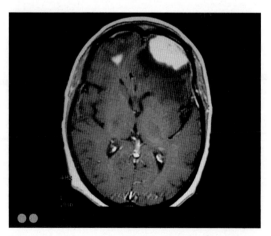

G4. Axial, post-contrast T1-weighted image shows an enhancing mass in the left frontal region with surrounding edema. Note a small enhancing intraparenchymal mass is seen in the right frontal lobe.

GANGLIOGLIOMA

Gangliogliomas are predominantly seen in children and young adults. They are the most common mixed glioneural tumors. They can appear as cystic mass with a mural nodule in up to 50% of the cases.

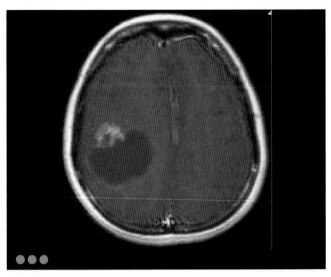

A. Axial, post-contrast T1-weighted image shows a cystic mass with an enhancing component seen in the right frontoparietal region.

RELATED PATTERNS

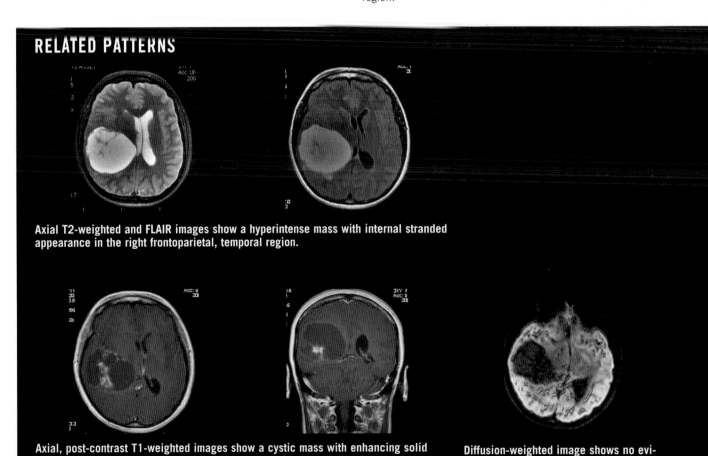

Axial T2-weighted and FLAIR images show a hyperintense mass with internal stranded appearance in the right frontoparietal, temporal region.

Axial, post-contrast T1-weighted images show a cystic mass with enhancing solid components.

Diffusion-weighted image shows no evidence of restricted diffusion in the solid component of the mass, indicating the solid component of the mass is not a highly cellular (malignant) tumor.

GANGLIOGLIOMA (CASE TWO)

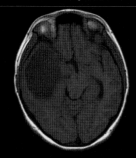

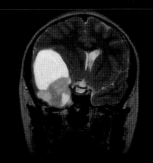

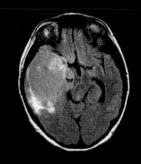

Axial T1-weighted image shows a large cystic mass with a small solid component anteromedially in the right temporal lobe. The cyst fluid is slightly hyperintense compared to CSF.

Coronal T2-weighted image demonstrates a large cystic mass in the right temporal lobe with a solid component at its anteroinferior portion

Axial T2-weighted FLAIR image shows the mass to be isointense and some surrounding edema is seen.

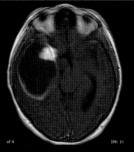

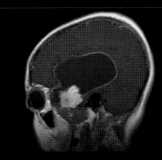

Axial and sagittal, post-contrast T1-weighted images demonstrate ring-like enhancement of the cystic mass in addition to the enhancement of the solid component.

DIFFERENTIAL DIAGNOSIS

At a Glance:

- *Cysticercosis*
- *Hydatid Disease*
- *Low-Grade Astrocytoma*
- *Metastatic Disease*
- *Neuroepithelial Cyst*
- *Oligodendroglioma*
- *Papillary Glioneuronal Tumor*
- *Pilocytic Astrocytoma*
- *Pleomorphic Xanthoastrocytoma*

CYSTICERCOSIS

Cysticercosis is the most common parasitic disease affecting the central nervous system. Cysticercosis affecting human is acquired by ingestion of eggs (encysted larvae) of the pork tapeworm, *T. solium*, either by ingestion of contaminated water or vegetable, or by autoinfection due to ano-oral contamination or reverse peristalsis in a patient who is infected with the tapeworm. Neurocysticercosis is a rare clinical entity in the United States. The condition is more endemic to Mexico, Central and South America, and parts of Asia.

There are four stages of parenchymal cysticercosis cysts, namely, vesicular, colloidal vesicular, granular nodular and nodular calcified stages. In the vesicular stage, the cysts show very thin wall and clear fluid with a scolex. No contrast enhancement or edema is seen in this stage. In the colloidal vesicular stage, the cyst fluid becomes turbid and a ring-like enhancement is seen with surrounding edema. Scolex may not be seen due to cyst degeneration. In the nodular calcified stage, an enhancing nodule is seen with surrounding edema. In the nodular calcified stage, a calcific area is seen as a residua of the lesion.

CYSTICERCOSIS (CASE ONE)

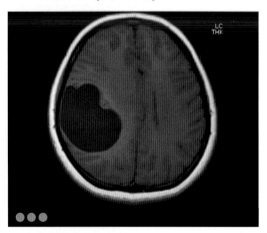

B1. Axial T1-weighted image shows a large cystic mass in the right frontoparietal region.

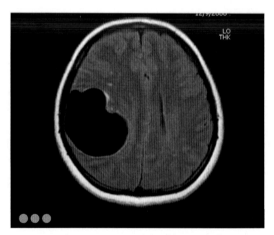

B2. Axial T2-weighted and FLAIR images show a large cystic mass in the left frontoparietal region.

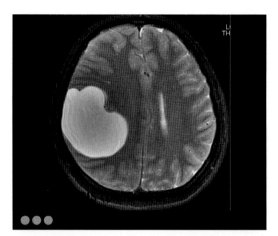

B3. Axial T2-weighted and FLAIR images show a large cystic mass in the left frontoparietal region.

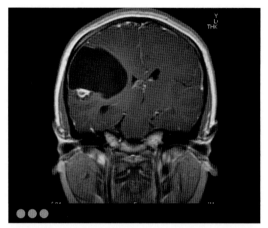

B4. Coronal, post-contrast T1-weighted image shows a large cytic mass with an adjacent small ring-like enhancing lesion.

CYSTICERCOSIS (CASE TWO)

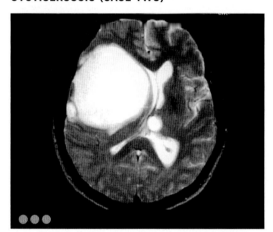

C1. Axial T2-weighted image shows three cysts, a large one in the right hemisphere, a small one lateral to it, and another small one in the left thalamus.

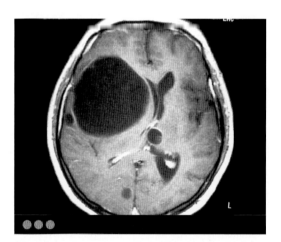

C2. Axial, post-contrast T1-weighted image demonstrates no enhancement of these cysts, A scolex is now seen within the cyst in left thalamus. A fourth cyst is partially seen in the right occipital lobe.

HYDATID DISEASE

Echinococcus is a parasitic disease and also known as **hydatid disease**. Echinococcus is the general term for three diseases caused by the larval stage of *Echinococcus* tape-worms. *Echinococcus granulosus* causes cystic echinococcus and is seen worldwide, in the rural areas. *Echinococcus multilocularis* causes alveolar disease and is seen only in the northern hemisphere. *Echinococcus vogeli* causes polycystic echinococcus and is seen in Central and South America.

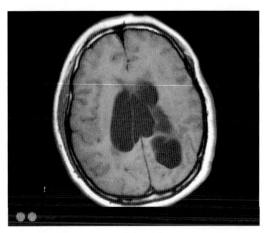

D1. Axial T1- and T2-weighted images demonstrate multicystic lesions in the region of lateral ventricles with surrounding edema in a patient with known echinococcus.

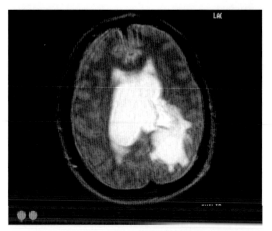

D2. Axial T1- and T2-weighted images demonstrate multicystic lesions in the region of lateral ventricles with surrounding edema in a patient with known echinococcus.

LOW-GRADE ASTROCYTOMA

Low-grade astrocytomas constitute about 25% of all cerebral gliomas. Peak incidence of low-grade astrocytoma is between the ages of 20 and 40 years and is generally 10 years below that for glioblastoma. Peritumoral edema is absent or minimal. Tumor calcification is detected in 20% of astrocytomas, but better seen on CT. The pattern of contrast enhancement is quite variable with 40% of low-grade astrocytomas exhibiting some degree of contrast enhancement.

Pathologically, low grade astrocytomas are hypercellular tumors with few mitoses and moderate pleomorphism. No vascular proliferation or necrosis is seen.

Strong affinity for glial fibrillary acidic protein (GFAP) is demonstrated. They usually arise in the white matter and grow by infiltration along the white matter tract.

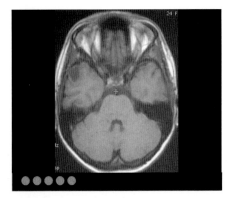

E1. Axial T1-weighted image demonstrates a hypointense cystic mass at the right temporal pole.

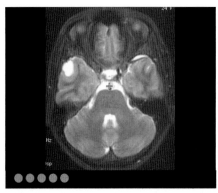

E2. Axial T2-weighted image reveals a hyperintense cystic mass at the right temporal pole.

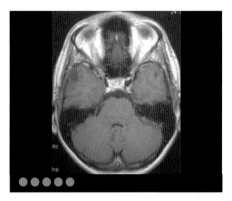

E3. Axial, post-contrast T1-weighted image shows no enhancement of the cystic mass.

METASTATIC DISEASE

Metastasis to the brain is the most feared complication of systemic neoplasms and the most common intracranial tumor in adults. The incidence of brain metastasis is rising with the increase in survival of cancer patients as a result of significant advances in cancer diagnosis and treatment. Approximately 40% of intracranial neoplasms are metastatic in nature. Multiple, large autopsy series suggest that, in order of decreasing frequency, lung, breast, melanoma, kidney and colon are the common primary sites. The most common location of brain metastasis is cerebrum (80–85%), followed by the cerebellum (10–15%), and the brain stem (3–5%). In more than half of the metastatic disease, lesions are multiple; solitary metastatic lesion is less common. Primary tumors that tend to produce multiple metastatic lesions include melanoma, lung and breast tumors. Intracranial metastases may be categorized by location as skull, dura, leptomeninges, and parenchymal brain metastases. Lesions of the brain and leptomeninges account for the majority (80%) of intracranial metastases.

Cystic metastases favor lung, breast, and gastrointestinal primary sites.

METASTATIC DISEASE (CASE ONE) (FROM LUNG CARCINOMA)

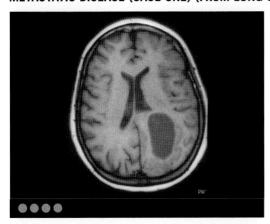

F1. Axial T1-weighted image reveals a large hypointnese, cystic mass in the left parietooccipital region.

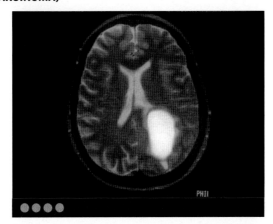

F2. Axial T2-weighted image shows a large, hyperintense, cystic mass in the left parietooccipital region.

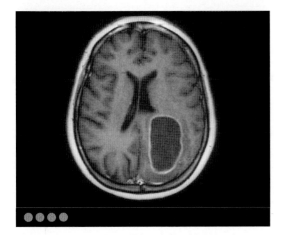

F3. Axial, post-contrast T1-weighted image shows ring-like enhancement of the cystic mass.

METASTATIC DISEASE (CASE TWO) (FROM OVARIAN CARCINOMA)

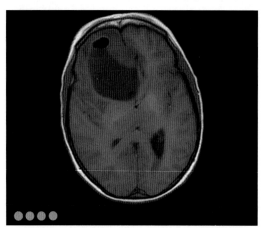

G1. Axial T1-weighted image shows a large cystic mass with a small solid component anteromedially in the right frontal lobe (air was introduced at the time of aspiration of cystic fluid).

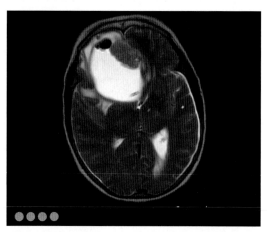

G2. Axial T2-weighted and FLAIR images demonstrate a large hyperintense cystic mass with a solid component anteromedially in the right frontal lobe.

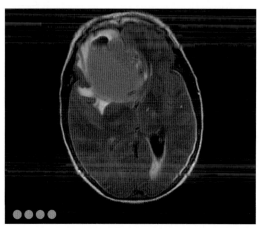

G3. Axial T2-weighted and FLAIR images demonstrate a large hyperintense cystic mass with a solid component anteromedially in the right frontal lobe.

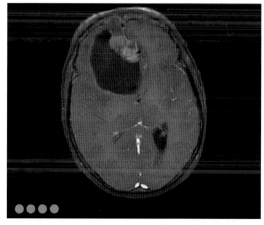

G4. Axial and coronal, post-contrast T1-weighted images reveal enhancement of the solid component of the mass.

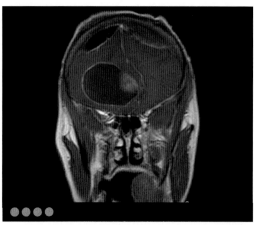

G5. Axial and coronal, post-contrast T1-weighted images reveal enhancement of the solid component of the mass.

NEUROEPITHELIAL CYST

Neuroepithelial cysts are a heterogenous group of cystic lesions of uncertain etiology. They most likely arise from sequestration of developing neural ectoderm and are lined by epithelial-like cells. Although neuroepithelial cysts are seen at any age, they are predominately seen in the older age group. These cysts may occur anywhere within the central nervous system, but are most commonly found in the choroid plexus, choroid fissure, cerebral ventricles, and occasionally within the intraaxial parenchyma.

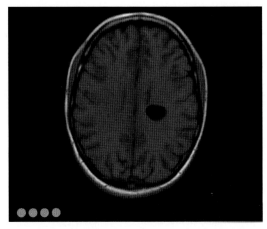

H1. Axial T1-weighted image shows a hypointense cystic lesion in the left frontal lobe.

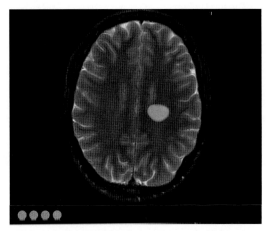

H2. Axial T2-weighted image shows a hyperintense cystic lesion in the left frontal lobe.

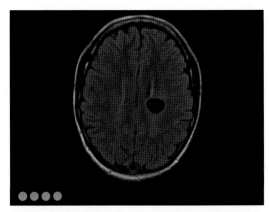

H3. Axial T2-weighted FLAIR image shows a hypointense cystic lesion in the left frontal lobe.

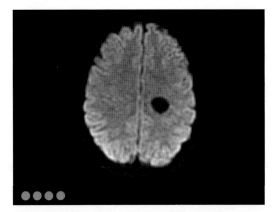

H4. Diffusion-weighted image shows the cystic lesion with no evidence of restricted diffusion.

OLIGODENDROGLIOMA

The majority of oligodendrogliomas occur in adults, with a peak incidence in the fourth or fifth decades of life. They are rarely seen in children. Only 6% of oligodendrogliomas arise during infancy and childhood. The tumor is predominantly seen in the supratentorial compartment (92%). In adults, oligodendrogliomas arise superficially within the cerebral cortex and extend into the white matter of the cerebral hemispheres. In tumors that are adjacent to the ventricular system or the subarachnoid spaces, seeding of the CSF pathways may occur. Occasionally, frontal lobe tumors may extend across the corpus callosum. Histopathologically, there are 2 grades for oligodendroglial tumors: WHO grade II for well-differentiated tumors and WHO grade III for anaplastic oligodendroglioma.

Cystic changes are frequently seen in **oligodendrogliomas**. Peritumoral edema is mild or absent.

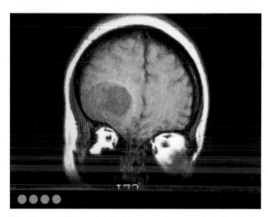

I1. Coronal T1-weighted image shows a left frontal mass with cystic and solid components.

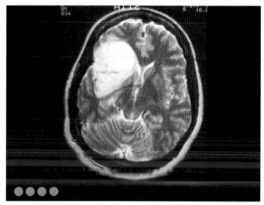

I2. Axial T2-weighted image shows a hyperintense mass in the left frontal region. Careful examination of the hyperintense mass reveals two areas of slightly different hyperintensity, one representing cystic compoent and the other solid component.

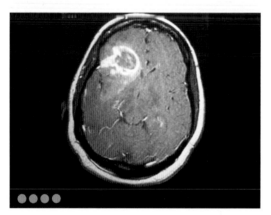

I3. Axial and coronal, post-contrast T1-weighted images show irregular ring-like enhancement of the mass with cystic component.

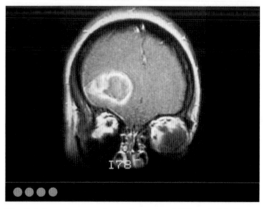

I4. Axial and coronal, post-contrast T1-weighted images show irregular ring-like enhancement of the mass with cystic component.

PAPILLARY GLIONEURONAL TUMOR

Papillary glioneuronal tumor is a recently identified low-grade mixed glial-neuronal neoplasm of juvenile and young adult patients. The WHO (2007) classification considers it as grade 1 tumor in the category of neuronal and mixed neuronal-glial tumor. Papillary glioneuronal tumor is a rare lesion first described in 1998. It is in the same class of tumors as gangliogliomas and dysembryoplastic neuroepithelial tumors.

The lesion is characterized pathologically by the presence of a pseudopapillary pattern with intervening neuronal cells. The male to female ratio is equal. Most patients present with seizures or headaches. The lesions are commonly partially cystic with an enhancing nodule. Complete resection is considered curative.

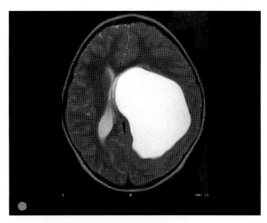

J1. Axial T2-weighted and FLAIR images show a large cystic mass in the left frontal region.

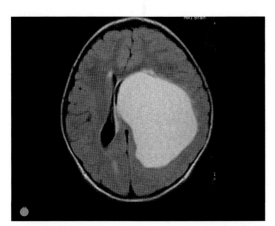

J2. Axial T2-weighted and FLAIR images show a large cystic mass in the left frontal region.

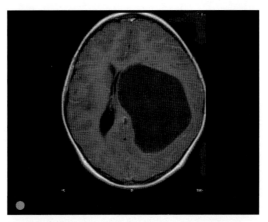

J3. Axial and coronal, post-contrast T1-weighted images demonstrate a large cystic mass with marginal enhancement seen posterosuperiorly.

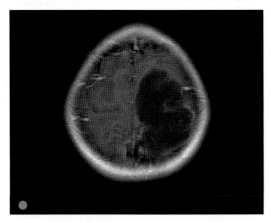

J4. Axial and coronal, post-contrast T1-weighted images demonstrate a large cystic mass with marginal enhancement seen posterosuperiorly.

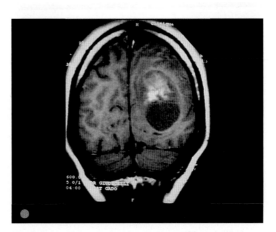

J5. Axial and coronal, post-contrast T1-weighted images demonstrate a large cystic mass with marginal enhancement seen posterosuperiorly.

PILOCYTIC ASTROCYTOMA

Primary intra-axial brain tumors account for approximately two thirds of all brain neoplasms, whereas the remaining one third is due to metastatic disease. As a group, gliomas are the most common brain tumors and include astrocytomas, ependymomas, choroid plexus tumors. Astrocytomas account for approximately 80% of intracranial gliomas and are the most common supratentorial tumor in all age groups.

Astrocytomas are often divided into circumscribed or infiltrating tumors. Pilocytic astrocytomas and subependymal giant-cell astrocytomas are in the circumscribed group because they do not invade the surrounding structures. Pilocytic astrocytomas are usually located infratentorially and generally well circumscribed and often cystic.

Most supratentorial **pilocytic astrocytomas** are solid and located in the region of hypothalamus. Cystic pilocytic astrocytomas in the cerebral hemisphere are rare.

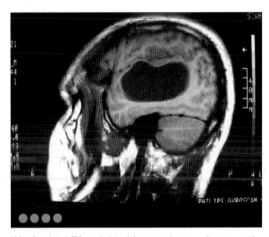

K1. Sagittal T1-weighted image shows a large cystic mass in the left cerebral hemisphere.

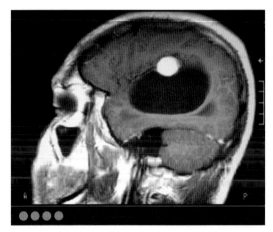

K2. Sagittal and coronal, post-contrast T1-weighted images demonstrate a large cystic mass with an enhancing mural nodule.

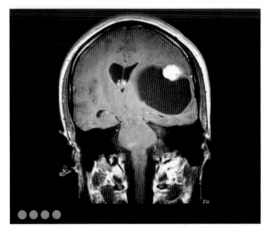

K3. Sagittal and coronal, post-contrast T1-weighted images demonstrate a large cystic mass with an enhancing mural nodule.

PLEOMORPHIC XANTHOASTROCYTOMA

Pleomorphic xanthoastrocytomas (PXAs) typically occur in children and young adults, occasionally they are seen in the fourth and fifth decades of life. Seizures is the classic clinical presentation. It is a rare benign subtype of astrocytoma.

PXA is typically a clearly marginated, cystic tumor with a discrete mural nodule in a superficial, cortical and subpial location. They may affect superficial cerebral cortex as well as the meninges. Occasionally, PXAs appear more diffuse and infiltrating.

They are WHO grade 2 neoplasms. On histology, there are pleomorphic tumor cells with abundant glassy cytoplasm and dark, multilobulated nuclei. There is a mixture of spindle-shaped cells, multinucleated giant cells, and foamy lipid-laden xanthomatous astrocytes in these tumors. Focal cystic changes are common. Mitosis are few and necrosis is absent. They are most commonly seen in temporal lobes, but may be seen in parietal, occipital, and frontal lobes.

PLEOMORPHIC XANTHOASTROCYTOMA (CASE ONE)

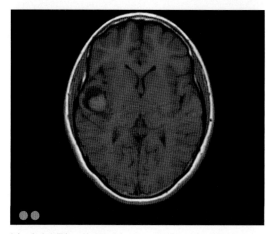

L1. Axial T1-weighted image shows a cystic mass with a mural nodule.

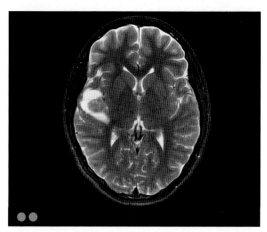

L2. Axial T2-weighted image demonstrates a cystic mass with a mural nodule.

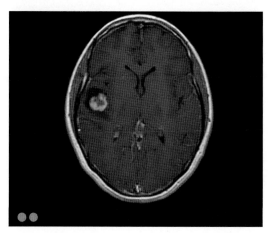

L3. Axial and coronal, post-contrast T1-weighted images demonstrate a cystic mass with enhancing mural nodule.

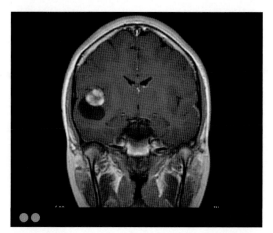

L4. Axial and coronal, post-contrast T1-weighted images demonstrate a cystic mass with enhancing mural nodule.

153

PLEOMORPHIC XANTHOASTROCYTOMA (CASE TWO)

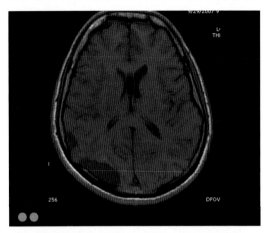

M1. Axial T1-weighted image shows a cortically located cystic mass with a solid nodule. Note the bony erosion of the adjacent calvarium by the solid nodule.

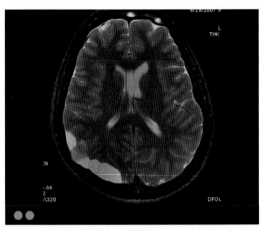

M2. Axial T2-weighted and FLAIR images reveal a cystic mass with a solid nodule on the cortical surface.

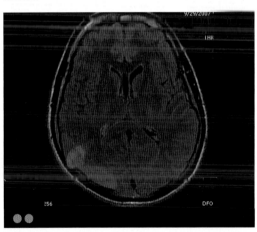

M3. Axial T2-weighted and FLAIR images reveal a cystic mass with a solid nodule on the cortical surface.

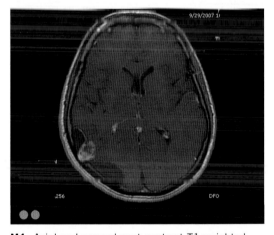

M4. Axial and coronal post-contrast T1-weighted images demonstrate avid enhancement of the solid nodule.

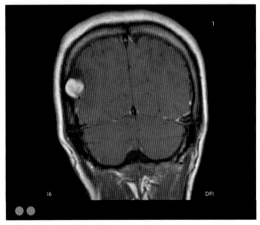

M5. Axial and coronal post-contrast T1-weighted images demonstrate avid enhancement of the solid nodule.

ANAPLASTIC EPENDYMOMA

Ependymomas comprise 8%–10% of all brain tumors occurring in young patients, with a peak incidence between two to three years of age. More than 90% of childhood ependymomas arise in the brain; approximately two-thirds are infratentorial and one-third supratentorial in location. Approximately half of the supratentorial tumors arise from the wall of the third ventricle; the remaining half arise in the area remote from the ventricular wall, presumably from fetal rests of the ectopic ependymal cells. Supratentorial extraventricular ependymoma is usually a slow-growing tumor that is often large at the time of presentation. Anaplastic ependymomas of the supratentorial compartment are aggressive tumors with high rates of recurrence even after gross total excision and irradiation.

Anaplastic ependymoma is considered WHO grade III. Tumor necrosis and hemorrhage are more frequently seen than lower grade ependymomas.

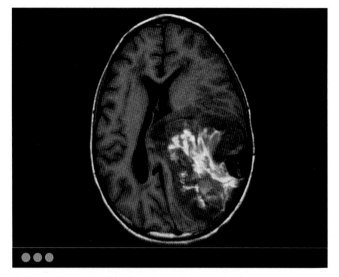

A. Axial T1-weighted image demonstrates a heterogeneously enhancing mass in the left temporal, parierooccipital region with surrounding edema and mass effect.

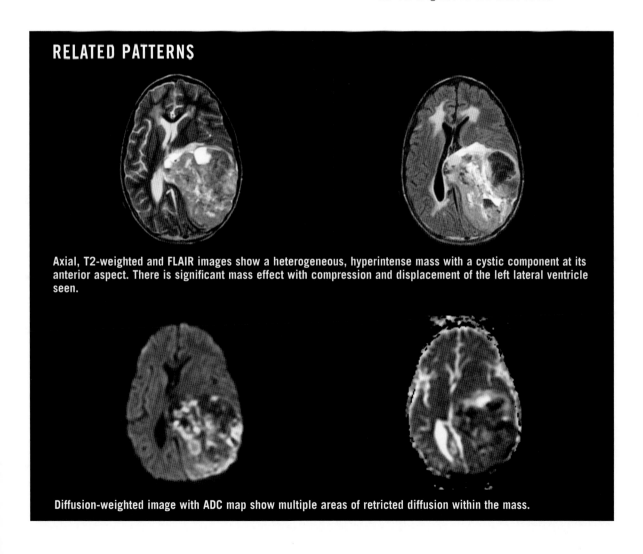

RELATED PATTERNS

Axial, T2-weighted and FLAIR images show a heterogeneous, hyperintense mass with a cystic component at its anterior aspect. There is significant mass effect with compression and displacement of the left lateral ventricle seen.

Diffusion-weighted image with ADC map show multiple areas of retricted diffusion within the mass.

DIFFERENTIAL DIAGNOSIS

At a Glance:

- Anaplastic Astrocytoma
- Atypical Teratoid/Rhabdoid Tumor (Atr Tumor)
- Calcified Oligodendroglioma
- Cavernous Angioma
- Glioblastoma Multiforme
- Low-Grade Glioma, Post-Radiation Therapy
- Metastatic Melanoma
- Necrotizing Encephalitis
- PNET
- Toxoplasmosis

ANAPLASTIC ASTROCYTOMA

Anaplastic astrocytomas occur most commonly in the fourth and fifth decade. They present as a mass in the white matter of cerebral hemisphere with ill-defined margins. Tumor hemorrhage is frequently seen. Necrosis could suggest malignant dedifferentiation of the tumor to glioblastoma multiforme. The pathological features of anaplastic astrocytomas consist of high cellularity, frequent mitoses, and foci of vascular proliferation. Tumor necrosis is usually absent.

It can occur as a result of progressive dedifferentiation of a previously low-grade astrocytoma.

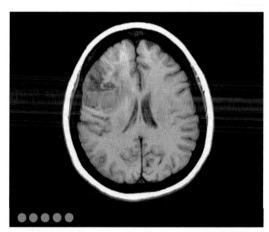

B1 Axial T1-weighted image shows a markedly heterogeneous mass in the right frontal lobe. Slight compression of the frontal horn of the right lateral ventricle is seen.

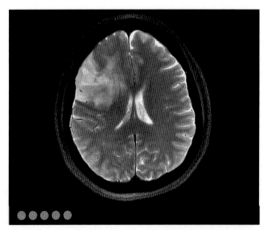

B2. Axial T2-weighted and FLAIR images show a heterogeneous mass in the right frontal lobe with surrounding edema.

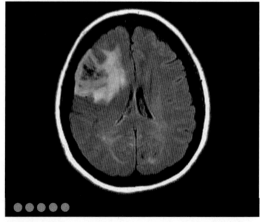

B3. Axial T2-weighted and FLAIR images show a heterogeneous mass in the right frontal lobe with surrounding edema.

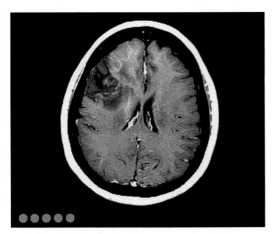

B4. Axial and coronal, post-contrast T1-weighted images demonstrate heterogeneous enhancement of the mass lesion.

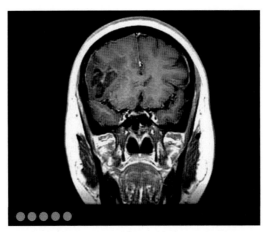

B5. Axial and coronal, post-contrast T1-weighted images demonstrate heterogeneous enhancement of the mass lesion.

ATYPICAL TERATOID/RHABDOID TUMOR (ATR TUMOR)

Atypical teratoid/rhabdoid tumors (AT/RTs) are rare malignant intracranial tumors, consisting of 1.3% of primary CNS tumors in the pediatric population and 6.7% of CNS tumors in children younger than 2 years. Malignant rhabdoid tumor can occur in many locations in the body with kidney and CNS the most common primary sites. They can occur in the supratentorial or infratentorial compartment. Imaging features of AT/RT are often variable secondary cystic/necrotic changes and/or hemorrhage. Disseminated tumor in the leptomeninges was seen with MR imaging in 24% of patients at initial diagnosis. Abnormalities involving chromosome 22 have been found in AT/RT. Deletion and/or mutation of hSNF5/INI1 genes is seen in approximately 70% of AT/RTs. Despite the fact that both the intracranial AT/RT and the malignant renal rhabdoid tumor may have inactivation of both hSNF5/INI1 tumor-suppressor genes, differing features may indicate that these two tumors are distinct primary lesions rather than metastases (will have similar histologic features and immunohistochemical profiles).

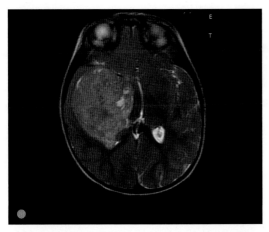

C1. Axial T2-weighted image shows a slightly heterogeneous mass in the right temporal region extending into the basal ganglia.

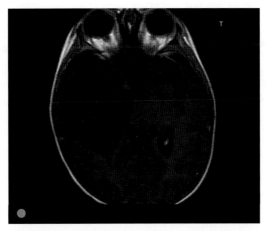

C2. Axial T1-weighted, post-contrast image shows a heterogeneously enhancing mass in the right temporal region extending into the basal ganglia.

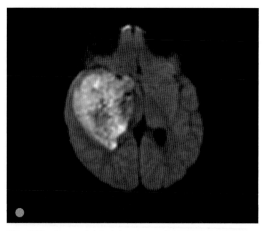

C3. Diffusion-weighted image and ADC map show a mass with restricted diffusion in the right temporal region extending into the basal ganglia.

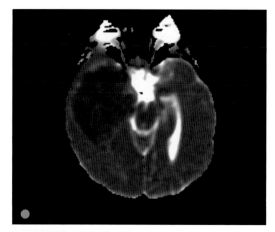

C4. Diffusion-weighted image and ADC map show a mass with restricted diffusion in the right temporal region extending into the basal ganglia.

CALCIFIED OLIGODENDROGLIUMA

Calcification is demonstrated in 50–90% of oligodendrogliomas. Calcification is seen as an area of hypointensity on T2-weighted images.

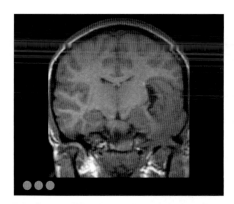

D1. Coronal T1-weighted image shows mixed iso- and hypointense mass in the right temporal region. The hypointensity is mainly due to calcification.

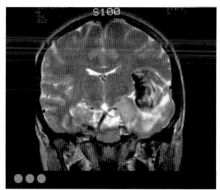

D2. Coronal and axial T2-weighted images demonstrate a heterogeneous mass in the right temporal region with surrounding edema. The hypointensity mimics a vascular pattern, but is due to calcification as demonstrated on CT.

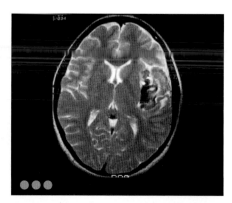

D3. Coronal and axial T2-weighted images demonstrate a heterogeneous mass in the right temporal region with surrounding edema. The hypointensity mimics a vascular pattern, but is due to calcification as demonstrated on CT.

CAVERNOUS ANGIOMA

Cavernous angiomas are developmental malformations of the vascular bed. These congenital abnormal vascular connections frequently enlarge over time. They can occur on a familial basis. The risk of hemorrhage of cavernous angiomas is estimated to be less than 2% per lesion per year. Cavernous angiomas are congenital vascular hamartomas composed of closely approximated endothelial-lined sinusoidal collections without significant amounts of interspersed neural tissue. Histopathologically, cavernous angiomas are characteristically lack of intervening neural tissue, whereas capillary telangiectasias exhibit significant amount of intervening neural tissue.

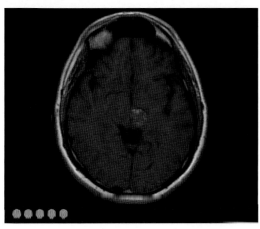

E1. Axial T1-weighted image shows a heterogeneous, predominantly hyperintense lesion in the left thalamus.

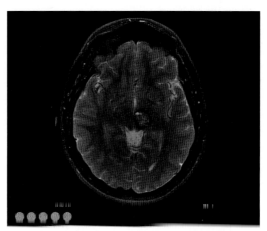

E2. Axial T2-weighted and FLAIR images show a heterogeneous, hyperintense lesion with a hypointense ring in the left thalamus.

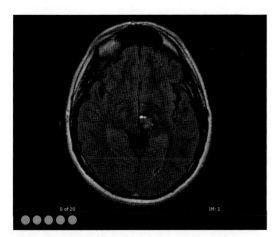

E3. Axial T2-weighted and FLAIR images show a heterogeneous, hyperintense lesion with a hypointense ring in the left thalamus.

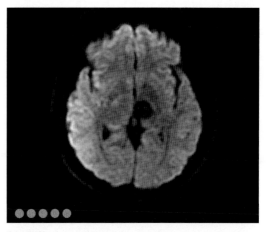

E4. Diffusion-weighted image shows a low signal lesion due to the presence of hemosiderin creating susceptibility artifact.

GLIOBLASTOMA MULTIFORME

Glioblastoma multiforme tends to occur in elderly patients and clinical course is short, usually a few months. Secondary GBMs that arise from malignant dedifferentiation of anaplastic astrocytomas or low-grade astrocytomas tend to occur in younger age group and have a more protracted course over a few years. Relative cerebral blood volume (rCBV) correlates with astrocytomas grade and vascularity on perfusion studies.

Glioblastoma multiforme is the most common primary tumor of the central nervous system. It characteristically involves the white matter, but infiltrates and destroys gray matter with loss of gray–white differentiation. Pathological features consist of areas of hypercellularity, cellular pleomorphism, endothelial proliferation, and intratumoral necrosis. Peritumoral edema and mass effect are always present.

GLIOBLASTOMA MULTIFORME (CASE ONE)

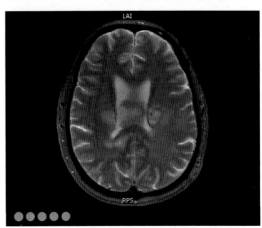

F1. Axial T2-weighted and FLAIR images show a heterogeneously hyperintense mass crossing the corpus callosum involving both hemispheres.

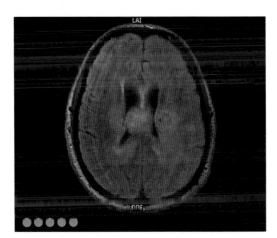

F2. Axial T2-weighted and FLAIR images show a heterogeneously hyperintense mass crossing the corpus callosum involving both hemispheres.

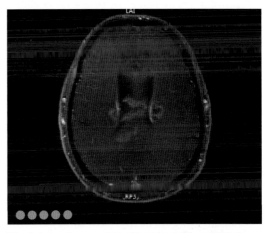

F3. Axial and coronal, post-contrast T1-weighted images show heterogeneous enhancement of the mass lesion.

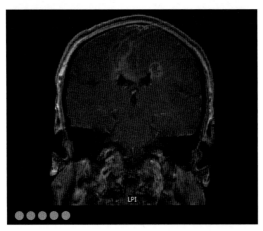

F4. Axial and coronal, post-contrast T1-weighted images show heterogeneous enhancement of the mass lesion.

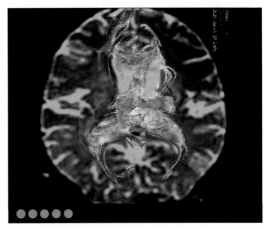

F5. Diffusion tensor imaging shows disruption of the white matter fibers at the corpus callosum.

GLIOBLASTOMA MULTIFORME (CASE TWO)

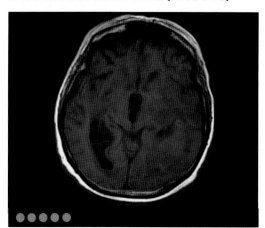

G1. Axial T1-weighted image shows a mixed hypointense, isointense mass in the left temporal, parietooccipital region with compression of the atrium and occipital horn of the left lateral ventricle.

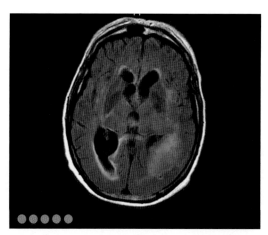

G2. Axial FLAIR image reveals a hyperintense mass with mixed signal intensity.

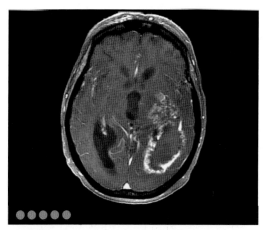

G3. Axial and coronal, post-contrast T1-weighted image show a heterogeneously enhancing mass in the left temporal, parietooccipital region.

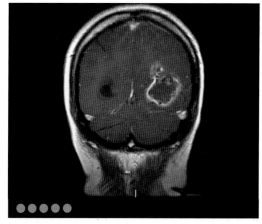

G4. Axial and coronal, post-contrast T1-weighted image show a heterogeneously enhancing mass in the left temporal, parietooccipital region.

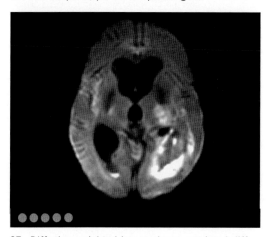

G5. Diffusion-weighted image shows restricted diffusion within the solid component of the mass.

161

LOW-GRADE GLIOMA, POST-RADIATION THERAPY

Necrotic change may be seen in **low-grade glioma** treated by radiation therapy. Proton MR Spectroscopy and Perfusion weighted images can be used to differentiate Post-radiation changes from Glioblastoma multiforme. On MR proton spectroscopy, an elevated choline peak is a surrogate marker of increased cell membrane turnover caused by tumor growth or normal cell destruction. This is seen in neoplasms, but not in post-radiation changes. A decreased NAA peak and elevated lipid and lactate peaks is seen in both high grade neoplasms and post-radiation changes. On perfusion weighted imaging, High grade tumor recurrence shows increased rCBV measurements whereas post-radiation changes reveal decreased rCBV.

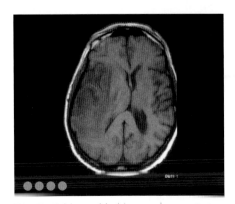

H1. Axial T1-weighted image shows a heterogeneous mass of mixed hypo- and isointensity in the right temporal region.

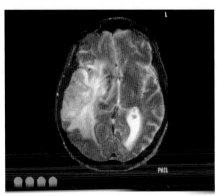

H2. Axial T2-weighted image reveals a heterogeneously hyperintense mass in the right temporal region with surrounding edema and mass effect.

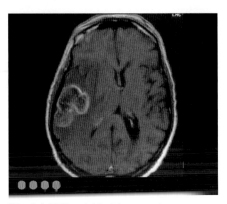

H3. Axial T2-weighted images show a hyperintense structure with remodeling of the inner table of the skull in the parasagittal region.

METASTATIC MELANOMA

Hemorrhage is commonly seen in **metastatic melanoma,** occurring in 30–50% of the metastases to the brain. Hemorrhagic lesions will present as hyperintense lesions on T1-weighted images on MRI.

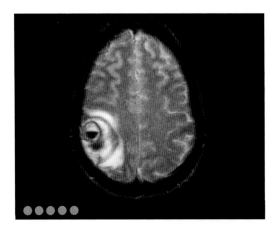

I1. Axial T2-weighted image shows a heterogeneous (due to intratumoral hemorrhage) mass with surrounding edema in the right parietal region.

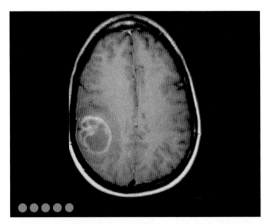

I2. Axial, post-contrast T1-weighted image shows a heterogeneously enhancing mass in the right parietal region.

NECROTIZING ENCEPHALITIS

Although the term "encephalitis" literally means "inflammation of the brain," it usually refers to brain inflammation resulting from a viral infection. Acute necrotizing encephalitis is an acute form of encephalitis, characterized by destruction of brain parenchyma; caused by herpes simplex and other viruses. Hemorrhage within the necrotic areas may be seen.

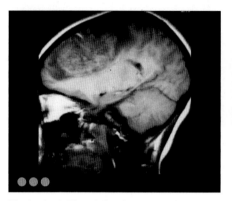
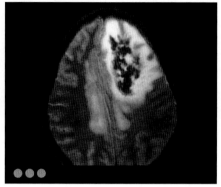
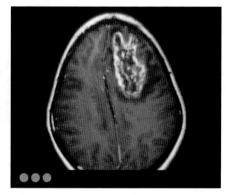

J1. Sagittal T1-weighted image shows a heterogeneous, mixed signal intensity mass-like lesion in the left frontal lobe.

J2. Axial T2-weighted image reveals a heterogeneous mass-like lesion with surrounding edema in the left frontal lobe. The hypointense areas are due to hemorrhage within the lesion.

J3. Axial, post-contrast T1-weighted image shows a heterogeneously enhancing lesion.

PNET

The term primitive neuroectodermal tumor or PNET is used to describe a group of tumors that exhibit similar cell types, but occur in different locations. Medulloblastoma, pineoblastoma, ependymoblastoma, retinoblastoma are all considered to be PNET. Medulloblastoma is the most common of all these tumors. PNETs generally occur in children. PNET of the brain can be divided grossly into infratentorial tumors (medulloblastoma) and supratentorial tumors (sPNET). The supratentorial tumors are much less common and are more likely to occur in young adults.

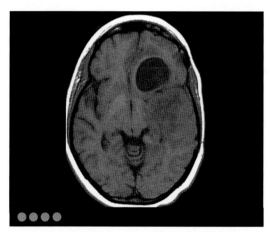
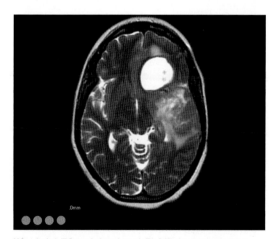

K1. Axial T1-weighted image shows an ill-defined hypointense mass with a large cystic component anteriorly in the left frontotemporal region.

K2. Axial T2-weighted and FLAIR images show a large heterogeneous mass with a large cystic component in the left frontotemporal region.

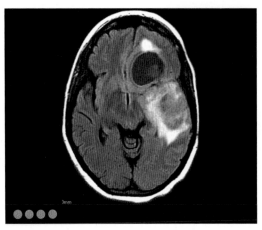

K3. Axial T2-weighted and FLAIR images show a large heterogeneous mass with a large cystic component in the left frontotemporal region.

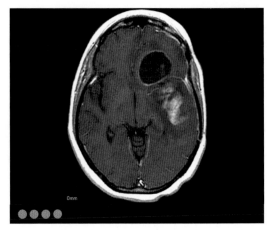

K4. Axial, post-contrast T1-weighted image reveals heterogeneously enhancing mass with a large cystic component.

TOXOPLASMOSIS

CNS **toxoplasmosis** is one of the more frequent opportunistic infections in AIDS patients. On imaging, toxoplasmosis presents as multiple lesions with various size and enhancement in the basal ganglia as well as corticomedullary junction. On MR proton spectroscopy, a de-creased *N*-acetylaspartate, moderately decreased choline, markedly increased lactate and lipid, and absent myoinositol peak may be seen in cerebral toxoplasmosis. Diffusion-weighted imaging usually demonstrates no evidence of restricted diffusion. Occasionally, the ring-like component may show a mild degree of restricted diffusion.

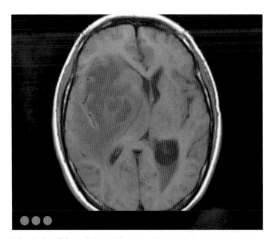

L1. Axial T1-weighted image shows a heterogeneous, hypointense mass in the region of right basal gnaglia with surrounding edema and mass effect.

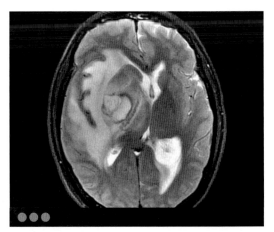

L2. Axial T2-weighted and FLAIR images show a heterogeneous, hyperintense mass with surrounding edema and mass effect.

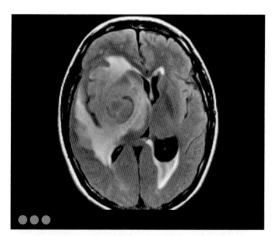

L3. Axial T2-weighted and FLAIR images show a heterogeneous, hyperintense mass with surrounding edema and mass effect.

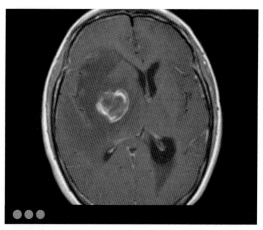

L4. Axial and coronal, post-contrast T1-weighted images demonstrate irregular ring-like enhancement of the mass with surrounding edema.

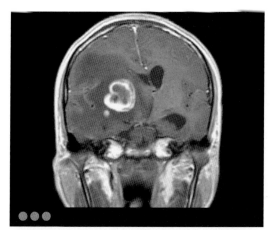

L5. Axial and coronal, post-contrast T1-weighted images demonstrate irregular ring-like enhancement of the mass with surrounding edema.

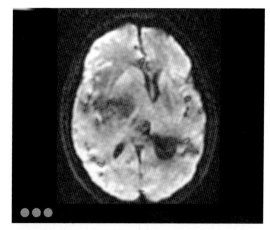

L6. Diffusion-weighted image demonstrate no evidence of restricted diffusion in the lesion.

CYSTICERCOSIS

Cysticercosis cysts can be divided according to their location into parenchymal, cisternal, ventricular, or spinal cysts. Mixed form may also be seen.

In the parenchymal form of neurocysticercosis, there are four stages in evolution of the disease process, namely, vesicular stage, colloidal vesicular stage, granular nodular stage, and nodular calcified stage. At the granular nodular stage, an enhancing nodule is seen on contrast-enhanced CT or MRI.

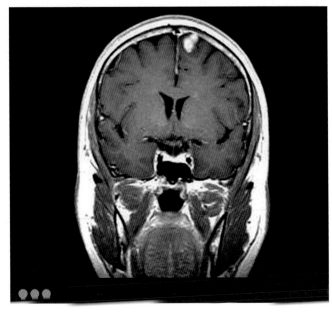

A. Coronal, post-contrast T1-weighted image shows a nodular enhancing lesion in the left frontal region.

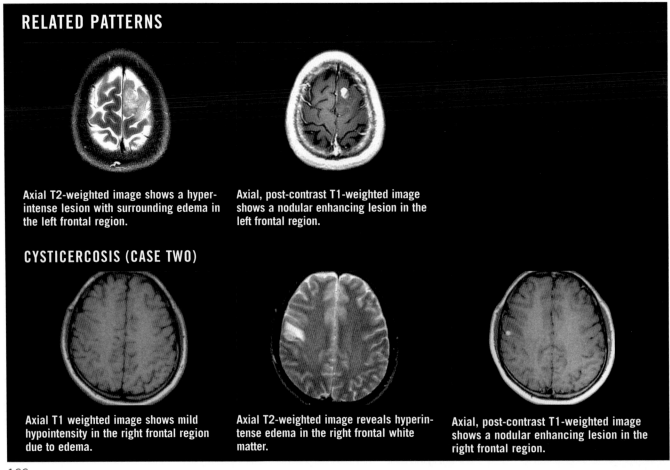

RELATED PATTERNS

Axial T2-weighted image shows a hyperintense lesion with surrounding edema in the left frontal region.

Axial, post-contrast T1-weighted image shows a nodular enhancing lesion in the left frontal region.

CYSTICERCOSIS (CASE TWO)

Axial T1 weighted image shows mild hypointensity in the right frontal region due to edema.

Axial T2-weighted image reveals hyperintense edema in the right frontal white matter.

Axial, post-contrast T1-weighted image shows a nodular enhancing lesion in the right frontal region.

DIFFERENTIAL DIAGNOSIS

At a Glance:

- *Lymphoma*
- *Metastatic Disease (Melanoma)*
- *Metastatic Disease (Breast Carcinoma)*
- *Pilocytic Astrocytoma*
- *Toxoplasmosis*
- *Whipple's Disease*
- *Tuberculosis* (not pictured)

LYMPHOMA

About 10% of the patients with systemic **lymphoma** develop CNS involvement in clinical series, and secondary CNS lymphoma may be found in up to 26% of the cases in autopsy series. Primary CNS lymphomas are more common than secondary CNS lymphoma. Approximately 20 to 40% of lesions are multiple.

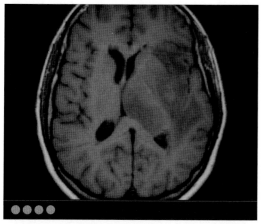

B1. Axial T1-weighted image shows a hypointense mass with surrounding edema and mass effect in the region of left basal ganglia.

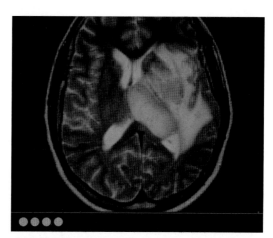

B2. Axial T2-weighted and FLAIR images reveal a hyperintense mass in the region of left basal ganglia with surrounding edema.

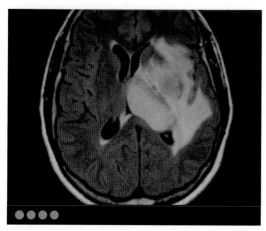

B3. Axial T2-weighted and FLAIR images reveal a hyperintense mass in the region of left basal ganglia with surrounding edema.

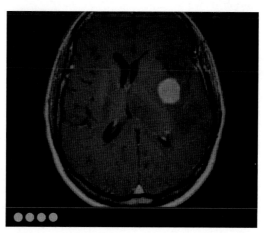

B4. Axial, post-contrast T1-weighted image shows a nodular enhancement within the mass lesion in the region of left basal ganglia.

METASTATIC DISEASE (MELANOMA)

Metastases are the most common masses in the supratentorial compartment in adults, consisting 40% of intracranial neoplasms supratentorially. Approximately half of the metastatic lesions are solitary and the other half are multiple. The primary site of neoplasm includes lung, breast, melanoma, kidney, and gastrointestinal tract.

Metastases are usually well defined, and sharply marginated. Metastatic lesions may be associated with extensive edema or minimal edema, especially those cortical metastases. Almost all the metastases show contrast enhancement due to the lack of blood brain barrier, but the pattern may be nodular, ring-like, irregular, homogeneous or heterogeneous.

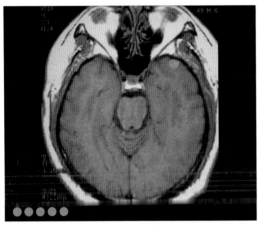

C1. Axial T1-weighted image shows a hyperintense mass at the anterior aspect of the left temporal lobe.

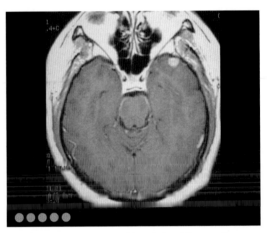

C2. Axial, post-contrast T1-weighted image demonstrates enhancement of the lef temporal nodular lesion.

METASTATIC DISEASE (BREAST CARCINOMA)

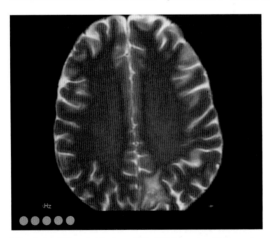

D1. Axial T2-weighted and FLAIR images show a hyperintense mass with surrounding edema in the left parietal region.

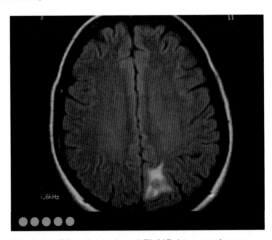

D2. Axial T2-weighted and FLAIR images show a hyperintense mass with surrounding edema in the left parietal region.

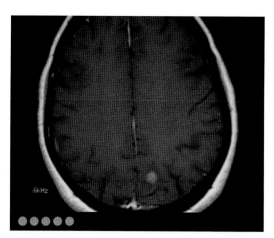

D3. Axial, post-contrast T1-weighted image demonstrates a nodular enhancing mass in the left parietal lobe.

PILOCYTIC ASTROCYTOMA

Cerebellar juvenile **pilocytic astrocytomas** are classified as WHO grade 1 astrocytoma. The majority of cerebellar astro-cytomas are of the pilocytic variety (85%) and they occur within the first decade of life. Supratentorial pilocytic astro-cytomas are usually solid masses and tend to occur in the hypothalamic region and are uncommon in other locations.

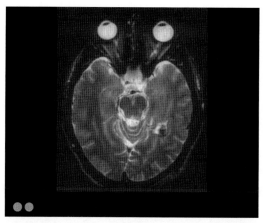

E1. Axial T2-weighted image shows a hypointense mass with surrounding edema in the medial, posterior left temporal lobe.

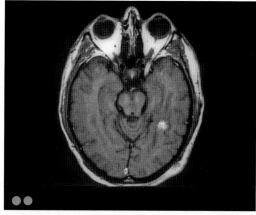

E2. Axial and coronal, post-contrast T1-weighted image shows a nodular enhancing lesion with surrounding edema.

169

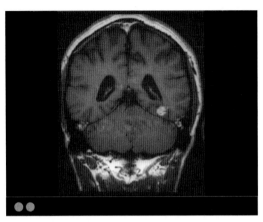

E3. Axial and coronal, post-contrast T1-weighted image shows a nodular enhancing lesion with surrounding edema.

TOXOPLASMOSIS

Toxoplasmosis is the most common complication encountered in HIV-infected immunocompromised patients. The challenge is to differentiate toxoplasmosis from lymphomas. Tosoplasmosis lesions tend to occur in the basal ganglia and cortical medullary junctions whereas lymphomas are more freuqnetly seen in the periventricualr white matter and corpus callosum. MR spectroscopy and diffusion weighted imaging have increased the ability to differentiate between these two lesions. On T1-weighted images, the lesions are hypointense relative to gray matter. On T2-weighted images, the foci of infection can be hyperintense, or occasionally isointense to hypointense. Surrounding edema is usually seen. Nodular or ring enhancement can be seen in approximately 70% of patients following intravenous injection of gadolinium.

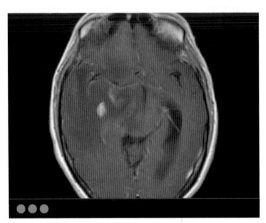

F1. Axial and coronal, post-contrast T1-weighted imag shows a nodular enhancing lesion within the right basal ganglia with surrounding edema.

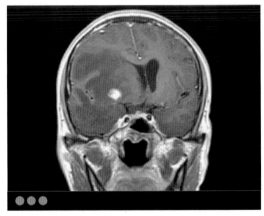

F2. Axial and coronal, post-contrast T1-weighted imag shows a nodular enhancing lesion within the right basal ganglia with surrounding edema.

WHIPPLE'S DISEASE

Clinically detectable involvement of the central nervous system ranges from 6% to 43% of patients suffering from Whipple disease. Focal abnormalities were found on imaging studies in approximately half of the cases. It has been postulated that multiple small circular or oval lesions, measuring an average of 2 mm in diameter, disseminated throughout the gray matter and characterized by the accumulation of macrophages. These lesions often show hypointensity on T1 weighted images and hyperintensity on T2 weighted images. Contrast enhancement is seen following the intravenous injection of Gadolinium. They are located in the medial part of the temporal lobes, in the hypothalamic region, or in the pons.

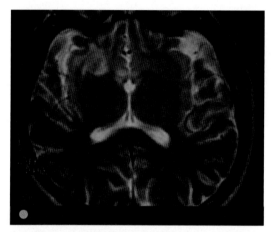

G1. Axial T2-weighted image shows an hyperintense area in the anterior right basal ganglia.

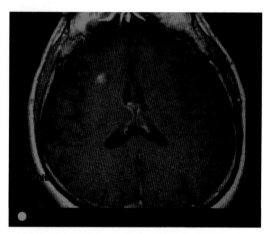

G2. Axial and coronal, post-contrast T1-weighted images show a nodular enhancing lesion at the anterior, inferior aspect of the right basal gnaglia.

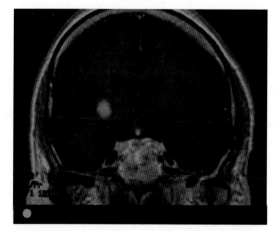

G3. Axial and coronal, post-contrast T1-weighted images show a nodular enhancing lesion at the anterior, inferior aspect of the right basal gnaglia.

ABSCESS

The most distinctive feature of abscess on imaging is the presence of a smooth, thin capsule with a moderate amount of cerebral edema. It is located at the corticomedullary junction and usually extends into the white matter. The abscess cavity has necrosis and liquefaction within its center. On MRI scans, the capsule is better visualized as compared with CT. The capsule is isointense to hyperintense to gray matter on T1-weighted images and hypointense on T2-weighted images. The hypointensity on the abscess capsule is consistently seen with abscess and may be useful in characterizing the lesion. However, other lesions, such as metastasis, glioma, and cysticercosis, may show a similar hypointense ring on T2-weighted images. The capsule enhances with intravenous administration of contrast material on MRI studies. The presence of satellite lesions is a unique feature of cerebral abscess. On diffusion-weighted images, the pus within the abscess cavity characteristically shows restricted diffusion.

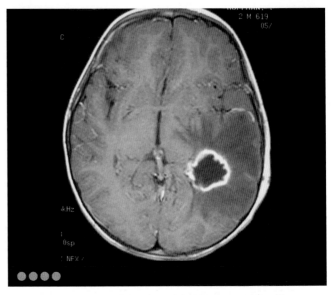

A. Axial, post contrast T1-weighted image shows a ring-like enhancing lesion in the region of left posterior temporal lobe.

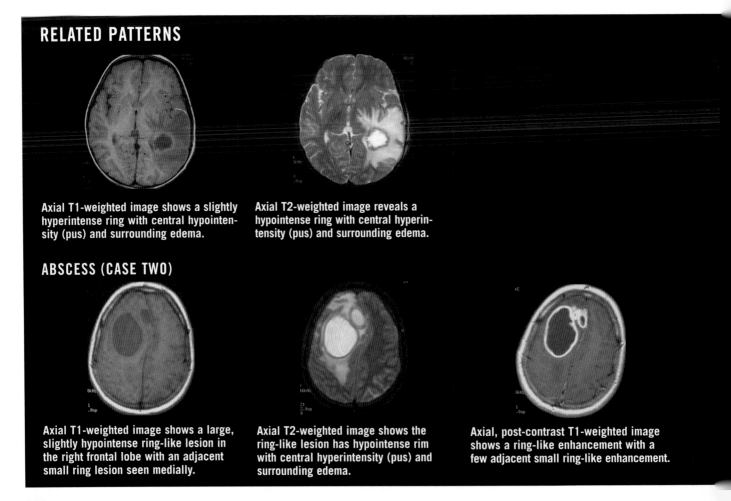

RELATED PATTERNS

Axial T1-weighted image shows a slightly hyperintense ring with central hypointensity (pus) and surrounding edema.

Axial T2-weighted image reveals a hypointense ring with central hyperintensity (pus) and surrounding edema.

ABSCESS (CASE TWO)

Axial T1-weighted image shows a large, slightly hypointense ring-like lesion in the right frontal lobe with an adjacent small ring lesion seen medially.

Axial T2-weighted image shows the ring-like lesion has hypointense rim with central hyperintensity (pus) and surrounding edema.

Axial, post-contrast T1-weighted image shows a ring-like enhancement with a few adjacent small ring-like enhancement.

ABSCESS (CASE THREE)

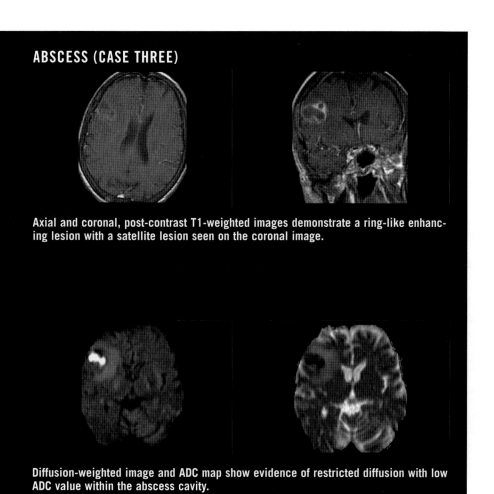

Axial and coronal, post-contrast T1-weighted images demonstrate a ring-like enhancing lesion with a satellite lesion seen on the coronal image.

Diffusion-weighted image and ADC map show evidence of restricted diffusion with low ADC value within the abscess cavity.

DIFFERENTIAL DIAGNOSIS

At a Glance:

- *Astrocytoma (Grade 2)*
- *Cysticercosis*
- *Echinococcus*
- *Glioblastoma Multiforme*
- *Lymphoma*
- *Metastasis*
- *Multiple Sclerosis*
- *Oligodendroglioma*
- *Pilocytic Astrocytoma*
- *Septic Emboli*
- *Toxoplasmosis*

ASTROCYTOMA (GRADE 2)

Grade 2 astrocytomas are considered to be low grade. On MRI, they are typically hypointense on T1 weighted images and hyperintense on T2-weighted images. Contrast enhancement may be absent or mild. Exceptions include the mural nodule of pilocytic astrocytoma and the strong heterogeneous enhancement of pleomorphic xanthoastrocytomas. Surrounding edema is usually mild. MRS may show an elevated Cho peak and decreased NAA peak. This is true for all high-grade tumors and many, but not all, low-grade tumors. Perfusion weighted MR imaging demonstrates no evidence of increased rCBV in low grade astrocytomas.

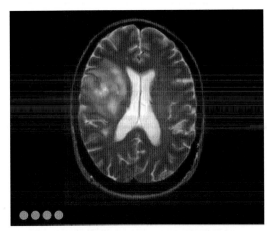

D1. Axial T2 weighted image shows a hyperintense lesion with mass effect in the right frontal region.

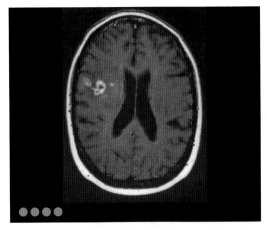

B2. Axial and coronal, post-contrast T1-weighted images show a small ring-like enhancing lesion with adjacent nodular enhancement.

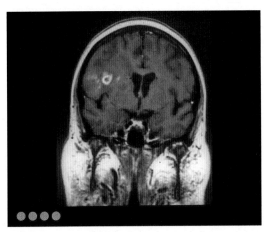

B3. Axial and coronal, post-contrast T1-weighted images show a small ring-like enhancing lesion with adjacent nodular enhancement.

CYSTICERCOSIS

In the colloidal vesicular stage of the parenchymal **neuro-cysticercosis**, a ring-like enhancing lesion is seen intra-parenchymally. Some surrounding edema may be seen depending on the stage of the disease. The scolex may not be identified due to its degeneration. The cyst fluid becomes more turbid.

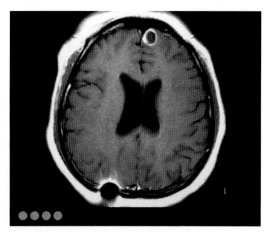

C. Axial T1 weighted, post-contrast image shows a ring-like enhancing lesion in the left frontal lobe.

ECHINOCOCCUS

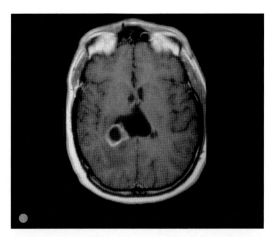

D. Axial, post-contrast T1-weighted image shows a ring-like enhancing lesion in the right periatrial region.

GLIOBLASTOMA MULTIFORME

Glioblastoma multiforme (GBM) is the most common and most malignant of all the gliomas. Of the estimated 17,000 primary brain tumors diagnosed in the United States each year, approximately 60% are gliomas. Gliomas comprise a heterogeneous group of neoplasms that differ in location, in age and sex distribution, in growth potential, in extent of invasiveness, in morphological features, in tendency for progression, and in response to treatments. Glioblastoma is composed of a heterogenous mixture of poorly differentiated neoplastic astrocytes. They primarily affect adults, and children are rarely affected. They are usually located in the cerebral hemispheres although brainstem involvement may be seen in children.

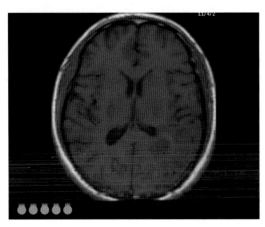

E1. Axial T1-weighted image shows a slightly hyperintense ring lesion with central hypointensity and surrounding edema in the left temporoparietal region.

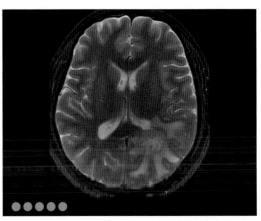

E2. Axial T2-weighted and FLAIR images show a ring-like lesion with central mixed hyperintensity and surrounding edema. Note the central mixed hyperintensity with the cystic area of the GBM is not as hyperintense as the pus seen in abscess cavity.

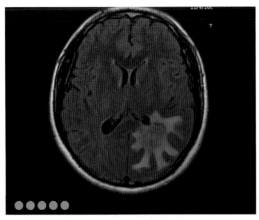

E3. Axial T2-weighted and FLAIR images show a ring-like lesion with central mixed hyperintensity and surrounding edema. Note the central mixed hyperintensity with the cystic area of the GBM is not as hyperintense as the pus seen in abscess cavity.

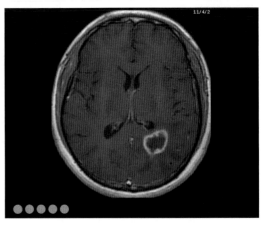

E4. Axial and coronal, post-contrast T1-weighted images demonstrate a ring-like enhancing mass.

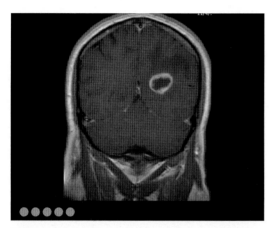

E5. Axial and coronal, post-contrast T1-weighted images demonstrate a ring-like enhancing mass.

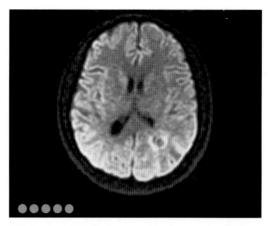

E6. Diffusion-weighted image shows restricted diffusion in the wall of the cystic mass. In contrast to abscess, which shows restricted diffusion in the pus within the cavity.

LYMPHOMA

Lymphoma of brain can be primary or secondary in nature. Primary lymphomas are more common than secondary lymphomas, consisting 70–80% of all lymphomas. Both primary and secondary lymphomas have similar imaging features on MR imaging. Meningeal involvement occurs more commonly in patients with secondary lymphoma than in patients with primary lymphoma. Of patients with primary lymphoma, 75–85% present with supratentorial tumor. Approximately 50% of patients present with multiple lesions.

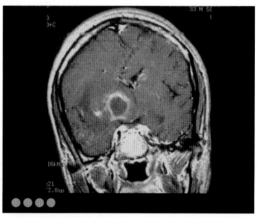

F. Coronal, post-contrast T1-weighted image shows a ring-like enhancing lesion in the right basal ganglia.

METASTASIS

Metastases are the most common masses in the supratentorial compartment in adults, consisting 40% of intracranial neoplasms supratentorially. Approximately half of the metastatic lesions is solitary and the other half is multiple.

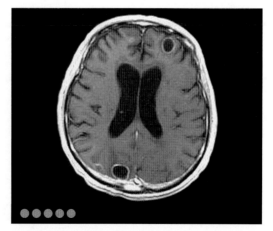

G. Axial, post-contrast T1-weighted image shows two ring-like enhancing lesions, one in the left frontal region and the other in the right occipital region.

MULTIPLE SCLEROSIS

Tumefactive **multiple sclerosis** are generally described as solitary lesions, greater than 2 cm in size, with imaging characteristics mimicking neoplasms, such as mass effect, edema and ring-like contrast enhancement. These lesions more commonly occur in women with an average age of 37 years. With rare exception, the tumefactive demyelinating lesions do not originate as a postinfectious or postvaccination response. Although the exact pathogenesis is not clearly understood, most patients respond favorably to corticosteroid therapy and may have a limited course. Symptoms are generally atypical for multiple sclerosis and usually relate to the presence of a focal mass lesion: focal neurologic deficit, seizure, or aphasia. Without a history of multiple sclerosis, the clinical presentation and radiographic appearance of these lesions often lead to biopsy.

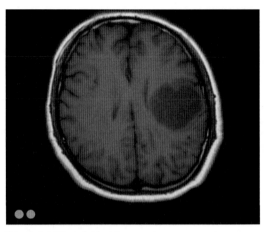

H1. Axial T1-weighted image shows a round, hypointense lesion in the left frontal region.

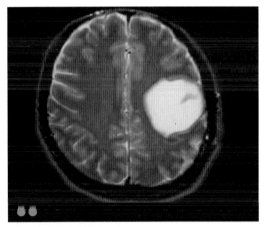

H2. Axial T2-weighted image reveals a hyperintense lesion in the left frontal region.

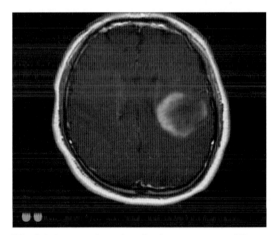

H3. Axial, coronal, and sagittal, post-contrast T1-weighted images demonstrate a ring-like enhancing lesion in the left frontal region.

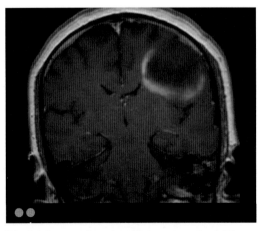

H4. Axial, coronal, and sagittal, post-contrast T1-weighted images demonstrate a ring-like enhancing lesion in the left frontal region.

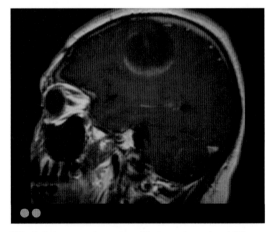

H5. Axial, coronal, and sagittal, post-contrast T1-weighted images demonstrate a ring-like enhancing lesion in the left frontal region.

OLIGODENDROGLIOMA

Oligodendrogliomas are primary glial tumors of the brain which can be divided into grade II oligodendrogliomas and grade III anaplastic oligodendrogliomas. Typically, oligo-dendrogliomas have an indolent course, and patients may have a long survive rate following initial diagnosis. Their relatively good prognosis probably is due to inherently less aggressive biological behavior and a favorable response to chemotherapy. Ring-like enhancement is uncommon in oligodendrogliomas.

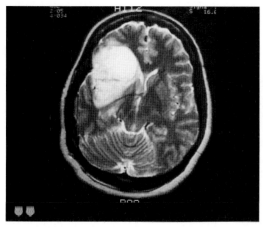

I1. Axial T2-weighted image shows a hyperintense mass in the right frontotemporal region.

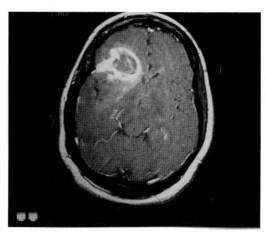

I2. Axial and coronal, post-contrast T1 weighted image shows a ring-like enahcing lesion with a focal enhancing solid component laterally.

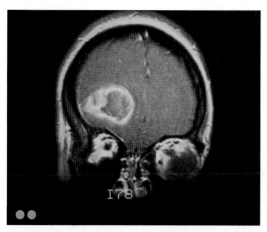

I3. Axial and coronal, post-contrast T1-weighted image shows a ring-like enahcing lesion with a focal enhancing solid component laterally.

PILOCYTIC ASTROCYTOMA

Pilocytic astrocytomas in the supratentorial compartment tend to occur in the region of diencephalon, including the hypothalamus, visual pathway, optic chiasm, and basal ganglia. Infratentorially, pilocytic astrocytoma tends to occur in the cerebellar vermis, hemispheres, and brainstem. Pilocytic astrocytomas are cystic or multicystic, with a mural nodule in 55% of the cases and solid in 45% of the cases. Chiasmati-Chypothalamic pilocytic astrocytomas are usually solid masses and are often associated with neurofibromatosis. MRI shows a cystic mass with a mural nodule or a solid mass. The mural nodule or the solid mass usually show intense contrast enhancement. The cyst wall does not enhance.

PILOCYTIC ASTROCYTOMA (CASE ONE)

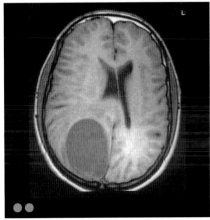

J1. Axial T1-weighted image shows a hypointense, cystic mass in the right parietooccipital region.

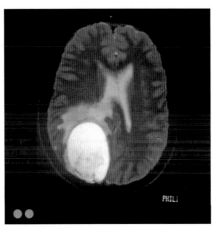

J2. Axial T2-weighted image shows a hyperintense, cystic mass in the right parietooccipital region.

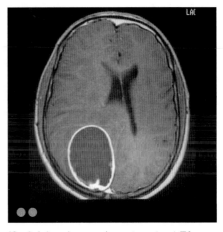

J3. Axial and coronal, post-contrast T1-weighted images show a ring-like enhancement of the cystic mass with a nodular enhancing areas.

PILOCYTIC ASTROCYTOMA (CASE TWO)

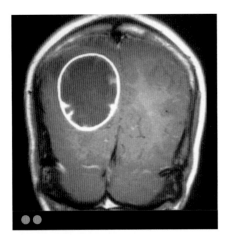

J4. Axial and coronal, post-contrast T1-weighted images show a ring-like enhancement of the cystic mass with a nodular enhancing areas.

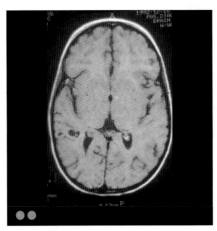

K1. Axial T1-weighted image shows a small ring lesion with adjacent small cyst in the right posterior temporal lobe.

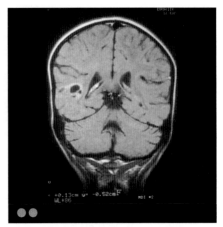

K2. Coronal, post-contrast T1-weighted image shows ring-like enhancing lesions with adjacent small cystic lesions. Note this finding is frequently seen in cerebral abscess, but can also be seen in pilocytic astrocytoma.

SEPTIC EMBOLI

Intracranial **septic emboli** are usually seen in patients with a history of intravenous drug abuse, cyanotic heart disease, and subacute bacterial endocarditis. Septic emboli may be solitary or multiple, and they usually involve middle cerebral artery branches. The relative frequency of middle cerebral artery branch involvement is probably explained by the likelihood of emboli being carried into this territory.

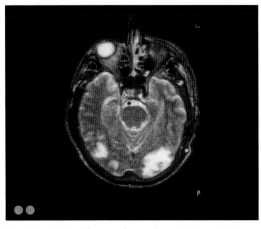

L1. T2-weighted image shows hyperintense lesions in both temporooccipital region.

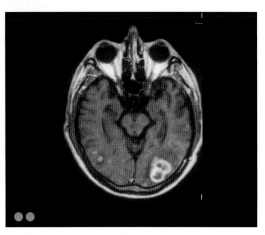

L2. Axial, post-contrast T1-weighted image reveals a multiring like enhancing lesion in the left temporooccipital region and a nodular enhancing lesion in the right posterior temporal region.

TOXOPLASMOSIS

Toxoplasmosis is caused by infestation with the parasite *Toxoplasma gondii*, a protozoan. The adult form usually occurs in immunocompromised patients or in patients with AIDS. Toxoplasmosis may appear as meningoencephalitis or as granulomas. In patients with AIDS, *Toxoplasma encephalitis* is the most common opportunistic infection. The granulomas may be situated at the corticomedullary junction or in the periventricular areas.

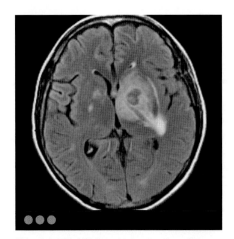

M1. Axial FLAIR image shows a hypointense ring-like lesion with central hyperintensity and peripheral edema in the left basal ganglia. A small hyperintensity is also seen in the right basal gnaglia.

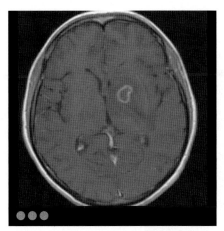

M2. Axial, post-contrast T1-weighted image shows a ring-like enhancing lesion in the left basal ganglia.

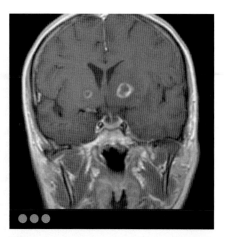

M3. Coronal, post-contrast T1-weighted image shows a ring-like enhancing lesion in the left basal ganglia and another small ring in the right basal ganglia.

METASTASIS

Primary lung cancers account for approximately 50% of all metastatic disease to the brain. Lung cancer is the most common origin of metastatic disease. Of lung cancer patients who survive for more than 2 years, 80% will have metastases involving the brain. Breast cancer is the main source of metastatic disease in women, followed by melanoma, renal, and colorectal cancers. Metastases are the most common masses in the supratentorial compartment in adults, consisting 40% of intracranial neoplasms supratentorially. Approximately half of the metastatic lesions are solitary and the other half are multiple.

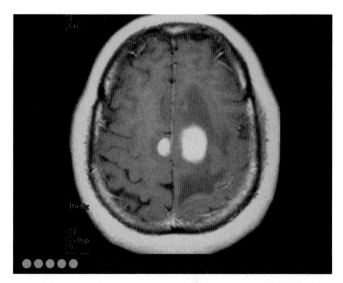

A. Axial, post-contrast T1-weighted image shows two nodular enhancing lesions, one in each frontal lobe in a patient with melanoma.

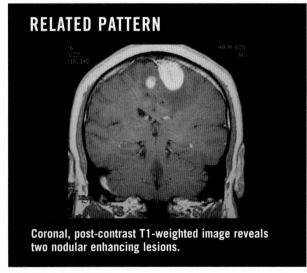

RELATED PATTERN

Coronal, post-contrast T1-weighted image reveals two nodular enhancing lesions.

DIFFERENTIAL DIAGNOSIS

At a Glance:

- *Lymphoma*
- *Multiple Sclerosis*
- *Cysticercosis* (not pictured)
- *Histoplasmosis* (not pictured)
- *Sarcoidosis* (not pictured)
- *Septic Emboli* (not pictured)
- *Tuberculosis* (not pictured)
- *Toxoplasmosis* (not pictured)

LYMPHOMA

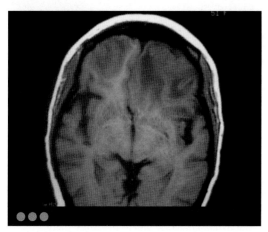

B1. Axial T1-weighted image shows bilateral frontal hypointense areas.

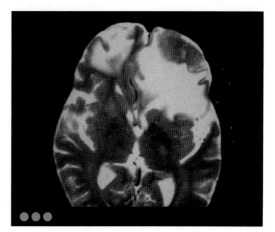

B2. Axial T2-weighted image shows bilateral frontal hyperintense areas.

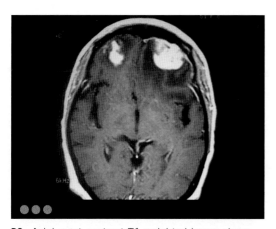

B3. Axial, post-contrast T1-weighted image shows two nodular enhancing lesions.

MULTIPLE SCLEROSIS

Multiple sclerosis is the most common inflammatory demyelinating disease of the central nervous system in young and middle-age people, but also can affect older people. According to the McDonald criteria for MS, the diagnosis requires objective evidence of lesions disseminated in time and space. As a consequence there is an important role for MRI in the diagnosis of MS, since MRI can show multiple lesions (dissemination in space), some of which can be clinically occult and MRI can show new lesions on follow up scans (dissemination in time). MS lesions have a typical distribution pattern in white matter, which includes involvement of corpus callosum, subcortical U fibers, brainstem, cerebellum and spinal cord. On MRI, MS lesions usually show hyperintensity on T2 weighted images and iso- to hypointensity on T1 weighted images. Following intravenous injection of Gadolinium, some lesions may show contrast enhancement whereas other may show no enhancement.

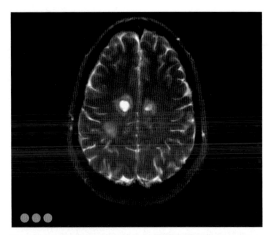

C1. Axial T2-weighted and FLAIR images show three hyperintense lesions in the white matter.

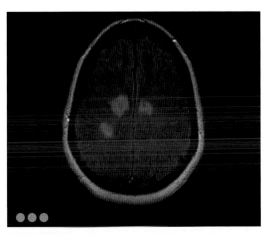

C2. Axial T2-weighted and FLAIR images show three hyperintense lesions in the white matter.

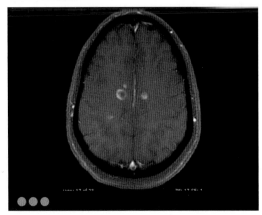

C3. Axial, post-contrast T1-weighted image demonstrate nodular and ring-like enhancing lesions in the white matter bilaterally.

METASTASIS

Metastases are the most common masses in the supra-tentorial compartment in adults, consisting 40% of intracranial neoplasms supratentorially. Approximately half of the metastatic lesions are solitary and the other half are multiple. Miliary type of contrast enhancement can be seen with multiple small metastatic lesions.

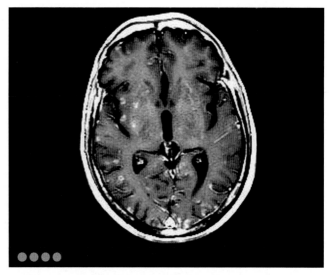

A. Axial, post-contrast T1-weighted image shows multiple small enhancing lesions in both hemispheres.

RELATED PATTERNS

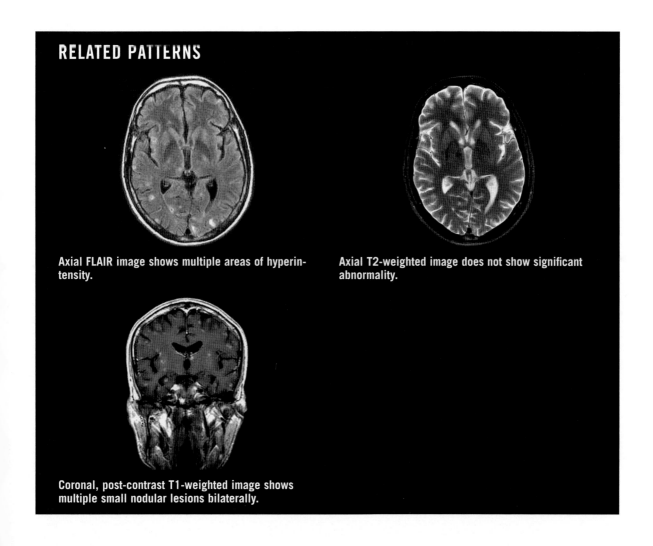

Axial FLAIR image shows multiple areas of hyperintensity.

Axial T2-weighted image does not show significant abnormality.

Coronal, post-contrast T1-weighted image shows multiple small nodular lesions bilaterally.

185

DIFFERENTIAL DIAGNOSIS

At a Glance:

- *Candida*
- *Coccidiomycosis*
- *Tuberculosis*
- *Cysticercosis* (not pictured)

CANDIDA

Central nervous system infections due to *Candida* species are rare and difficult to diagnose. The two primary forms are exogenous infection and endogenous infection. Exogenous infection results from postoperative infection, trauma, lumbar puncture, or shunt placement. Endogenous infection results from candidomia, thus involving the brain parenchyma with multiple small microabscesses. The primary site of involvement is usually esophagus.

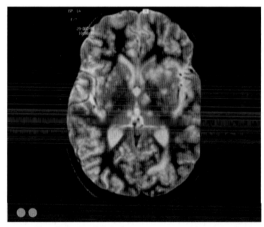

B1. Axial T2-weighted image shows multiple small hyperintense areas through the cerebrum.

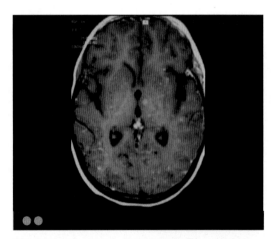

B2. Axial and coronal, post-contrast T1-weighted images demonstrate multiple miliary type of enhancing lesions in both hemisphere.

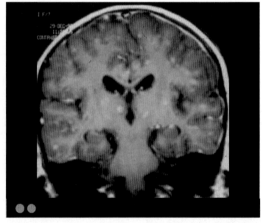

B3. Axial and coronal, post-contrast T1-weighted images demonstrate multiple miliary type of enhancing lesions in both hemisphere.

COCCIDIOMYCOSIS

There is an increase in the frequency of this rare disease (**coccidiomycosis**), in part due to the increase in antibiotics use and in part due to the increasing number of immuno-compromised individuals. Some fungal infection can present as military type of enhancing lesions.

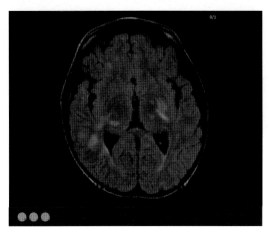

C1. Axial FLAIR image shows multiple areas of hyperintensity.

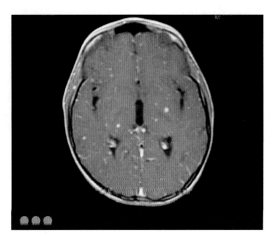

C2. Axial, post-contrast T1-weighted image shows multiple small nodular enhancing lesions.

TUBERCULOSIS

Over 90% of the military **tuberculosis** occurs in multiple organs including lung, liver, spleen, and brain. Up to 25% of patients with military tuberculosis may have meningeal disease. If unrecognized and untreated, it can be a fatal disease.

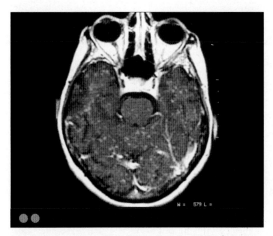

D1. Axial, post-contrast T1-weighted images show multiple military type of enhancing lesions.

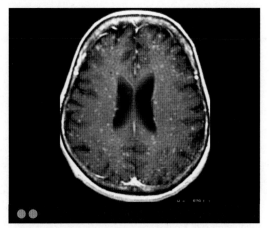

D2. Axial, post-contrast T1-weighted images show multiple military type of enhancing lesions.

187

ANAPLASTIC ASTROCYTOMA

For patients with anaplastic astrocytomas, the tumor growth rate and interval between onset of symptoms and diagnosis is situated between low-grade astrocytomas and glioblastomas. Although highly variable, an interval of approximately 1.5–2 years between onset of symptoms and diagnosis is frequently reported. They can also occur as malignant dedifferentiation of a low grade tumor. Involvement of the corpus callosum is not as common as glioblastoma multiforme.

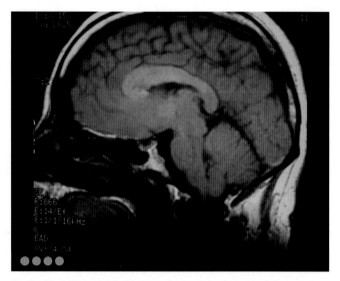

A. Sagittal T1-weighted image shows enlargement of the genu of the corpus callosum due to infiltration by the anaplastic astrocytoma.

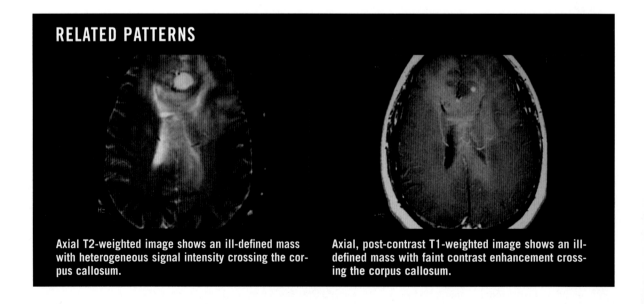

RELATED PATTERNS

Axial T2-weighted image shows an ill-defined mass with heterogeneous signal intensity crossing the corpus callosum.

Axial, post-contrast T1-weighted image shows an ill-defined mass with faint contrast enhancement crossing the corpus callosum.

DIFFERENTIAL DIAGNOSIS

At a Glance:

1. NEOPLASTIC PROCESSES

- *Glioblastoma Multiforme*
- *Gliomatosis*
- *Lymphoma*
- *Metastasis* (not pictured)

2. NONNEOPLASTIC LESIONS INVOLVING CORPUS CALLOSUM

- *Diffuse Axonal Injury*
- *Focal Hyperintensity in Splenium (in a Patient with Seizure)*

- *Infarct*
- *Multiple Sclerosis*
- *Progressive Multifocal Leukoencephalopathy (PML)*
- *Vascular Malformation* (not pictured)
- *HIV Infection* (not pictured)
- *Hypoglycemia/Electrolyte Abnormality* (not pictured)
- *Marchiafava–Bignami Disease* (not pictured)

3. CONGENITAL MALFORMATIONS OF CORPUS CALLOSUM

- *Agenesis of Corpus Callosum*
- *Lipoma of Corpus Callosum*
- *Pericallosal Lipoma*

GLIOBLASTOMA MULTIFORME

Glioblastoma multiforme differs from anaplastic astrocytoma by the presence of tumor necrosis on microscopy. At least 2 genetic pathways have been documented in its development: de novo (primary) glioblastomas and secondary glioblastomas. De novo glioblastomas are more common. De novo GBM develops in patients in their sixties or seventies and demonstrates a high rate of epidermal growth factor receptor (EGFR) overexpression, chromosome 10 (*PTEN*) mutations, and *p16INK4A* deletions. In contrast, secondary GBM develops in younger patients and develops from a malignant transformation of a previously diagnosed lower grade tumor. *TP53* and retinoblastoma gene (*RB*) mutations are more common in the development of secondary glioblastomas.

GLIOBLASTOMA MULTIFORME (CASE ONE)

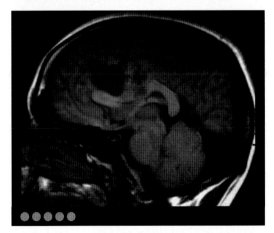

B1. Sagittal T1-weighted image shows a large, heterogeneous multicystic mass involving the corpus callosum.

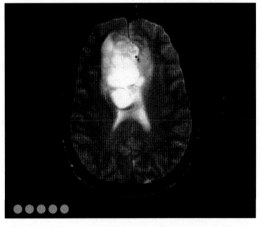

B2. Axial T2-weighted image demonstrates a large hyperintense mass with surrounding edema.

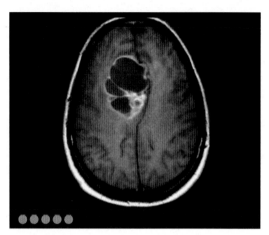

B3. Axial, post-contrast T1-weighted image reveals heterogeneous enhancement of the mass.

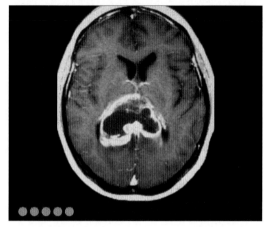

C. Axial, post-contrast T1-weighted image shows a butterfly-like mass with necrotic center and peripheral rim enhancement.

GLIOMATOSIS

Gliomatosis cerebri is a diffuse, frequently bilateral, glial neoplasm which infiltrates the brain parenchyma, and usually involves more than two lobes in the cerebrum. It may extend to the posterior fossa to involve the cerebellum and even the spinal cord. According to the current WHO classification of brain tumors, gliomatosis cerebri is a distinct malignant neuroepithelial neoplasm of uncertain origin. The tumor tends to infiltrate the white diffusely and may have a multifocal appearance on MR imaging.

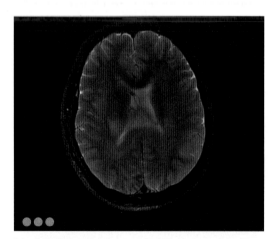

D1. Axial T2-weighted and FLAIR images show ill-defined hyperintense lesions in both corona radiate extending into the corpus callosum.

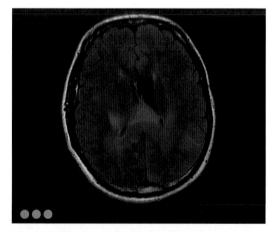

D2. Axial T2-weighted and FLAIR images show ill-defined hyperintense lesions in both corona radiate extending into the corpus callosum.

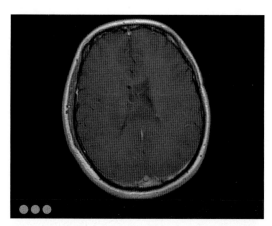

D3. Axial, post-contrast T1-weighted image reveals no abnormal contrast enhancement.

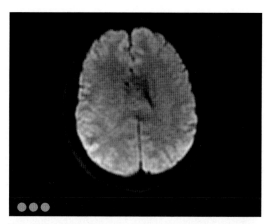

D4. Diffusion-weighted image demonstrates no evidence of restricted diffusion in the lesion, indicating it is a relatively benign lesion.

LYMPHOMA

Primary lymphomas of the central nervous system are rare aggressive neoplasms, accounting for less than 2% of malignant primary brain tumors. They are almost always of the B-cell non-Hodgkin's type. Common locations include the corpus callosum, deep gray matter structures, and the periventricular region. Lymphomas usually show less peritumoral edema than GBM, are more commonly multifocal.

They are less likely to be necrotic, are highly radiosensitive. There is a high tendency of necrosis of lymphomas that occur in immunocompromised patients as compared to immunocompetent patients. Lymphomas may temporarily respond dramatically to steroid treatment producing "vanishing tumors". They are usually iso- or hypointense on T1-weighted images and iso- to slightly hyperintense on T2-weighted images. Contrast enhancement is usually present.

LYMPHOMA (CASE ONE)

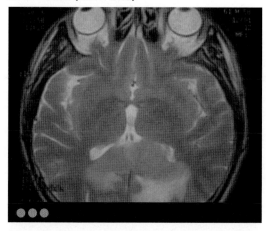

E1. Axial T2-weighted image shows a hyperintense mass crossing the splenium of the corpus callosum with surrounding edema.

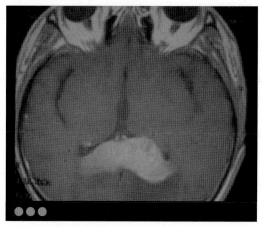

E2. Axial, post-contrast T1-weighted image shows an enhancing mass crossing the corpus callosum.

LYMPHOMA (CASE TWO)

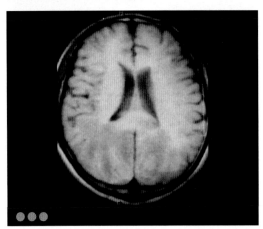

F1. Axial T1-weighted image shows a focal mass in the region of splenium of corpus callosum.

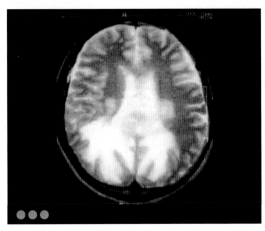

F2. Axial T2-weighted image reveals a mass in the corpus callosum with edema seen bilaterally in both parietooccipital regions.

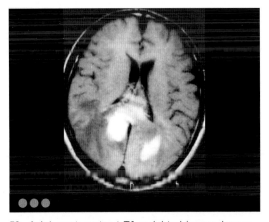

F3. Axial, post-contrast T1-weighted image demonstrates enhancing mass lesions involving the corpus callosum as well as parietooccipital region bilaterally.

DIFFUSE AXONAL INJURY

Diffuse axonal injury (DAI) is a frequent result of traumatic deceleration injuries and a frequent cause of persistent vegetative state in patients. DAI is the most significant cause of morbidity in patients with traumatic brain injuries, which most commonly result from high-speed motor vehicle accidents. Sudden acceleration–deceleration impact can produce rotational forces that can cause injury to the brain. The injury causes the greatest damage in those areas where the density difference is the greatest, namely at the gray–white matter junction. Corpus callosum is also frequently involved.

Traumatic injury to the brain with resultant shearing injury of the corpus callosum can exhibit as focal hemorrhage or edema within the splenium of the corpus callosum.

DIFFUSE AXONAL INJURY (CASE ONE)

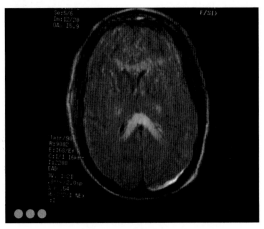

G. Axial T2-weighted FLAIR image reveals hyperintensity in the splenium of the corpus callosum.

DIFFUSE AXONAL INJURY (CASE TWO)

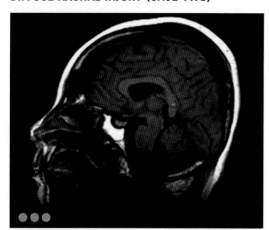

H1. Sagittal T1-weighted image shows a focal hyper-intensity in the splenium of the corpus callosum.

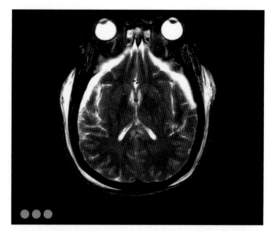

H2. Axial T2-weighted and FLAIR images reveal hyperintensity in the splenium of corpus callosum.

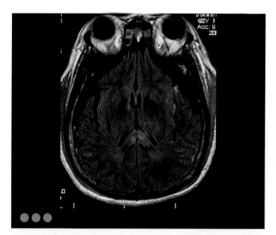

H3. Axial T2-weighted and FLAIR images reveal hyperintensity in the splenium of corpus callosum.

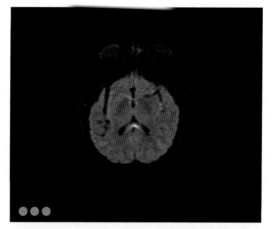

H4. Diffusion-weighted image shows restricted diffusion in the splenium of corpus callosum.

FOCAL HYPERINTENSITY IN SPLENIUM (IN A PATIENT WITH SEIZURE)

It is important to be aware that a reversible focal lesion in the splenium of corpus callosum may occur in patients with epilepsy, particularly those receiving antiepileptic medication, such as dilatin and vigabatrin , because it may help avoid unnecessary diagnostic and therapeutic intervention.

A discrete, focal, ovoid, nonhemorrhagic **hyperintense lesion in the splenium** of the corpus callosum may be seen on T2-weighted images of patients with epilepsy. The lesion is considered to be reversible demyelination related to antiepilepsy drug toxicity or transient edema caused by generalized seizure. Some lesions exhibited restricted diffusion, which is also reversible.

FOCAL HYPERINTENSITY IN SPLENIUM (IN A PATIENT WITH SEIZURE) (CASE ONE)

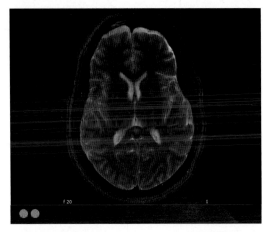

I1. Axial T2-weighted and coronal FLAIR images show a focal hyperintense lesion in the region of splenium of corpus callosum.

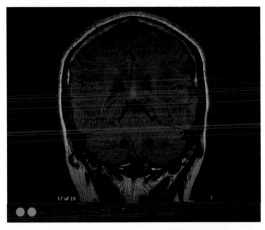

I2. Axial T2-weighted and coronal FLAIR images show a focal hyperintense lesion in the region of splenium of corpus callosum.

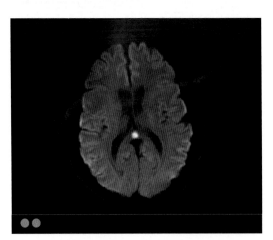

I3. Diffusion-weighted image shows focal area of restricted diffusion in the selenium of the corpus callosum.

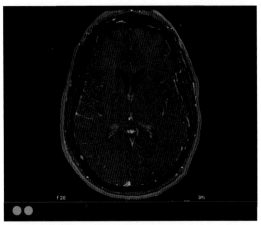

I4. Axial, post-contrast T1-weighted, fat-suppressed image shows no evidence of abnormal enhancement.

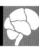

FOCAL HYPERINTENSITY IN SPLENIUM (IN A PATIENT WITH SEIZURE) (CASE TWO)

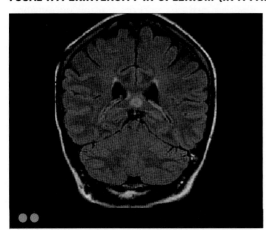

J1. Coronal T2-weighted FLAIR image shows a hyperintense lesion in the splenium of the corpus callosum in a patient with seizure disorder.

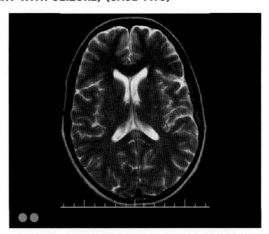

J2. Axial T2-weighted image shows a hyperintense lesion.

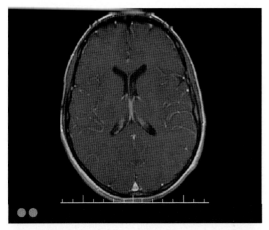

J3. Axial, post-contrast T1-weighted image shows no abnormal contrast enhancement.

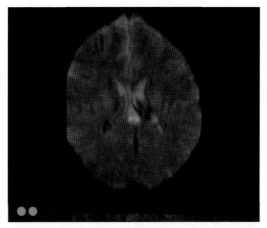

J4. Diffusion-weighted image shows restricted diffusion involving the lesion in the splenium.

INFARCT

Infarcts involving the corpus callosum are uncommon, because it is a dense white matter tract and therefore is less sensitive to ischemic insults than gray matter. The anterior and posterior cerebral arteries provide the major blood supply of the corpus callosum via the anterior and posterior pericallosal arteries and their small penetrating branches. On MR imaging, infarcts have the same imaging features as strokes elsewhere. Diffusion weighted images are critical in the early detection of acute infarcts.

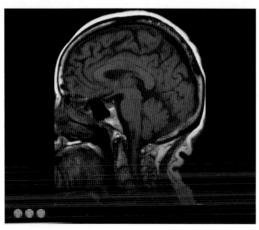

K1. Sagittal T1-weighted image shows slight hypointensity involving the body of corpus callosum.

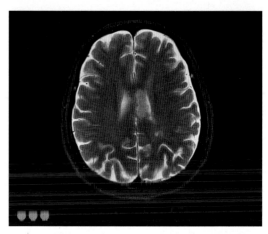

K2. Axial T2-weighted and FLAIR images show an ovoid hyperintense area in the body of corpus callosum.

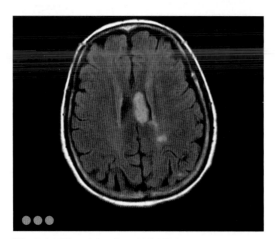

K3. Axial T2-weighted and FLAIR images show an ovoid hyperintense area in the body of corpus callosum.

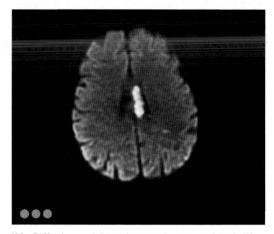

K4. Diffusion-weighted image shows restricted diffusion of the lesion, consistent with an acute infarct.

MULTIPLE SCLEROSIS

Multiple sclerosis (MS) is a demyelinating disease that has a tendency to affect young women. Lesions of MS characteristically involve the periventricular white matter, internal capsule, corpus callosum, and pons, although MS plaques can be found anywhere in the white matter and even in gray matter abnormalities have been documented. The plaques involving the corpus callosum can be focal or confluent nodular lesions and have a tendency to affect the callosal–septal interface. On MR imaging, the prevalence of plaquess in the corpus callosum has been reported to be up to 93% in the literature. Long-standing multiple sclerosis may result in atrophy of the brain as well as atrophy of the corpus callosum. The lesions are hyperintense on T2 weighted and T2 weighted fluid-attenuated inversion recovery (FLAIR) sequences. Contrast enhancement may be seen in acute lesions. Some lesions (acute) show evidence of restricted diffusion with low Apparent Diffusion Coefficient (ADC) values whereas others (chronic) do not show restricted diffusion.

MULTIPLE SCLEROSIS (CASE ONE)

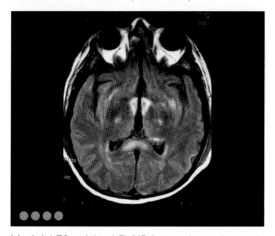

L1. Axial T2-weighted FLAIR image shows abnormal hyperintense lesions in the splenium of the corpus callosum as well as in the hypothalamus.

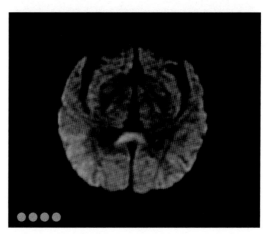

L2. Diffusion-weighted image shows evidence of restricted diffusion in the splenium of the corpus callosum.

MULTIPLE SCLEROSIS (CASE TWO)

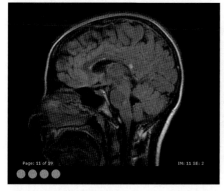

M1. Sagittal T2-weighted and FLAIR images show a focal hyperintense lesion in the splenium of corpus callosum.

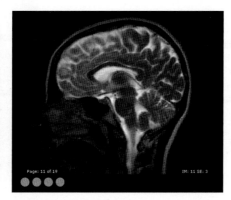

M2. Sagittal T2-weighted and FLAIR images show a focal hyperintense lesion in the splenium of corpus callosum.

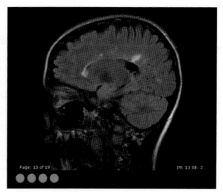

M3. Parasagittal T2-weighted FLAIR images show multiple lesions in the periventricular white matter.

PROGRESSIVE MULTIFOCAL LEUKOENCEPHALOPATHY (PML)

PML occurs in immuno-compromised patients and is caused by JC papovavirus. It is a rapidly progressive disease that can be fatal. The virus affects the myelin sheath of the oligodendrocytes, thus involving white matter of the brain and spine. The lesions are often multifocal and asymmetric, most commonly involving the subcortical white matter and corpus callosum. In the corpus callosum, small, focal lesions can enlarge and coalesce, resulting in a confluent lesions as the disease progresses. They are usually hypointense on T1 weighted images and hyperintense on T2 weighted images. They usually do not show contrast enhancement, although some lesions may enhance faintly at the periphery, especially in patients under treatment with improved immunity.

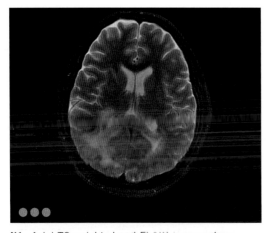

N1. Axial T2-weighted and FLAIR images show hyperintense lesion crossing the corpus callosum extending into parietal white matter bilaterally.

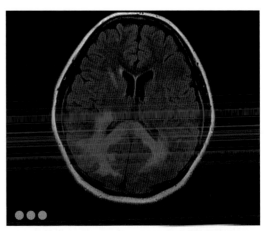

N2. Axial T2-weighted and FLAIR images show hyperintense lesion crossing the corpus callosum extending into parietal white matter bilaterally.

AGENESIS OF THE CORPUS CALLOSUM

Agenesis of the corpus callosum is an anomaly that may occur in isolation or in association with other central nervous system or systemic malformations. Because the corpus callosum may be partially or completely absent, the term dysgenesis has also been used to describe the spectrum of callosal anomalies. Dysgenesis of the corpus callosum is usually a sporadic event, although there are reports that their incidence is increased in patients with trisomy 18, trisomy 13, and trisomy 8. Fibers of the corpus callosum arise from the superficial layers of the cerebral cortex; they project to the homotypic region of the contralateral cerebral cortex by passing through the corpus callosum, which crosses the midline. Disturbance of embryogenesis in the first trimester of gestation by various insults lead to failure of the formation of callosal axons across the midline. These arrested fibers form the longitudinally oriented bundles of Probst that are situated medial to the lateral ventricles in patients with callosal agenesis.

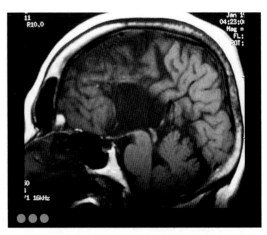

O. Sagittal T1-weighted image shows absence of the corpus callosum with dysplastic cingulated gyrus.

198

LIPOMA OF THE CORPUS CALLOSUM

Lipomas are rare developmental lesions of the central nervous system, which are usually asymptomatic and found incidentally. Their common locations are in the region of the corpus callosum and the pericallosal cistern, consisting of up to 65% of all intracranial lipomas. Callosal dysgenesis is frequently associated with lipoma of the corpus callosum. On MR imaging, they show characteristic hyperintensity on both T1 and T2 weighted sequences. The hyperintensity associated with fat is suppressed with fat-suppression technique.

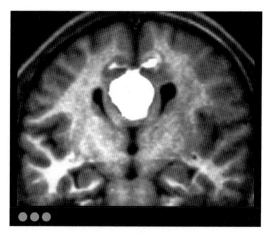

P. Coronal T1-weighted image shows a hyperintense lipoma in the region of the corpus callosum associated with agenesis of the corpus callosum.

PERICALLOSAL LIPOMA

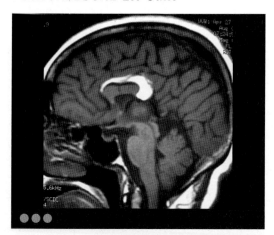

Q1. Sagittal and coronal T1-weighted images demonstrate a hyperintense mass in the region of corpus callosum associated with partial agenesis of the corpus callosum.

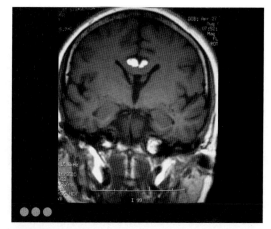

Q2. Sagittal and coronal T1-weighted images demonstrate a hyperintense mass in the region of corpus callosum associated with partial agenesis of the corpus callosum.

4-9 Cystic Mass with an Enhancing Mural Nodule

HEMANGIOBLASTOMA

Hemangioblastomas are rare and they account for 1–2.5% of all intracranial neoplasms. The peak age of presentation is 30–40 years. They can be associated with Von Hippel Lindau syndrome and the patients are usually younger. They are most commonly seen in the cerebellum, but can be found in the medulla and spinal cord. Approximately 60% are cystic and 40% are solid masses. Cyst fluid may contain erythropoietin and cause erythrocythemia in patients. About half of the cystic lesions consist of a thin wall cyst with an eccentrically located mural nodule and the other half are masses with cystic areas seen within it.

VHL is characterized by a predisposition to bilateral and multicentric retinal angiomas, central nervous system hemangioblastomas; renal cell carcinomas; pheochromocytomas; islet cell tumors of the pancreas; endolymphatic sac tumors; and renal, pancreatic, and epididymal cysts. Central nervous system hemangioblastoma (Lindau tumor) is the most commonly recognized manifestation of VHL and occurs in 40% of patients. They are seen in cerebellum (65%), medulla oblongata (20%), and spinal cord (15%). Supratentorial hemangioblastomas are very rare. Multiple hemangioblastomas are seen in 10–15% of the cases. Endolymphatic sac tumors are very rare in the general population. In people with von Hippel Lindau syndrome, they are seen in 11–16% of the cases on imaging studies.

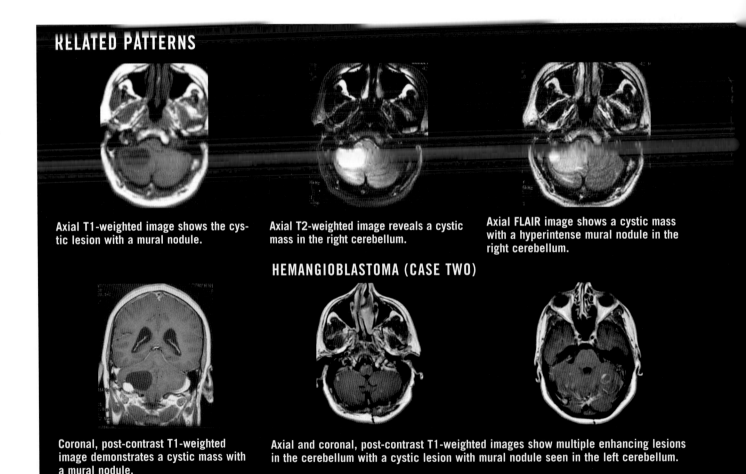

RELATED PATTERNS

Axial T1-weighted image shows the cystic lesion with a mural nodule.

Axial T2-weighted image reveals a cystic mass in the right cerebellum.

Axial FLAIR image shows a cystic mass with a hyperintense mural nodule in the right cerebellum.

HEMANGIOBLASTOMA (CASE TWO)

Coronal, post-contrast T1-weighted image demonstrates a cystic mass with a mural nodule.

Axial and coronal, post-contrast T1-weighted images show multiple enhancing lesions in the cerebellum with a cystic lesion with mural nodule seen in the left cerebellum.

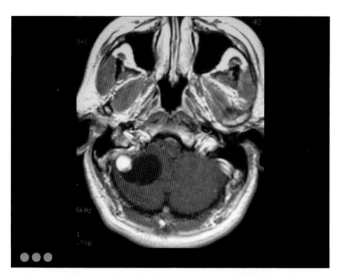

A. Axial, post-contrast T1-weighted image shows a cystic mass with an enhancing mural nodule seen in the right cerebellum. Note the enhancing mural nodule is located at the pial surface of the cerebellum

HEMAGNGIOBLASTOMA (CASE TWO)-CONTINUED

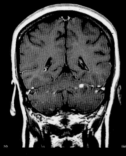

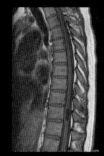

Axial and coronal, post-contrast T1-weighted images show multiple enhancing lesions in the cerebellum with a cystic lesion with mural nodule seen in the left cerebellum.

Sagittal T1-weighted, T2-weighted and post-contrast T1-weighted with fat-suppression images show a cystic lesion with enhancing mural nodule in the lower thoracic cord.

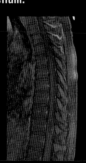

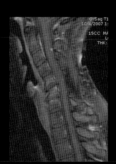

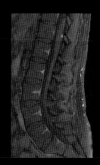

Sagittal T1-weighted, T2-weighted and post-contrast T1-weighted with fat-suppression images show a cystic lesion with enhancing mural nodule in the lower thoracic cord.

Sagittal, post-contrast T1-weighted images demonstrate a nodular enhancing lesion on the surface of the cord at C3 level.

Sagittal, post-contrast T1-weighted images demonstrate a nodular enhancing lesion on the surface of the cord at T12 level.

DIFFERENTIAL DIAGNOSIS

At a Glance:

- *Metastatic Disease (Adenocarcinoma)*
- *Pilocytic Astrocytoma*

METASTATIC DISEASE (ADENOCARCINOMA)

Metastatic disease is more commonly seen in the supratentorial compartment; infratentorial metastatic disease is less common. However, a single lesion in the cerebellum in a patient over 50 years of age, the most likely diagnosis is metastatic disease. The detection of cerebellar metasta-tic disease is critical because neurosurgical removal of the solitary lesion is considered as the treatment of choice. When a cystic lesion with a mural nodule is seen in the cerebellum, the differential diagnosis includes juvenile pilocytic astrocytoma (in children and young adults), hemangioblastoma (in patients 30–40 years of age) and metastatic disease (in patients older than 50 years).

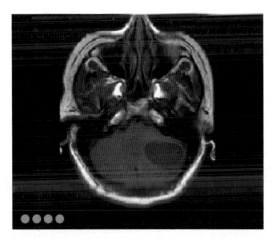

B1. Axial T1-weighted image shows a cystic lesion in the left cerebellum.

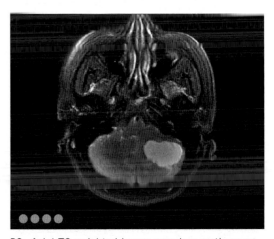

B2. Axial T2-weighted image reveals a cystic mass in the left cerebellum.

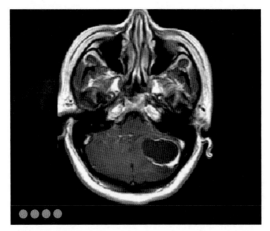

B3. Axial, post-contrast T1-weighted image demonstrates a cystic mass with irregular, partial enhancement in the cyst wall.

PILOCYTIC ASTROCYTOMA

Cerebellar juvenile **pilocytic astrocytomas** are classified as WHO grade 1 astrocytoma. The majority of cerebellar astrocytomas are of the pilocytic variety (85%) and they occur within the first decade of life. Cerebellar pilocytic astrocytomas are well-circumscribed cystic masses with a small mural nodule. Cyst walls usually do not enhance and merely represent compressed brain tissue.

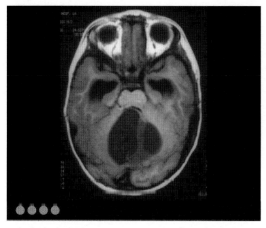

C1. Axial T1-weighted image reveals a cystic mass with an internal septum.

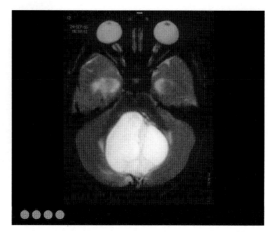

C2. Axial T2-weighted image shows a cystic mass with an internal septum.

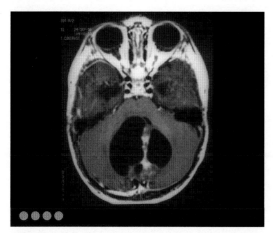

C3. Axial, post-contrast T1-weighted image shows a large cystic mass with an enhancing internal septum.

EPENDYMOMA

Ependymomas constitute 2–6% of all gliomas. About 60% of intracranial ependymomas occur in the infratentorial compartment. Ependymomas are 4–6 times more common in children than in adults. MRI shows a heterogeneous mass lesion that is hypointense on T1-weighted images and hyperintense on T2-weighted images with dense punctate calcification, areas of necrosis or cystic changes. Hemorrhage may also be seen. Contrast enhancement is variable, from heterogeneous to homogeneous.

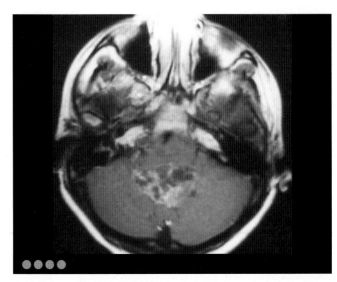

A. Axial, post-contrast T1-weighted image shows a heterogeneously enhancing mass with multiple small cystic areas within the mass seen in the fourth ventricle.

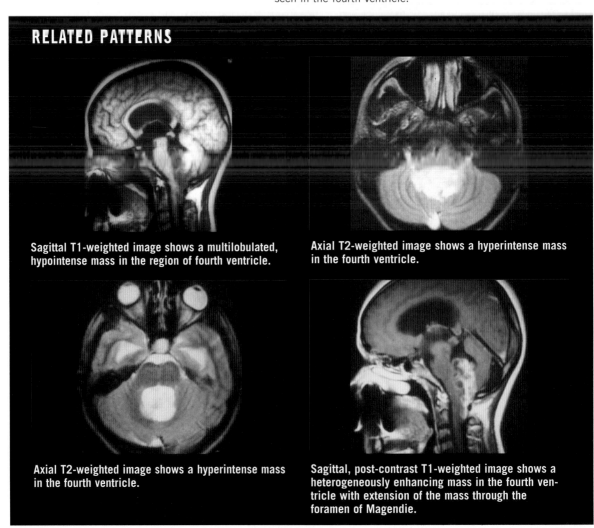

RELATED PATTERNS

Sagittal T1-weighted image shows a multilobulated, hypointense mass in the region of fourth ventricle.

Axial T2-weighted image shows a hyperintense mass in the fourth ventricle.

Axial T2-weighted image shows a hyperintense mass in the fourth ventricle.

Sagittal, post-contrast T1-weighted image shows a heterogeneously enhancing mass in the fourth ventricle with extension of the mass through the foramen of Magendie.

DIFFERENTIAL DIAGNOSIS

At a Glance:

- *Glioblastoma Multiforme*
- *Hemorrhagic PNET*
- *Anaplastic Astrocytoma* (not pictured)
- *Metastatic Disease* (not pictured)

GLIOBLASTOMA MULTIFORME

Approximately 70% of the posterior fossa glioblastoma multiforme are seen in adults whereas 30% of the tumors are seen in children. Approximately 80% of the tumors occur in the lateral aspect of the cerebellum and the remaining 20% are seen near the midline.

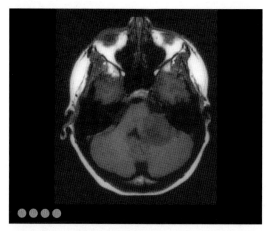

B1. Axial T1 weighted image shows a mixed, hypo- to isointense lesion in the region of left brachium pontis.

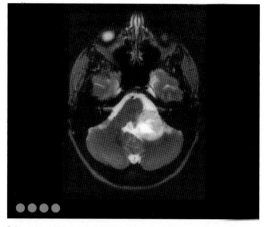

B2. Axial T2-weighted image reveals a heterogeneously hyperintense lesion.

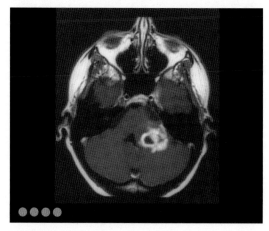

B3. Axial, post-contrast T1-weighted image shows a heterogeneously enhancing mass in the left brachium pontis.

HEMORRHAGIC PNET

PNETs represent a variety of tumors that include medulloblastomas, neuroblastomas, pineoblastomas, and retinoblastomas. PNETs are the most common primary malignant brain tumors in children, consisting of approximately 30 percent of all brain tumors in children. They are thought to arise from primitive (undifferentiated) nerve cells left over from the gestational development of the nervous system. Because the tumors are malignant, they tend to spread easily through the cerebrospinal fluid (CSF) pathway. Up to 30% of the medulloblastomas are found to have metastatic seeding into the subarachnoid space at the time of initial diagnosis.

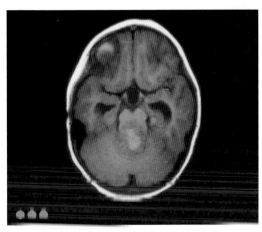

C1. Axial T1-weighted image shows a heterogeneous, mixed iso- and hyperintense mass in the region of vermis. Note the presence of obstructive hydrocephalus.

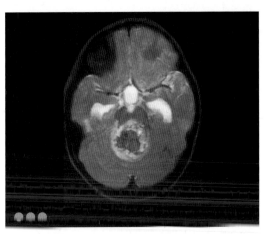

C2. Axial T2-weighted image shows a heterogeneous mass with hypointense center and hyperintense periphery.

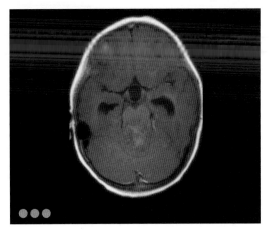

C3. Axial and sagittal, post-contrast T1-weighted images show a faintly enhancing mass in the region of vermis.

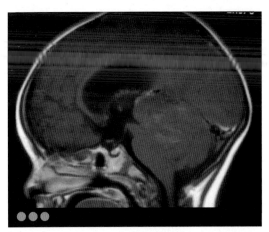

C4. Axial and sagittal, post-contrast T1-weighted images show a faintly enhancing mass in the region of vermis.

HEMANGIOBLASTOMA

Hemangioblastoma represents approximately 8–12% of all posterior fossa primary neoplasms. The peak age of presentation is 30–40 years. They can be associated with Von Hippel Lindau syndrome and the patients are usually younger. They are most commonly seen in the cerebellum, but can be found in the medulla and spinal cord. Approximately 60% are cystic and 40% are solid masses.

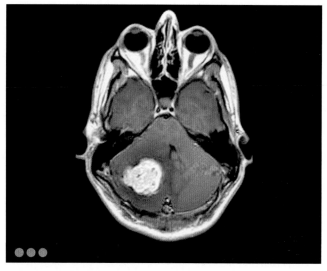

A. Axial, postcontrast T1-weighted image shows an enhancing mass in the right cerebellum with mild surrounding edema.

RELATED PATTERNS

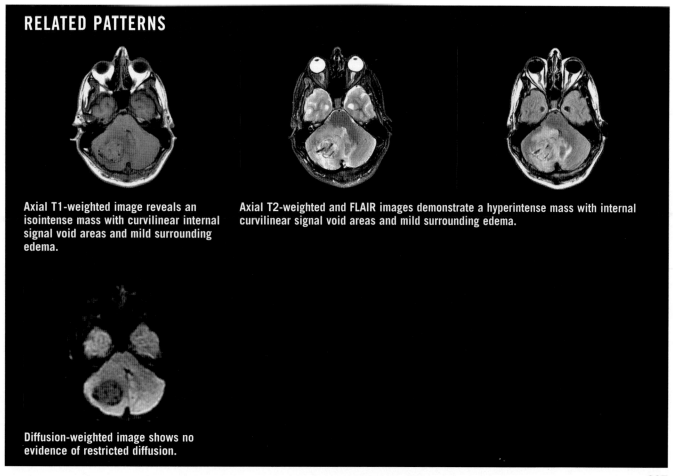

Axial T1-weighted image reveals an isointense mass with curvilinear internal signal void areas and mild surrounding edema.

Axial T2-weighted and FLAIR images demonstrate a hyperintense mass with internal curvilinear signal void areas and mild surrounding edema.

Diffusion-weighted image shows no evidence of restricted diffusion.

ATYPICAL TERATOID/RHABDOID TUMOR (AT/RT)

Atypical teratoid/rhabdoid tumor is a rare tumor of the central nervous system. They are very aggressive tumor seen in very young children, usually less than 3 years of age and quite rarely, in older children and young adults. Due to the rarity and rapidly growing nature of this tumor, it is very important to differentiate this tumor from primitive neuroectodermal tumors.

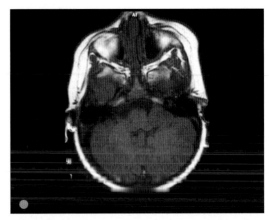

B1. Axial T1-weighted image shows an isointense mass at the left middle cerebellar peduncle.

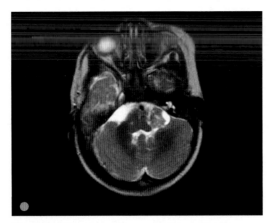

B2. Axial T2-weighted image reveals a slightly hyperintense mass at the left middle cerebellar peduncle.

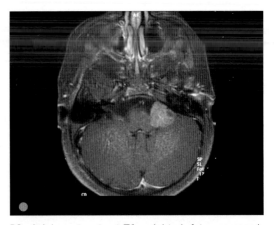

B3. Axial, postcontrast T1-weighted, fat-suppressed image demonstrates slightly heterogeneous enhancement of the mass lesion.

LYMPHOMA

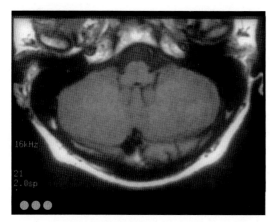

C1. Axial T1-weighted image shows a hypointense lesion in the left cerebellum.

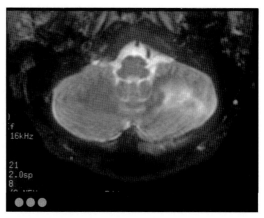

C2. Axial T2-weighted image reveals a hyperintense lesion in the left cerebellum.

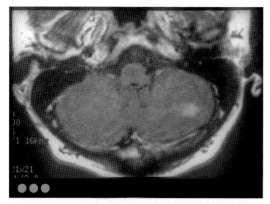

C3. Axial, post-contrast T1-weighted image demonstrates a faintly enhancing mass in the left cerebellum.

METASTASIS

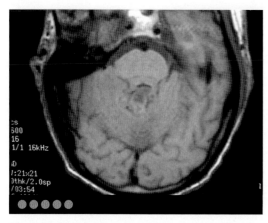

D1. Axial T1-weighted image shows mixed signal intensity mass in the region of vermis extending into the right cerebellum.

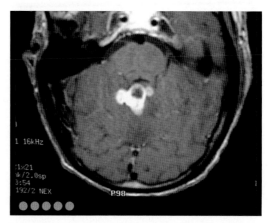

D2. Axial, post-contrast T1-weighted image shows an enhancing mass in the region of vermis extending into the right cerebellum.

PNET (MEDULLOBLASTOMA)

The **medulloblastoma** originates from poorly differentiated germinative cells of the roof of the fourth ventricle that migrate superiorly and laterally to the external granular layer of the cerebellar hemisphere. The medulloblastoma can occur anywhere along the path of migration. Midline vermian medulloblastomas are seen in children whereas laterally situated medulloblastomas are seen in young adults. Up to 30% of the cases exhibit seeding of the neoplasm into the CSF pathway, more commonly in the spine than brain, at the time of initial diagnosis.

PNET (CASE ONE)

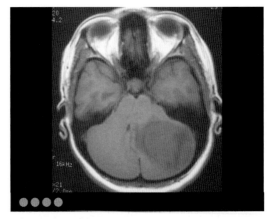

E1. Axial T1-weighted image shows a hypointense mass with focal cystic changes in the left cerebellum.

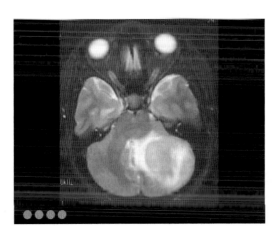

E2. Axial T2-weighted image reveals a slightly hyperintense mass with cystic changes and surrounding edema in the left cerebellum.

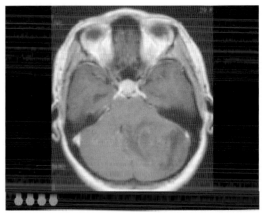

E3. Axial, coronal, sagittal, post-contrast T1-weighted images demonstrate a hypointense mass with faint, patchy enhancement.

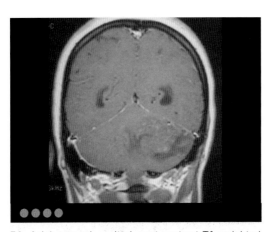

E4. Axial, coronal, sagittal, post-contrast T1-weighted images demonstrate a hypointense mass with faint, patchy enhancement.

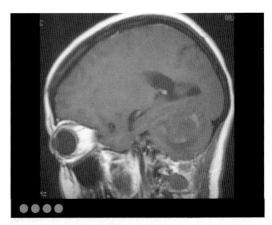

E5. Axial, coronal, sagittal, post-contrast T1-weighted images demonstrate a hypointense mass with faint, patchy enhancement.

PNET (CASE TWO)

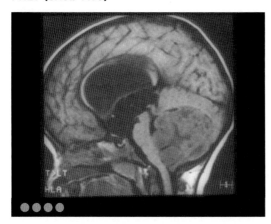

F1. Sagittal and axial T1-weighted images show a slightly hypointense lesion in the region of vermis.

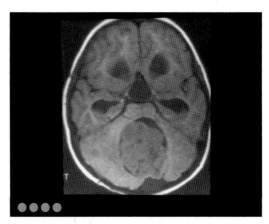

F2. Sagittal and axial T1-weighted images show a slightly hypointense lesion in the region of vermis.

PNET (CASE THREE)

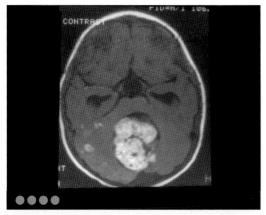

F3. Axial, post-contrast T1-weighted image demonstrates an intensely enhancing mass with some heterogeneity.

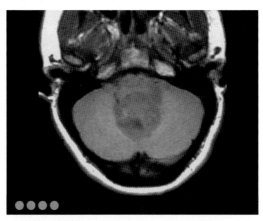

G1. Axial T1-weighted image shows a slightly hypointense mass in the vermis with compression of the fourth ventricle. Note the presence of small cystic areas within the mass.

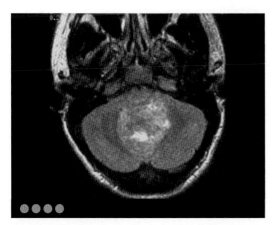

G2. Axial T2-weighted image reveals a slightly hyperintense mass with cystic changes in the vermis.

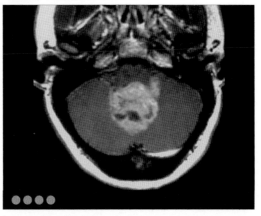

G3. Axial, post-contrast T1-weighted image demonstrates avid enhancement of the mass with small cystic areas.

PNET (CASE FOUR)

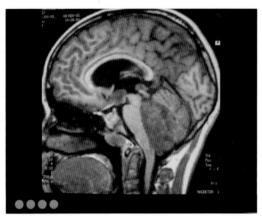

H1. Sagittal and axial T1-weighted images show a slightly heterogeneous, hypointense mass in the region of vermis with compression of the fourth ventricle.

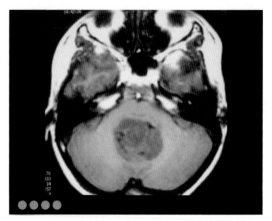

H2. Sagittal and axial T1-weighted images show a slightly heterogeneous, hypointense mass in the region of vermis with compression of the fourth ventricle.

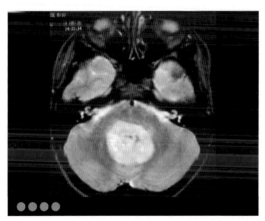

H3. Axial T2-weighted image reveals a slightly heterogeneous, hyperintense mass.

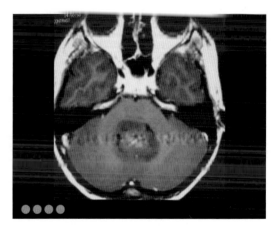

H4. Axial and coronal, post-contrast T1-weighted images demonstrate a heterogeneously enhancing mass in the vermis.

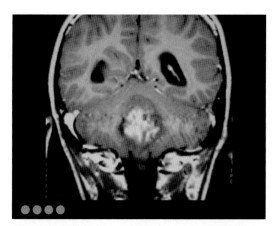

H5. Axial and coronal, post-contrast T1-weighted images demonstrate a heterogeneously enhancing mass in the vermis.

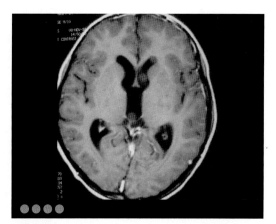

H6. Axial and coronal, post-contrast T1-weighted images show multiple nodular lesions in the lateral and third ventricles, consistent with seeding of PNET.

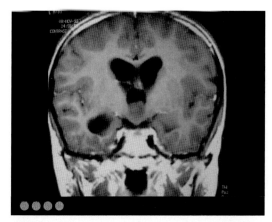

H7. Axial and coronal, post-contrast T1-weighted images show multiple nodular lesions in the lateral and third ventricles, consistent with seeding of PNET.

ABSCESS

The most distinctive feature of abscess on imaging is the presence of a smooth, thin capsule with a moderate amount of cerebral edema. It is located at the corticomedullary junction and usually extends into the white matter. The abscess cavity has necrosis and liquefaction within its center. The abscess capsule enhances with intravenous administration of contrast material on MRI studies. The presence of satellite lesions is a unique feature of cerebral abscess. On diffusion-weighted images, the pus within the abscess cavity characteristically shows restricted diffusion.

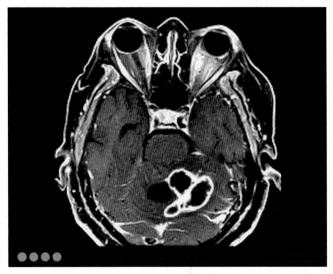

A. Axial, post-contrast T1-weighted, fat-suppressed image shows a left cerebellar lesion with multiring-like enhancement.

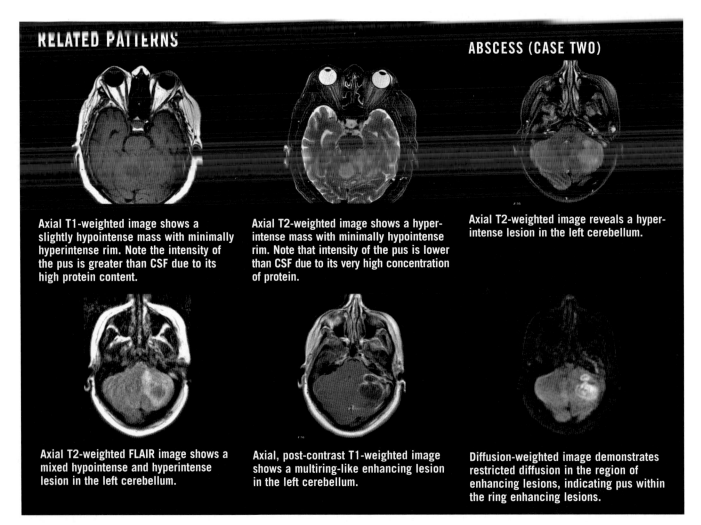

RELATED PATTERNS

ABSCESS (CASE TWO)

Axial T1-weighted image shows a slightly hypointense mass with minimally hyperintense rim. Note the intensity of the pus is greater than CSF due to its high protein content.

Axial T2-weighted image shows a hyperintense mass with minimally hypointense rim. Note that intensity of the pus is lower than CSF due to its very high concentration of protein.

Axial T2-weighted image reveals a hyperintense lesion in the left cerebellum.

Axial T2-weighted FLAIR image shows a mixed hypointense and hyperintense lesion in the left cerebellum.

Axial, post-contrast T1-weighted image shows a multiring-like enhancing lesion in the left cerebellum.

Diffusion-weighted image demonstrates restricted diffusion in the region of enhancing lesions, indicating pus within the ring enhancing lesions.

DIFFERENTIAL DIAGNOSIS

At a Glance:

- *Hemangioblastoma*
- *Metastatic Melanoma*
- *Toxoplasmosis*
- *Astrocytoma* (not pictured)
- *Cysticercosis* (not pictured)
- *Multiple Sclerosis* (not pictured)
- *Tuberculoma* (not pictured)

HEMANGIOBLASTOMA

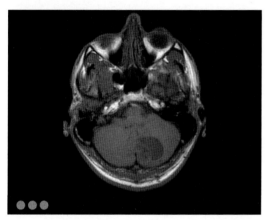

B1. Axial T1-weighted image shows a cystic mass with isointense mural nodule in the left cerebellum.

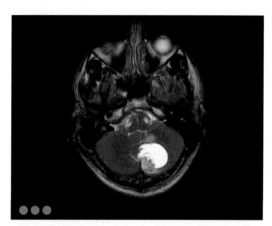

B2. Axial T2-weighted image shows a cystic mass with a mural nodule in the left cerebellum.

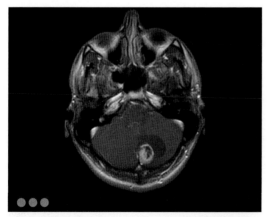

B3. Axial and coronal, post-contrast T1-weighted images demonstrate a cystic mass with an enhancing mural nodule. Note the mural nodule has necrotic center and shows ring-like enhancement.

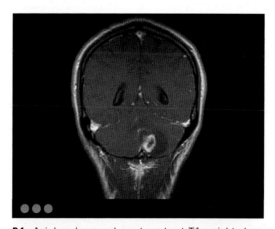

B4. Axial and coronal, post-contrast T1-weighted images demonstrate a cystic mass with an enhancing mural nodule. Note the mural nodule has necrotic center and shows ring-like enhancement.

METASTATIC MELANOMA

METASTATIC MELANOMA (CASE ONE)

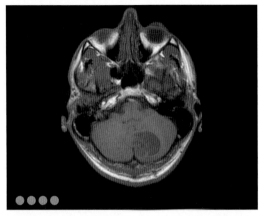

C1. Axial T1-weighted image shows a hypointense lesion in the right cerebellum

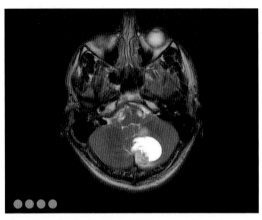

C2. Axial T2-weighted FLAIR image demonstrates hyperintense edema with a central cystic area in the right cerebellum.

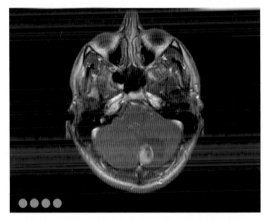

C3. Axial, post-contrast T1-weighted image reveals a ring-like enhancing lesion in the right cerebellum.

METASTASIS (CASE TWO)

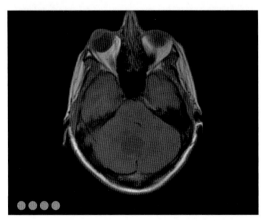

D1. Axial T1-weighted image shows a hypointense lesion just posterior to fourth ventricle.

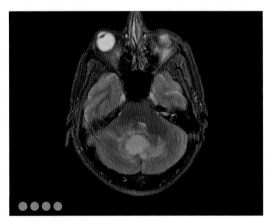

D2. Axial T2-weighted and FLAIR images show a hyperintense lesion in the region of vermis with surrounding edema.

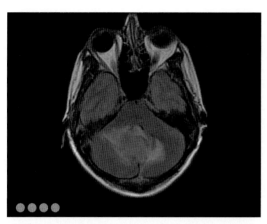

D3. Axial T2-weighted and FLAIR images show a hyperintense lesion in the region of vermis with surrounding edema.

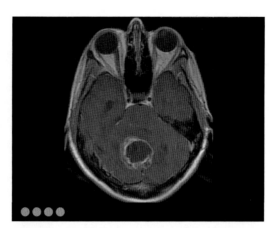

D4. Axial, post-contrast T1-weighted image demonstrates a ring-like enhancing lesion in the cerebellar vermis, jsut behind the fourth ventricle.

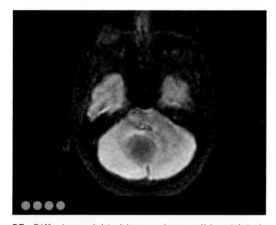

D5. Diffusion-weighted image shows mild restricted diffusion in the wall of the cystic lesion. Note the center of the lesion does not show restricted diffusion (in contrast to abscess).

TOXOPLASMOSIS

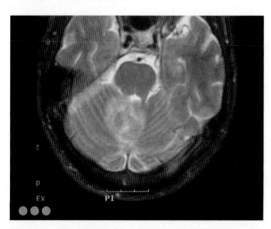

E1. Axial T2-weighted image shows a heterogeneously hyperintense mass with edema.

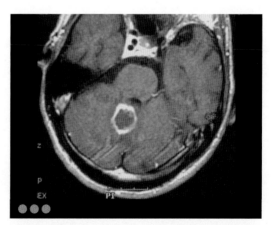

E2. Axial, post-contrast T1-weighted image shows a ring-like enhancing mass with surrounding edema in the left cerebellum.

METASTATIC MELANOMA

Melanoma commonly metastasizes to the brain. About 40–60% of patients with melanoma will develop brain metastasis. Melanoma cells are closely related to cells in the central nervous system due to their embryonic origin, and they share common antigens such as MAG-1 and MAG-2. Approximately 14% of cases have no identifiable primary tumor. Melanoma can also involve the pia, the subarachnoid space, the dura or the skull. The cerebral or cerebellar lesions are usually multiple, but occasionally a solitary lesion may be seen. Melanotic melanomas contain melanin whereas amelanotic melanomas do not have melanin. Melanoma can present as hyperintense lesions on T1-weighted images due to the presence of melanin or hemorrhage, or both, in the tumor.

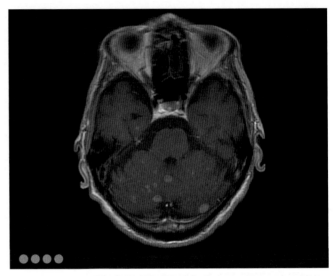

A. Axial, post-contrast T1-weighted image shows multiple small nodular enhancing lesions throughout the cerebellum.

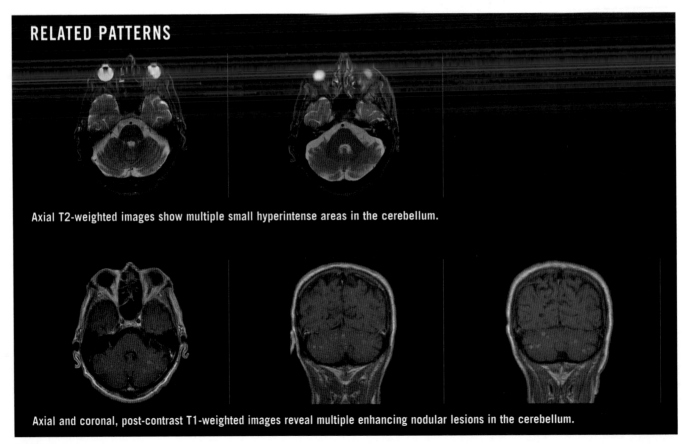

Axial T2-weighted images show multiple small hyperintense areas in the cerebellum.

Axial and coronal, post-contrast T1-weighted images reveal multiple enhancing nodular lesions in the cerebellum.

DIFFERENTIAL DIAGNOSIS

At a Glance:

- *Hemangioblastoma*
- *Other Metastatic Disease* (not pictured)

HEMANGIOBLASTOMA

Hemangioblastoma represents approximately 8–12% of all posterior fossa primary neoplasms. The peak age of presentation is 30–40 years. Most hemangioblastomas arise sporadically. However, in approximately one quarter of all cases, they are associated with von Hippel-Lindau (VHL) disease, an autosomal dominant hereditary syndrome involving chromosome 3 that includes retinal angiomatosis, central nervous system hemangioblastomas, and various visceral tumors involving the kidneys and adrenal glands. In some patients with VHL disease, hemangioblastomas may produce erythropoietin-like substances into their cystic components, causing polycythemia. Patients with von Hippel-Lindau disease are usually younger than those with hemangioblastomas.

HEMANGIOBLASTOMA (CASE ONE)

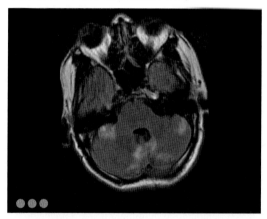

B1. Axial T2-weighted FLAIR image shows multiple hyperintense foci in the cerebellum.

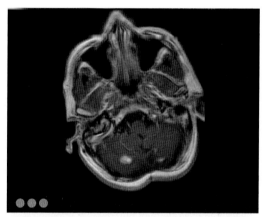

B2. Axial and coronal, post-contrast T1-weighted images demonstrate multiple enhancing nodules in the cerebellum.

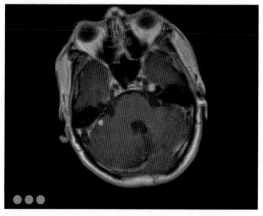

B3. Axial and coronal, post-contrast T1-weighted images demonstrate multiple enhancing nodules in the cerebellum.

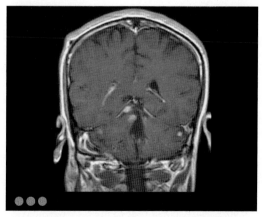

B4. Axial and coronal, post-contrast T1-weighted images demonstrate multiple enhancing nodules in the cerebellum.

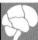

HEMANGIOBLASTOMA (CASE TWO)

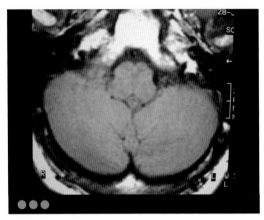

C1. Axial T1-weighted image is unremarkable.

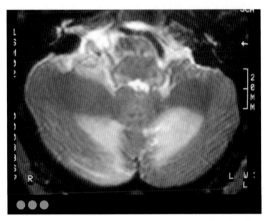

C2. Axial T2-weighted images shows multiple areas of hyperintensity.

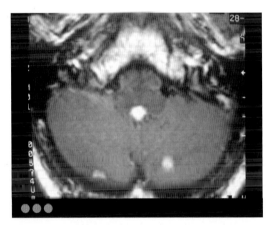

C3. Axial and sagittal, post-contrast T1-weighted images demonstrate multiple, nodular enhancing lesions.

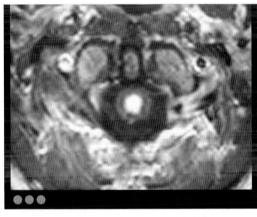

C4. Axial and sagittal, post-contrast T1-weighted images demonstrate multiple, nodular enhancing lesions.

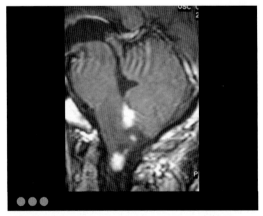

C5. Axial and sagittal, post-contrast T1-weighted images demonstrate multiple, nodular enhancing lesions.

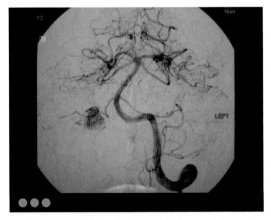

C6. Vertebral angiogram demonstrates multiple hyper-vascular nodules on arterial phase of the angiogram.

BRAINSTEM INFARCT

Brainstem infarct is a devastating ischemic event, usually due to basilar artery thrombosis. It is usually associated with abrupt onset of symptoms such as dizziness, vertigo, diplopia, dysarthria, tingling around the mouth, sudden loss of consiousness, weakness of limbs and blindness. Occlusion of the pontine perforating arteries can result in paramedian pontine infarction. Paramedian pontine infarcts consist of approximately 28% of infarcts of the vertebrobasilar system. Occlusion of the posterior inferior cerebellar artery can cause lateral medullary infarct (Wallenberg syndrome). On MR imaging, infarctions demonstrate hypointensity on T1 weighted images and hyperintenisty on T2 weighted images. The overall mass effect for infarcts is usually less than neoplastic process. The maximum mass effect is seen between 5–7 days after onset. Diffusion weighted images can provide early detection of small infarcts.

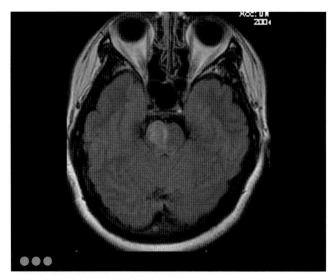

A. Axial T2-weighted FLAIR image shows a focal hyperintensity over the right side of pons.

RELATED PATTERNS

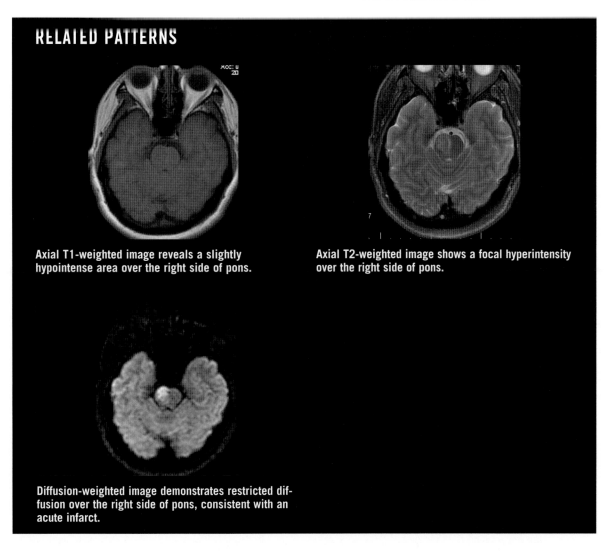

Axial T1-weighted image reveals a slightly hypointense area over the right side of pons.

Axial T2-weighted image shows a focal hyperintensity over the right side of pons.

Diffusion-weighted image demonstrates restricted diffusion over the right side of pons, consistent with an acute infarct.

BEHCET'S SYNDROME

Behcet's syndrome involves the CNS in approximately 5–10% of cases. Behcet's syndrome is classically characterized as a triad of symptoms that include recurring crops of mouth ulcers (aphthous ulcers), genital ulcers, and uveitis. The disease is more prevalent and severe in patients from Asia and the Eastern Mediterranean region. Both inherited (genetic) and environmental factors, such as microbe infections, are suspected to contribute to the development of Behcet's syndrome. Behcet's syndrome is also sometimes referred to as Behcet's disease. Behcet's disease is a multisystemic inflammatory disorder with relapsing courses. There are two main patterns of central nervous system involvement, namely, parenchymal and nonparenchymal. The neuropathology of the parenchymal form is that of multifocal necrotizing lesions with marked inflammatory cell reactions, secondary to vasculitis, mainly with small venule disease.

BEHCET'S SYNDROME (CASE ONE)

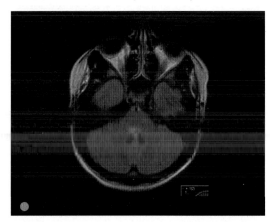

B. Axial T2-weighted FLAIR image shows focal hyperintense lesion in the pons in a patient with Behcet's syndrome.

BEHCET'S SYNDROME (CASE TWO)

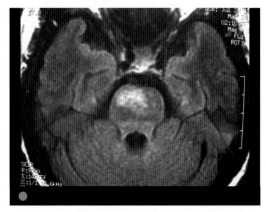

C1. Axial FLAIR image shows hyperintensity involving the pons on the right side.

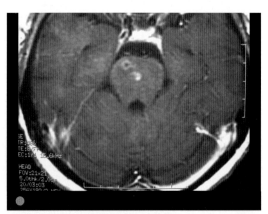

C2. Axial, post-contrast T1-weighted image demonstrates curvilinear and ring-like enhancement involving the right side of the pons.

BRAINSTEM ENCEPHALITIS

Brainstem encephalitis can be caused by a host of viruses or can be a postinfectious demyelinating process. MRI usually shows T1-hypointense and T2-hyperintense lesion in the brainstem. Contrast enhancement may be seen.

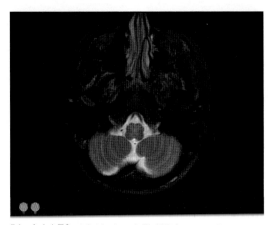

D1. Axial T2-weighted and FLAIR images show abnormal hyperintensity in the region of medulla in a patient with viral encephalitis.

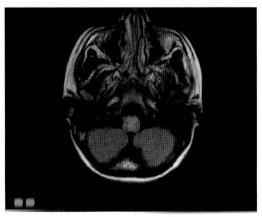

D2. Axial T2-weighted and FLAIR images show abnormal hyperintensity in the region of medulla in a patient with viral encephalitis.

LUPUS ENCEPHALITIS

Systemic lupus erythematosus (SLE) is a multi-system autoimmune disease involving multiple organs with a wide variety of immunological and clinical manifestations. It is featured by an autoantibody response to nuclear and cytoplasmic antigens. The skin, joints, kidneys, blood cells, and nervous system are mainly involved. The neuropsychiatric symptoms vary from overt neurologic and psychiatric disorders to more subtle signs such as headache, mood disorders, and defects in cognitive function. MR imaging is the imaging modality of choice for evaluating SLE patients. Large infarcts, cortical atrophy, and multifocal gray matter and/or white matter lesions can be detected at MR imaging in patients with SLE; the most common finding is the presence of multiple focal lesions in the white matter.

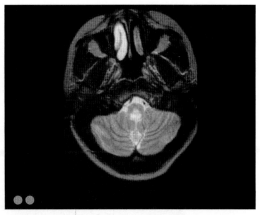

E1. Axial, sagittal and coronal T2-weighted images demonstrate abnormal hyperintensity involving the medulla in a patient with brainstem lupus encephalitis.

223

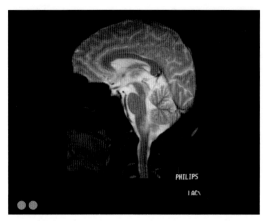

E2. Axial, sagittal and coronal T2-weighted images demonstrate abnormal hyperintensity involving the medulla in a patient with brainstem lupus encephalitis.

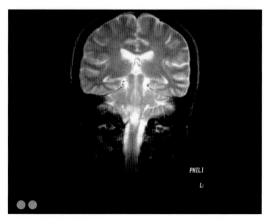

E3. Axial, sagittal and coronal T2-weighted images demonstrate abnormal hyperintensity involving the medulla in a patient with brainstem lupus encephalitis.

SYPHILIS

The incidence of Syphilis has been on the rise along with the incidence of AIDS. The imaging manifestations of neurosyphilis can be broadly classified into meningeal and parenchymal. Meningeal manifestations range from various forms of meningitis and meningoencephalitis to the formation of well circumscribed masses (gumma). Parenchymal manifestations are the results of vasculitis, which may involve large as well as small vessels.

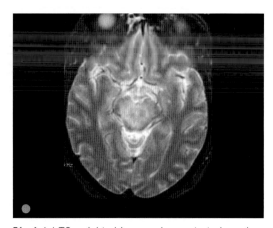

F1. Axial T2-weighted images demonstrate hyperintense lesion involving the brainstem.

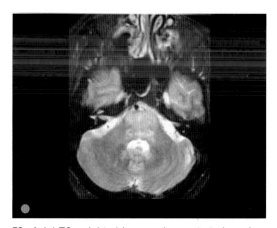

F2. Axial T2-weighted images demonstrate hyperintense lesion involving the brainstem.

TUBERCULOSIS

Mycobacterium tuberculosis has infected humans for thousands of years. Tuberculosis of the central nervous system is a granulomatous infection caused by Mycobac- terium tuberculosis. The disease predominantly involves the brain and meninges resulting in meningitis or tuberculoma, but occasionally it can affect the spinal cord. Clinical symptomology may include headache, fever, mental deterioration, and seizures.

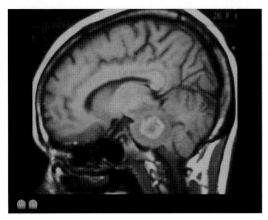

G1. Sagittal and axial T1-weighted images show a hyperintense ring with central low intensity and peripheral edema.

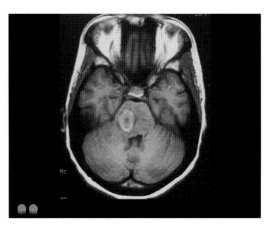

G2. Sagittal and axial T1-weighted images show a hyperintense ring with central low-intensity and peripheral edema.

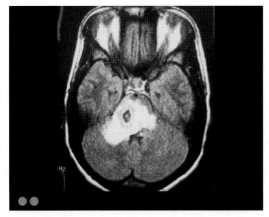

G3. Axial T2-weighted FLAIR image demonstrates a mixed intensity lesion with surrounding edema in the brainstem.

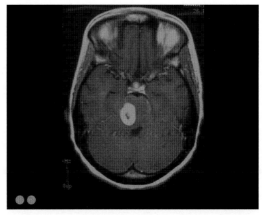

G4. Axial, post-contrast T1-weighted image shows a ring-like enhancing lesion with surrounding edema over the right side of pons.

BRAINSTEM CONTUSION

Diffuse axonal injury is a type of brain damage which is secondary to trauma by rotational acceleration/deceleration force. Centripetal forces, usually generated by high-speed impact, lead to cortico-medullary shearing. As the severity of such forces increases, deeper areas of the brain are progressively involved, with eventual involvement of the corpus callosum and the brainstem.

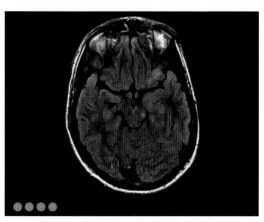

H. Axial T2-weighted FLAIR image shows a focal hyperintensity over the left side of midbrain.

BRAINSTEM HEMORRHAGE

Brainstem hemorrhage may be due to direct injury such as in the case of diffuse axonal injury or Duret hemorrhage. Duret hemorrhage consists of small areas of hemorrhage in the ventral and paramedian parts of the upper brain stem secondary to transtentorial herniation. The mechanism of hemorrhage is probably due to stretching and laceration of the pontine perforating arteries.

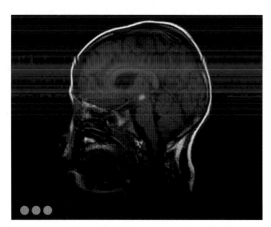

I1. Sagittal T1-weighted image reveals a focal hyperintensity in the midbrain.

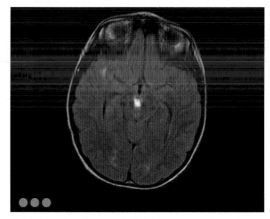

I2. Axial T2-weighted FLAIR image demonstrates a focal hyperintensity in the midbrain.

INFILTRATIVE BRAINSTEM ASTROCYTOMA

Astrocytomas are typically found in certain locations in the brain. In adults infiltrative astrocytomas are most often located in the cerebral hemispheres (75%). In children,

infiltrative astrocytomas are typically within the brainstem, and pilocytic astrocytoma in the cerebellum. Infiltrative astrocytomas usually infiltrate the brain stem, but does not cause its destruction. Malignant dedifferentiation may occur.

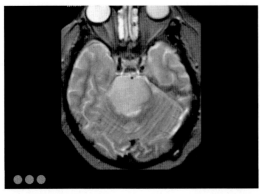

J1. Axial T2-weighted FLAIR image shows a hyper-intense mass involving the pons.

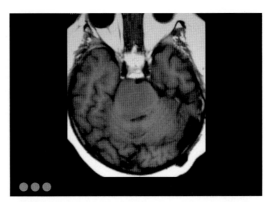

J2. Axial and sagittal, post-contrast T1-weighted images show an expanding mass involving the pons with extension into the midbrain and medulla without contrast enhancement.

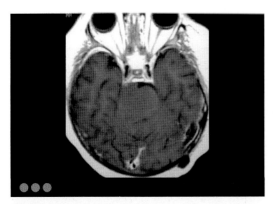

J3. Axial and sagittal, post-contrast T1-weighted images show an expanding mass involving the pons with extension into the midbrain and medulla without contrast enhancement.

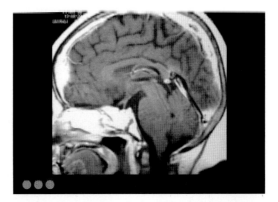

J4. Axial and sagittal, post-contrast T1-weighted images show an expanding mass involving the pons with extension into the midbrain and medulla without contrast enhancement.

METASTATIC DISEASE

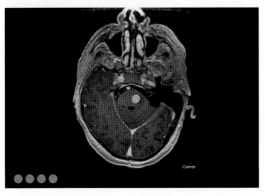

K. Axial, post-contrast T1-weighted image shows a nodular enhancing lesion in the pons.

227

PILOCYTIC ASTROCYTOMA

Pilocytic astrocytoma is the most common glial neoplasm in the pediatric patients and the most common pediatric neoplasm involving the cerebellum. This tumor has a noteworthy benign biologic behavior with an extremely high survival rate 94% at 10 years. Most patients are children in the first 2 decades of life. The cerebellum, optic nerve and chiasm, and hypothalamic region are the most common locations, but the tumor can also be found in the cerebral hemisphere, ventricles, and brainstem. MR imaging often demonstrates a cystic mass with an enhancing mural nodule and occasionally a solid mass without surrounding edema. In the brainstem, they tend to involve the midbrain and medulla whereas infiltrative glioma has a tendency to involve pons.

PILOCYTIC ASTROCYTOMA (CASE ONE)

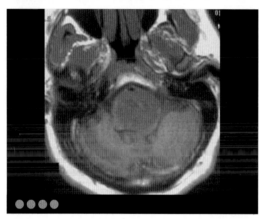

L1. Axial T1-weighted image reveals a hypointense mass involving the pontomedullary junction.

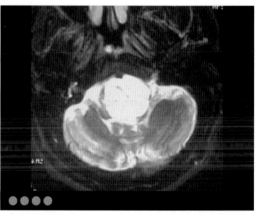

L2. Axial T2-weighted and FLAIR images show a hyperintense mass at the pontomedullary junction.

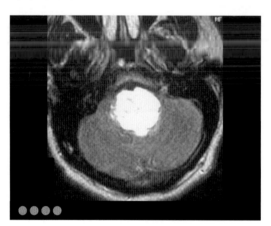

L3. Axial T2-weighted and FLAIR images show a hyperintense mass at the pontomedullary junction.

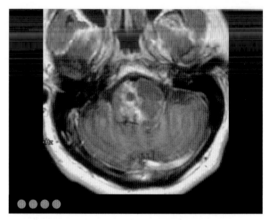

L4. Axial, coronal, sagittal, post-contrast T1-weighted images demonstrate a patchy, irregular, partially enhancing mass involving the pontomedullary junction.

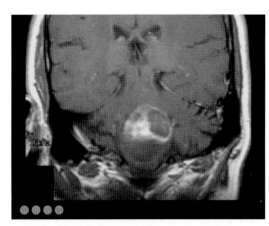

L5. Axial, coronal, sagittal, post-contrast T1-weighted images demonstrate a patchy, irregular, partially enhancing mass involving the pontomedullary junction.

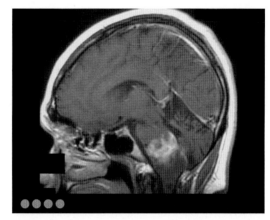

L6. Axial, coronal, sagittal, post-contrast T1-weighted images demonstrate a patchy, irregular, partially enhancing mass involving the pontomedullary junction.

PILOCYTIC ASTROCYTOMA (CASE TWO)

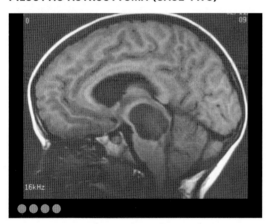

M1. Sagittal and axial T1-weighted images show a cystic mass involving the midbrain and upper pons with a mural nodule.

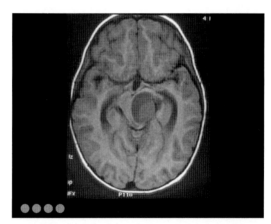

M2. Sagittal and axial T1-weighted images show a cystic mass involving the midbrain and upper pons with a mural nodule.

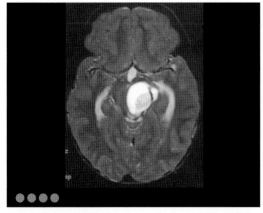

M3. Axial T2-weighted image shows a cystic mass with a mural nodule.

CENTROPONTINE MYELINOLYSIS (OSMOTIC MYELINOLYSIS)

Osmotic myelinolysis is a demyelinating disorder in alcoholic, malnourished patients and others with electrolyte abnormalities, including children. The disorder is commonly associated with electrolyte disturbances, particularly rapid correction of hyponatremia. While many patients may be asymptomatic, some demonstrate quadriparesis, pseudobulbar palsy, and acute changes in mental status. The pontine lesion is classically centrally located. T2 hyperintense lesion is seen in the central basis pontis, which may improve with treatment.

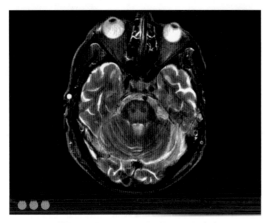

N1 Axial T2-weighted and FLAIR images demonstrate hyperintensity in the region of pons.

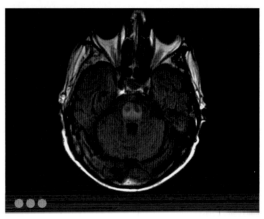

N2. Axial T2 weighted and FLAIR images demonstrate hyperintensity in the region of pons.

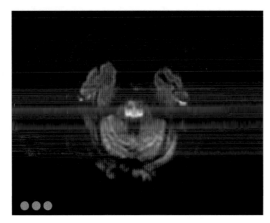

N3. Diffusion-weighted image shows restricted diffusion in the pons corresponding to the hyperintense area seen on T2-weighted images.

LEIGH'S DISEASE

The differential diagnosis for abnormal signal intensity involving the periaqueductal gray matter includes **Leigh's disease** and Wernicke–Korsakoff syndrome. Leigh's disease is a mitochondrial encephalomyopathy and is a hereditary disease transmitted as an autosomal recessive disorder. It is also called subacute necrotizing encephalomyelopathy. The disease present earlier in infancy and has poor prognosis. On MRI abnormal signal intensity areas are detected in basal ganglia, thalamus, brainstem, cerebellar white matter, cerebellar cortex, and cerebral white matter.

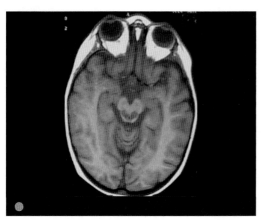

01. Axial T1-weighted image shows hypointnensity in the periaqueductal gray matter

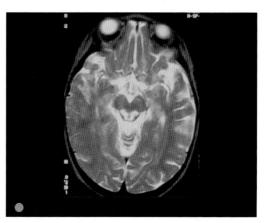

02. Axial T2-weighted and FLAIR images show hyperintensity in the periaqueductal gray matter.

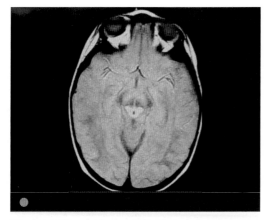

03. Axial T2-weighted and FLAIR images show hyperintensity in the periaqueductal gray matter.

MULTIPLE SCLEROSIS

Multiple sclerosis (MS) is characterized clinically by exacerbations and remissions of neurologic dysfunction. Causative factors include infection, trauma, pregnancy, emotional stress, and allergic reactions. Abnormal findings on MR are seen in 70% to 95% of patients with definite clinical MS. MR findings have become an important factors in the diagnosis of MS. Frequent involvement of the brain stem and spinal cord are seen in young patients with MS. At autopsy, MS lesions are typically found scattered through the cerebrum, brainstem, and spinal cord and both gray and white matter are involved.

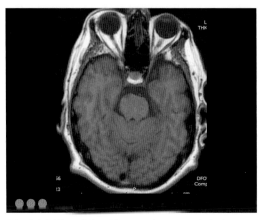

P1. Axial T1-weighted image shows a subtle hypointense lesion at the right anterior aspect of the pons.

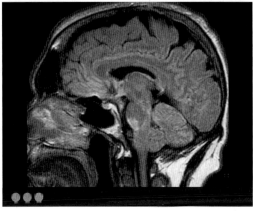

P2. Sagittal and axial T2-weighted FLAIR, and axial T2 weighted images show focal hyperintensity at the right anterior aspect of pons.

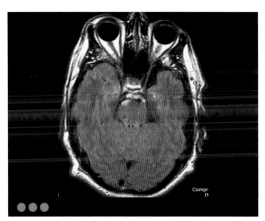

P3. Sagittal and axial T2-weighted FLAIR, and axial T2-weighted images show focal hyperintensity at the right anterior aspect of pons.

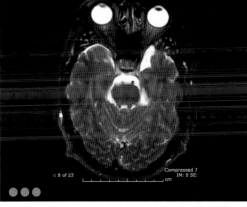

P4. Sagittal and axial T2-weighted FLAIR, and axial T2-weighted images show focal hyperintensity at the right anterior aspect of pons.

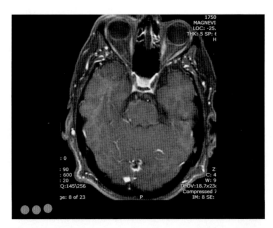

P5. Axial, post-contrast, fat-suppressed T1-weighted image demonstrates faintly enhancing lesion at the right anterior aspect of the pons.

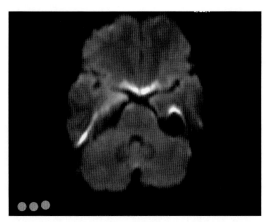

P6. Diffusion-weighted image shows restricted diffusion.

PROGRESSIVE MULTIFOCAL LEUKOENCEPHALOPATHY (PML)

PML is a demyelinating disease caused by JC virus. The JC virus infects the oligodendrocytes, causing cytolytic destruction with resultant demyelination. In patients with HIV and subcortical white matter lesions, PML is more likely than other HIV-related infections. Clinically, the disease is a progressive one with death commonly occurs within 9 months after the onset of clinical symptoms. CT shows low-density lesions in the white matter, in the parietooccipital and frontal locations. Posterior fossa lesions are also seen. PML can involve the myelinated fibers in the deep gray matter. PML may be difficult to differentiate from HIV related demyelination. White matter lesions in HIV related encephalopathy are more diffuse and periventricular, whereas those in PML are more often multifocal, with a greater tendency for subcortical location.

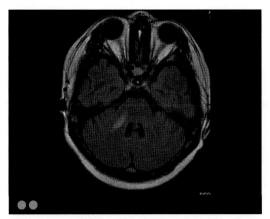

Q. Axial T2 weighted, FLAIR image shows a hyperintense lesion involving the right brachium pontis.

RADIATION CHANGES

Postradiation injury to the brain can be divided into early delayed **radiation injury** and late radiation injury. Early delayed radiation injury usually occurs in the second month postradiation and improves within 6 weeks. On MRI, there is transient hyointensity on T1-weighted and hyperintensity on T2-weighted images. Late radiation injury occurs between 1 and 10 years postradiation. Changes in the white matter may be localized or diffuse. Contrast enhancement and focal mass effect may be seen.

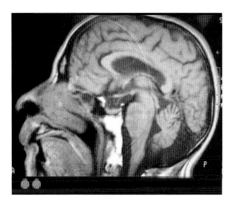

R1. Sagittal T1-weighted image reveals swelling of the pons. Note the hyperintense fatty replacement of the marrow of the clivus secondary to previous radiation.

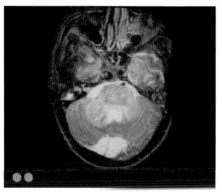

R2. Axial T2-weighted image shows hyperintensity in the pons with surrounding hyperintense edema.

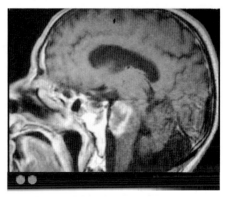

R3. Sagittal, post-contrast T1-weighted image shows an ovoid ring like enhancement involving the pons.

CAVERNOUS ANGIOMA

There are four types of vascular malformation, namely, arteriovenous malformation, cavernous angioma, capillary telangiectasia, and developmental venous anomaly. MRI findings of parenchymal cavernous angiomas demonstrate typical, popcornlike, smoothly circumscribed, well-delineated complex lesions. The center core is formed by multiple foci of mixed signal intensities, which represents hemorrhage in various stages of evolution, surrounded by a hypointense ring due to the presence of hemosiderin.

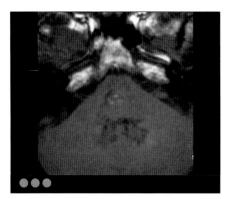

S1. Axial T1-weighted image shows a heterogeneous, slightly hyperintense lesion in the pons.

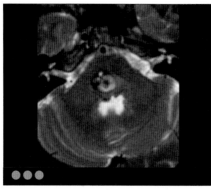

S2. Axial and coronal T2-weighted images show a hyperintense lesion with hypointense center and peripheral rim in the pons.

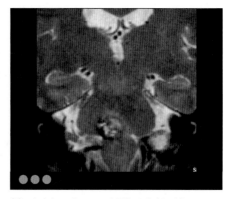

S3. Axial and coronal T2-weighted images show a hyperintense lesion with hypointense center and peripheral rim in the pons.

Chapter 5

Mass Lesions in the Region of the Ventricular System

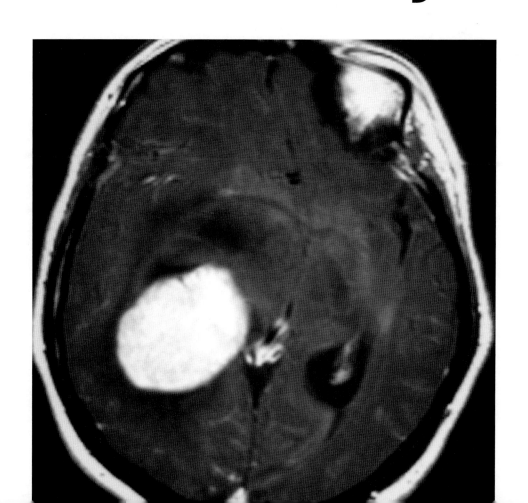

MENINGIOMA

Meningiomas arising within the ventricular system are uncommon, constituting approximately 0.5% to 2% of all intracranial meningiomas. They most commonly arise in the trigone of the lateral ventricle and slightly more common on the left side. There is a female predominance of approximately 2:1. Intraventricular meningioma can occur in age group, there is a wide age range, they are most common over the age of 30 years. Meningiomas rarely may arise in the third ventricle or fourth ventricle. When intraventricular meningioma is seen in children, neurofibromatosis type II should be considered. It is uncertain regarding the origin of intraventricular meningiomas. They appear to arise either from the stroma of the choroid plexus or from rests of arachnoid cells within the choroid plexus.

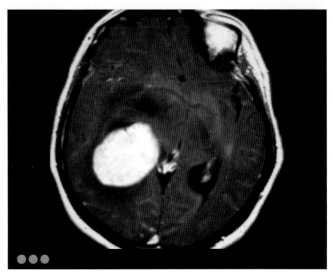

A. Axial, post-contrast T1-weighted image shows an intensely enhancing mass in the atrium of right lateral ventricle.

RELATED PATTERNS

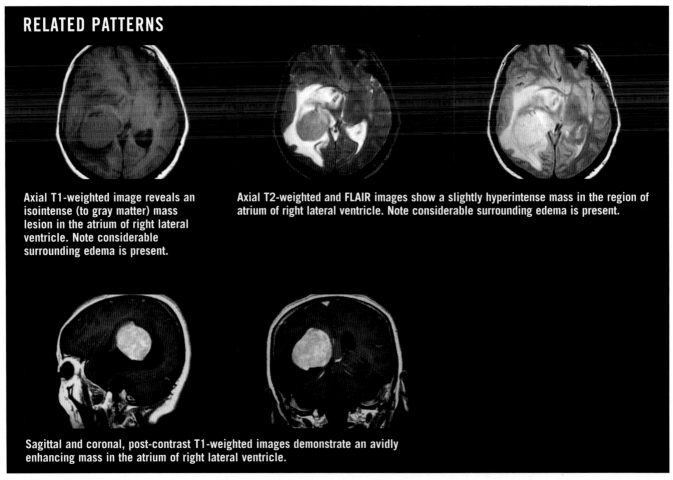

Axial T1-weighted image reveals an isointense (to gray matter) mass lesion in the atrium of right lateral ventricle. Note considerable surrounding edema is present.

Axial T2-weighted and FLAIR images show a slightly hyperintense mass in the region of atrium of right lateral ventricle. Note considerable surrounding edema is present.

Sagittal and coronal, post-contrast T1-weighted images demonstrate an avidly enhancing mass in the atrium of right lateral ventricle.

DIFFERENTIAL DIAGNOSIS

At a Glance:

- *Central Neurocytoma*
- *Choroid Plexus Carcinoma*
- *Choroid Plexus Papilloma*
- *Cysticercosis*
- *Ependymal Cyst*
- *Ependymoma*
- *Juvenile Pilocytic Astrocytoma*
- *Pleomorphic Xanthoastrocytoma*
- *PNET*
- *Subependymal Giant Cell Astrocytoma*
- *Subependymoma*
- *Metastasis* (not pictured)

CENTRAL NEUROCYTOMA

Central neurocytomas are seen in young adults and consist of 0.5% of primary brain tumors. They present as mass lesions in the body of lateral ventricle with cystic, necrotic change and broad-based attachment of the superolateral ventricular wall. Tumor calcification is common. Homogeneous or heterogeneous mass with heterogeneous contrast enhancement is seen on MRI.

CENTRAL NEUROCYTOMA (CASE ONE)

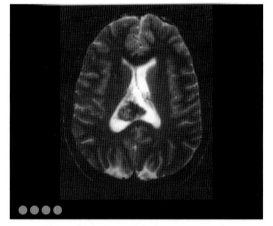

B1. Axial T2-weighted image shows a mixed signal intensity mass in the body of right lateral ventricle.

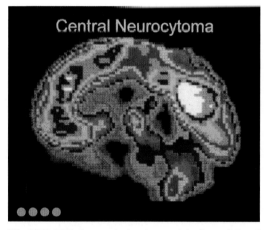

B2. FDG-PET demonstrates low metabolic activity of the tumor mass.

CENTRAL NEUROCYTOMA (CASE TWO)

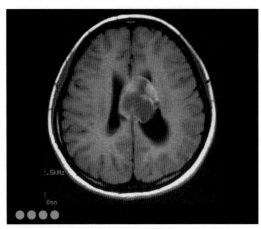

C1. T1-weighted image shows mixed signal intensity, predominantly hypointense mass in the lateral ventricle.

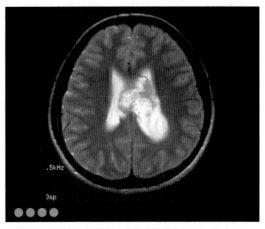

C2. Axial T2-weighted image reveals mixed signal intensity, predominantly hyperintense mass in the lateral ventricle.

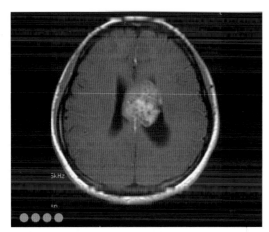

C3. Axial and sagittal, post-contrast T1-weighted image demonstrates a heterogeneously enhancing mass in the lateral ventricle.

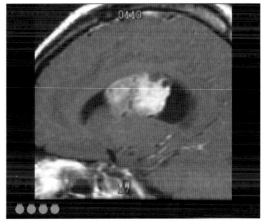

C4. Axial and sagittal, post-contrast T1-weighted image demonstrates a heterogeneously enhancing mass in the lateral ventricle.

CENTRAL NEUROCYTOMA (CASE THREE)

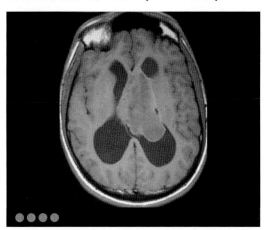

D1. Axial T1-weighted image shows an iso- to hypointense mass in the left lateral ventricle.

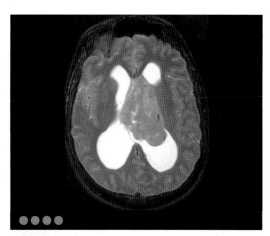

D2. Axial T2-weighted image reveals a predominantly isointense mass with small hyperintense areas.

CENTRAL NEUROCYTOMA (CASE FOUR)

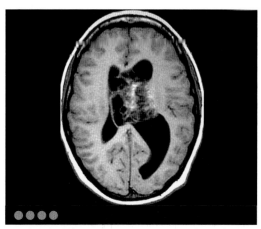

E1. Axial T1-weighted image shows a heterogeneous mass with multiple cystic areas.

D3. Axial, post-contrast T1-weighted image shows a minimally enhancing mass.

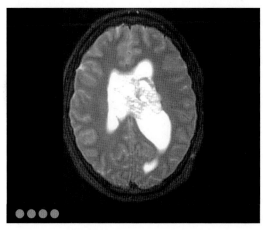

E2. Axial T2-weighted image shows a heterogeneous mass with multiple cystic areas.

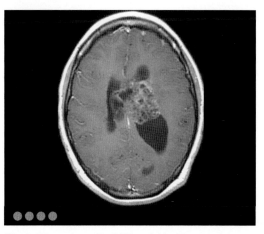

E3. Axial, post-contrast T1-weighted image demonstrates a patchy enhancing mass with multiple cystic areas.

239

CHOROID PLEXUS CARCINOMA

Choroid plexus carcinoma (CPC) is a malignant tumor. There may be hydrocephalus due to a combination of factors including overproduction of CSF, decreased absorption, and mechanical obstruction, and there is usually less overproduction of CSF from carcinoma than from papilloma. The majority (80%) of CPC arises in children, usually within the first 5 years of life and is equally distributed between male and female. Microscopic examination can differentiate CPC from papilloma in that carcinoma is hypercellular, pleomorphic, with increased mitotic activity, cysts, necrosis, hemorrhage, microcalcifications, and brain invasion.

Immunohistochemical characteristics include expression of cytokeritan, but minimal expression of glial fibrillary acid protein, transthyretin, and S100. CPC is a rapidly growing tumor that may seed the CSF pathways. Prognosis is poor with only 40% surviving at 5 years. It is difficult to distinguish CPP from CPC with imaging studies as the two types of tumors have similar imaging characteristics. Therefore, tissue biopsy is usually required in order to make a definitive diagnosis. Generally speaking, CPC usually presents as a more heterogeneous lesion on imaging studies.

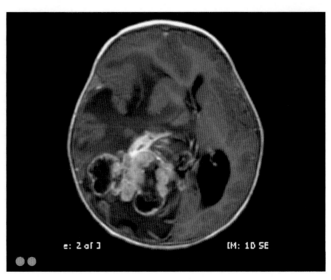

F. Axial, post-contrast T1-weighted image shows a large heterogeneously enhancing mass with cystic changes in the region of atrium of the right lateral ventricle. A siginficant amount of surrounding edema is seen.

CHOROID PLEXUS PAPILLOMA

Choroid plexus papillomas consist of less than 1% of all brain tumors. They are among the most common brain tumors in children below 2 years of age and represent 40% of all brain tumors in the first 60 days of life. Lateral ventricular tumors tend to occur in children whereas fourth ventricular tumors are seen predominantly in adults. Choroid plexus papillomas are predominantly well-circumscribed, smoother lobulated masses that may display frondlike margin. They are of mixed intensity with intense contrast enhancement on MRI. Calcification and hemorrhage are commonly seen.

Pathologically, they consist of well-differentiated proliferation of both the surface epithelium of the choroid plexus and the underlying vascular connective tissue.

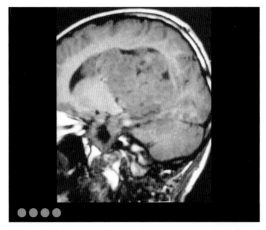

G1. Sagittal T1-weighted image shows a lobulated, mixed signal intensity mass in the atrium of the right lateral ventricle.

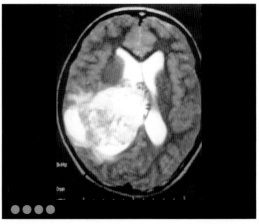

G2. Axial T2-weighted image reveals a heterogeneously hyperintense mass in the atrium of the right lateral ventricle.

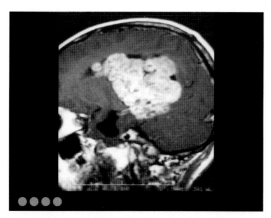

G3. Sagittal and axial, post-contrast T1-weighted images demonstrate a heterogeneously enhancing mass with a small cystic component laterally in the atrium of right lateral ventricle.

G4. Sagittal and axial, post-contrast T1-weighted images demonstrate a heterogeneously enhancing mass with a small cystic component laterally in the atrium of right lateral ventricle.

CYSTICERCOSIS

Neurocysticercossis can be divided into parenchymal, intraventricular, cisternal and mixed types. Intraventricular cysticercosis lesions are more commonly seen in the lateral ventricle, followed by fourth, and third ventricle. Cyst migration can occur in the ventricles. Lateral ventricular cysts can migrate to third ventricle. Third ventricular cysts can migrate into fourth ventricle and fourth ventricular cysts can migrate into cisterna magna. An isolated live cyst can be removed surgically. Enhancing (degenerative) cysts in the ventricles are difficult to remove due to adhesion of the cyst wall to the ependyma.

CYSTICERCOSIS (CASE ONE)

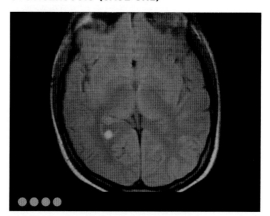

H1. Axial T2-weighted FLAIR image shows a cystic lesion with and eccentric hyperintense nodule situated posteriorly. Note the cyst fluid is slightly more hyperintense than CSF.

CYSTICERCOSIS (CASE TWO)

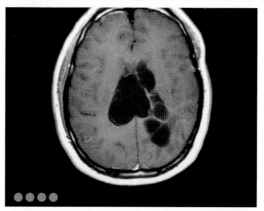

H2. Axial, post-contrast T1-weighted image demonstrates a cyst with enhancing scolex situated posteriorly. Note the enhancing structure anteriorly is the glomus of choroid plexus of the lateral ventricle.

I. Axial T1-weighted image shows multiple cystic lesions in the lateral ventricles bilaterally due to cysticercosis.

241

EPENDYMAL CYST

Ependymal cysts are rare, benign, ependymal-lined cysts of the lateral ventricle. Less frequently, they are seen in juxtaventricular region of the temporoparietal region and frontal lobe. Ependymal cysts are thought to arise from sequestration of developing neuroectoderm during embryogenesis. Ependymal cysts are thin-walled cysts filled with clear serous fluid secreted from ependymal cells.

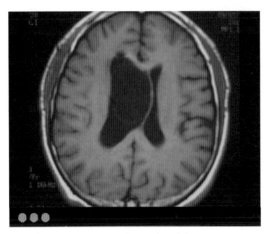

J1. Axial T1 weighted image shows a hypointense cystic mass in the frontal horn of the right lateral ventricle.

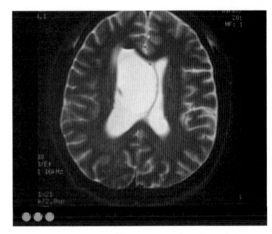

J2. Axial T2-weighted image reveals a hyperintense cyst in the frontal horn of the right lateral ventricle.

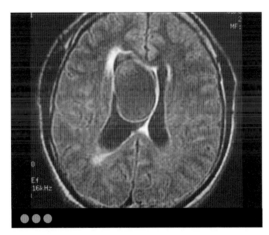

J3. Axial T2-weighted FLAIR image reveals a cystic mass which is slightly hyperintense as compared to CSF.

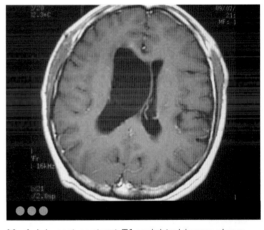

J4. Axial, post-contrast T1-weighted image shows no abnormal contrast enhancement.

EPENDYMOMA

Ependymomas constitute 2–6% of all gliomas. Only 40% of intracranial ependymomas occur in the supratentorial compartment. The reported incidence of parenchymal origin of the ependymomas varies from 55–85%. Parenchymal ependymomas are more commonly seen in the supratentorial compartment. Ependymomas are 4–6 times more common in children than in adults. MRI shows a heterogeneous mass lesion that is T1-hypointense and T2-hyperintense with dense punctate calcification, areas of necrosis, or cystic changes. Hemorrhage may also be seen. Contrast enhancement is variable, from heterogeneous to homogeneous.

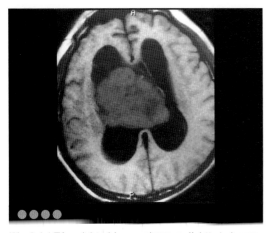

K1 Axial T1-weighted image shows a slightly heterogeneous, hypointense mass in the right lateral ventricle.

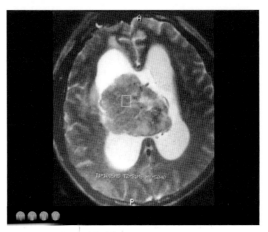

K2. Axial T2-weighted image reveals a heterogeneously hyperintense mass in the right lateral ventricle.

JUVENILE PILOCYTIC ASTROCYTOMA

Juvenile pilocytic astrocytomas may be seen anywhere in the central nervous system including the supratentorial compartment, the infratentorial compartment and spinal canal. In the supratentorial compartment, they can occasionally be intraventricular in location. They are lower-grade tumors which tend to be homogeneous and well circumscribed. On contrast-enhanced MR images, Juvenile pilocytic astrocytoma shows avid contrast enhancement. Peritumoral edema is mild, and usually no hemorrhage is present.

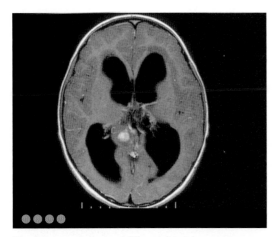

L1. Axial, post-contrast T1-weighted image shows a partially enhancing mass.

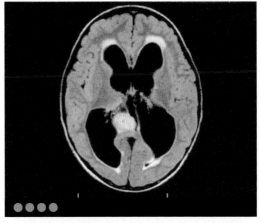

L2. Axial T2-weighted FLAIR image shows a hyperintense mass in the right lateral ventricle with associated hydrocephalus.

PLEOMORPHIC XANTHOASTROCYTOMA

Pleomorphic xanthoastrocytoma is a rare glial neoplasm thought to originate from subpial astrocytes, representing a distinct form of supratentorial astrocytoma. They are super- ficial cortical tumors with extensive leptomeningeal involvement, usually involving the temporal lobe. They are seen equally in males and females, with a predominance in young adults. Intraventricular location of this tumor is extremely unusual.

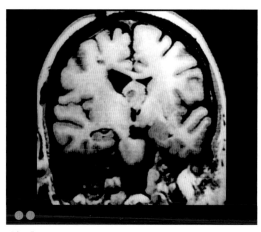

M1. Coronal and sagittal T1-weighted images show a heterogeneous mass at the anterior third ventricle.

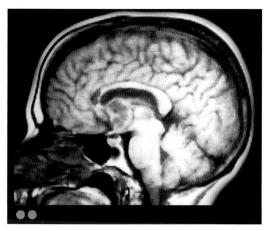

M2. Coronal and sagittal T1-weighted images show a heterogeneous mass at the anterior third ventricle.

PNET

The term primitive neurectodermal tumor (PNET) represents a group of small cell embryonal tumors of the central nervous system that exhibit divergent differentiation. Supratentorial PNETs are highly malignant tumors in infants and young children. Despite the rarity of these lesions, they represent the most common congenital brain tumor. The majority of PNETs occur before the age of 5 years, with many presenting during infancy. Most PNETs are paraventricular masses, located in the deep white matter of the frontal or parietal lobes. The lesions that are intraventricular often involve the body of the lateral ventricle and can reach significant size at the time of presentation. These tumors are large, bulky hemispheric masses that appear well circumscribed on imaging studies.

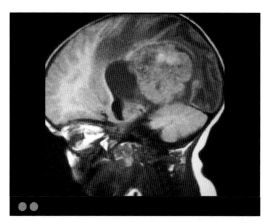

N1. Axial T1-weighted image shows a mixed signal intensity, predominantly isointense mass in the atrium and occipital horn of the right lateral ventricle.

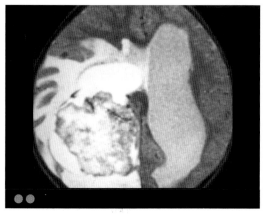

N2. Axial T2-weighted image shows a predominantly hyperintense, heterogeneous mass in the right lateral ventricle with adjacent parenchymal edema.

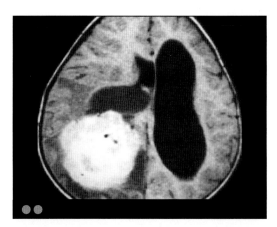

N3. Axial and coronal, post-contrast T1-weighted image shows a heterogeneously enhancing mass in the lateral ventricle.

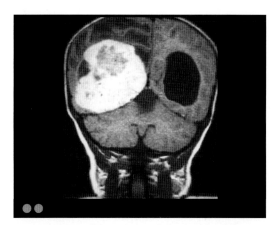

N4. Axial and coronal, post-contrast T1-weighted image shows a heterogeneously enhancing mass in the lateral ventricle.

SUBEPENDYMAL GIANT CELL ASTROCYTOMA

Subependymal giant cell astrocytomas are found in 10–15% of patients with tuberous sclerosis and are usually seen in patients below 20 years of age. They usually occur in the wall of the lateral ventricle near the foramen of Monro. The roof of the third ventricle is involved if the tumor extends inferiorly. Calcification and cysts are commonly seen on CT or MRI. On MRI, T1 hypointensity and T2-hyperintensity are seen with heterogeneous contrast enhancement

SUBEPENDYMAL GIANT CELL ASTROCYTOMA (CASE ONE)

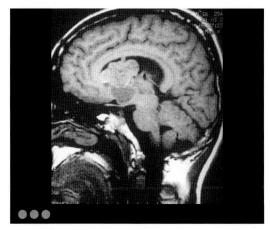

01. Sagittal T1-weighted image shows a mixed signal, predominantly isointense mass with a cystic component in the lateral ventricle near the foramen of Monro.

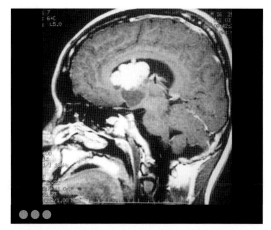

02. Sagittal, post-contrast T1-weighted image demonstrates an enhancing mass with a cystic component in the lateral ventricle near the foramen of Monro.

SUBEPENDYMAL GIANT CELL ASTROCYTOMA (CASE TWO)

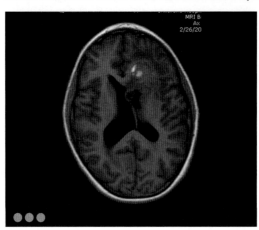

P1. Axial T1-weighted image shows a heterogeneous mass with foci of hyperintensity, consistent with hemorrhage, in the region of frontal horn of the left lateral ventricle near foramen of Monro.

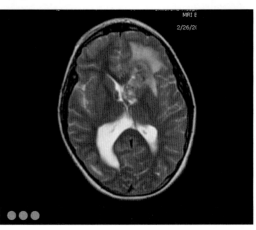

P2. Axial T2-weighted image shows a heterogeneous, iso- to hyperintense mass in the region of frontal horn of the left lateral ventricle with adjacent edema.

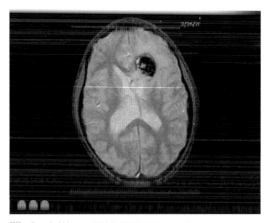

P3. Axial T2-weighted gradient-echo image demonstrates hypointensity within the mass, consistent with hemorrhage.

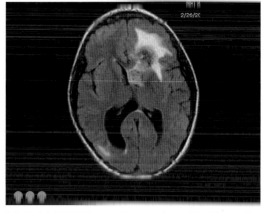

P4. Axial FLAIR image shows mixed signal intensity mass with adjacent edema.

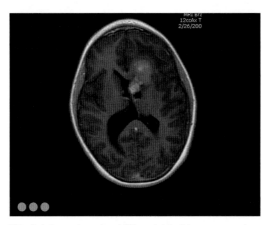

P5. Axial, post-contrast T1-weighted image reveals enhancement of the mass lesion in the frontal horn of the left lateral ventricle.

SUBEPENDYMOMA

Subependymomas are relatively rare tumors found in middle-aged and elderly patients. Subependymomas can be discovered incidentally or due to obstruction of the CSF pathway. They most frequently arise from the lower medulla and project into the fourth ventricle. They also have been found in the frontal horn of the lateral ventricles and along the septum pellucidum. Subependymomas are well-circumscribed, lobulated isointense mass on both T1- and T2-weighted images that may or may not exhibit contrast enhancement.

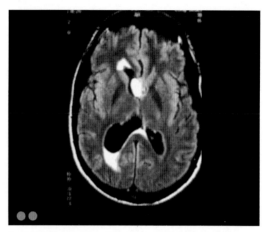

Q. Axial T2-weighted FLAIR image shows a hyperintense mass in the frontal horn of the right lateral ventricle. Note the presence of hydrocephalus with periventricular edema.

COLLOID CYST

Colloid cysts are congenital in origin, but only 1–2% present before the age of 10 years. Most colloid cysts become symptomatic between the third and fifth decade. Colloid cysts occur most frequently in the anterior third ventricle, originating from the roof near the foramen of Monro. Colloid cysts are thought to enlarge due to increase in their contents. The epithelial lining of the cell wall secretes a mucinous fluid. In addition, cyst cavities filled with blood degradation products and cholesterol crystals have been reported. These lesions are most often hyperintense but variable due to cyst content on T1-weighted images. They are most often hyperintense but rarely circumferentially hyperintense with a profoundly hypointnese center on T2-weighted images. There is occasional peripheral enhancement.

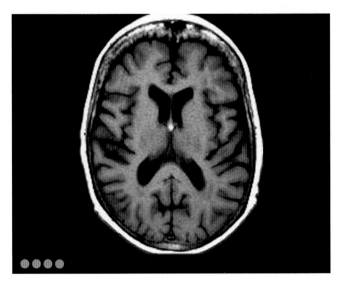

A. Axial T1-weighted image shows a hyperintense mass at the anterior third ventricle.

RELATED PATTERNS

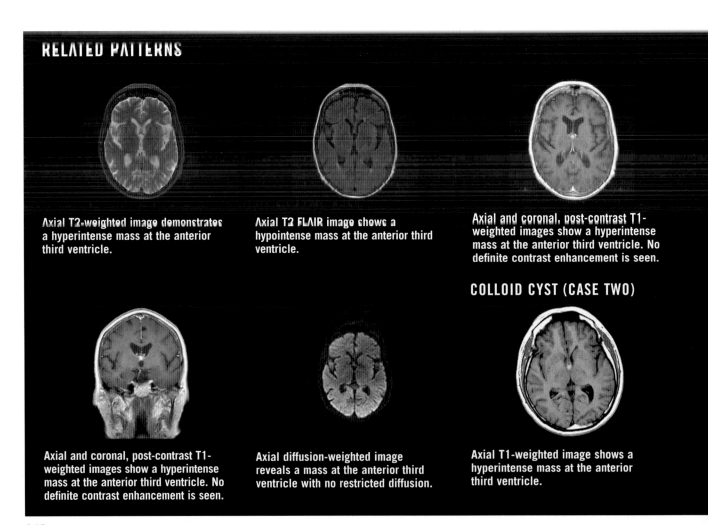

Axial T2-weighted image demonstrates a hyperintense mass at the anterior third ventricle.

Axial T2 FLAIR image shows a hypointense mass at the anterior third ventricle.

Axial and coronal, post-contrast T1-weighted images show a hyperintense mass at the anterior third ventricle. No definite contrast enhancement is seen.

COLLOID CYST (CASE TWO)

Axial and coronal, post-contrast T1-weighted images show a hyperintense mass at the anterior third ventricle. No definite contrast enhancement is seen.

Axial diffusion-weighted image reveals a mass at the anterior third ventricle with no restricted diffusion.

Axial T1-weighted image shows a hyperintense mass at the anterior third ventricle.

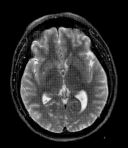
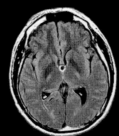
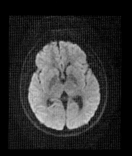

Axial T2-weighted and FLAIR images reveal a hyperintense mass with a hypointense center.

Axial diffusion-weighted image demonstrates no restricted diffusion.

COLLOID CYST (CASE THREE)

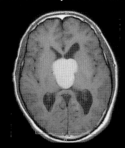
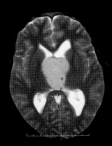

Axial T1-weighted image shows a large hyperintense mass at the anterior third ventricle.

Axial T2-weighted and FLAIR images reveal a large hyperintense mass at the anterior third ventricle.

RELATED PATTERNS (continued)
COLLOID CYST (CASE THREE) (continued)

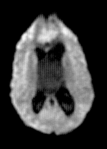

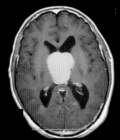

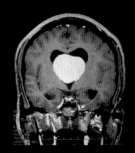

Diffusion-weighted image shows no evidence of restricted diffusion.

Axial and coronal, post-contrast T1-weighted images demonstrate no definite enhancement of the mass lesion.

COLLOID CYST (CASE FOUR)

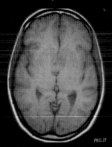

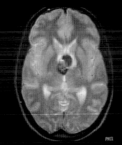

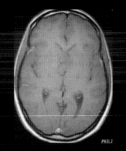

Axial T1-weighted image shows a mixed, hypo- to isointensity mass at the anterior third ventricle.

Axial T2-weighted image demonstrates a heterogeneously hypo-intense mass in the region of foramen of Monro, consistent with hemorrhage seen at surgical pathology.

Axial, post-contrast T1-weighted image shows no abnormal enhancement of the mass

DIFFERENTIAL DIAGNOSIS

At a Glance:

- *Central Neurocytoma*
- *Ependymoma*
- *Meningioma*
- *Metastatic Adenocarcinoma (from Colon)*

- *Oligodendroglioma*
- *Tanycytic Ependymoma*
- *Choroid Plexus Papilloma* (not pictured)
- *Craniopharyngioma* (not pictured)
- *Cysticercosis* (not pictured)
- *Subependymoma* (not pictured)

CENTRAL NEUROCYTOMA

Central neurocytomas are seen in young adults and consist of 0.5% of primary brain tumors. They present as mass lesions in the body of lateral ventricle with cystic, necrotic change, and broad-based attachment of the superolateral ventricular wall. Third ventricular location is less common. Tumor calcification is common. Homogeneous or heterogeneous mass with heterogeneous contrast enhancement is seen on MRI.

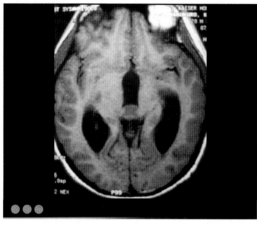

B1. Axial T1-weighted image shows a hypointense mass in the posterior third ventricle. Note the third ventricle is dilated.

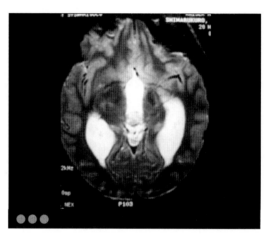

B2. Axial T2-weighted image reveals the mass to be of similar signal intensity as CSF.

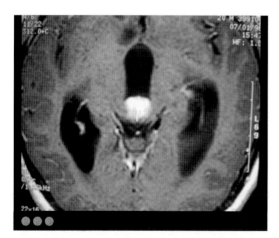

B3. Axial and sagittal, post-contrast T1-weighted image demonstrates an avidly enhancing mass in the posterior third ventricle.

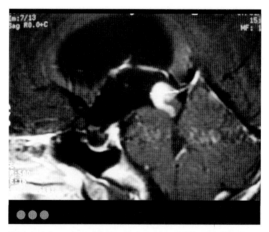

B4. Axial and sagittal, post-contrast T1-weighted image demonstrates an avidly enhancing mass in the posterior third ventricle.

EPENDYMOMA

Ependymomas constitute 2–6% of all gliomas. Only 40% of intracranial ependymomas occur in the supratentorial compartment. Ependymomas are 4–6 times more common in children than in adults. MRI shows a heterogeneous mass lesion with dense punctate calcification, areas of necrosis or cystic changes. Hemorrhage may also be seen. Contrast enhancement is variable, from heterogeneous to homogeneous.

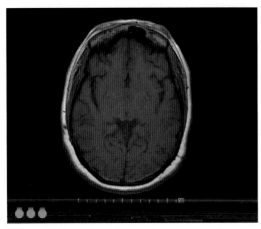

C1. Axial T1-weighted image shows an isointense mass in the third ventricle.

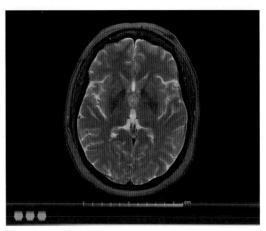

C2. Axial T2-weighted and FLAIR images show a hyperintense mass in the third ventricle.

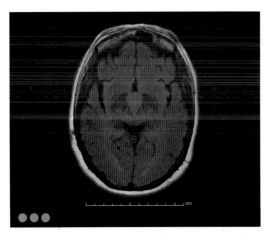

C3. Axial T2-weighted and FLAIR images show a hyperintense mass in the third ventricle.

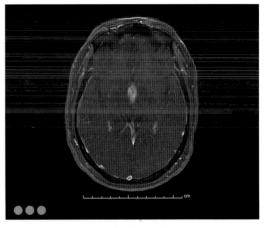

C4. Axial, post-contrast T1-weighted image demonstrates an enhancing mass in the third ventricle.

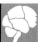

MENINGIOMA

Intraventricular meningiomas are uncommon neoplasms. The origin of these tumors can be explained by embryological invagination of arachnoid cells into the choroid plexus. Since the choroid plexus has a more bulky presence in the lateral ventricles, the incidence of lateral ventricular meningiomas is higher than those in the third or fourth ventricles. These tumors are usually asymptomatic in the early stage of the disease because ventricles of the brain provide space for tumor expansion, and until the cerebrospinal fluid pathways are mechanically occluded. The MR imaging features of intraventricular meningiomas are similar to dural based meningiomas. Avid contrast enhancement is usually seen following intravenous injection of gadolinium. The MR proton spectroscopy and perfusion weighted imaging may help to increase the certainty of preoperative diagnosis. An increased alanine level has been reported as a MR proton spectroscopic finding for meningiomas. Increased rCBV is seen in meningioma on perfusion weighted imaging.

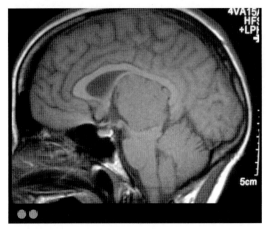

D1. Sagittal T1-weighted image shows an isointense mass in the third ventricle.

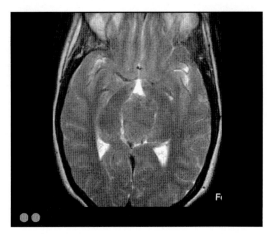

D2. Axial T2-weighted image reveals an isointense mass in the third ventricle.

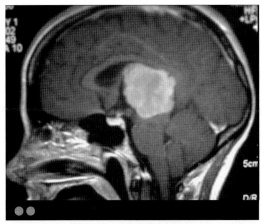

D3. Axial and sagittal, post-contrast T1-weighted images demonstrate an intensely enhancing mass in the third ventricle.

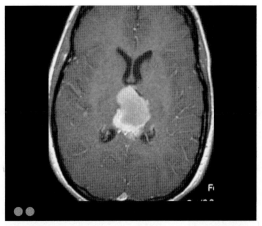

D4. Axial and sagittal, post-contrast T1-weighted images demonstrate an intensely enhancing mass in the third ventricle.

METASTATIC ADENOCARCINOMA (FROM COLON)

The neoplasms of lateral ventricle usually arise from the walls of the ventricle or tissues within and around the ventricle notably choroid plexus, septum pellucidum and thalamus. Most of the tumors are low grade and slow growing such as astrocytoma, oligodendroglioma, choroid plexus papilloma, subependymoma, meningioma. Few of them are highly malignant like malignant ependymoma and choroid plexus carcinoma. Metastasis is a rare differential diagnosis for intraventricular mass. Single intraventricular metastases are seen in 0.14% of cases in an autopsy series of cancer patients. Metastasis is more likely seen in lateral ventricles as compared to third and fourth ventricle. The most common location in the lateral ventricle is atrium where the glomus of the choroid plexus is located.

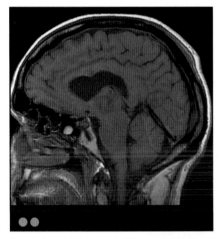

E1. Sagittal T1-weighted image shows a hypointense mass in the region of third ventricle.

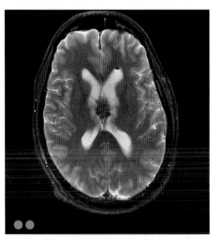

E2. Axial T2-weighted and FLAIR images demonstrate a hypointense mass in the thrid vetricle with surrounding edema.

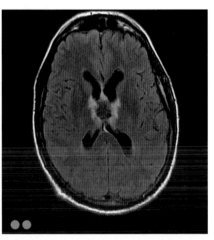

E3. Axial T2-weighted and FLAIR images demonstrate a hypointense mass in the thrid vetricle with surrounding edema.

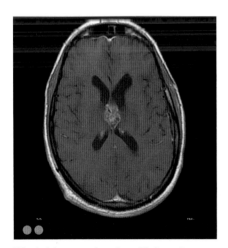

E4. Axial, coronal and sagittal, post-contrast T1-weighted images reveal an enhancing mass in the thrid ventricle.

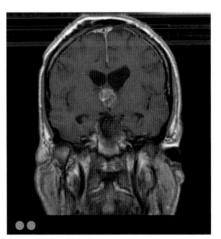

E5. Axial, coronal and sagittal, post-contrast T1-weighted images reveal an enhancing mass in the thrid ventricle.

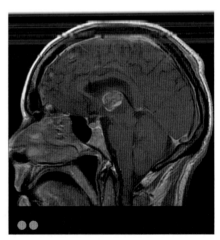

E6. Axial, coronal and sagittal, post-contrast T1-weighted images reveal an enhancing mass in the thrid ventricle.

OLIGODENDROGLIOMA

Oligodendroglioma comprise 5–9% of all primary intracranial gliomas and are usually found in the cerebral hemispheres; primary intraventricular oligodendroglioma is quite rare. The intraventricular oligodendrogliomas are slightly more common in females whereas intraparenchymal ones shows a slight male predominance. There is no age difference between the intraventricular and parenchymal varieties of oligodendrogliomas. They are most commonly found in the anterior parts of the lateral ventricles. Third ventricular oligodendrogliomas are extremely rare.

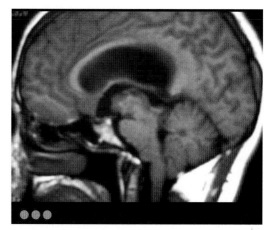

F1. Sagittal and axial T1-weighted images show an isointense mass in the third ventricle. There is associated hydrocephalus.

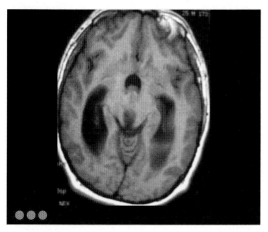

F2. Sagittal and axial T1-weighted images show an isointense mass in the third ventricle. There is associated hydrocephalus.

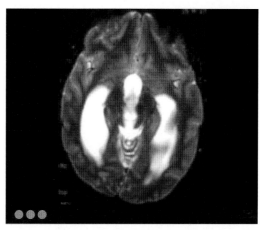

F3. Axial T2-weighted image reveals a hyperintense mass in the third ventricle.

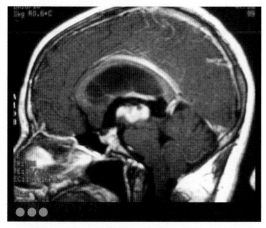

F4. Sagittal and axial, post-contrast T1-weighted images demonstrate intense enhancement of the mass.

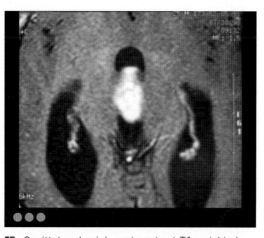

F5. Sagittal and axial, post-contrast T1-weighted images demonstrate intense enhancement of the mass.

TANYCYTIC EPENDYMOMA

The World Health Organization (WHO) classification scheme for **ependymomas** includes three grades based on histologic appearance: WHO grade I, myxopapillary ependymoma and subependymoma; WHO grade II, ependymoma (with cellular, papillary, tanycytic, and clear cell variants); WHO grade III, anaplastic ependymoma. Tanycytes were first described by Horstmann in 1954 and are found in the floor of the fourth ventricle, aqueduct of Sylvius, circumventricular organs and most commonly in the infralateral walls of the floor of the third ventricle. These tumor cells have similar microscopic features of the tanycyte. On the electron microscopy, these tumor cells have more epithelial-type features that are not seen in astrocytomas.

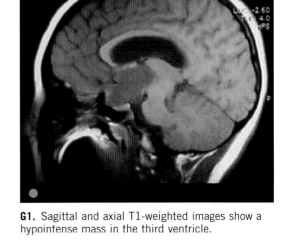

G1. Sagittal and axial T1-weighted images show a hypointense mass in the third ventricle.

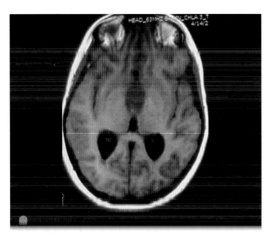

G2. Sagittal and axial T1-weighted images show a hypointense mass in the third ventricle.

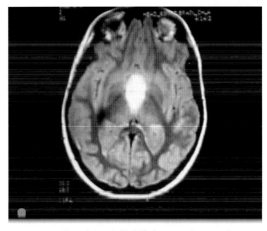

G3. Axial T2-weighted FLAIR image shows a hyperintense mass in the third ventricle.

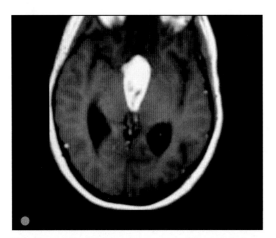

G4. Axial and sagittal, post-contrast T1-weighted images demonstrate an intensely enhancing mass in the third ventricle.

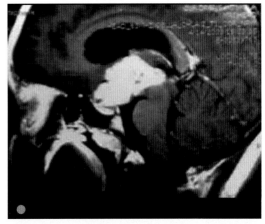

G5. Axial and sagittal, post-contrast T1-weighted images demonstrate an intensely enhancing mass in the third ventricle.

CHOROID PLEXUS PAPILLOMA

Choroid plexus papillomas are predominantly well-circumscribed, smoothly lobulated masses that may display frondlike margin. They are of mixed intensity with intense contrast enhancement on MRI. Calcification and hemorrhage are common. Choroid plexus papillomas in the fourth ventricle are predominantly seen in adults.

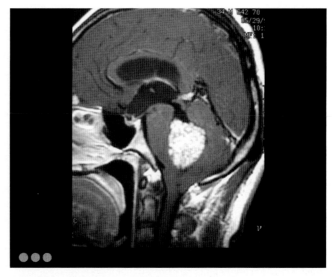

A. Sagittal, post-contrast T1-weighted image shows an enhancing mass with cauliflower-like margin in the fourth ventricle.

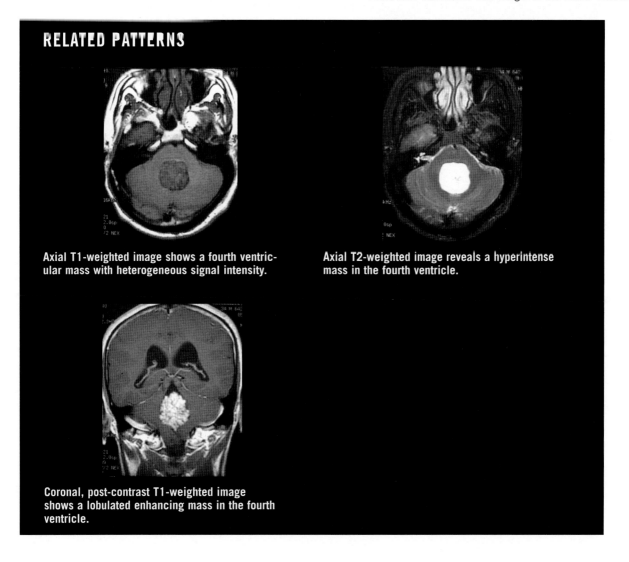

RELATED PATTERNS

Axial T1-weighted image shows a fourth ventricular mass with heterogeneous signal intensity.

Axial T2-weighted image reveals a hyperintense mass in the fourth ventricle.

Coronal, post-contrast T1-weighted image shows a lobulated enhancing mass in the fourth ventricle.

RELATED PATTERNS (continued)

CHOROID PLEXUS PAPILLOMA (CASE TWO)

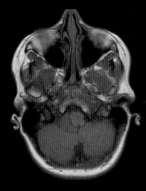

Axial T1-weighted image shows a slightly hypointense mass in the right lateral recess of fourth ventricle.

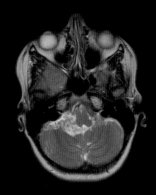

Axial T2-weighted image reveals a hyperintense mass in the right lateral recess of fourth ventricle.

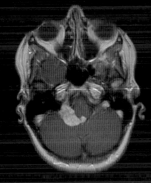

Axial and coronal, post contrast T1-weighted images demonstrate an avidly enhancing mass in the right lateral recess of fourth ventricle. Note the corrugated appearance of contour of the mass.

DIFFERENTIAL DIAGNOSIS

At a Glance:

- *Cysticercosis*
- *Ependymoma*
- *Subependymoma*
- *Metastasis* (not pictured)

CYSTICERCOSIS

Intraventricular cysticercosis cysts may or may not cause obstruction of the CSF pathway. Obstructive hydrocephalus can be a serious complication of intraventricular cysticercosis. When intraventricualr cysts exhibit contrast enhancement, underlying ependymitis is seen around the cyst. This would indicate surgical removal of the cyst might be a difficult task due to underlying adhesion of the cyst wall to the ventricular wall.

CYSTICERCOSIS (CASE ONE)

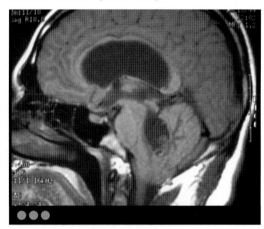

B1. Sagittal T1-weighted image shows a cystic lesion in the fourth ventricle with a hyperintense scolex seen.

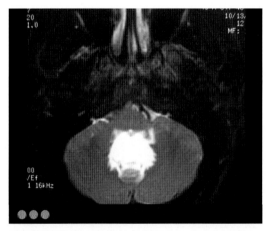

B2. Axial T2-weighted image reveals a hyperintense lesion in the fourth ventricle.

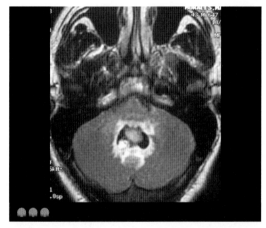

B3. Axial T2-weighted FLAIR image reveals a cystic lesion with a hyperintense scolex in the fourth ventricle. Note the presence of hyperintense surrounding edema.

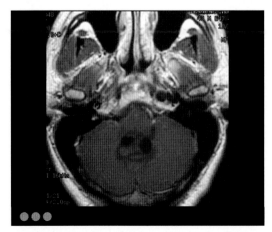

B4. Axial and coronal, post-contrast T1-weighted images demonstrate a cystic lesion with a scolex in the fourth ventricle.

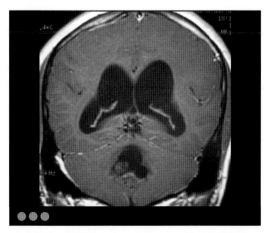

B5. Axial and coronal, post-contrast T1-weighted images demonstrate a cystic lesion with a scolex in the fourth ventricle.

259

CYSRICERCOSIS (CASE TWO)

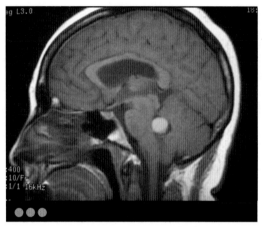

C1. Sagittal and axial T1-weighted images show a hyperintense lesion in the fourth ventricle. This proved to be the scolex of a cysticercosis cyst.

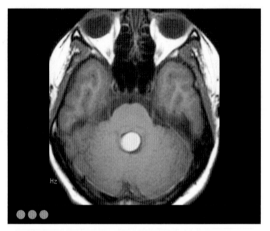

C2. Sagittal and axial T1-weighted images show a hyperintense lesion in the fourth ventricle. This proved to be the scolex of a cysticercosis cyst.

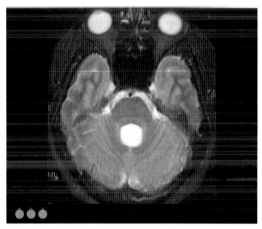

C3. Axial T2-weighted image shows a hyperintense lesion in the fourth ventricle.

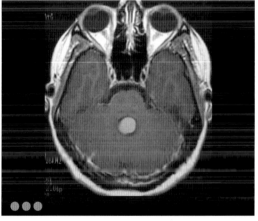

C4. Axial, post-contrast T1-weighted image reveals no definite enhancement of the lesion.

EPENDYMOMA

Ependymomas constitute 2–6% of all gliomas. Approximately 60% of intracranial ependymomas occur in the infratentorial compartment. Ependymomas are 4–6 times more common in children than in adults. MRI shows a heterogeneous mass lesion with dense punctate calcification, areas of necrosis or cystic changes. Hemorrhage may also be seen. Contrast enhancement is variable, from heterogeneous to homogeneous.

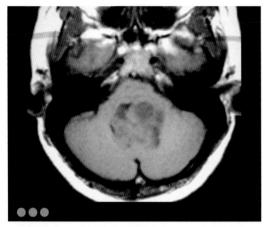

D1. Axial T1-weighted image shows a slightly heterogeneous, hypointense mass in the fourth ventricle.

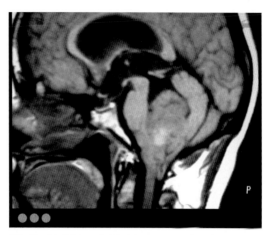

D2. Sagittal T1-weighted image reveals a heterogeneous mass with a focal hyperintense area, consistent with hemorrhage.

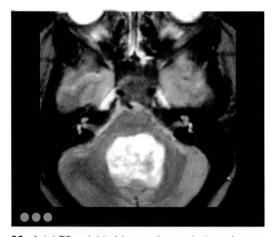

D3. Axial T2-weighted image demonstrates a hyperintense mass in the fourth ventricle.

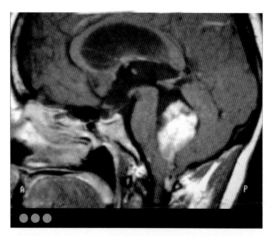

D4. Sagittal, post-contrast T1-weighted image demonstrates a heterogeneously enhancing mass. Note extension of the mass through the foramen of Majendie.

SUBEPENDYMOMA

Subependymomas are relatively rare tumors found in middle-aged and elderly patients. Subependymomas can be discovered incidentally or due to obstruction of the CSF pathway. They most frequently arise from the lower medulla and project into the fourth ventricle. They also have been found in the frontal horn of the lateral ventricles and along the septum pellucidum. Subependymomas are well-circumscribed, lobulated, isointense mass on MRI that may or may not exhibit contrast enhancement.

SUBEPENDYMOMA (CASE ONE)

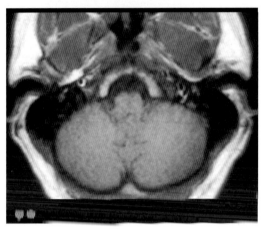

E1. Axial T1-weighted image shows an isointense mass in the midline recess of the fourth ventricle.

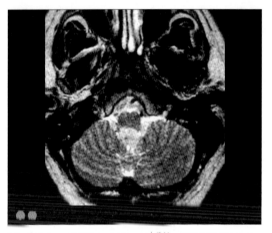

E2. Axial, sagittal and coronal T2-weighted images demonstrate a slightly hyperintense mass in the midline recess of the fourth ventricle.

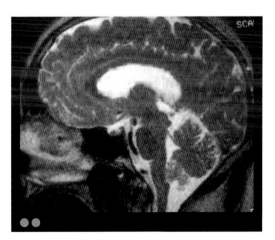

E3. Axial, sagittal and coronal T2-weighted images demonstrate a slightly hyperintense mass in the midline recess of the fourth ventricle.

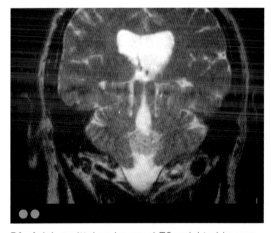

E4. Axial, sagittal and coronal T2-weighted images demonstrate a slightly hyperintense mass in the midline recess of the fourth ventricle.

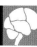

SUBEPENDYMOMA (CASE TWO)

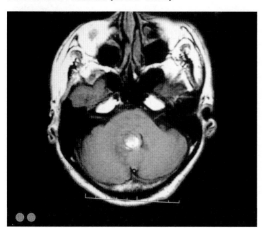

F1. Axial T1-weighted image shows a hyperintense mass in the fourth ventricle

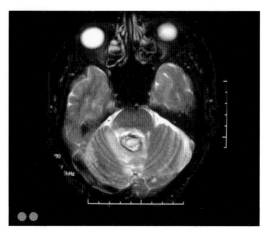

F2. Axial fat-suppressed T2-weighted image demonstrates a hyperintense mass with a hypointense rim and surrounding edema in the fourth ventricle.

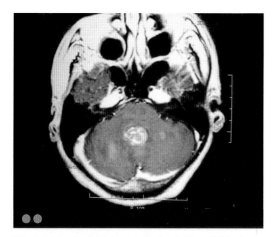

F3. Axial and sagittal post contrast T1-weighted images show heterogenously enhancing mass.

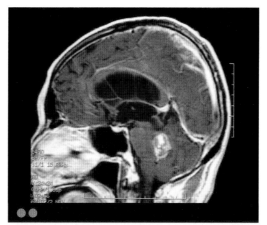

F4. Axial and sagittal post contrast T1-weighted images show heterogenously enhancing mass.

GERMINOMA

Germinoma is the most common pineal region neoplasm. They are seen in young males with a 9:1 male to female ratio. Occasionally, a pineal region mass may be seen in association with a suprasellar mass.

Tumor calcification is not seen, although the tumor may engulf a calcified pineal gland. On MRI, they are usually isointense on both T1- and T2-weighted images. Occasionally, they may show a slight hyperintensity on T2-weighted images. Small cystic areas may be seen. Contrast enhancement is usually intense.

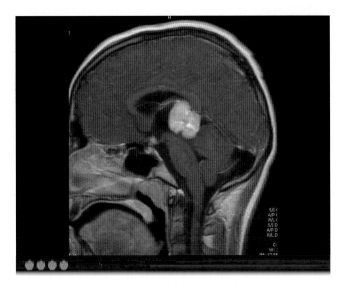

A. Sagittal, post contrast T1 weighted image shows an avidly enhancing mass in the pineal region as well as a small enhancing mass in the suprasellar region.

RELATED PATTERNS

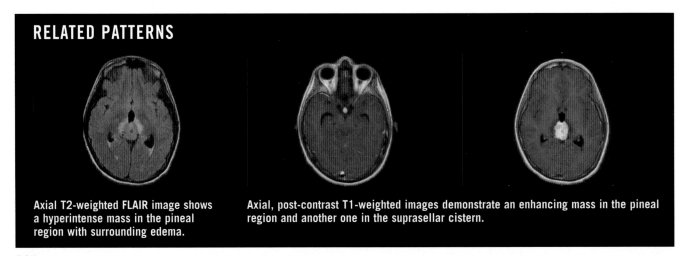

Axial T2-weighted FLAIR image shows a hyperintense mass in the pineal region with surrounding edema.

Axial, post-contrast T1-weighted images demonstrate an enhancing mass in the pineal region and another one in the suprasellar cistern.

DIFFERENTIAL DIAGNOSIS

At a Glance:

- *Anaplastic Astrocytoma of Tectum*
- *Astrocytoma of Tectum*
- *Epidermoid*
- *Meningioma*
- *Metastasis*
- *Pineal Cyst*

- *Pineal Parenchymal Tumor of Intermediate Differentiation*
- *Pineoblastoma*
- *Pineocytoma*
- *Teratoma*
- *Trilateral Retinoblastoma*
- *Vein of Galen Malformation*

ANAPLASTIC ASTROCYTOMA OF TECTUM

Since the normal pineal gland contains fibrillary astrocytes, an astrocytoma may arise from the pineal gland. The majority of pineal region **astrocytomas** arise from the quadrigeminal plate or the thalamus.

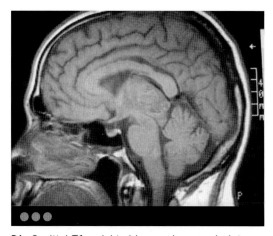

B1. Sagittal T1-weighted image shows an isointense mass arising from the tectum of the midbrain.

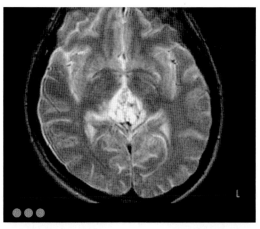

B2. Axial T2-weighted image reveals a heterogeneously hyperintense mass in the pineal region.

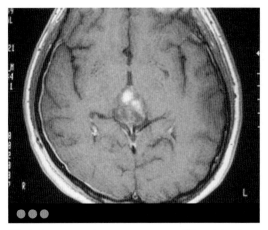

B3. Axial and sagittal, post-contrast T1-weighted image demonstrates a patchy enhancing mass arsing from the tectum.

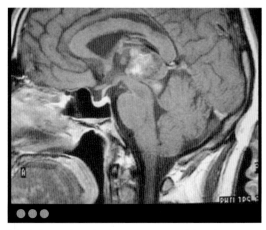

B4. Axial and sagittal, post-contrast T1-weighted image demonstrates a patchy enhancing mass arsing from the tectum.

ASTROCYTOMA OF TECTUM

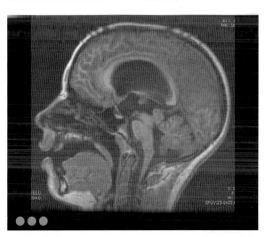

C1. Sagittal T1-weighted image shows an isointense mass arising from the tectum.

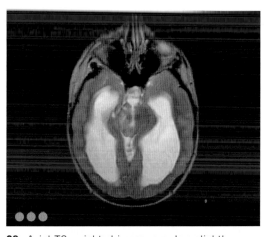

C2. Axial T2-weighted image reveals a slightly hyperintense mass in the tectal region.

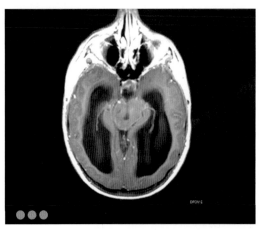

C3. Axial, post-contrast T1-weighted image reveals the mass to be nonenhancing.

EPIDERMOID

Intracranial epidermoid tumors are congenital neoplasms that constitute about 1% of all intracranial tumors. They tend to occur in basal subarachnoid cisterns and ventricles, especially in cerebellopontine angles, parasellar regions, and the fourth ventricles. They tend to insinuate themselves through the cerebrospinal fluid space with causing significant mass effect. On conventional MR imaging, they are of similar signal intensity to cerebrospinal fluid (CSF) and sometime, they may exhibit so called "dirty CSF" appearance. Diffusion weighted imaging is a useful technique to differentiate epidermoid tumors from arachnoid cysts, by revealing the solid nature of epidermoid tumors as opposed to the pure fluid of arachnoid cysts according to their apparent diffusion coefficients.

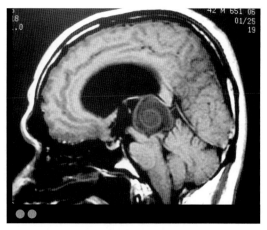

D1. Sagittal and axial T1-weighted images show a heterogeneous, hypointnese mass in the pineal region.

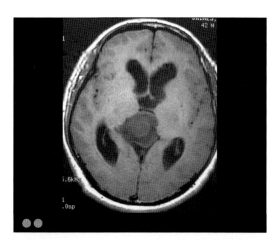

D2. Sagittal and axial T1-weighted images show a heterogeneous, hypointnese mass in the pineal region.

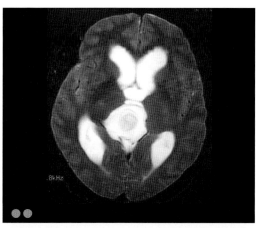

D3. Axial T2-weighted and FLAIR images show a hyperintense mass in the pineal region.

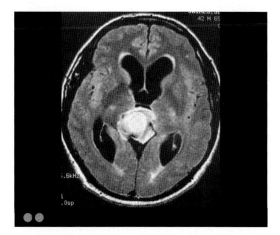

D4. Axial T2-weighted and FLAIR images show a hyperintense mass in the pineal region.

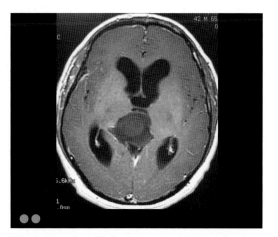

D5. Axial and sagittal, post-contrast T1-weighted images show no evidence of enhancement.

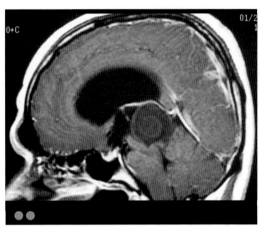

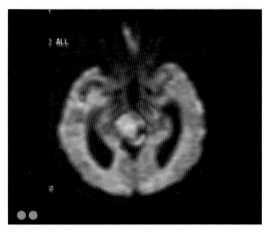

D6. Axial and sagittal, post-contrast T1-weighted images show no evidence of enhancement.

D7. Diffusion-weighted image demonstrates a hyper-intense lesion, consistent with restricted diffusion.

MENINGIOMA

Meningioma in the pineal region arises from the velum interpositum or from the free edge of the tentorium. Rarely, they arise from the arachnoid cell inclusions in the pineal gland.

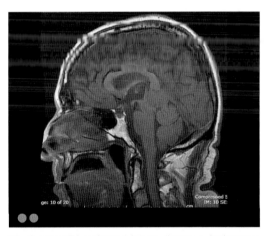

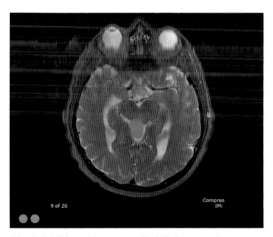

E1. Sagittal T1-weighted image shows an isointense mass in the pineal region.

E2. Axial T2-weighted and FLAIR images show slightly hyperintense mass in the pineal region.

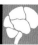

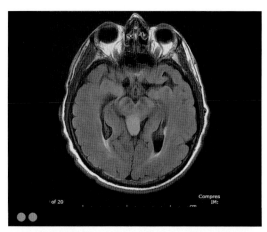

E3. Axial T2-weighted and FLAIR images show slightly hyperintense mass in the pineal region.

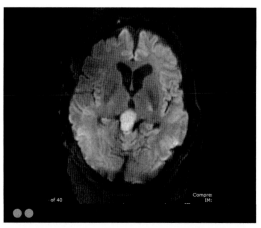

E4. Diffusion-weighted image shows hyperintensity with low ADC value, consistent with restricted diffusion. This was a case of atypical meningioma.

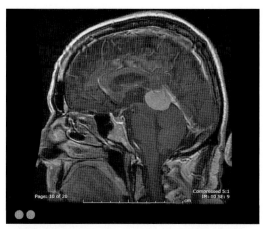

E5. Sagittal, axial and coronal, post-contrast T1-weighted images demonstrate intense enhancement of the mass with a dural tail seen along the right tentorium.

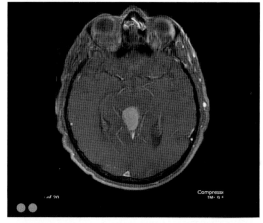

E6. Sagittal, axial and coronal, post-contrast T1-weighted images demonstrate intense enhancement of the mass with a dural tail seen along the right tentorium.

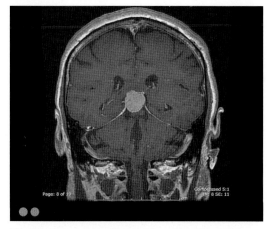

E7. Sagittal, axial and coronal, post-contrast T1-weighted images demonstrate intense enhancement of the mass with a dural tail seen along the right tentorium.

METASTASIS

Intracranial metastatic disease occurs more frequently than primary brain tumors, but metastasis to pineal gland are rare. The main treatment goals for patients with brain metastases in this region include relief of neurological symptoms with cerebrospinal fluid diversion for relief of hydrocephalus, and long-term control of metastatic lesion.

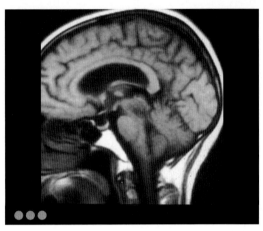

F1. Sagittal T1-weighted image shows a mass lesion involving the tectum of the midbrain (contrast enhancement of the mass is seen on the post-contrast study).

PINEAL CYST

Pineal cysts are commonly seen and are present in approximately 5% of MRIs and 20–40% of autopsy series. They are typically small in size (80% less than 1 cm) and are largely asymptomatic, especially when small. When larger they can present with mass effect on the tectum leading to compression of the superior colliculi and parinaud syndrome. Aqueductal compression by a large pineal cyst can cause obstructive hydrocephalus. Rarely hemorrhage into a pineal cyst can cause rapid expansion of the cyst.

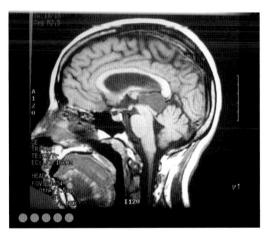

G1. Sagittal and axial T1-weighted images show a cystic mass in the pineal region. The lesion is of slightly higher signal intensity as compared to CSF, probably due to its protein content.

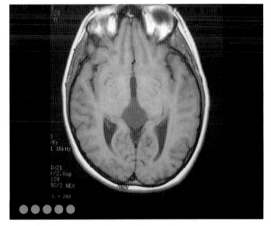

G2. Sagittal and axial T1-weighted images show a cystic mass in the pineal region. The lesion is of slightly higher signal intensity as compared to CSF, probably due to its protein content.

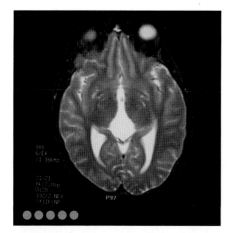

G3. Axial T2-weighted and FLAIR images reveal a hyperintense cystic lesion in the pineal region.

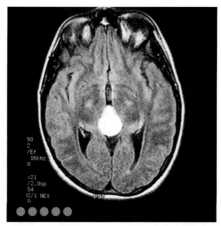

G4. Axial T2-weighted and FLAIR images reveal a hyperintense cystic lesion in the pineal region.

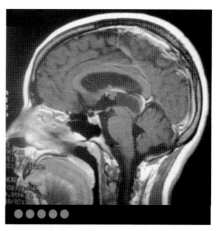

G5. Sagittal, post-contrast T1-weighted image shows no enhancement of the cyst. Enhancement of the adjacent veins is seen.

PINEAL PARENCHYMAL TUMOR OF INTERMEDIATE DIFFERENTIATION

Pineal parenchymal tumor of intermediate differentiation are highly cellular tumors. They may exhibit mild nuclear atypia with occasional mitotic figures. Pineocytomatous rosettes are absent. Unlike pineoblastomas, metastasis is uncommon in pineal paranchymal tumor of intermediate differentialion.

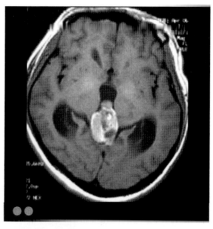

H1. Axial T1-weighted image shows a hyperintense mass in the pineal region.

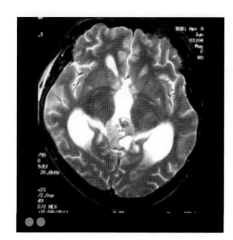

H2. Axial T2-weighted and FLAIR images show a hyperintense mass in the pineal region.

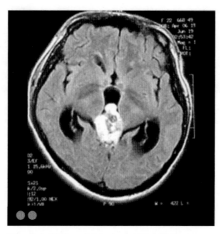

H3. Axial T2-weighted and FLAIR images show a hyperintense mass in the pineal region.

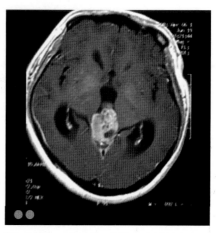

H4. Axial, post-contrast T1-weighted image demonstrates some enhancement of the pineal region mass.

271

PINEOBLASTOMA

Pineoblastomas affect male and female equally and are predominantly seen in the first and second decade. They are about six times more common than pineocytomas. The association of bilateral retinoblastoma with a pineoblas-toma was called trilateral retinoblastoma. Calcification may be seen in pineoblastoma. On MRI, they show hypointensity on T1-weighted images and hyperintensity on T2-weighted images. Contrast enhancement is seen.

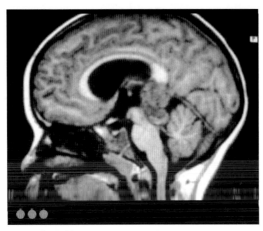

I1. Sagittal T1-weighted image shows a hypointense mass in the pineal region in a 12-year-old child.

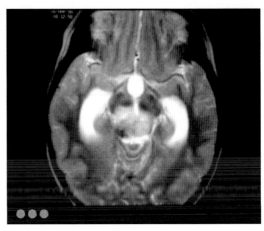

I2. Axial T2-weighted image shows a hyperintense mass with a focal area of hypointensity on the right side, which represents calcification. Note there is associated hydrocephalus.

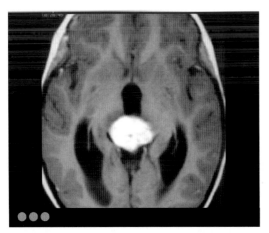

I3. Axial and sagittal, post-contrast T1-weighted images demonstrate intense enhancement of the mass.

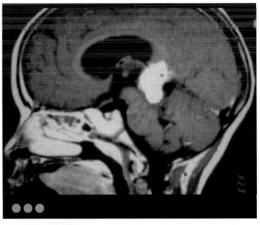

I4. Axial and sagittal, post-contrast T1-weighted images demonstrate intense enhancement of the mass.

PINEOCYTOMA

Pineocytmas are seen in males and females equally. They can be seen in any age group, but patients with pineocytma are generally older than patients with pineoblastomas. They are isointense to hyperintense on T1-weighted image and hyperintense on T2-weighted image. Contrast enhancement is seen. Tumor calcification may be seen.

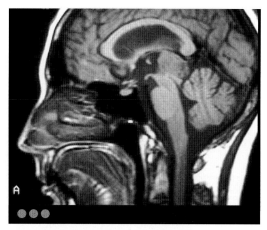

J1. Sagittal and axial T1-weighted image shows a slightly hypointense mass in the pineal region.

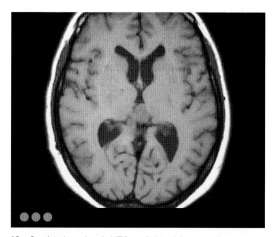

J2. Sagittal and axial T1-weighted image shows a slightly hypointense mass in the pineal region.

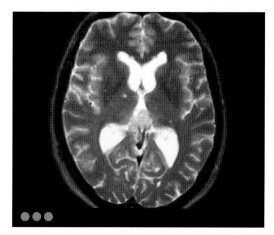

J3. Axial T2-weighted image demonstrates a hyperintense mass in the pineal region.

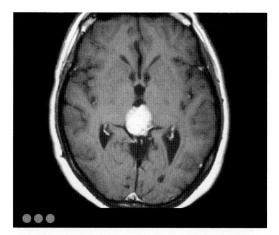

J4. Axial and sagittal, post-contrast T1-weighted image shows avid enhancement of the mass lesion.

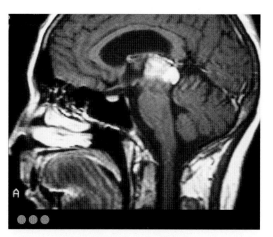

J5. Axial and sagittal, post-contrast T1-weighted image shows avid enhancement of the mass lesion.

TERATOMA

The pineal region is the most common site of **intracranial teratoma.** Pineal teratomas are seen exclusively in young males. MRI shows heterogeneous signal intensity mass on both T1- and T2-weighted images. Focal fat can be seen as high signal intensity area on T1-weighted images.

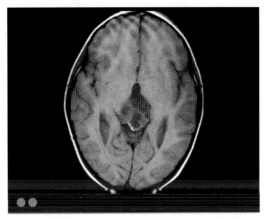

K1 Axial T1-weighted image shows heterogeneous mass with multicystic changes. Note the presence of a focal hyperintensity posteriorly on the right side, consistent with fat. Calcification is seen on CT, but not appreciated on MRI.

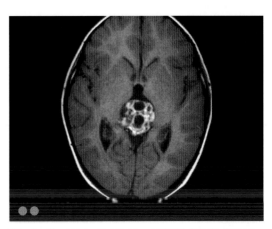

K2 Axial, post-contrast T1-weighted image demonstrates multiring-like enhancement of the mass.

TRILATERAL RETINOBLASTOMA

Retinoblastoma is the most common malignant intraocular neoplasm of childhood. The tumor is usually diagnosed during infancy, usually before the age of 3 years. Calcification in the globe is seen on CT scans. Calcification is seen in approximately 95% of retinoblastoma examined histologically and this explains the high incidence of calcification seen on CT scans.

The term trilateral retinoblastoma is used to refer to the presence of bilateral retinoblastomas with an associ-

ated midline, primary intracranial neoplasm of primitive type (usually in the pineal region but occasionally in the suprasellar or parasellar region). Such a coexistent intracranial neoplasm is found in approximately 2–11% of patients with bilateral retinoblastoma. The intracranial tumor is considered a lesion distinct from the intraocular neoplasms, not a metastasis. There is usually a latent period between diagnosis of the intraocular tumor and a coexistent intracranial tumor, usually about one year.

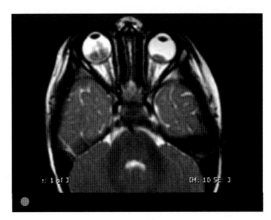

L1. Axial T2-weighted image shows abnormal signal in the posterior aspect of the globes bilaterally.

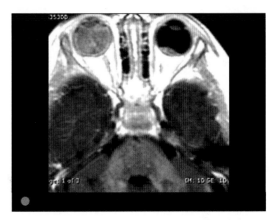

L2. Axial, post-contrast T1-weighted image shows abnormal enhancement involving both globes.

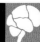

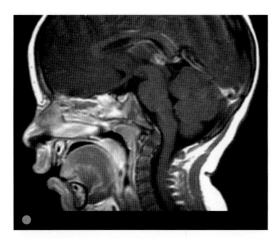

L3. Sagittal, post-contrast T1-weighted image shows an enhancing mass in the pineal region, consistent with pineoblastoma.

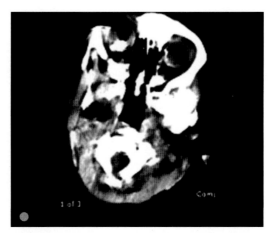

L4. Axial CT shows calcifications in the posterior aspect of both globes.

VEIN OF GALEN MALFORMATION

The vein of Galen malformation is a choroidal type of arteriovenous malformation involving the vein of Galen. It results from an aneurysmal malformation with an arteriovenous shunting of blood. The congenital malformation develops during weeks 6–11 of gestational age as a persistent embryonic prosencephalic vein of Markowski. Vein of Galen malformation is actually a misnomer. The vein of Markowski actually drains into the vein of Galen.

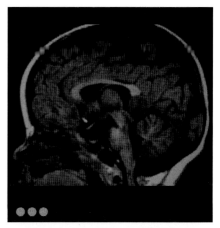

M1. Sagittal T1-weighted image shows a hypointense mass in the pineal region.

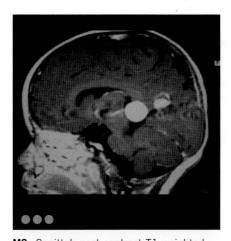

M2. Sagittal, post-contrast T1-weighted image reveals an avidly enhancing mass lesion in the pineal region.

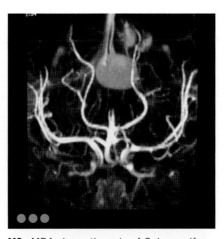

M3. MRA shows the vein of Galen malformation.

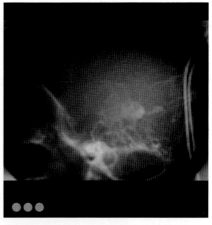

M4. Lateral view of cerebral angiogram shows a faintly filling vein of Galen malformation.

275

LYMPHOMA

Ependymal enhancement due to lymphoma is usually more irregular as compared to infectious etiology. Ependymal enhancement is more likely due to lymphoma in patients infected with human immunodeficiency virus although infectious etiology can also cause ependymal enhancement.

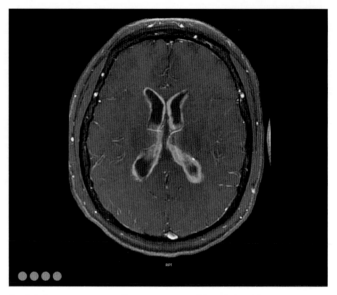

A. Axial, post-contrast, fat-suppressed T1-weighted image shows diffuse periventricular enhancement in a patient with lymphoma

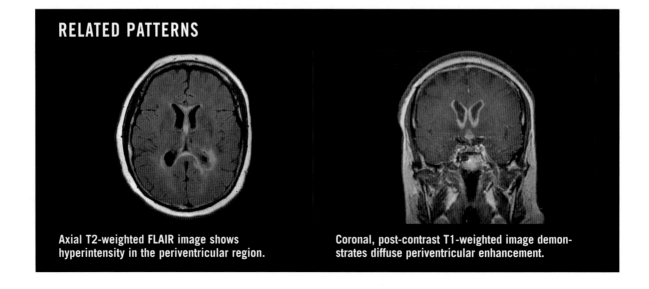

RELATED PATTERNS

Axial T2-weighted FLAIR image shows hyperintensity in the periventricular region.

Coronal, post-contrast T1-weighted image demonstrates diffuse periventricular enhancement.

At a Glance:

- *Metastatic Disease (Breast Carcinoma)*
- *Subependymal Spread of GBM*
- *Ventriculitis*

METASTATIC DISEASE (BREAST CARCINOMA)

Metastatic disease to the ependyma may arise through hematogenous spread of tumor to the brain and ventricles, or dissemination of malignant cells by cerebrospinal fluid (CSF) pathways. The ependymal enhancement due to metastatic disease is usually more nodular and irregular in contour as compared to the infectious etiology.

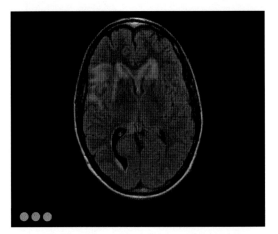

B1. Axial T2 FLAIR image shows periventricular hyperintensity. A focal hypointense lesion with surrounding edema is seen in the right frontal region.

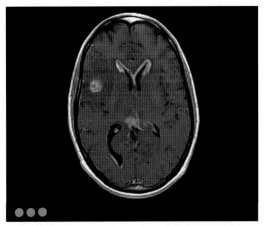

B2. Axial, post-contrast T1-weighted image shows diffuse periventricular enhancement. In addition, an enhancing lesion is seen in the right frontal region.

SUBEPENDYMAL SPREAD OF GBM

Glioblastoma multiforme (GBM) is the most common intracranial primary malignant glioma. It may spread via cerebrospinal fluid pathways. Only less than 2% of GBMs exhibit cerebrospinal fluid seeding, either within the central nervous system or through ventriculoperitoneal shunts into the abdomen. Subependymal spread of GBM is an uncommon but characteristic pattern of dissemination that correlates with a poor prognosis.

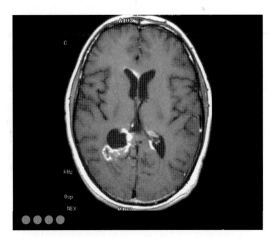

C. Axial, post-contrast T1-weighted image shows irregular enhancment in the periventricular region with focal nodular lesion in the right periatrial region.

VENTRICULITIS

Ventriculitis, or ependymitis, is an inflammation of the ependymal lining of the ventricular system. Spread of infection to the ventricles may result from rupture of a periventricular abscess or from retrograde spread of infection from the basal cisterns by way of the fourth ventricle. MRI studies may show marginal ventricular abnormality or only slightly increased signal intensity in the region of affected ependyma on T2-weighted FLAIR images. The fluid within the ventricles may show slightly increased intensity, indicating the presence of cells and inflammatory debris as well as increased protein concentration in the CSF.

Contrast-enhanced MRI studies show uniform, thin ependymal enhancement.

VENTRICULITIS (CASE ONE)

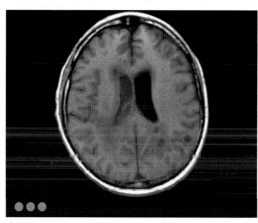

D1. Axial T1-weighted image shows mixed signal intensity in the right lateral ventricle. In addition, three small low signal areas are seen in the left parietal region.

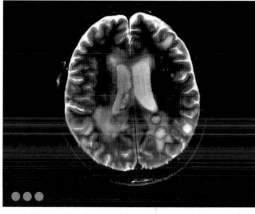

D2. Axial T2-weighted image shows periventricular hyperintensity. Three round cystic areas are seen in the left parietal region.

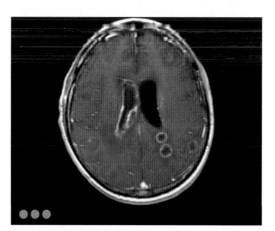

D3. Axial and coronal, post-contrast T1-weighted image demonstrates diffuse periventricular enhancement involving the right lateral ventricle. In addition, three ring-like enhancing lesions are seen in the left parietal region, consistent with abscesses. A fourth abscess is seen in the right parietal region.

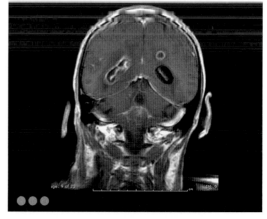

D4. Axial and coronal, post-contrast T1-weighted image demonstrates diffuse periventricular enhancement involving the right lateral ventricle. In addition, three ring-like enhancing lesions are seen in the left parietal region, consistent with abscesses. A fourth abscess is seen in the right parietal region.

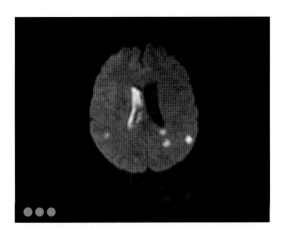

D5. Diffusion-weighted image shows right lateral ventricle containing pus with restricted diffusion. The three small abscesses also contain pus with restricted diffusion and a single very small abscess shows some restricted diffusion.

VENTRICULITIS (CMV) (CASE TWO)

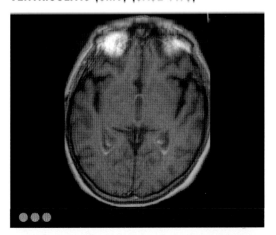

E1. Axial and coronal, post-contrast T1-weighted images show diffuse periventricular enhancement.

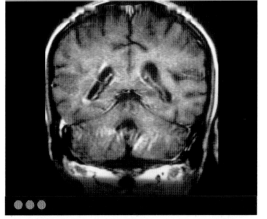

E2. Axial and coronal, post-contrast T1-weighted images show diffuse periventricular enhancement.

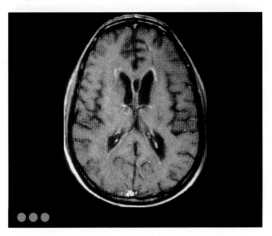

E3. Axial and coronal, post-contrast T1-weighted images show diffuse periventricular enhancement.

Chapter 6

Sellar and Parasellar Masses

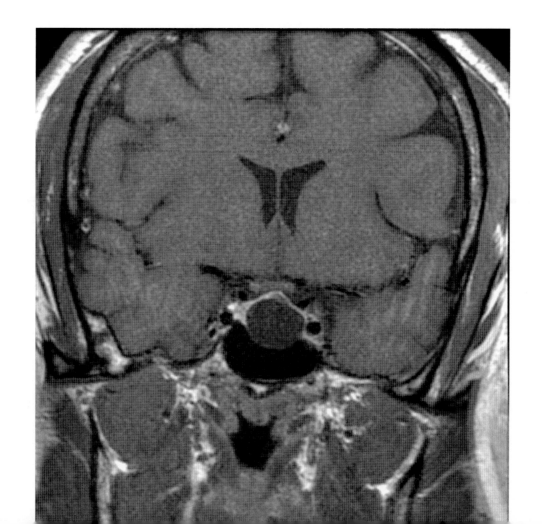

RATHKE'S CLEFT CYST

Rathke's cleft cysts are lined by columnar or cuboidal epithelium. Cystic fluid within the Rathke's cleft cysts varies from serous to mucoid. Therefore, they are of variable signal intensity on MRI studies. Cyst with low protein content appears hypointense on T1-weighted images and hyperintense on T2-weighted images. Cyst fluid containing free methemoglobin or high protein concentration shows hyperintensity on both T1- and T2-weighted images. A cyst containing very high protein concentration appears hyperintense on T1-weighted images and hypointense on T2-weighted images. A mild rim of contrast enhancement is occasionally seen following the administration of contrast material. Approximately 70% of the Rathke's cleft cysts are both intra- and suprasellar; 25% are intrasellar; and 5% are completely suprasellar.

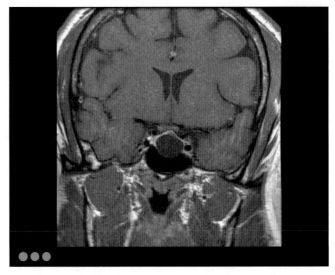

A. Coronal, post-contrast T1-weighted image shows a hypointense, cystic mass with peripheral rim enhancement in the sellar turcica.

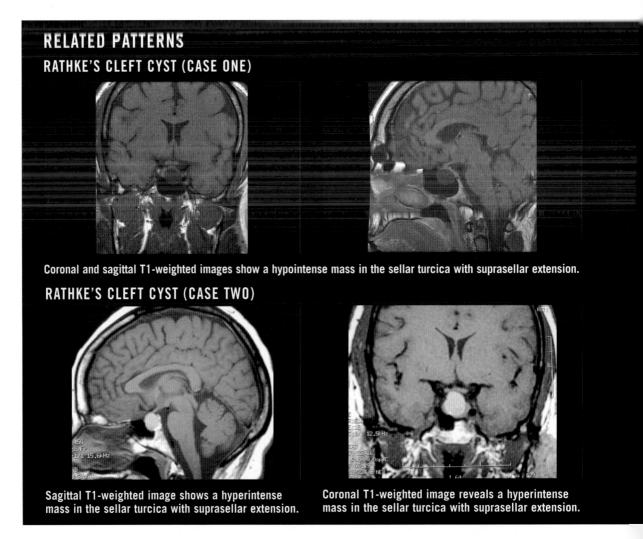

RELATED PATTERNS

RATHKE'S CLEFT CYST (CASE ONE)

Coronal and sagittal T1-weighted images show a hypointense mass in the sellar turcica with suprasellar extension.

RATHKE'S CLEFT CYST (CASE TWO)

Sagittal T1-weighted image shows a hyperintense mass in the sellar turcica with suprasellar extension.

Coronal T1-weighted image reveals a hyperintense mass in the sellar turcica with suprasellar extension.

RATHKE'S CLEFT CYST (CASE TWO) (continued)

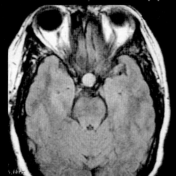

Axial T2-weighted FLAIR image shows a hyperintense mass in the sellar turcica with suprasellar extension

RATHKE'S CLEFT CYST (CASE THREE)

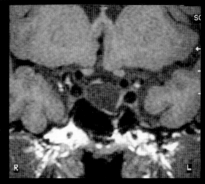

Coronal T1-weighted images show a hypointense mass in the sellar turcica with suprasellar extension.

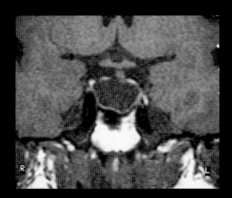

Coronal T1-weighted images show a hypointense mass in the sellar turcica with suprasellar extension.

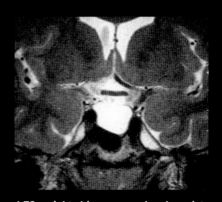

Coronal T2-weighted image reveals a hyperintense mass in the sellar turcica with suprasellar extension.

ABSCESS

Pituitary abscess is a rare disease and its clinical presentations are often non-specific. Pituitary abscess can occur denovo in an otherwise normal pituitary gland or less frequently in a pre-existing pathology. Its intensity on T1 weighted or T2 weighted MRI images is variable probably related to its protein content. Enhancement of the abscess capsule and residual pituitary gland may be seen on the post-contrast images and it often shows an incomplete ring-like enhancement.

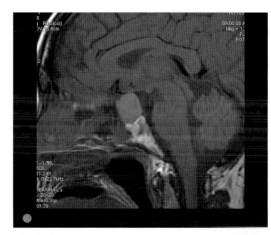

B1. Sagittal and coronal T1 weighted images show a hyperintense mass in the sellar and suprasellar region with enlargement of the sellar turcica and compression of the optic chiasm.

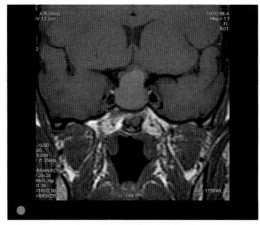

B2. Sagittal and coronal T1 weighted images show a hyperintense mass in the sellar and suprasellar region with enlargement of the sellar turcica and compression of the optic chiasm.

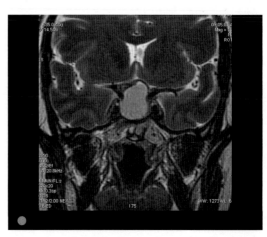

B3. Coronal T2 weighted image shows a hyperintense mass in the sellar and suprasellar region.

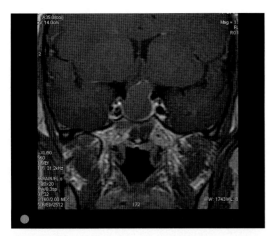

B4. Sagittal and coronal, post-contrast T1 weighted images demonstrate an incomplete ring enhancement of the sellar and suprasellar lesion.

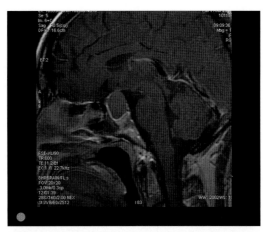

B5. Sagittal and coronal, post-contrast T1 weighted images demonstrate an incomplete ring enhancement of the sellar and suprasellar lesion.

ANEURYSM

Intracranial aneurysms are classified into saccular and nonsaccular types on the based on their shape and etiology. Nonsaccular aneurysms include atherosclerotic, fusiform, traumatic, and mycotic types. Saccular, or berry, aneurysms are considered to be developmental and have several anatomic characteristics that distinguish them from other types of intracranial aneurysms. Typically, saccular aneurysms arise at a bifurcation or along a curve of the parent vessel, or they point in the direction in which flow would proceed if the curve were not present. The incidence of intracranial aneurysms is increased in patients with connective tissue disorders, such as Marfan's syndrome, Ehlers Danlos syndrome, polycystic kidney disease, coarctation of the aorta, and intracranial arteriovenous malformations. Saccular aneurysms are seen most frequently at the anterior communicating artery (35%), followed by internal carotid/posterior communicating artery (35%), middle cerebral artery (20%), basilar tip (5%) and other vertebrobasilar arteries (5%).

A giant aneurysm is defined as one larger than 2.5 cm in diameter. There is increased morbidity and mortality associated with the treatment of giant aneurysms as compared to smaller ones. Giant aneurysms are thought to represent approximately 5–8% of all intracranial aneurysms. About 25% of giant aneurysms present with subarachnoid hemorrhage and the remaining present with focal mass effect with consequent visual failure, cranial nerve dysfunction, hemiparesis, seizure or headache. Thombus formation may be seen in giant aneurysms. Stroke can occur as embolus from the breakdown of the thrombus within the giant aneurysm can cause occlusion of small arteries. 60% of giant aneurysm occur on the Internal carotid artery, 10% in the anteior communicating artery region, 10% in the middle cerebral artery, 15% at the tip of basilar artery, and the remaining 5% at the vertebral artery.

ANEURYSM (CASE ONE)

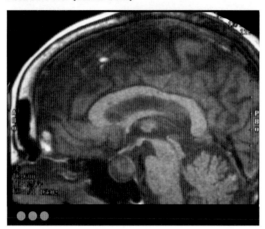

C1. Sagittal T1-weighted image shows a mixed hypointense to isointense lesion in the sellar region.

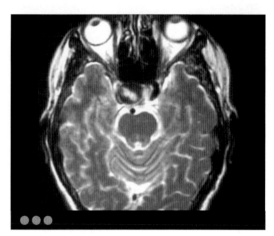

C2. Axial T2-weighted image shows a round lesion with central hyperintensity and peripheral hypointensity in the sellar region.

ANEURYSM (CASE TWO)

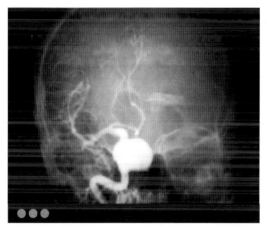

C3. Cerebral angiogram demonstrates an aneurysm in the sellar region.

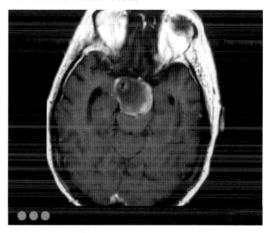

D1. Axial and sagittal T1-weighted image shows a sellar and suprasellar mass with hypointense center and hyperintense rim.

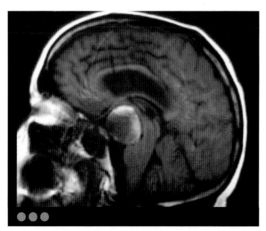

D2. Axial and sagittal T1-weighted image shows a sellar and suprasellar mass with hypointense center and hyperintense rim.

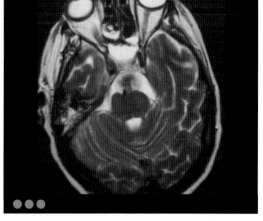

D3. Axial T2-weighted image shows mixed signal intensity lesion in the sellar region.

CRANIOPHARYNGIOMAS

Craniopharyngiomas can be histologically classified into three types: adamantinomatous, papillary, and mixed. The adamantinomatous type is predominantly seen in children (92–96%). Grossly, these tumors usually have both solid and cystic components. The fluid within the cysts has been historically described as "crankcase oil" because of its frequently dark and oily intraoperative appearance. The papillary type of craniopharyngiomas is more frequently seen in adults. They are well-circumscribed, pure, and solid masses. On MRI, the solid component of the tumor is inhomogeneous and shows variable contrast enhancement, whereas the cystic component may be lined by similar epithelial cells containing desquamated keratin, cellular debris, cholesterol crystals, and lipids in solution, blood products, and protein. Various signal intensity patterns on T1- and T2-weighted MRI images have been attributed to the various composition of cyst fluid. Hemorrhage within the cystic component of the craniopharyngioma can occasionally occur.

CRANIOPHARYNGIOMA (CASE ONE)

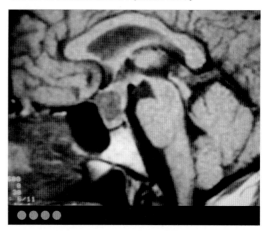

E1. Sagittal and coronal T1-weighted images show a cystic mass in the sellar turcica with suprasellar extension and compression of the optic chiasm.

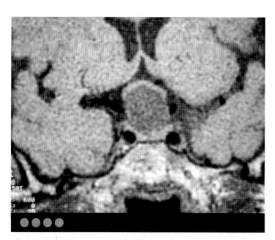

E2. Sagittal and coronal T1-weighted images show a cystic mass in the sellar turcica with suprasellar extension and compression of the optic chiasm.

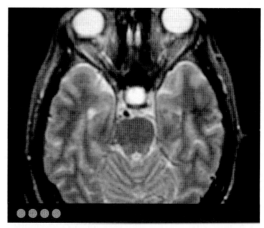

E3. Axial T2-weighted image reveals a hyperintense cystic mass in the sellar turcica.

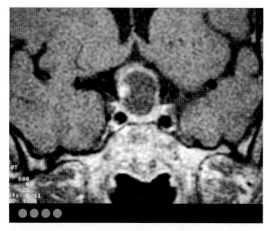

E4. Coronal and sagittal, post-contrast T1-weighted image demonstrates peripheral enhancement of the mass with a nodular area on the right side.

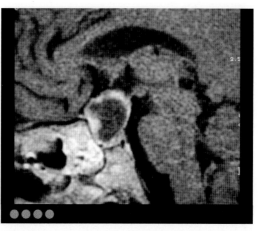

E5. Coronal and sagittal, post-contrast T1-weighted image demonstrates peripheral enhancement of the mass with a nodular area on the right side.

CRANIOPHARYNGIOMA (CASE TWO)

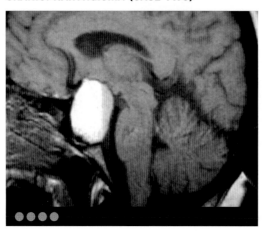

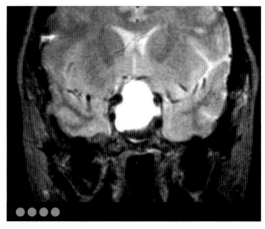

F1. Sagittal T1-weighted image shows a hyperintense mass in the sellar suprasellar region. Note there is a fluid–fluid level within the cystic mass.

F2. Coronal T2-weighted image reveals a hyperintense sellar and suprasellar mass.

CRANIOPHARYNGIOMA (CASE THREE)

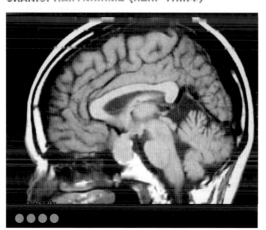

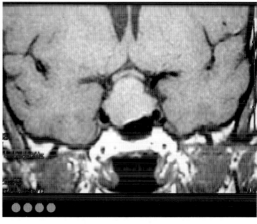

G1. Sagittal and coronal T1-weighted images show a slightly hyperintense mass in the sellar and suprasellar region.

G2. Sagittal and coronal T1-weighted images show a slightly hyperintense mass in the sellar and suprasellar region.

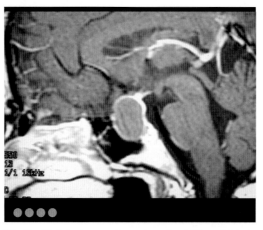

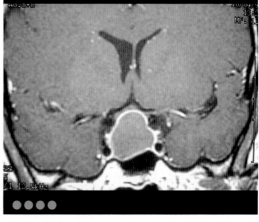

G3. Sagittal and coronal, post-contrast T1-weighted images show rim enhancement of the mass lesion.

G4. Sagittal and coronal, post-contrast T1-weighted images show rim enhancement of the mass lesion.

PITUITARY ADENAOMA

Most pituitary adenomas are slow-growing and tend to grow in an upward direction into the suprasellar cistern. Intrasellar expansion of these adenomas may erode the sellar turcica and compress the cavernous sinuses laterally. Most expanding adenomas demonstrate a globular configuration. The diaphragm sellae may cause a waistline indentation between the intrasellar and suprasellar components of large adenoma, resulting in "hourglass" configuration. In some cases, nodular outgrowth of the suprasellar component of the adenoma result in a multilobulated adenoma that can further extend in a subfrontal, middle cranial fossa or retrosellar direction. Nodular outgrowth arising from the intrasellar component of the adenoma may destroy adjacent structures by invading them. Occasion-ally, cystic component of the adenoma may be seen. Pituitary adenomas can be defined by their sizes. Microade-nomas are defined as intrasellar adenomas up to 10 mm in diameter without sellar enlargement or suprasellar extension. Macroadenomas cause symptoms of mass effect, such as headache or visual loss and measure greater than 10 mm in diameter.

The word apoplexy is defined as a sudden onset of neurologic impairment, usually caused by a vascular process. Pituitary apoplexy is characterized by a sudden onset of headache, visual field and visual acuity impair-ment, altered mental status, and hormonal dysfunction due to acute hemorrhage or infarction of a pre-existing pituitary adenoma. Diffusion weighted imaging has been advocated by some authors for early detection of pituitary tumor infarction.

RELATED PATTERNS
CASE ONE (LARGE MACROADENOMA)

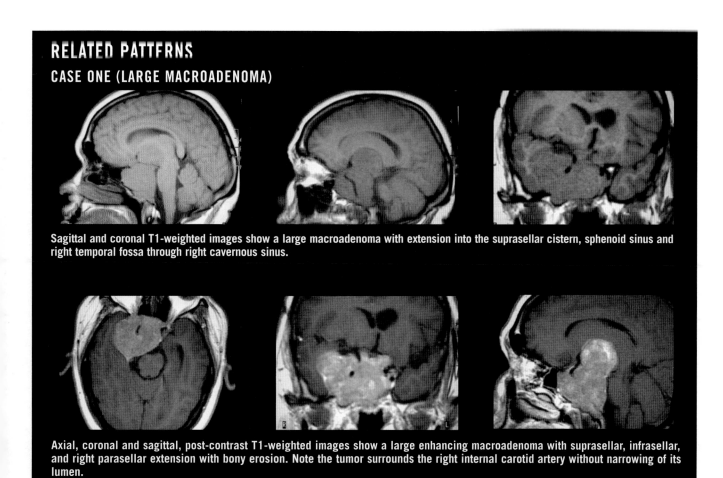

Sagittal and coronal T1-weighted images show a large macroadenoma with extension into the suprasellar cistern, sphenoid sinus and right temporal fossa through right cavernous sinus.

Axial, coronal and sagittal, post-contrast T1-weighted images show a large enhancing macroadenoma with suprasellar, infrasellar, and right parasellar extension with bony erosion. Note the tumor surrounds the right internal carotid artery without narrowing of its lumen.

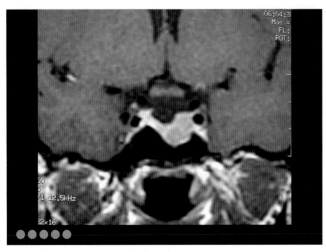

A. Coronal, post-contrast T1-weighted image shows a pituitary microadenoma on the left side of sella turcica, which shows less contrast enhancement than the normal pituitary. The patient had elevated level of prolectin.

RELATED PATTERNS (oontinuod)

CASE TWO (PITUITARY ADENOMA DISPLACING THE GLAND SUPERIORLY)

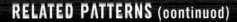

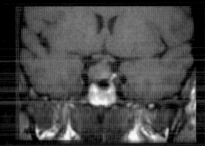

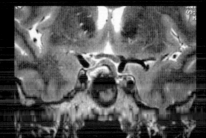

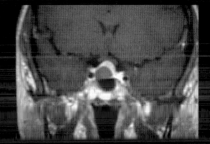

Coronal T1-weighted image shows an isointense mass in the sellar turcica.

Coronal T2-weighted image reveals a hyperintense mass displacing the gland superiorly.

Coronal, post-contrast T1-weighted image shows intense enhancement of the pituitary gland and relatively less enhancement of the tumor.

CASE THREE (PITUITARY ADENOMA WITH INFRASELLAR LOCATION)

PITUITARY APOPLEXY (CASE ONE)

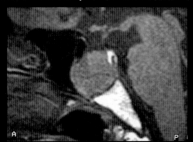

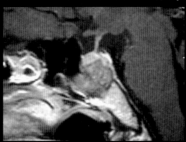

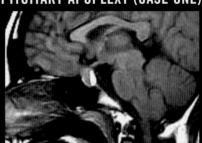

Sagittal T1-weighted image shows an isointense mass in the enlarged sellar turcica.

Sagittal, post-contrast T1-weighted image shows infrasellar location of the pituitary tumor with the more prominantly enhancing pituitary gland situated superiorly.

Sagittal, coronal and axial T1-weighted images demonstrate hyperintensity posteriorly in the pituitary tumor presenting a blood–fluid level.

PITUITARY APOPLEXY (CASE ONE) (continued)

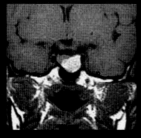

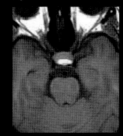

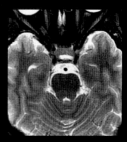

Sagittal, coronal and axial T1-weighted images demonstrate hyperintensity posteriorly in the pituitary tumor presenting a blood–fluid level.

Axial T2-weighted image shows hyperintenisty posteriorly in the pituitary tumor in conjunction with the hyperintensity seen on T1-weighted images, indicating the presence of hemorrhage within the pituitary tumor in the stage of extracellular methemoglobin.

PITUITARY APOPLEXY (CASE TWO)

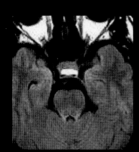

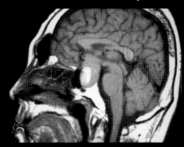

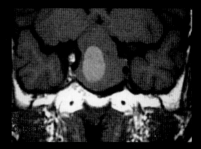

Axial FLAIR image shows hyperintensity posteriorly in the pituitary tumor as seen on T2 weighted image.

Sagittal and coronal T1 weighted images show a large pituitary adenoma with enlargement of the sellar turcica and suprasellar extension. Note the presence of an ovoid hyperintense area at the anterior, inferior aspect of the tumor, indicating the presence of hemorrhage.

RELATED PATTERNS (continued)
PITUITARY APOPLEXY (CASE TWO) (continued)

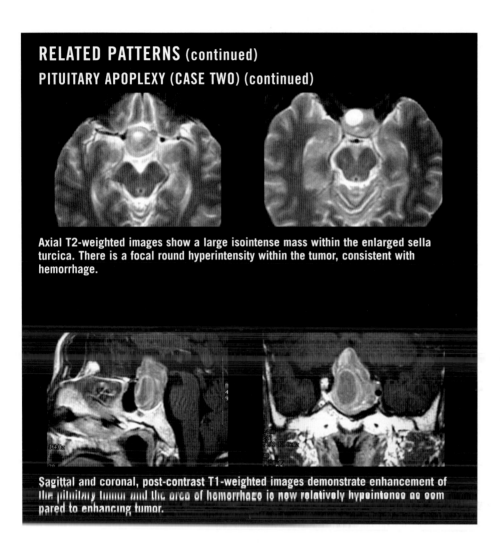

Axial T2-weighted images show a large isointense mass within the enlarged sella turcica. There is a focal round hyperintensity within the tumor, consistent with hemorrhage.

Sagittal and coronal, post-contrast T1-weighted images demonstrate enhancement of the pituitary tumor and the area of hemorrhage is now relatively hypointense as compared to enhancing tumor.

DIFFERENTIAL DIAGNOSIS

At a Glance:

- Craniopharyngioma
- Hemangiopericytoma
- Lymphocytic Adenohypophysistis
- Meningioma
- Metastatic Prostate Carcinoma
- Mixed Germ Cell Tumor
- Pituitary Carcinoma
- Sarcoid (not pictured)
- Fungal Infection (not pictured)
- Tuberculosis (not pictured)

CRANIOPHARYNGIOMA

Craniopharyngioma is a slow-growing, extra-axial, epithelial-squamous, calcified cystic tumor arising from remnants of the craniopharyngeal duct and/or Rathke cleft. They are seen in the sellar and suprasellar region. The most common type is adamantinomatous type and is frequently seen in children. The papillary type is more frequently seen in adults (40–60 years of age) and is formed of masses of metaplastic squamous cells. They tend to be solid in appearance, and less likely to calcify.

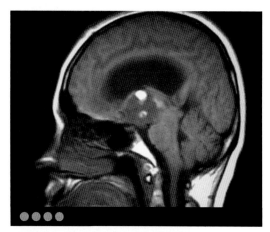

B1. Sagittal T1-weighted image shows a hypointense mass with focal hyperintense areas (fat) in the suprasellar cistern.

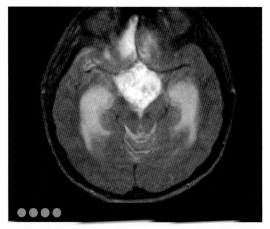

B2. Axial T2-weighted image shows a hyperintense mass in the suprasellar cistern.

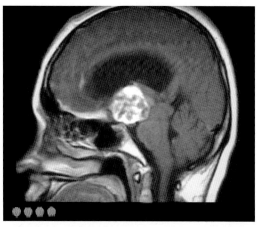

B3. Sagittal, coronal, axial, post-contrast T1-weighted images demonstrate a patchy enhancing mass in the suprasellar cistern.

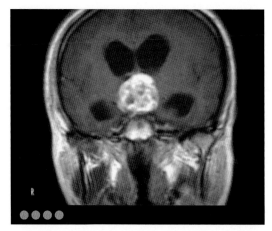

B4. Sagittal, coronal, axial, post-contrast T1-weighted images demonstrate a patchy enhancing mass in the suprasellar cistern.

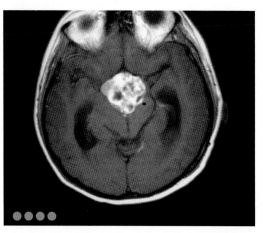

B5. Sagittal, coronal, axial, post-contrast T1-weighted images demonstrate a patchy enhancing mass in the suprasellar cistern.

HEMANGIOPERICYTOMA

Hemangiopericytoma is a neoplasm assumed to originate from pericytes. Pericytes are cells of mesodermal origin surrounding blood capillaries. Hemangiopericytoma is a potentially malignant vascular neoplasm that rarely occur intracranially. When they do occur in the intracranial com- partment, they are most often meningeal in origin. Hemangiopericytoma arising within the sellar turcica is an even more sporadic event. Morphologically, these are well-circumscribed tumors characterized by a thin walled branching vascular pattern surrounded by closely packed plump to spindled tumor cells with usually ovoid nuclei and indistinct cytoplasmic margins.

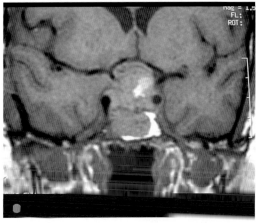

C1. Coronal and sagittal T1-weighted images show a large, isointense sellar mass with suprasellar exten- sion and focal hyperintense areas consistent with hemorrhage. Compression of the optic chiasm is seen.

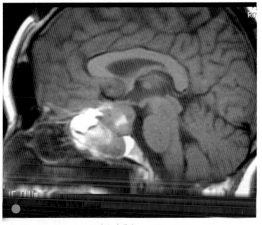

C2. Coronal and sagittal T1-weighted images show a large, isointense sellar mass with suprasellar exten- sion and focal hyperintense areas consistent with hemorrhage. Compression of the optic chiasm is seen.

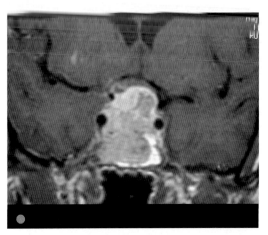

C3. Coronal and sagittal, post-contrast T1-weighted images demonstrate enhancement of the mass.

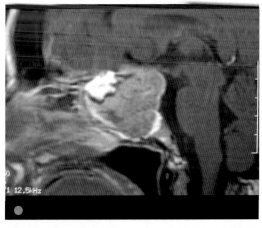

C4. Coronal and sagittal, post-contrast T1-weighted images demonstrate enhancement of the mass.

LYMPHOCYTIC ADENOHYPOPHYSISTIS

Lymphocytic adenohypophysistis is presumably an autoimmune disorder; it has been diagnosed primarily in women who were or had recently been pregnant. It may also present in women with no recent history of pregnancy, in postmenopausal women, and even in men. Pathologic study of the involved gland reveals a varying degree of infiltration by lymphocytes and other inflammatory cells as well as associated fibrotic changes.

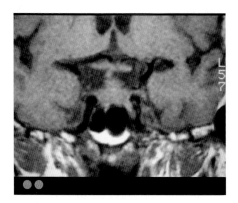

D1. Coronal T1-weighted image shows a sellar mass with suprasellar extension.

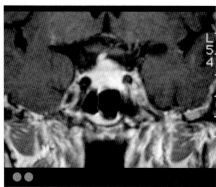

D2. Coronal and sagittal, post-contrast T1-weighted images demonstrate avid enhancement of the mass extending into the pituitary stalk.

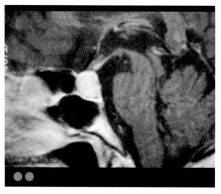

D3. Coronal and sagittal, post-contrast T1 weighted images demonstrate avid enhancement of the mass extending into the pituitary stalk.

MENINGIOMA

Meningiomas account for approximately 15% of the intracranial neoplasms. They are benign, encapsulated tumors attached to the dura. Suprasellar meningiomas usually arise from the tuberculum sellae or the sulcus chiasmatis. Due to its proximity to the optic chiasm, suprasellar meningiomas frequently cause compression of the chiasm or nerves even when the tumors are still small in size.

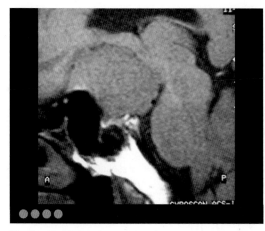

E1. Sagittal T1-weighted image shows an isointense suprasellar mass extending toward the planum sphenoidale. Note the brainstem is displaced posteriorly.

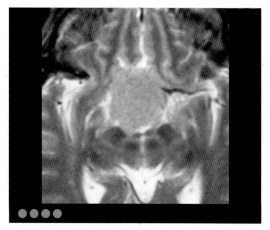

E2. Axial T2-weighted image reveals an isointense mass in the suprasellar cistern.

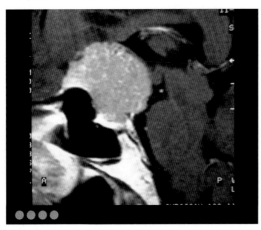

E3. Sagittal and coronal, post-contrast T1-weighted images demonstrate a homogeneously enhancing mass in the suprasellar cistern.

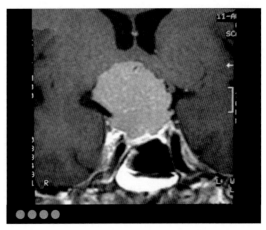

E4. Sagittal and coronal, post-contrast T1-weighted images demonstrate a homogeneously enhancing mass in the suprasellar cistern. Compression of the optic chiasm and nerves is clearly seen.

METASTATIC PROSTATE CARCINOMA

The pituitary gland is an uncommon site for metastasis. In surgical series, it is detected in less than 1% of patients subjected to transsphenoidal surgery for sellar or parasellar tumors. In autopsy series, pituitary metastasis is seen in approximately 5% of patients with known malignancy. In breast cancer patients, the incidence is significantly higher. Neoplasms from almost every tissue have been reported to metastasize to the pituitary. Breast and lung cancer account for approximately two thirds of all metastatic tumors to the pituitary.

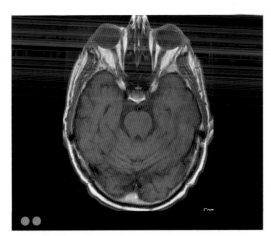

F1. Axial T1-weighted images show a hyperintense lesion in the sellar and suprasellar region.

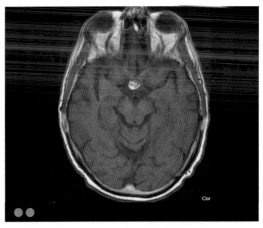

F2. Axial T1-weighted images show a hyperintense lesion in the sellar and suprasellar region.

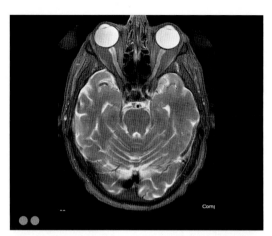

F3. Axial T2-weighted images reveal a hypointense mass in the sellar and suprasellar region.

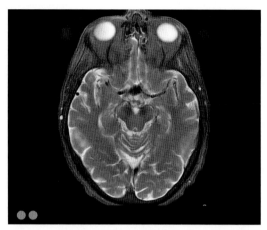

F4. Axial T2-weighted images reveal a hypointense mass in the sellar and suprasellar region.

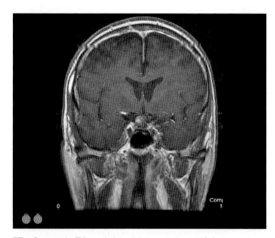

F5. Coronal, T1-weighted image shows faint enhancement of the mass lesion

MIXED GERM CELL TUMOR

Germ cell tumors make up 0.3–3% of pediatric brain tumors. There is a higher incidence in the Japanese and Chinese population. The majority of germ cell tumors (45%) are germinomas. Mixed germ cell tumors are uncommon. The suprasellar region is the second most common location for these tumors, second only to the pineal region. Germinomas in the pineal region, the third ventricle are predominantly seen in males whereas suprasellar Germinomas are equally seen in males and females. Suprasellar germinomas cause three symptoms: diabetes insipidus, visual disturbances, and pituitary dysfunction.

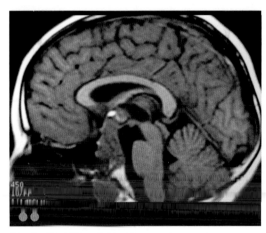

G1. Sagittal T1-weighted image shows a hypo-intense mass in the enlarged sellar turcica with suprasellar extension.

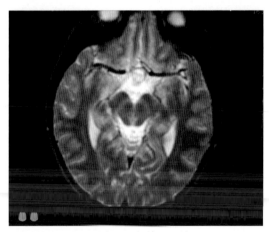

G2. Axial T2-weighted image reveals a hyperintense mass in the suprasellar cistern.

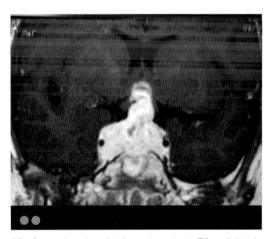

G3. Coronal and sagittal, post-contrast T1-weighted images demonstrate an enhancing mass in the enlarged sellar turcica with suprasellar extension.

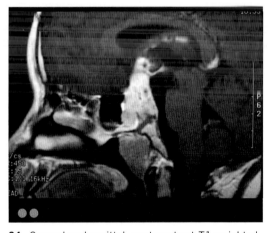

G4. Coronal and sagittal, post-contrast T1-weighted images demonstrate an enhancing mass in the enlarged sellar turcica with suprasellar extension.

PITUITARY CARCINOMA

The great majority of **pituitary tumors** are noninvasive benign pituitary adenomas that either remain within the sella or may exhibit invasive growth to surrounding tissue. Approximately 45–55% of the cases, can become invasive, infiltrating dura, bone, and/or surrounding structures.

However, such pituitary tumors are not considered to be malignant, even when extensive dural invasion is seen; true carcinomas are defined only by the presence of craniospinal and/or systemic metastases. A number of studies have suggested an incidence of pituitary carcinoma of less than 0.5% of symptomatic pituitary tumors, probably in the region of 0.2%.

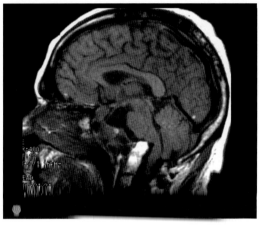

H1. Sagittal and coronal T1-weighted images show an irregular, heterogeneous mass in the region of sellar turcica with extension into the sphenoid sinus and bone destruction of the clivus.

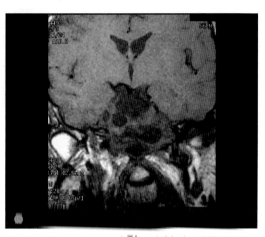

H2. Sagittal and coronal T1-weighted images show an irregular, heterogeneous mass in the region of sellar turcica with extension into the sphenoid sinus and bone destruction of the clivus.

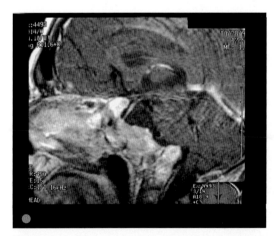

H3. Sagittal and coronal, post-contrast T1-weighted images show an irregular, heterogeneously enhancing mass in the region of sellar turcica with extension into the sphenoid sinus and bone destruction of the clivus.

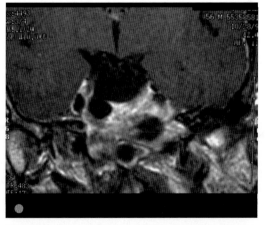

H4. Sagittal and coronal, post-contrast T1-weighted images show an irregular, heterogeneously enhancing mass in the region of sellar turcica with extension into the sphenoid sinus and bone destruction of the clivus.

MENINGIOMA

Meningiomas are the most common nonglial primary neoplasm of the central nervous system. Women are preferentially involved by a ratio of 2:1. Meningiomas arising from the tuberculum or diaphragma sellae may grow downward into the pituitary fossa, or grow upward into the suprasellar cistern. On MRI, an enhancing suprasellar mass associated with thickened and/or depressed diaphragma sellae is suggestive of meningioma. A separate normal pituitary gland can usually be identified.

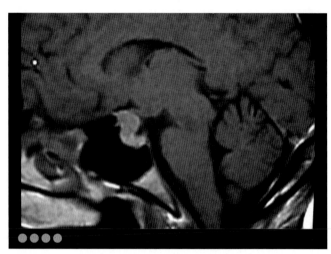

A. Sagittal, post-contrast T1-weighted image shows a small suprasellar mass with contrast enhancement. Note there is compression of the optic chiasm by the mass.

RELATED PATTERNS

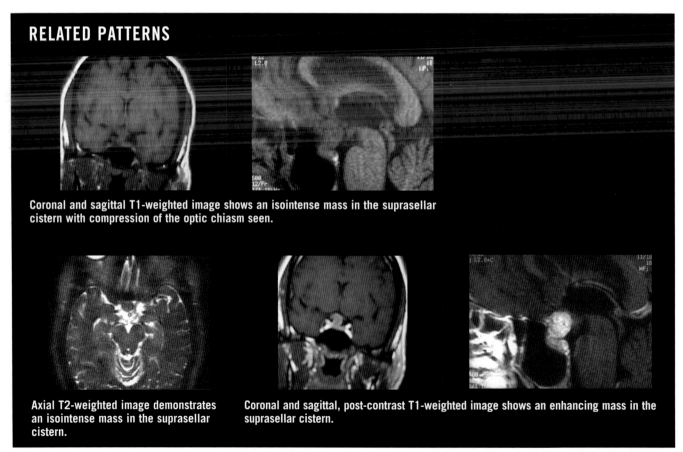

Coronal and sagittal T1-weighted image shows an isointense mass in the suprasellar cistern with compression of the optic chiasm seen.

Axial T2-weighted image demonstrates an isointense mass in the suprasellar cistern.

Coronal and sagittal, post-contrast T1-weighted image shows an enhancing mass in the suprasellar cistern.

DIFFERENTIAL DIAGNOSIS

At a Glance:

- *Aneurysm*
- *Cavernous Angioma*
- *Chordoid Glioma*
- *Craniopharyngiomas*
- *Germinoma*
- *Glioblastoma Multiforme (GBM)*
- *Hypothalamic Anaplastic Astrocytoma*
- *Hypothalamic Pilocytic Astrocytoma*
- *Hypothalamic Pilocytic Astrocytoma with Seeding*
- *Lymphoma*
- *Metastatic Disease (Renal Cell Carcinoma)*
- *Sarcoidosis*
- *Schistosomiasis*
- *Tuberculosis*

ANEURYSM

An **aneurysm** arising from the circle of Willis or cavernous internal carotid artery may project into the suprasellar cistern and/or sellar turcica. On MRI, most aneurysms appear as a well circumscribed, round mass in the sellar and suprasellar region. The MRI signal intensity of the aneurysm can be variable depending on the velocity of the flow in the aneurysm, and the presence or absence of the blood clot within the aneurysm.

A nonthrombosed aneurysm is readily detected on MRI as a typical flow void mass. However, the flow void may not be seen with gradient-echo T1-weighted images as in this case. Heterogeneous rings inside rings may be seen in the thrombosed aneurysm

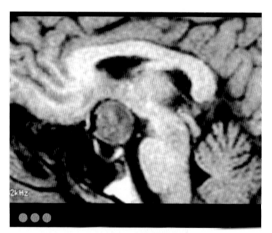

B1. Sagittal T1-weighted, gradient-echo image shows a hypointense suprasellar mass.

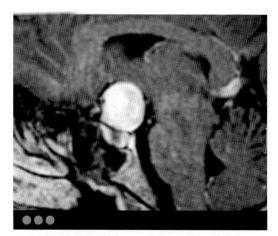

B2. Sagittal, post-contrast T1-weighted image shows intense enhancement of the mass.

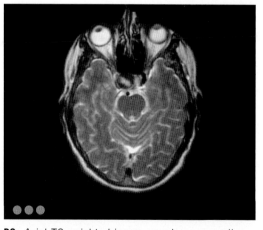

B3. Axial T2-weighted image reveals a suprasellar mass with mixed hypo- and hyperintensity.

301

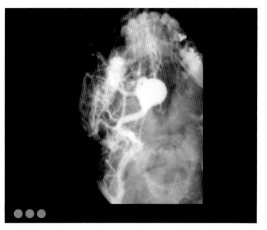

B4. Cerebral angiogram shows a suprasellar aneurysm.

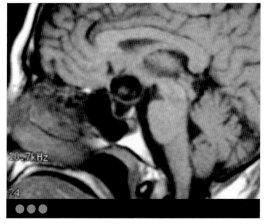

B5. Sagittal T1-weighted image shows a suprasellar mass with flow void.

CAVERNOUS ANGIOMA

Cavernous angiomas are developmental malformations of the vascular bed. A familial basis of this malformation has been reported. Cavernous angiomas are considered to be congenital vascular hamartomas composed of closely approximated endothelial-lined sinusoidal collections without significant amounts of interspersed normal neural tissue. These congenital abnormal vascular connections frequently enlarge over time. Approximately 80–90% of the malformations are supratentorial in location. The common supratentorial sites include the deep cerebral white matter, corticomedullary junction, and basal ganglia, the common posterior fossa sites include pons and cerebellar hemispheres. Intracranial extracerebral cavernous angiomas can also occur, but these are less common. They typically originate from the cavernous sinus and involve the middle cranial fossa. Suprasellar location is rare.

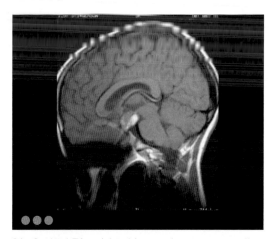

C1. Sagittal T1-weighted image shows a suprasellar mass with areas of hyperintensity, consistent with hemorrhage.

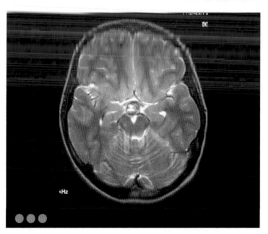

C2. Axial T2-weighted image reveals a heterogeneously hyperintense lesion in the suprasellar region.

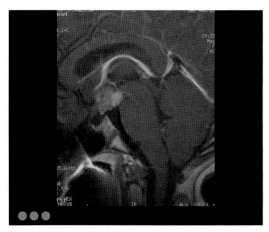

C3. Sagittal and coronal, post-contrast T1-weighted images demonstrate an enhancing mass in the suprasellar region.

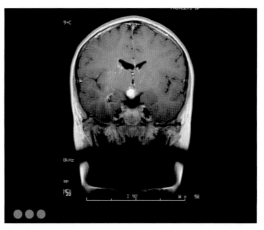

C4. Sagittal and coronal, post-contrast T1-weighted images demonstrate an enhancing mass in the suprasellar region.

CHORDOID GLIOMA

Chordoid glioma is an uncommon neoplasm subject to the hypothalamic, anterior third ventricular region. It is named chordoid glioma because of its distinctive histologic appearance, reminiscent of chordoma, and its avid staining with GFAP. On imaging, it appears as an ovoid, well-circumscribed mass with uniform and intense enhancement. It is isointense on T1-weighted images and iso- to slightly hyperintense on T2-weighted images.

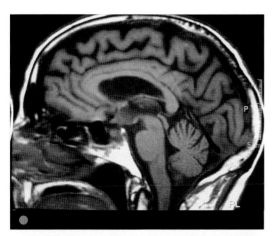

D1. Sagittal T1-weighted image shows an isointense mass in the suprasellar region.

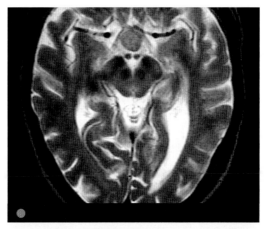

D2. Axial T2-weighted image shows an isointense lesion in the suprasellar region.

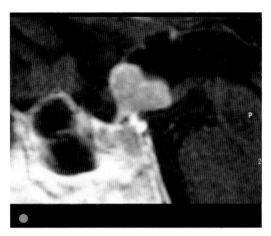

D3. Sagittal and coronal, post-contrast T1-weighted images demonstrate an enhancing mass in the suprasellar, hypothalamic region.

D4. Sagittal and coronal, post-contrast T1-weighted images demonstrate an enhancing mass in the suprasellar, hypothalamic region.

CRANIOPHARYNGIOMAS

Craniopharyngiomas originate from the remnants of Rathke's pouch. They represent 3–5% of primary intracranial neoplasms. They have a bimodal age distribution; more than half occur in children and young adults. A second smaller peak occurs in the fifth and sixth decade. Craniopharyngiomas are both intra- and suprasellar in about 70% of cases. They are suprasellar in only about 20% and intrasellar in 10% of cases. They are well-circumscribed, multilobulated masses with cystic and solid components. Calcification is present in 90% of the pediatric cases and 50% of the adult cases. Cystic masses are more frequently seen in children while the solid masses are seen predominantly in adult patients.

CRANIOPHARYNGIOMA (CASE ONE)

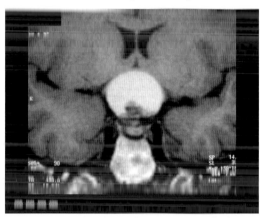

F1. Coronal and axial T1 weighted images show a hyperintense cystic mass in the suprasellar cistern with a small sold component seen at its inferior portion. Note the fluid–fluid level on the axial image.

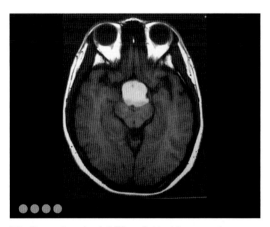

E2. Coronal and axial T1-weighted images show a hyperintense cystic mass in the suprasellar cistern with a small sold component seen at its inferior portion. Note the fluid–fluid level on the axial image.

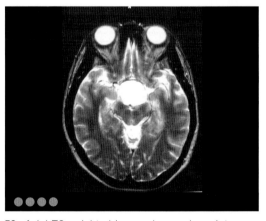

E3. Axial T2-weighted image shows a hyperintense, cystic lesion.

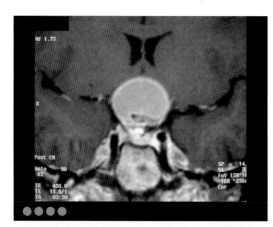

E4. Coronal and axial, post-contrast T1-weighted images demonstrate a rim enhancement of the cystic mass with enhancement of the inferiorly located solid component of the mass.

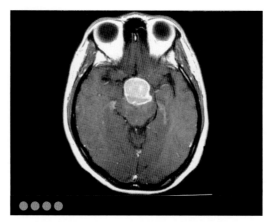

E5. Coronal and axial, post-contrast T1-weighted images demonstrate a rim enhancement of the cystic mass with enhancement of the inferiorly located solid component of the mass.

CRANIOPHARYNGIOMA (CASE TWO)

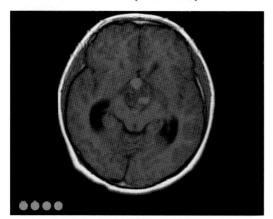

F1. Axial T1-weighted image shows a hypointense suprasellar mass with foci of hyperintensity, consistent with cystic areas containing proteinaceous fluid.

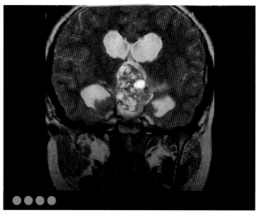

F2. Coronal T2-weighted image reveals a suprasellar mass with mixed signal intensity. Areas of hyperintensity are consistent with cystic areas.

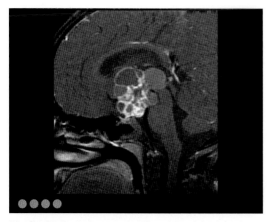

F3. Sagittal, post-contrast T1-weighted images demonstrate a large, suprasellar, enhancing mass with multiple cystic areas.

305

GERMINOMA

Germ cell tumors make up 0.3–3% of pediatric brain tumors of which 45% are **germinomas**. The suprasellar region is the second most common location for these tumors, next to pineal region. On MR imaging, germinomas appear isointense on T1-weighted images and iso- to slightly hyperintense on T2-weighted images. Marked contrast enhancement is seen on the post-contrast images. Of note, the hypothalamic stalk is often involved and thus thickened.

GERMINOMA (CASE ONE)

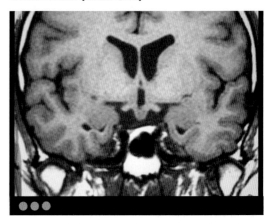

G1. Coronal T1-weighted image shows a small isointense mass along the pituitary stalk.

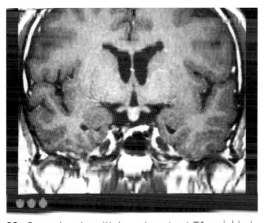

G2. Coronal and sagittal, post-contrast T1-weighted images demonstrate an enhancing mass along the pituitary stalk.

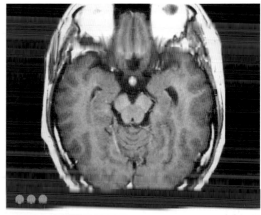

G3. Coronal and sagittal, post-contrast T1-weighted images demonstrate an enhancing mass along the pituitary stalk.

GERMINOMA (CASE TWO)

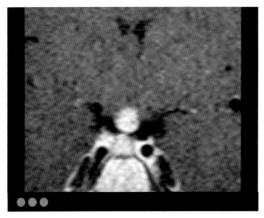

G4. Coronal, post-contrast T1-weighted image shows an enhancing mass in the suprasellar region.

GLIOBLASTOMA MULTIFORME (GBM)

Glioblastoma multiforme (GBM) is the most common and most aggressive type of primary glial tumors. Its peak incidence is in the 5th and 6th decade. It accounts for 52% of all parenchymal brain tumor cases and 20% of all intracranial tumors. Glioblastomas multiforme are characterized by the presence of small areas of necrotizing tissue surrounded by anaplastic cells (so called pseudopalisading necrosis). This characteristic, as well as the presence of angiogenesis, differentiates GBM from anaplastic astrocytomas, which do not have these features. Suprasellar, hypothalamic location is not common.

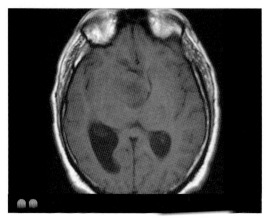

H1 Axial T1 weighted image shows a mixed signal intensity mass in the suprasellar region.

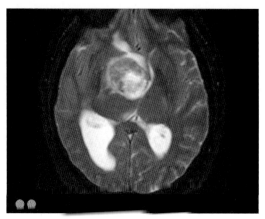

H2. Axial T2-weighted image reveals a mixed signal, predominantly hyperintense mass with a cystic area.

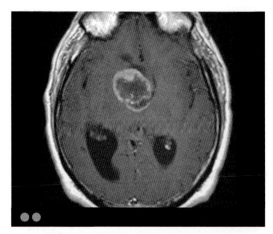

H3. Axial, coronal and sagittal, post-contrast T1-weighted images demonstrate an enhancing mass with central cystic, necrotic areas in the suprasellar, hypothalamic region.

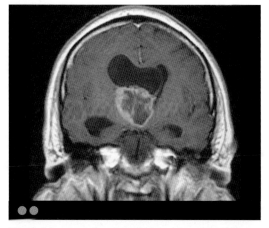

H4. Axial, coronal and sagittal, post-contrast T1-weighted images demonstrate an enhancing mass with central cystic, necrotic areas in the suprasellar, hypothalamic region.

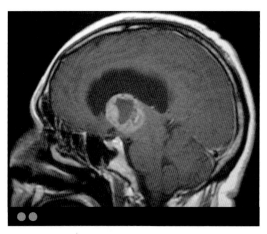

H5. Axial, coronal and sagittal, post-contrast T1-weighted images demonstrate an enhancing mass with central cystic, necrotic areas in the suprasellar, hypothalamic region.

HYPOTHALAMIC ANAPLASTIC ASTROCYTOMA

The criteria for WHO grading scheme for gliomas include nuclear atypia, mitotic activity, cellularity, vascular proliferation, and necrosis. WHO grade I corresponds to pilocytic astrocytoma, WHO grade II corresponds to low-grade (diffuse) astrocytoma, WHO grade III corresponds to anaplastic astrocytoma, and WHO grade IV corresponds to glioblastoma multiforme (GBM). Suprasellar, hypothalamic anaplastic astrocytomas are uncommon.

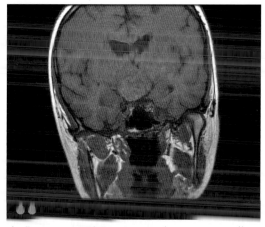

I1. Coronal T1-weighted image shows a suprasellar, hypothalamic, and isointense mass.

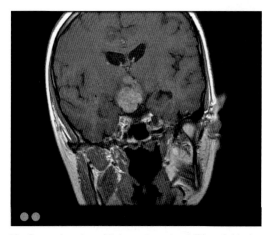

I2. Coronal and sagittal, post-contrast T1-weighted image demonstrates an enhancing mass in the suprasellar, hypothalamic region. Small cystic, necrotic areas are seen within the mass.

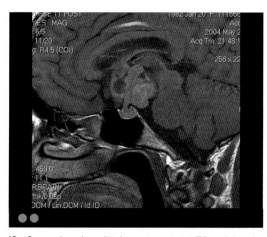

I3. Coronal and sagittal, post-contrast T1-weighted image demonstrates an enhancing mass in the suprasellar, hypothalamic region. Small cystic, necrotic areas are seen within the mass.

HYPOTHALAMIC PILOCYTIC ASTROCYTOMA

Hypothalamic/chiasmatic glioma presents as a mass lesion in the suprasellar cistern. It is isointense on T1-weighted images and hyperintense on T2-weighted images. The hyperintensity may extend along the entire visual pathway. Homogeneous contrast enhancement of the tumor mass is seen. Calcification of untreated tumor is rare. Bilateral optic nerve astrocytomas are associated with neurofibromatosis.

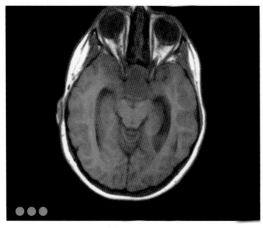

J1. Axial T1-weighted image shows a hypointense mass in the suprasellar region.

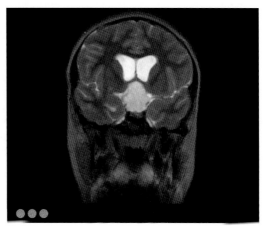

J2. Coronal T2-weighted image reveals a hyperintense mass in the suprasellar cistern.

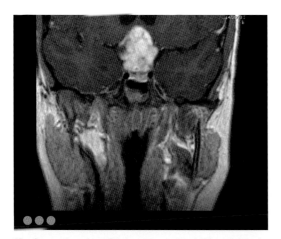

J3. Coronal and sagittal, post-contrast T1-weighted image demonstrates an enhancing mass in the suprasellar, hypothalamic region.

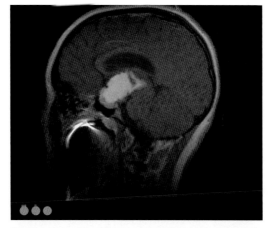

J4. Coronal and sagittal, post-contrast T1-weighted image demonstrates an enhancing mass in the suprasellar, hypothalamic region.

HYPOTHALAMIC PILOCYTIC ASTROCYTOMA WITH SEEDING

Pilocytic astrocytomas are WHO grade I astrocytomas and rarely exhibit seeding into the subarachnoid space or ventricle. Seeding may be seen at the time of presentation or following surgical intervention. Dissemination of the tumor cells through the CSF pathway is probably the primary mechanism of central nervous system spread.

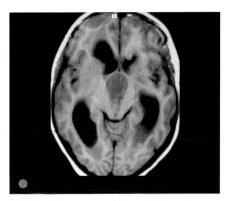 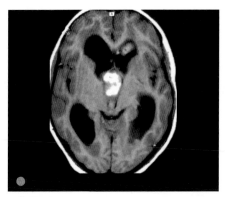 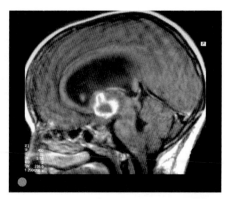

K1. Axial T1-weighted image shows a hypointense mass in the suprasellar, hypothalamic region. Note there is an additional isointense mass at the frontal horn of the left lateral ventricle

K2. Axial and sagittal T1-weighted images demonstrate an enhancing mass in the hypothalamic region. The enhancing nodule seen in the frontal horn of the left lateral ventricle is due to metastatic seeding

K3. Axial and sagittal T1-weighted images demonstrate an enhancing mass in the hypothalamic region. The enhancing nodule seen in the frontal horn of the left lateral ventricle is due to metastatic seeding

LYMPHOMA

Non Hodgkin's lymphoma may involve the central nervous system either as a primary tumor or hematogenously from a systemic lymphoma. Primary CNS lymphoma is more common. The occurrence of malignant lymphoma in the suprasellar region is rare. On MR imaging, lesions tend to be round, oval, or, rarely, gyriform in appearance. They are iso- to hypointense in signal intensity to the gray matter on T_1-weighted images and are typically iso- to hypointense to gray matter on T_2-weighted images. Due to the high cellularity and decreased water content from a high nucleus-to-cytoplasm ratio, these tumors tend to exhibit iso- to hypointensity on T_2 weighted images and high signal intensity (restricted diffusion) on diffusion weighted images.

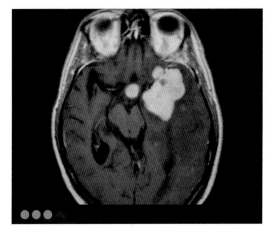 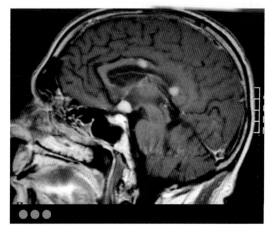

L1. Axial and sagittal, post-contrast T1-weighted images demonstrate an enhancing mass in the suprasellar cistern. In addition, other enhancing masses are seen involving the corpus callosum and left temporal lobe.

L2. Axial and sagittal, post-contrast T1-weighted images demonstrate an enhancing mass in the suprasellar cistern. In addition, other enhancing masses are seen involving the corpus callosum and left temporal lobe.

METASTATIC DISEASE (RENAL CELL CARCINOMA)

Metastasis to the brain is a frequent complication of many systemic cancers, occurring in approximately one third of all cancer patients. Brain metastasis represents the most common form of intracranial neoplasms, more frequently seen than primary brain neoplasms. The incidence of metastasis to the brain appears to have recently increased, possibly due to the more aggressive clinical management, resulting in improved survival. In addition, the modern imaging modalities and new techniques allow for better detection of metastatic lesions to the brain. In adults, the most common primary sites of metastatic lesions to the brain include the lung (50–60%), breast (15–20%), skin (5–10%), and gastrointestinal tract (4–6%). Metastasis to the hypothalamic region is uncommon.

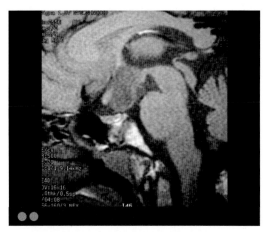

M1. Sagittal and coronal T1-weighted images show a slightly hypointense mass in suprasellar region.

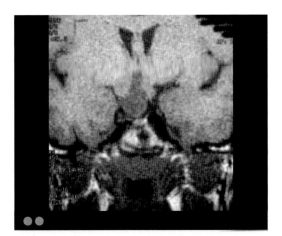

M2. Sagittal and coronal T1-weighted images show a slightly hypointense mass in suprasellar region

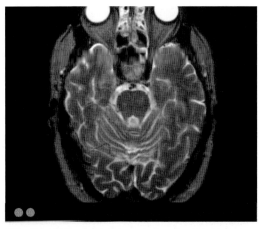

M3. Axial T2-weighted image shows a hyperintense mass in the suprasellar region.

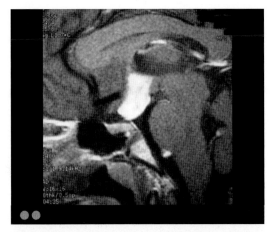

M4. Sagittal and coronal, post-contrast T1-weighted images show enhancement of the mass with an irregular margin.

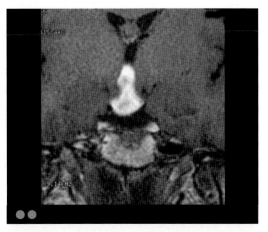

M5. Sagittal and coronal, post-contrast T1-weighted images show enhancement of the mass with an irregular margin.

SARCOIDOSIS

Sarcoidosis of the central nervous system has a predilection for the leptomeninges. Hypothalamus, optic chiasm, and pituitary gland may be involved.

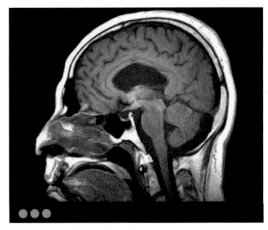

N1. Sagittal T1-weighted image shows a slightly hyperintense lesion in the suprasellar, hypothalamic region.

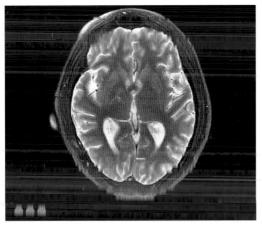

N2. Axial T2-weighted image reveals the lesion to be hypointense.

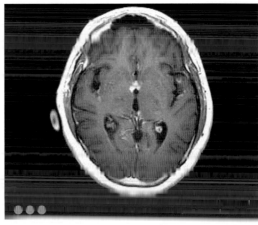

N3. Axial and coronal, post-contrast T1-weighted images show an enhancing lesion in the suprasellar, hypothalamic region.

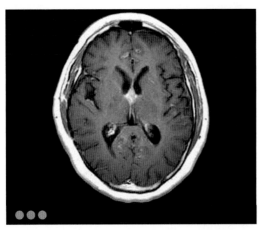

N4. Axial and coronal, post-contrast T1-weighted images show an enhancing lesion in the suprasellar, hypothalamic region.

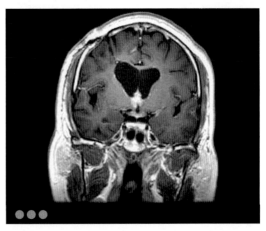

N5. Axial and coronal, post-contrast T1-weighted images show an enhancing lesion in the suprasellar, hypothalamic region.

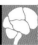

SCHISTOSOMIASIS

Human **schistosomiasis** is principally caused by one of the six species of parasitic worms. Schistosomes are blood flukes and belong to the class Trematoda. Unlike other trematodes, schistosomes are elongated but become round as they adept to residing in blood vessels of the genitourinary or GI tract of human beings. They require a vertebrate and an intermediate water-dwelling snail host to complete their life cycle. Geographic distribution and maintenance of human infection by schistosomes depends on and is limited by the presence of a suitable snail host. Schistosome eggs are usually excreted from the body, but approximately 50% of the eggs can embolize to other parts of the body, leading to a host immune reaction and granuloma formation. Granulomas begin to form with maturation of the miracidium at 6 days and become focal within 2 weeks. The most common sites are the liver and the bladder. Other areas less commonly affected include the lungs, CNS, and kidneys.

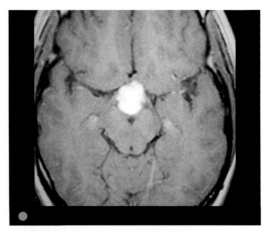

01. Axial, post-contrast T1-weighted image shows an enhancing mass in the suprasellar region.

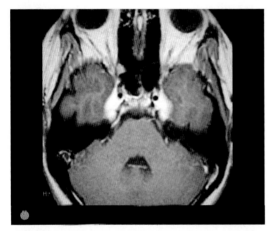

02. Axial, post-contrast T1-weighted image shows extension of the enhancing mass into the cavernous sinuses bilaterally.

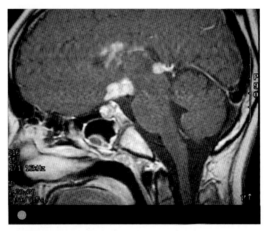

03. Sagittal, post-contrast T1-weighted image shows an enhancing mass in the suprasellar region as well as in the pineal region.

TUBERCULOSIS

Intracranial tuberculosis has two related pathologic processes, tuberculous meningitis, and intracranial tuberculoma. The intracranial tuberculomas present as a nodule that can be hypointense on T1-weighted images and hyperintense on T2-weighted images. Contrast enhancement is usually present. These nodules may be solitary or multiple, associated with mass effect and surrounding edema. Calcification is seen in less than 20% of the cases. As it grows, tuberculomas can adhere to the dura, causing hyperostosis of the adjacent bony calvarium.

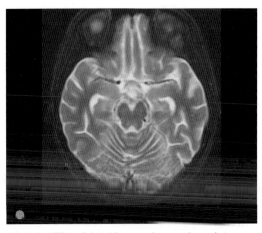

P1. Axial T2-weighted image shows a hyperintense lesion in the suprasellar cistern.

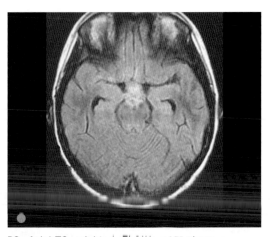

P2. Axial T2-weighted, FLAIR image shows a slightly hyperintense lesion.

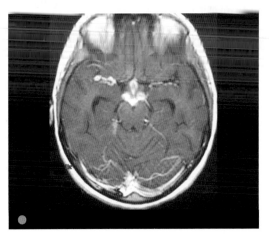

P3. Axial and coronal, post-contrast T1-weighted images demonstrate an enhancing mass in the suprasellar cistern with involvement of the pituitary stalk.

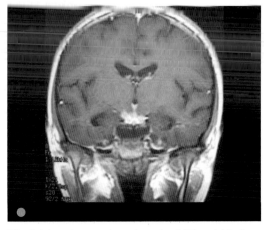

P4. Axial and coronal, post-contrast T1-weighted images demonstrate an enhancing mass in the suprasellar cistern with involvement of the pituitary stalk.

EPIDERMOIDS

Epidermoids are congenital masses, but their clinical presentation usually is in the third or fourth decade. They are predominantly located in basal cisterns and are usually lateral in location as opposed to the midline location of dermoids. Common locations include cerebellopontine angle, middle cranial fossa, suprasellar, and fourth ventricle. Epidermoids are composed of ectodermal elements and are lined with stratified squamous epithelium containing epithelial keratinaceous debris and cholesterol crystals. Epidermoids have similar signal intensity features to those of CSF on both T1-weighted and T2-weighted images. Sometimes, an internal stranded appearance can be seen, giving a "dirty-CSF" appearance. Diffusion-weighted images can be useful in differentiating epidermoids from arachnoid cysts. Epidermoids show restricted diffusion whereas arachnoid cysts do not show restricted diffusion.

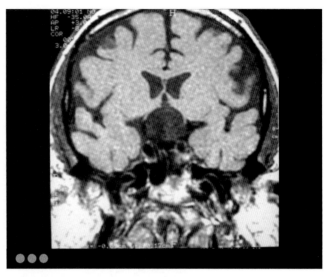

A. Coronal T1-weighted image shows a suprasellar mass with similar signal intensity to CSF.

RELATED PATTERNS

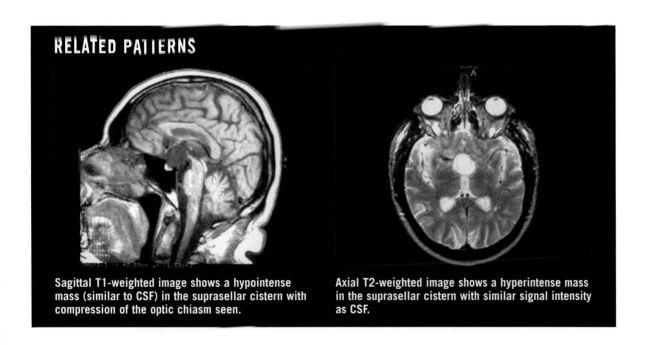

Sagittal T1-weighted image shows a hypointense mass (similar to CSF) in the suprasellar cistern with compression of the optic chiasm seen.

Axial T2-weighted image shows a hyperintense mass in the suprasellar cistern with similar signal intensity as CSF.

DIFFERENTIAL DIAGNOSIS

At a Glance:

- Arachnoid Cyst
- Cysticercosis
- Dermoid
- Hamartoma of the Tuber Cinerium
- Lipoma
- Sphenoid Mucocele

ARACHNOID CYST

Arachnoid cysts consist of 1% of all intracranial masses. There is a male predominance with 3:1 ratio. Arachnoid cysts can be seen in any age group, but mostly in children.

Common locations include middle cranial fossa, suprasellar cistern, and convexity. Focal bony erosion may be seen on imaging studies. They are of similar signal intensity to CSF on both T1-weighted and T2-weighted images. No contrast enhancement is seen.

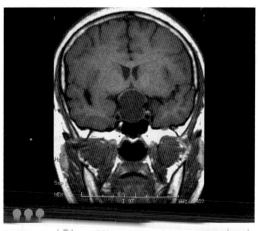

B1. Coronal T1-weighted image shows a CSF signal intensity lesion in the suprasellar cistern.

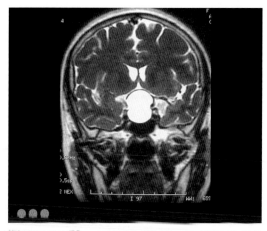

B2. Coronal T2-weighted image demonstrates a CSF signal intensity lesion in the suprasellar cistern.

CYSTICERCOSIS

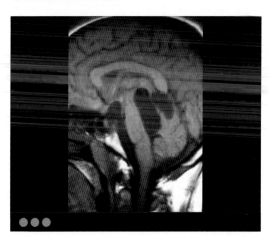

C. Sagittal T1-weighted image shows cysticercosis cysts in the region of suprasellar cistern, superior vermian cistern, and along the aqueduct.

DERMOID

Dermoid cysts are inclusion cysts composed of ectodermal elements. They are uncommon lesions, accounting for approximately 0.3% of all brain masses. Dermoid tumors are thought to arise from misplaced ectodermal elements during the third to fifth week of embryonic life, when the neural tube closes at the midline. This may explain the fre-

quent midline location of dermoid cysts. In contrast, epidermoid cysts are often located lateral to the midline of the cranium. Dermoid cysts are often seen within the posterior cranial fossa near midline, in suprasellar cistern, and in the subfrontal region. Epidermoid tumors are more frequently seen in the cerebellopontine angle cistern, in the suprasellar and parasellar regions, in choroidal, sylvian, and interhemispheric fissures and within the ventricles.

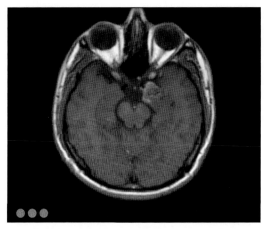

D1. Axial T1-weighted images show a hyperintense lesion in the left parasellar region. Multiple small hyperintense lesions in the sylvian fissure, more on the left, are due to rupture of the dermoid.

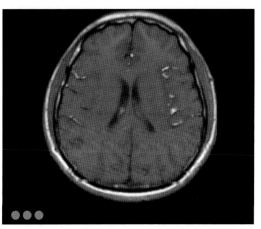

D2. Axial T1-weighted images show a hyperintense lesion in the left parasellar region. Multiple small hyperintense lesions in the sylvian fissure, more on the left, are due to rupture of the dermoid.

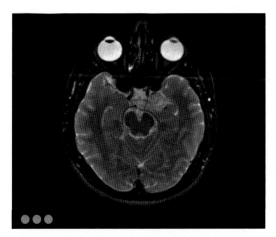

D3. Axial T2-weighted image demonstrates a hyperintense lesion in the left parasellar region.

HAMARTOMA OF THE TUBER CINERIUM

Hamartomas of the tuber cinerium consist of hyperplastic hypothalamic glial and neural tissue. Patients characteristically present with gelastic seizures and precocious puberty due to disruption of the normal hypothalamic inhibition of gonadotropin production during the prepuberty years.

HAMARTOMA OF THE TUBER CINERIUM (CASE ONE)

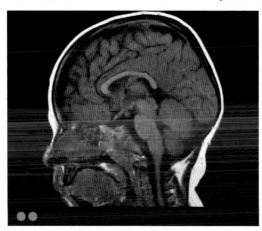

E1. Sagittal T1-weighted image shows an isointense mass in the hypothalamus.

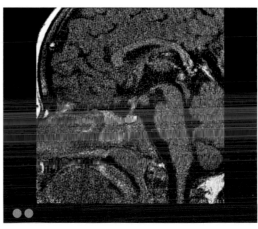

E2. Sagittal and coronal, post-contrast T1 weighted images show an isointense mass in the hypothalamus without contrast enhancement

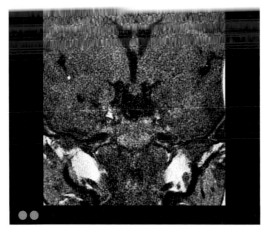

E3. Sagittal and coronal, post-contrast T1-weighted images show an isointense mass in the hypothalamus without contrast enhancement.

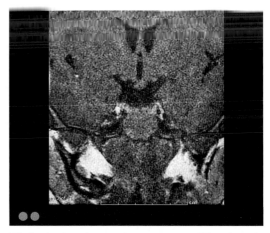

E4. Sagittal and coronal, post-contrast T1-weighted images show an isointense mass in the hypothalamus without contrast enhancement.

HAMARTOMA OF THE TUBER CINERIUM (CASE TWO)

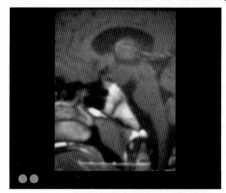

F1. Sagittal T1-weighted image shows an isointense mass in the region of hypothalamus.

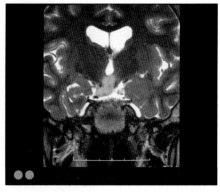

F2. Coronal T2-weighted image shows an isointense mass in the region of hypothalamus.

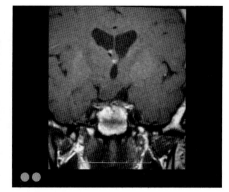

F3. Coronal, post-contrast T1-weighted image reveals no enhancement of the mass lesion.

LIPOMA

Although magnetic resonance imaging (MRI) has proven to be superior to computed tomography (CT) in almost all areas of neuroimaging. However, this one case proves that CT can still be a useful adjunct to MR imaging. Detection of fat and blood can rarely pose problems on MRI since both may exhibit hyperintensity on T1 weighted images, which could be solved by performing a CT

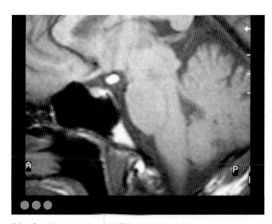

G1. Sagittal and axial T1-weighted images show a hyperintense lesion in the suprasellar/hypothalamic region.

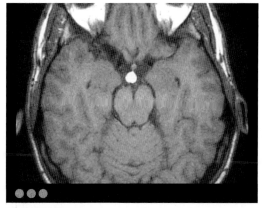

G2. Sagittal and axial T1-weighted images show a hyperintense lesion in the suprasellar/hypothalamic region.

SPHENOID MUCOCELE

Mucoceles are benign, expansile, cyst-like lesions lined with a secretory respiratory mucosa of pseudostratified columnar epithelium in the paranasal sinuses. A mucocele is formed due to blockage of the draining ostium of the sinus. The mucocele slowly enlarges as the mucosa secrets, expanding and eroding the adjacent bony structures. The most commonly involved paranasal sinuses are the frontal and anterior ethmoid sinuses. Sphenoid sinus mucoceles are the least common. On MR imaging, the signal intensity of mucoceles varies depending on the fluid content and its protein concentration, presence of hemorrhage.

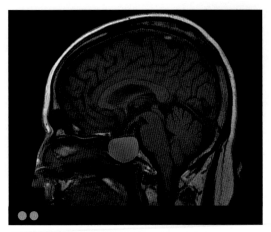

H1. Sagittal and coronal T1-weighted images show a large cystic, hyperintense lesion in the sphenoid sinus extending into the sellar turcica.

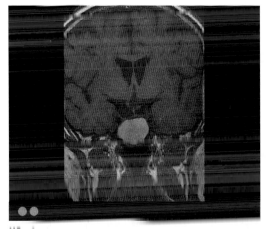

H2. Sagittal and coronal T1-weighted images show a large cystic, hyperintense lesion in the sphenoid sinus extending into the sellar turcica.

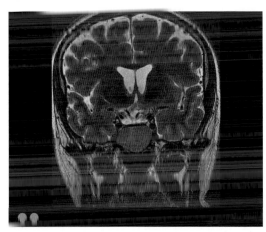

H3. Coronal T2-weighted image shows an isointense lesion in the sphenoid sinus extending into the sellar turcica.

CAVERNOUS ANGIOMA

Parasellar cavernous hemangiomas are hypointense on T1-weighted images and hyperintense on T2-weighted images. Avid contrast enhancement is seen following the intravenous injection of the contrast material. Occasionally, heterogeneous contrast enhancement is seen.

Parasellar cavernous hemangiomas are difficult to remove surgically and tend to be adherent to the cavernous sinus and may also bleed profoundly.

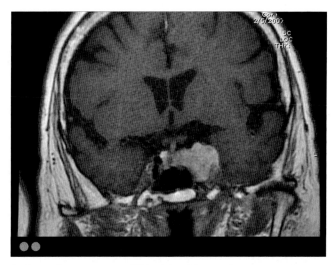

A. Coronal, post-contrast T1-weighted image demonstrates an enhancing mass in the left cavernous sinus. Note extension of the mass into the left side of the sella turcica.

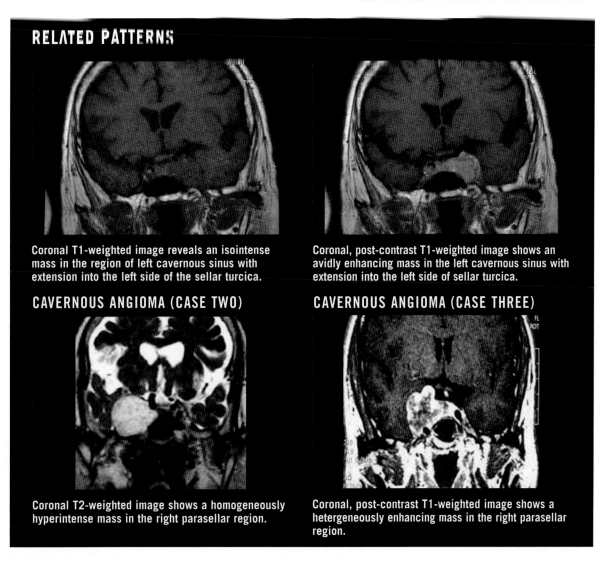

RELATED PATTERNS

Coronal T1-weighted image reveals an isointense mass in the region of left cavernous sinus with extension into the left side of the sellar turcica.

Coronal, post-contrast T1-weighted image shows an avidly enhancing mass in the left cavernous sinus with extension into the left side of sellar turcica.

CAVERNOUS ANGIOMA (CASE TWO)

CAVERNOUS ANGIOMA (CASE THREE)

Coronal T2-weighted image shows a homogeneously hyperintense mass in the right parasellar region.

Coronal, post-contrast T1-weighted image shows a hetergeneously enhancing mass in the right parasellar region.

DIFFERENTIAL DIAGNOSIS

At a Glance:

- *Aneurysm*
- *Carotid-Cavernous Fistula*
- *Chondrosarcoma*
- *Dermoid*
- *Tolossa–Hunt Syndrome*
- *Lymphoma*
- *Meningioma*
- *Metastasis*
- *Pituitary Adenoma*
- *Sarcoid*
- *Schwannoma (Fifth Nerve)*
- *Teratoma*
- *Cavernous Sinus Thrombosis* (not pictured)
- *Chordoma* (not pictured)

ANEURYSM

Aneurysms in the cavernous sinus are extradural in location. A carotid cavernous sinus fistula is produced when they rupture. Since they are extradural in location, there is no subarachnoid hemorrhage.

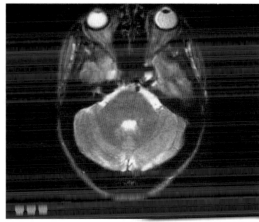

B1. Axial T2-weighted image shows a round lesion with hyperintense center and hypointense periphery in the region of left cavernous sinus.

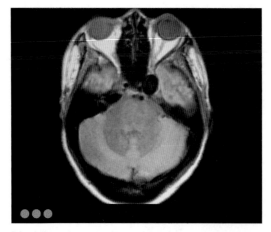

B2. Axial proton density-weighted image shows a hypointense lesion in the region of left cavernous sinus.

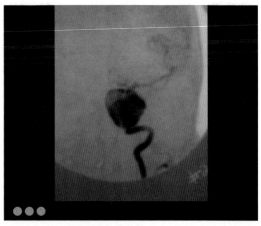

B3. AP view of left carotid angiogram reveals a large aneurysm in the region of left cavernous sinus.

CAROTID-CAVERNOUS FISTULA

Spontaneous or traumatic rupture of the wall of the intracavernous segment of the internal carotid artery or its dural branches results in sudden shunting of the arterial blood into the cavernous sinus. Tortuosity and dilatation of the superior ophthalmic vein is the hallmark on CT or MRI for the diagnosis of **carotid-cavernous fistula**. Focal bulging or expansion of the cavernous sinus is another sign of C-C fistula.

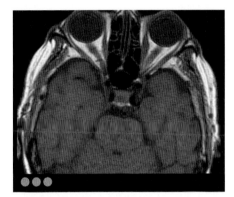

C1. Axial T1-weighted image shows a prominent left cavernous sinus.

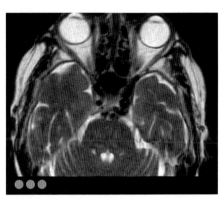

C2. Axial T2-weighted image shows flow void within the prominet left cavernous sinus.

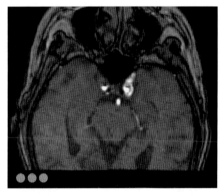

C3. Axial MR angiogram source image shows prominent vascularture in the left cavernous sinus.

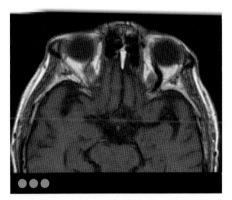

C4. Axial T1-weighted, T2-weighted and MRA images demonstrate a prominent left superior ophthalmic vein.

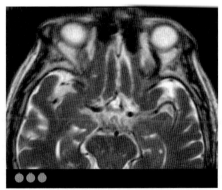

C5. Axial T1-weighted, T2-weighted and MRA images demonstrate a prominent left superior ophthalmic vein.

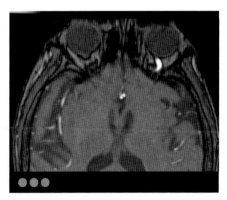

C6. Axial T1-weighted, T2-weighted and MRA images demonstrate a prominent left superior ophthalmic vein.

CHONDROSARCOMA

Most of the sellar region tumors are pituitary adenomas. Nonpituitary sellar and parasellar masses are uncommon. About 10% of such nonpituitary sellar masses are cartilaginous tumors originating from the skull base. Chordomas are more frequently seen than chondrosarcomas. Chondrosarcomas are malignant tumors of cartilage-forming cells that occur mainly in the axial part of the skeleton, consisting of less than 5% of skull base tumors with approximately 75% arising in the parasellar region.

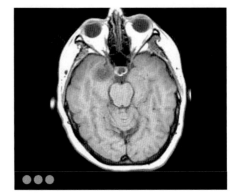

D1. Axial T1-weighted imge shows a hypointense mass in the region of right cavernous sinus.

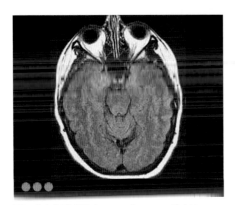

D2. Axial FLAIR image shows a slightly hyperintense mass

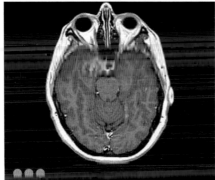

D3. Axial and coronal, post-contrast T1-weighted images show a heterogeneously enhancing mass in the right cavernous sinus.

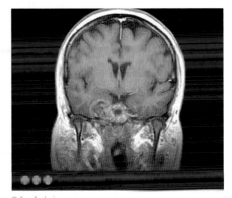

D4. Axial and coronal, post-contrast T1-weighted images show a heterogeneously enhancing mass in the right cavernous sinus

DERMOID

Intracranial **dermoids** are rare lesions. Common locations include fourth ventricle, suprasellar, parasellar, subfrontal, and in the facial region. Due to their fat content, they are high signal intensity lesions with focal heterogeneity on T1-weighted images.

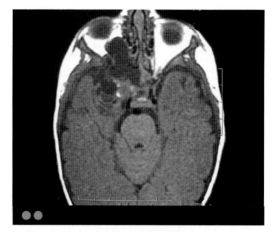

E1. Axial T1-weighted image shows a mixed signal intensity mass in the region of right cavernous sinus with extension into the right orbit. Small hyperintense areas are due to fat and hypointense areas are due to cystic changes.

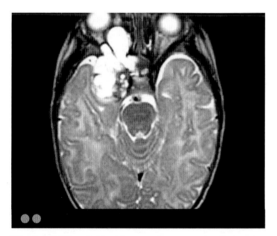

E2. Axial T2-weighted image shows a mixed signal intensity mass.

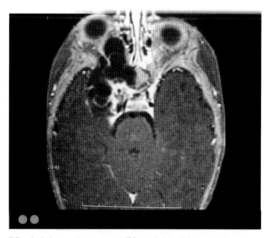

E3. Axial, post-contrast T1-weighted image demonstrates partial enhancement of the mass.

TOLOSSA–HUNT SYNDROME

It is a painful ophthalmoplegia caused by nonspecific inflammation in the cavernous sinus. It responds to steroid treatment. Abnormal signal and contrast enhancement may be seen in the cavernous sinus. Subtle enlargement of the cavernous sinus may be seen. Extension of the granulomatous mass into the orbit may be seen.

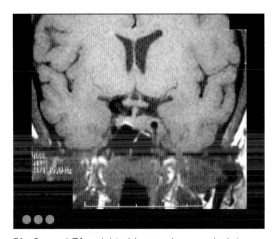

F1. Coronal T1-weighted image shows an isointense mass in the left cavernous sinus.

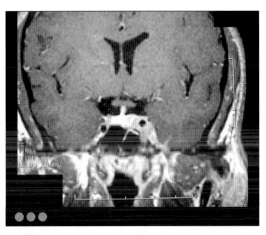

F2. Coronal, post-contrast T1-weighted image shows an enhancing mass in the left cavernous sinus.

LYMPHOMA

Primary CNS lymphoma may involve the cavernous sinus and should be considered in the differential diagnosis of cavernous sinus lesions.

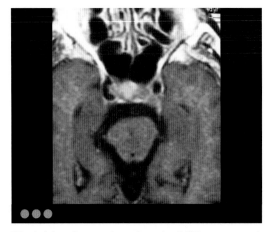

G1. Axial and coronal, post-contrast CT scans reveal an enhancing mass in the left cavernous sinus, displacing the internal carotid artery.

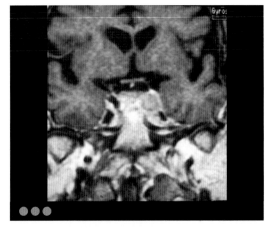

G2. Axial and coronal, post-contrast CT scans reveal an enhancing mass in the left cavernous sinus, displacing the internal carotid artery.

MENINGIOMA

Meningiomas may involve the cavernous sinus region. They are usually isointense to gray matter on both T1 weighted and T2 weighted images, but their signal intensity may be variable as illustrated by the following cases.

MENINGIOMA (CASE ONE)

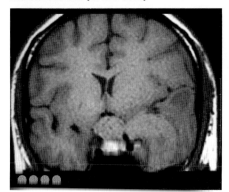

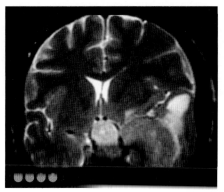

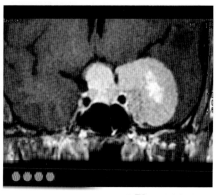

H1. Coronal T1 weighted image shows an isointense, left parasellar, cavernous sinus mass as well as a suprasellar mass.

H2. Coronal T2-weighted image shows an isointense, left parasellar mass and a hyperintense, suprasellar mass. At surgery, It proved to be a meningioma with two different histopathological components. The left parasellar mass turned out to be a meningothelial type and the suprasellar component turned out to be angioblastic type.

II3. Coronal, post contrast T1-weighted image demonstrates avid enhancement of the tumor. There is encasement of the left internal carotid artery seen.

MENINGIOMA (CASE TWO)

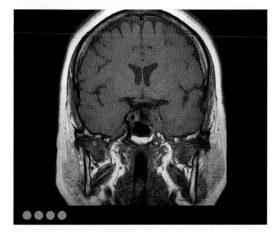

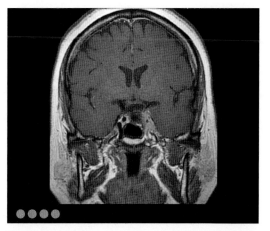

I1. Coronal T1-weighted image shows an isointense mass in the left cavernous sinus. Note the narrowing of the lumen of the left internal carotid artery due to encasement.

I2. Coronal, post-contrast T1-weighted image shows intense enhancement of the mass lesion in the left cavernous sinus.

MENINGIOMA (CASE THREE)

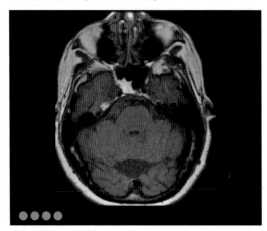

J1. Axial T1-weighted image shows an isointense, right cavernous sinus mass with extension into the right ambien cistern.

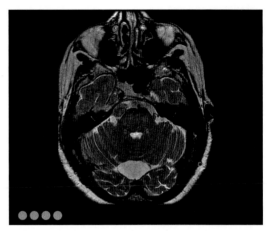

J2. Axial T2-weighted image shows an inhomogenous isointense, right cavernous sinus mass with extension into the right ambien cistern.

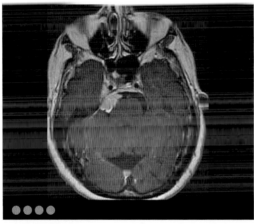

J3. Axial and coronal post-contrast T1-weighted image demonstrates avid, homogenous enhancement of the tumor.

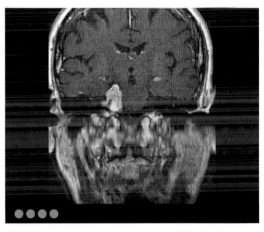

J4. Axial and coronal post-contrast T1-weighted image demonstrates avid, homogenous enhancement of the tumor.

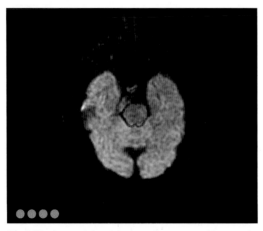

J5. Diffusion-weighted image shows no evidence of restricted diffusion lesion.

METASTASIS

Metastatic disease involving the cavernous sinus may result from extension from adjacent neoplasms or hematogenous spread. A number of skull base tumors can cause perineural spread of the neoplasms.

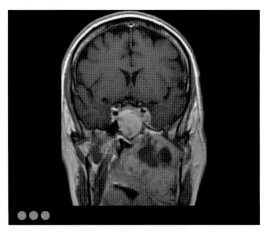

K. Coronal, post-contrast T1-weighted image shows an enhancing tumor (small cell neuroendocrine tumor) from the sphenoid sinus invading the pituitary and left cavernous sinus. Note the necrotic mass in the left masticator space and skull base.

PITUITARY ADENOMA

Invasion of the cavernous sinus by pituitary tumor is not uncommon. The pituitary tumor usually does not encase the internal carotid artery whereas a meningioma involving the cavernous sinus frequently encase the internal carotid artery and result in narrowing of the vascular lumen.

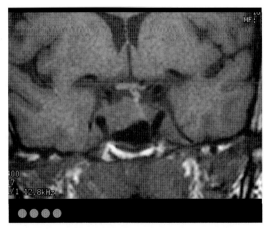

L1. Coronal T1-weighted image shows a pituitary tumor extending into the right cavernous sinus.

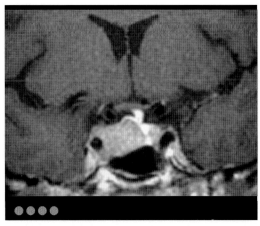

L2. Coronal, post-contrast T1-weighted image shows enhancement of the tumor, which involves the right cavernous sinus.

SARCOID

Sarcoid can involve the cavernous sinus as other granulo-matous lesions do. The appearances of sarcoid on neu-roimaging is quite variable and it can mimic anything.

SARCOID (CASE ONE)

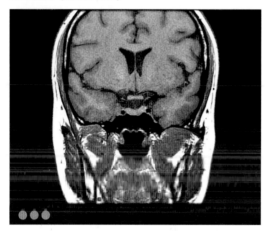

M1. Coronal T1-weighted image shows an isointense mass in the right cavernous sinus.

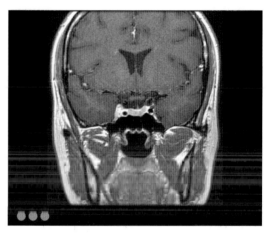

M2. Coronal, post-contrast T1-weighted image shows avid enhancement of the mass.

SARCOID (CASE TWO)

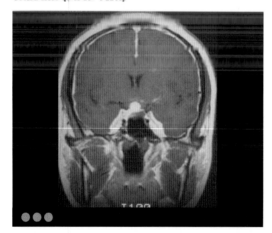

N. Coronal, post-contrast T1-weighted image shows enhancing lesion involving both cavernous sinuses, suprasellar region. In addition, there is diffuse pachymeningeal thickening seen.

SCHWANNOMA (FIFTH NERVE)

Schwannomas of the parasellar region are uncommon and usually arise from trigeminal nerve. Intracranial schwannomas account for 8–10% of all primary intracranial tumors. Intracranial schwannomas occur predominantly in associ- ation with the vestibular portion of the VIII cranial nerve in the cerebellopontine angle. Schwannomas are benign, slowly growing encapsulated tumors. Trigeminal schwannomas can present as prepontine posterior fossa, middle fossa, or a combined posterior-middle fossa lesions.

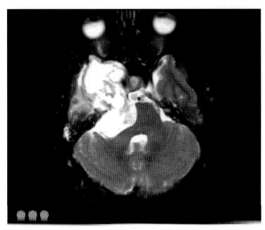

01. Axial T2-weighted and FLAIR images show a hyperintense, heterogeneous mass involving the right medial middle fossa, right cavernous sinus and right CPA cistern.

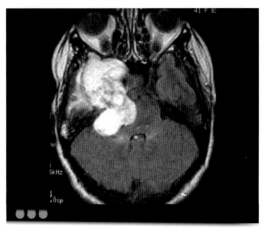

02. Axial T2-weighted and FLAIR images show a hyperintense, heterogeneous mass involving the right medial middle fossa, right cavernous sinus and right CPA cistern.

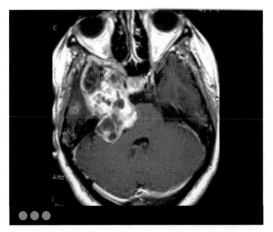

03. Axial and coronasl, post-contrast T1-weighted images show enhancement of the bilobular mass with multiple internal cystic areas.

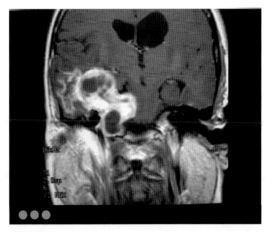

04. Axial and coronasl, post-contrast T1-weighted images show enhancement of the bilobular mass with multiple internal cystic areas.

SCHWANNOMA (CASE TWO)

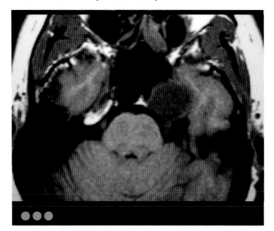

P1. Axial T1-weighted image shows a hypointense lesion in the left cavernous sinus and parasellar region.

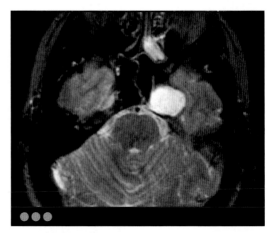

P2. Axial T2-weighted image shows a hyperintense mass in the left parasellar region.

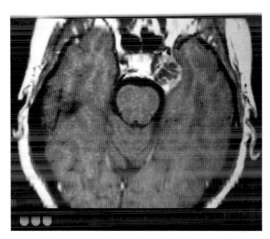

P3. Axial and coronal, post-contrast T1-weighted images demonstrate a heterogeneouly enhancing mass with cystic areas in the left parasellar region.

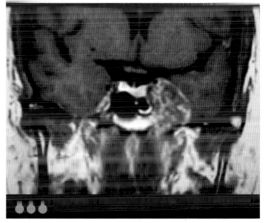

P4. Axial and coronal, post-contrast T1-weighted images demonstrate a heterogeneouly enhancing mass with cystic areas in the left parasellar region.

SCHWANNOMA (CASE THREE)

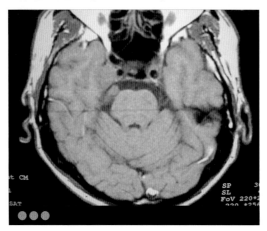

Q1. Axial T1-weighted image shows a isointense lesion in the right cavernous sinus extending posteriorly into the ambien cistern.

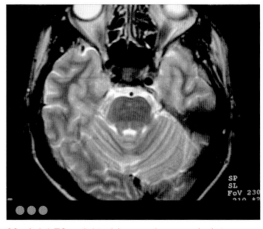

Q2. Axial T2-weighted image shows an isointense mass in the right parasellar region.

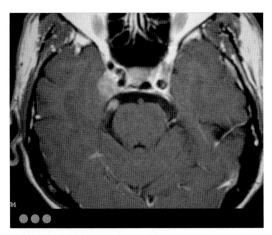

Q3. Axial, post-contrast T1-weighted images demonstrate an enhancing mass in the right parasellar region extending into the posterior fossa.

TERATOMA

Teratomas arise from multipotential cells that produce tissue consisting of a mixture of two or more layers of embryological tissues including ectoderm, mesoderm and endoderm. They can be benign or malignant in nature. They are commonly seen in the pineal region or sacroccocygeal region. Parasellar location is uncommon. There is a slight male predominance. Teratomas are heterogeneous lesions on MRI due to the presence of soft tissue, lipid, and CSF within the mass lesions.

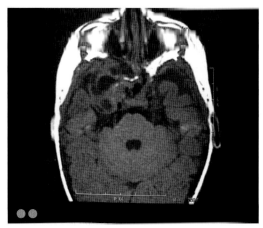

R1. Axial T1-weighted image shows a heterogeneous mass with mixed iso- and hypointensity and speckles of hyperintensity in the right parasellar region involving the right cavernous sinus.

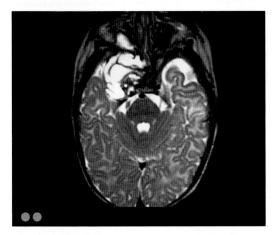

R2. Axial T2-weighted image reveals a perdominantly hyperintense mass in the right parasellar region.

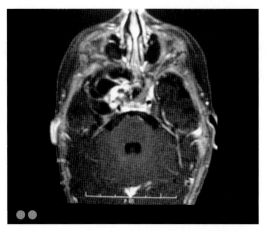

R3. Axial, post-contrast T1-weighted image shows a heterogeneously enhancing mass in the right parasellar region involving the cavernous sinus.

GERMINOMA

The infundibulum is usually 3- to 3.5-mm wide superiorly near the medial eminence and 2-mm wide inferiorly near its insertion to the pituitary gland. A number of diseases can enlarge the infundibulum. In many cases, these lesions usually involve the hypothalamus as well. Diabetes insipidus is a common finding in lesions affecting the stalk and hypothalamus. In children, Langerhans' cell histiocytosis, germinomas, and chronic meningitis are the common causes of thickened infundibulum. In adults, sarcoidosis, germinomas, metastasis, and lymphoma are the common causes of thicken pituitary stalk.

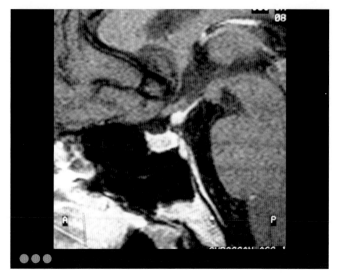

A. Sagittal, post-contrast T1-weighted image demonstrates enhancement of the thickened pituitary stalk.

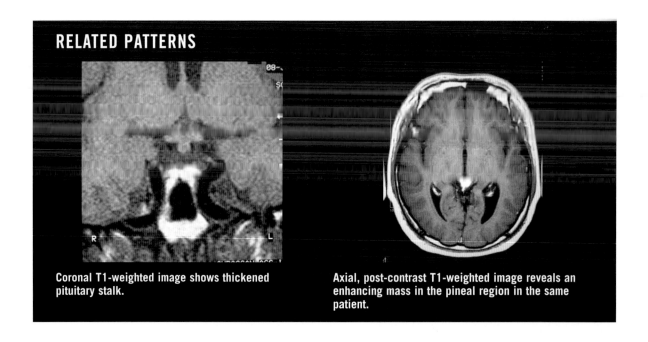

RELATED PATTERNS

Coronal T1-weighted image shows thickened pituitary stalk.

Axial, post-contrast T1-weighted image reveals an enhancing mass in the pineal region in the same patient.

DIFFERENTIAL DIAGNOSIS

At a Glance:

- *Histiocytosis*
- *Lymphocytic Adenohyphophysitis*
- *Lymphoma*
- *Sarcoidosis*
- *Chronic Meningitis* (not pictured)
- *Infiltration by Adjacent Neoplasm* (not pictured)
- *Metastasis* (not pictured)

HISTIOCYTOSIS

In children, Langerhans'cell **histiocytosis,** germinomas are the common causes of thickened infundibulum.

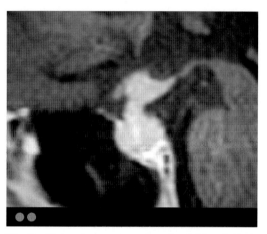

B1. Sagittal and coronal, post-contrast T1-weighted images show a thickened pituitary stalk with a mass in the hypothalamus.

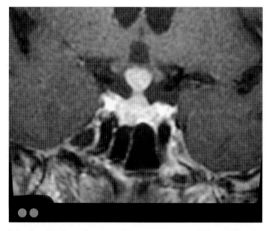

B2. Sagittal and coronal, post-contrast T1-weighted images show a thickened pituitary stalk with a mass in the hypothalamus.

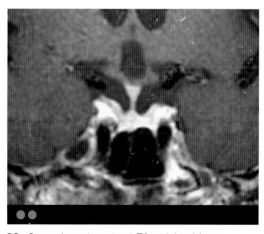

B3. Coronal, post-contrast T1-weighted image shows a significant decrease in the size of pituitary stalk following treatment.

LYMPHOCYTIC ADENOHYPHOPHYSITIS

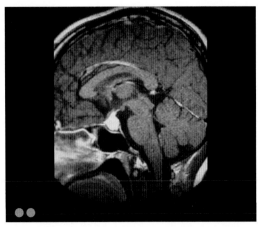

C1. Sagittal and coronal, post-contrast T1-weighted Images demonstrate enlargement of the pituitary gland and thickening of the pituitary stalk.

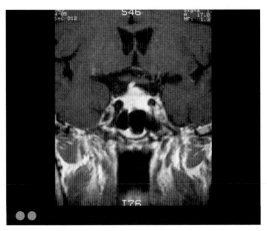

C2. Sagittal and coronal, post-contrast T1-weighted Images demonstrate enlargement of the pituitary gland and thickening of the pituitary stalk.

LYMPHOMA

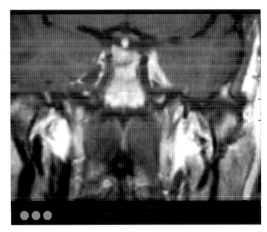

D. Coronal, post-contrast T1-weighted image shows thickened pituitary stalk and an enhancing lesion in the left cavernous sinus.

SARCOIDOSIS

In adults, **sarcoidosis,** germinomas, metastasis, and lymphoma are the common causes of thickened pituitary stalk.

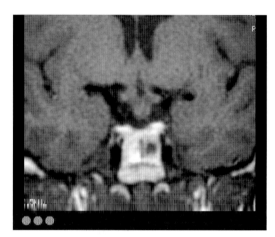

E1. Coronal pre and post contrast T1-weighted images show a thickened pituitary stalk with contrast enhancement.

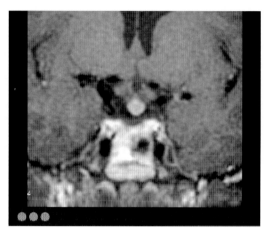

E2. Coronal pre- and post-contrast T1-weighted images show a thickened pituitary stalk with contrast enhancement.

Chapter 7

Vascular Lesions

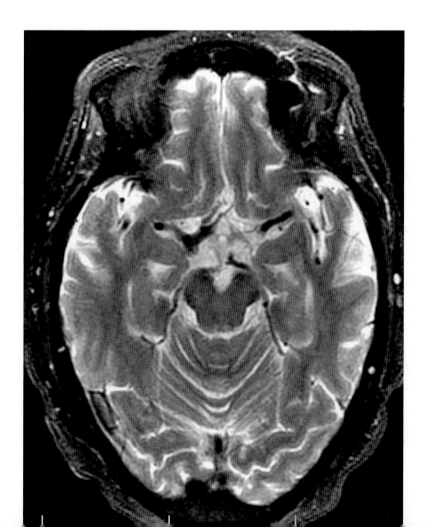

ANEURYSM

Intracranial developmental aneurysms are usually seen at an arterial bifurcation. The muscularis and elastic laminae terminate at the aneurysm neck and the sac or dome of the aneurysm consists of intima, adventitia, and occasionally thrombus. MR demonstrates focal signal void for nonthrombosed aneurysm. MRA can be used to detect intracranial aneurysms, although CTA is the imaging modality of choice.

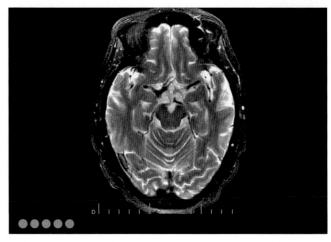

A. Axial T2-weighted image shows a nodular low signal intensity area adjacent to right internal carotid artery.

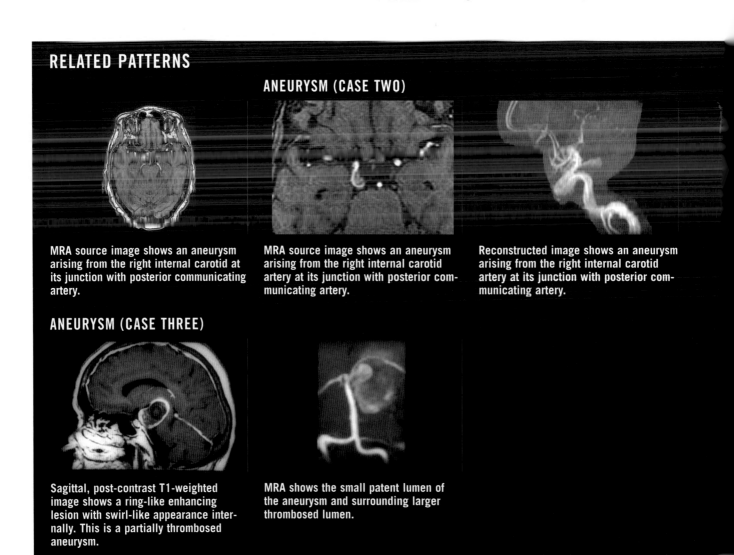

RELATED PATTERNS

ANEURYSM (CASE TWO)

MRA source image shows an aneurysm arising from the right internal carotid at its junction with posterior communicating artery.

MRA source image shows an aneurysm arising from the right internal carotid artery at its junction with posterior communicating artery.

Reconstructed image shows an aneurysm arising from the right internal carotid artery at its junction with posterior communicating artery.

ANEURYSM (CASE THREE)

Sagittal, post-contrast T1-weighted image shows a ring-like enhancing lesion with swirl-like appearance internally. This is a partially thrombosed aneurysm.

MRA shows the small patent lumen of the aneurysm and surrounding larger thrombosed lumen.

ANEURYSM (CASE FOUR)

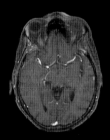 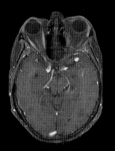

Axial, post-contrast T1-weighted images show a nodular enhancing lesion in the region of left middle cerebral artery bifurcation.

MRA demonstrates an aneurysm at the left middle cerebral artery bifurcation, corresponding to the nodular enhancing area seen on contrast enhanced MRI.

AMYLOID

Amyloid was first described by Virchow. It is an eosinophilic, insoluble, extracellular protein that stains with Congo red. Amyloid in tissue is identified by the following three parameters: 1. positive Congo red staining with apple green birefringence under polarized light, 2. distinct fibrillar ultrastructure on electron microscopy, 3. crossed beta pleated sheets on x ray diffraction. Amyloid may be present as a part of a systemic disease or as a focal deposition. Systemic amyloid deposition, also known as amyloidosis, is found in patients with gammopathies or plasma cell dyscrasias. Localized amyloid deposition is seen within the media and intima of the arteries and arterioles of the brain and meninges, which is known as cerebral amyloid angiopathy. Cerebral amyloid angiopathy appears to have slight predilection for the temporal, parietal, and occipital lobes. It predominantly affects the elderly patients and there is no sex predilection. Superficial cortical hemorrhages are seen. The amyloid within the vessel walls presumably leads to increased vascular fragility or rupture of microaneurysms of these vessels.

Hemorrhages due to **amyloid** angiopathy are usually lobar, involving frontal and parietal lobes. Subarachnoid and subdural hemorrhages have also been reported. There is a tendency for recurrent or multiple hemorrhages. MRI may exhibit multiple areas of low signal intensity, consistent with chronic hemorrhage.

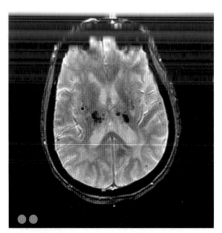

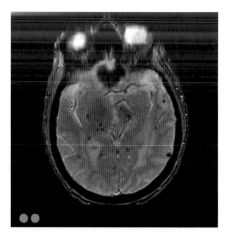

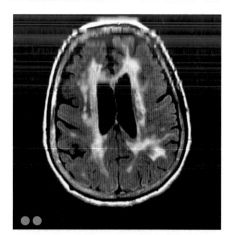

B1. Axial T2-weighted gradient-echo images demonstrate multiple low signal intensity areas in the brain, consistent with multiple sites of old hemorrhage. The deep gray matter lesions are probably due to hypertensive hemorrhage as Amyloid hemorrhages tend to occur in the superficial cortical region.

B2. Axial T2-weighted gradient-echo images demonstrate multiple low signal intensity areas in the brain, consistent with multiple sites of old hemorrhage.

B3. Axial T2-weighted FLAIR image shows extensive periventricular white matter ischemic changes.

ARTERIOVENOUS FISTULA WITH VARIX (AVF WITH VARIX)

They are high-flow lesions with arteriovenous shunting. Dural **arteriovenous fistulas** make up to 10–15% of intracranial vascular malformations, and one-third of posterior fossa AVMs is dural. Most dural AV fistulas are clinically manifest between 40 and 60 years of age. Women are affected more than men, especially in cases of dural malformation involving the cavernous sinus. Enlarged draining veins are more likely to be identified than enlarged feeding arteries on MRI.

MRI is more useful than CT. The identification of enlarged cortical veins without any AVM nidus suggests a dural AV fistula. Complications, such as infarction, sinus thrombosis, and hydrocephalus are well seen on MRI.

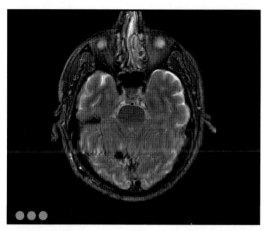

C1. Axial T2-weighted image shows a round low signal area near the torcular with adjacent serpiginous vessels.

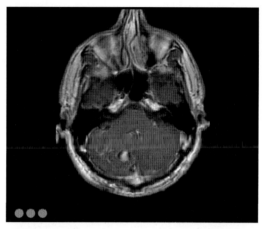

C2. Axial post-contrast T1-weighted image shows enhancement of the nodular lesion with some tortuous vessels. The nodular lesion is actually a varix due to dural arteriovenous fistula.

CAVERNOUS ANGIOMA

Cavernous angiomas are the most common types of vascular malformations. There is a tendency for multiplicity and a familial predisposition. They may be discovered incidently or present with seizures or neurological symptoms, particularly if they are associated with hemorrhage. MR is the imaging modality of choice for cavernous angioma. The angioma is a round, well-circumscribed area that has mixed signal intensity due to the presence of various blood products. It has been described as "popcornlike" in appearance. There is a circumscribed ring of hemosiderin that is dark and has a blooming effect on T2-weighted

images and particularly on T2*-weighted gradient-echo images. Occasionally, a low signal nodular lesion is seen. Contrast enhancement is usually present on MRI. The differentiation of a cavernous hemangioma from a hemorrhagic tumor may be challenging, but the evolution of hemorrhage in a tumor contrasts with the static appearance of the angioma. A complete hemosiderin ring and lack of mass effect and edema favor a cavernous angioma. If the angioma has an acute hemorrhage, it is more difficult to differentiate from a hemorrhagic tumor; with time, however, it will evolve to the typical appearance of an angioma. They are seen intraparenchymally or extradurally.

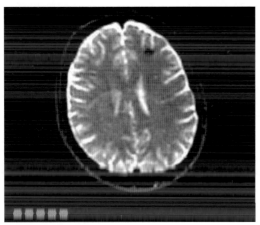

D1. Axial T2-weighted images show a low signal lesion in the left frontal lobe.

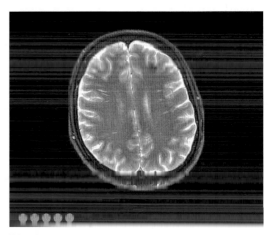

D2. Axial T2-weighted images show a low signal lesion in the left frontal lobe

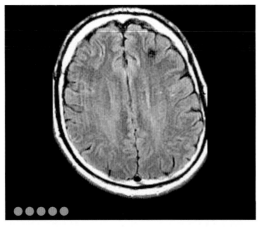

D3. Axial T2-weighted FLAIR image reveals a low signal intensity lesion in the left frontal lobe.

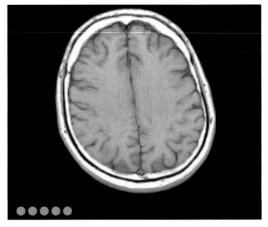

D4. Axial T1-weighted image shows no definite abnormality.

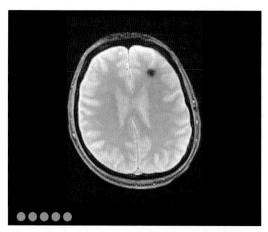

D5. Axial T2-weighted gradient-echo image shows a prominent low signal lesion in the left frontal lobe.

MYCOTIC ANEURYSM

Infection weakens the arterial wall and causes **mycotic aneurysms.** *Streptococcus viridans* is the most common bacterial cause. *Aspergillus* is the most common fungal cause. Most mycotic aneurysms are due to infective emboli that lodge in branch arteries; thus they are typically found on the peripheral branches of the middle cerebral artery. They are actually pseudoaneurysms and are associated with high incidence of intracranial bleed and high mortality. A signal void may be seen on MRI.

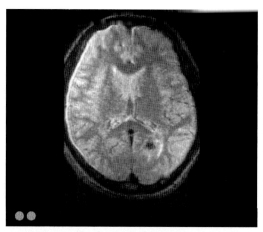

E1. Axial and sagittal T2-weighted images show a focal nodular, low signal lesion in the left parietal region.

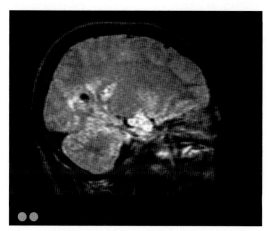

E2. Axial and sagittal T2-weighted images show a focal nodular, low signal lesion in the left parietal region.

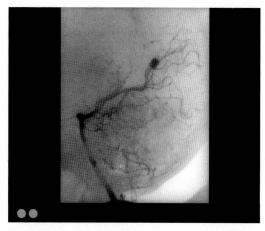

E3. A lateral view angiogram shows an aneurysm arising from the parieto-occipital branch of the left posterior cerebral artery.

VEIN OF GALEN MALFORMATION

Vein of Galen malformation has multiple causes. It can be a pial AVM with deep venous drainage, a direct arteriovenous fistula, or a combination of both. The common arterial supply is from dilated thalamoperforating arteries, anterior cerebral branches, and branches from the posterior cerebral arteries. Steal phenomenon and parenchymal loss may be seen in children with untreated vein of Galen malformation. Hydrocephalus is commonly seen. MRI demonstrates flow void in the dilated vein of Galen and torcular due to the increased flow velocity in the veins secondary to AV shunting.

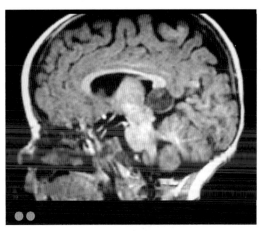

F1. Sagittal T1-weighted image shows a low signal lesion in the region of vein of Galen.

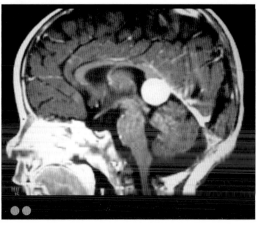

F2. Sagittal and coronal, post-contrast T1-weighted images show an enhancing mass in the region of vein of Galen.

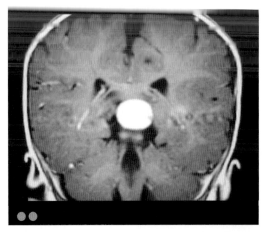

F3. Sagittal and coronal, post-contrast T1-weighted images show an enhancing mass in the region of vein of Galen.

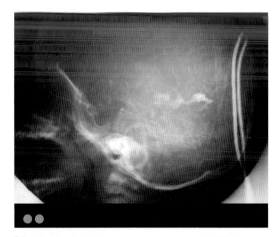

F4. Cerebral angiogram shows a contrast filled vein of Galen malformation.

ARTERIOVENOUS MALFORMATION

They are usually solitary, but occasionally they may be multiple (2%). When they are multiple, they may be associated with Rendu—Osler–Weber or Wyburn–Mason syndrome. These lesions are congenital and at least 25% of patients have symptoms in childhood. Approximately 80–90% of arteriovenous malformations are supratentorial. The classic appearance of the malformation is a wedge-shaped lesion with base toward the brain surface. Typically, there is little or no mass effect. MRI offers many advantages for imaging AVMs. The presence of flow-void within the nidus, enlarged feeding and draining vessels are characteristic of AVMs. Gradient-echo images may be used to differentiate flowing blood from calcifications and hemosiderin since they all exhibit low signal on T1- and T2-weighted images. Blood flow has bright signal on gradient-echo sequences, but calcification and hemosiderin will remain dark.

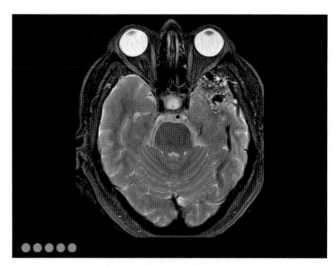

A. Axial T2-weighted image shows a left temporal lesion with multiple tiny low signal areas (flow voids) mixed with adjacent high signal intensity. In addition, nodular and curvilinear low signal areas (flow voids) are seen, which represent dilated draining veins

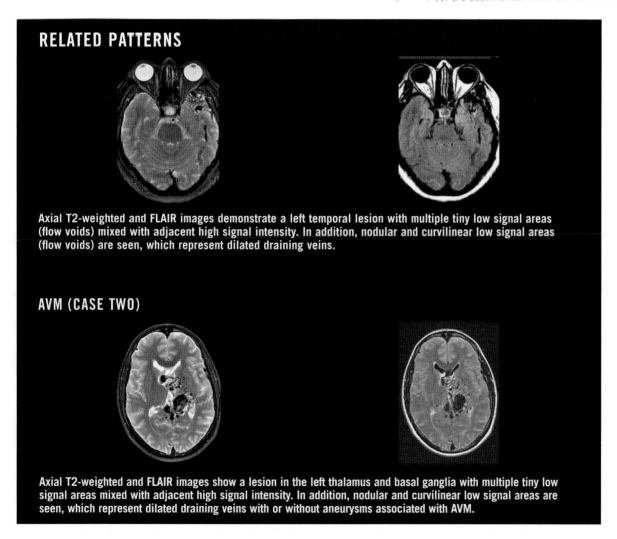

RELATED PATTERNS

Axial T2-weighted and FLAIR images demonstrate a left temporal lesion with multiple tiny low signal areas (flow voids) mixed with adjacent high signal intensity. In addition, nodular and curvilinear low signal areas (flow voids) are seen, which represent dilated draining veins.

AVM (CASE TWO)

Axial T2-weighted and FLAIR images show a lesion in the left thalamus and basal ganglia with multiple tiny low signal areas mixed with adjacent high signal intensity. In addition, nodular and curvilinear low signal areas are seen, which represent dilated draining veins with or without aneurysms associated with AVM.

RELATED PATTERNS (continued)
AVM (CASE TWO) (continued)

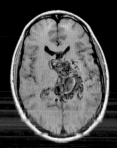

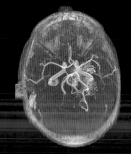

Axial, post-contrast T1-weighted image shows partial enhancement within the low intensity areas of this lesion.

Magnetic resonance angiogram demonstrates the arteriovenous malformation.

AVM (CASE THREE)

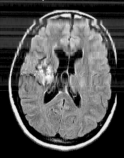

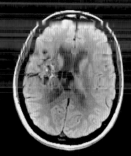

Axial T2-weighted and FLAIR images show a lesion in the right basal ganglia with multiple tiny low signal areas mixed with adjacent high signal intensity. In addition, nodular and curvilinear low signal areas are seen, which represent dilated draining veins.

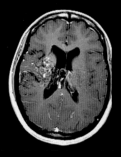

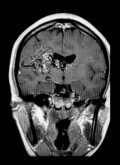

Axial and coronal, post-contrast T1-weighted images show partial enhancement of the lesion.

AVM (CASE FOUR)

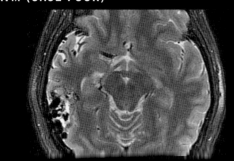

Axial T2 weighted image shows multiple curvilinear flow voids in the right frontal, temporal region.

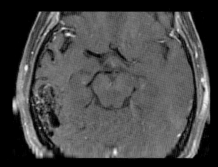

Axial, post-contrast T1-weighted image reveals multiple curvilinear flow voids in the right frontal, temporal region. Patchy contrast enhancement is seen.

AVM (CASE FIVE)

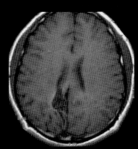

Axial T1-weighted image shows a lesion with serpiginous flow void in the right occipital region.

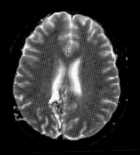

Axial T2-weighted image reveals heterogeneous signal intensity in the right occipital region.

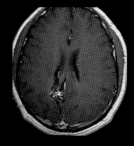

Axial, post-contrast T1-weighted image shows patchy contrast enhancement.

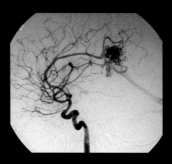

A lateral angiogram shows an arteriovenous malformation with a vascular nidus fed by pericallosal artery and an early draining vein.

DIFFERENTIAL DIAGNOSIS

At a Glance:

- *Dural Arteriovenous Fistula*
- *Wyburn–Mason Syndrome*

DURAL ARTERIOVENOUS FISTULA

Abnormal arteriovenous fistula (AVF) that occur within the dural leaflets (essential for the Dx), and they are usually related to dural sinuses. The nidus of the AV shunt is located within the dura. The arterial supply is recruited from dural arteries and from the pachymeningeal branches of cerebral arteries. The nidus is often located near a venous sinus. Dural AVFs represent 10–15% of cerebral AVMs. Although 20% of cerebral AVMs may acquire dural arterial supply, DAVFs are distinct entities.

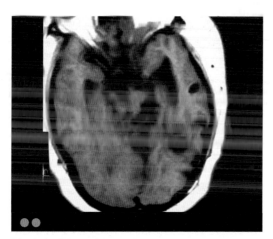

B1. Axial T1-weighted image shows multiple areas of low signal flow void in left temporal region as well as along the tentorium.

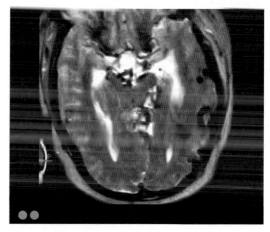

B2. Axial T2-weighted image shows multiple areas of flow void in the left temporal region as well as along the tentorium.

WYBURN–MASON SYNDROME

Wyburn–Mason syndrome is a rare condition characterized by arteriovenous malformations (AVMs) on one or both sides of the brain, especially involving the face, orbit, retina, and along the optic pathway to the optic chiasm in the suprasellar region. This condition is considered to be congenital, nonhereditary, and without sex or race predilection. Other vascular malformations may be present elsewhere in the body.

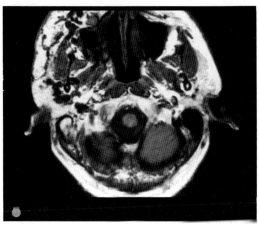

C1. Axial T1-weighted images show a lesion involving the right face, orbit, and suprasellar region with a mixture of multiple tiny low signal areas and serpiginous low signal areas.

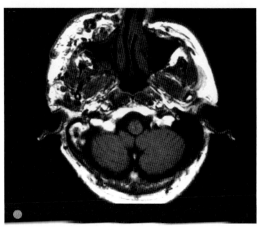

C2. Axial T1-weighted images show a lesion involving the right face, orbit, and suprasellar region with a mixture of multiple tiny low signal areas and serpiginous low signal areas.

351

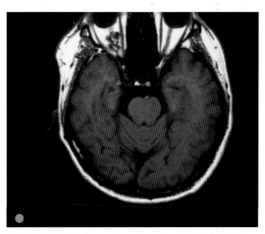

C3. Axial T1-weighted images show a lesion involving the right face, orbit, and suprasellar region with a mixture of multiple tiny low signal areas and serpiginous low signal areas.

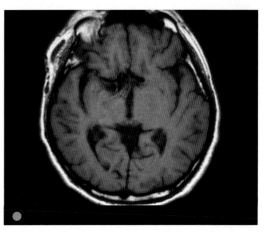

C4. Axial T1-weighted images show a lesion involving the right face, orbit, and suprasellar region with a mixture of multiple tiny low signal areas and serpiginous low signal areas.

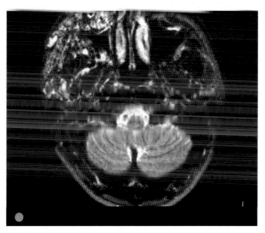

C5. Axial T2-weighted image demonstrates a mixture of low and high signal areas involving the right face.

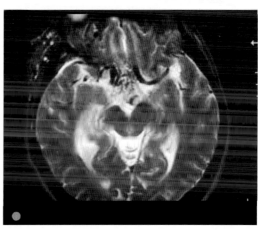

C6. Axial T2-weighted image shows abnormal flow-voids involving the Right suprasellar region. Not the presence of curvilinear and nodular high signal areas in the subcutaneous tissue in right temporal region.

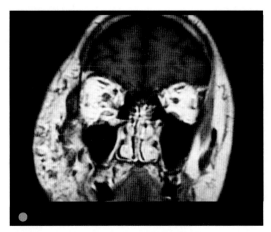

C7. Coronal, post-contrast T1-weighted image shows partial enhancement of the lesion.

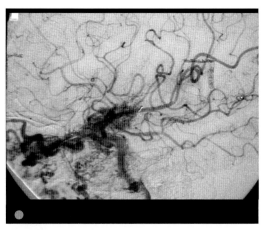

C8. Cerebral angiograms demonstrate the arteriovenous malformation involves the face, orbit, and around the optic chiasm.

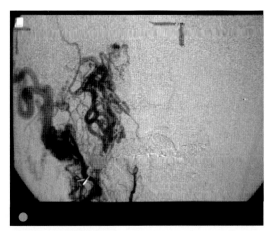

C9. Cerebral angiograms demonstrate the arteriovenous malformation involves the face, orbit, and around the optic chiasm.

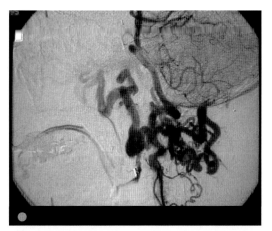

C10. Cerebral angiograms demonstrate the arteriovenous malformation involves the face, orbit, and around the optic chiasm.

VENOUS MALFORMATION

Venous malformations are probably developmental venous anomalies rather than true vascular malformation. They are the most common vascular malformation of the brain at autopsy and have been reported to occur in 26% of the population. They are usually solitary. They are usually seen incidently on MRI. The typical location of the lesions is the deep white matter of the cerebrum or cerebellum. They are frequently seen adjacent to the frontal horns of the lateral ventricle.

MRI shows flow within the draining transcerebral vein, which is usually fast enough to have a flow void. After contrast administration, the draining vein and tributaries are usually enhanced.

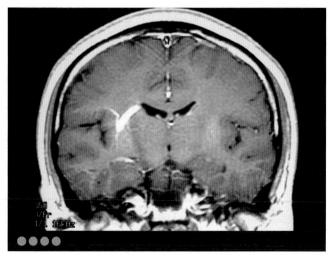

A. Coronal, post contrast T1 weighted image shows a linear enhancing lesion with small tributaries in the region of right basal ganglia adjacent to the lateral ventricle.

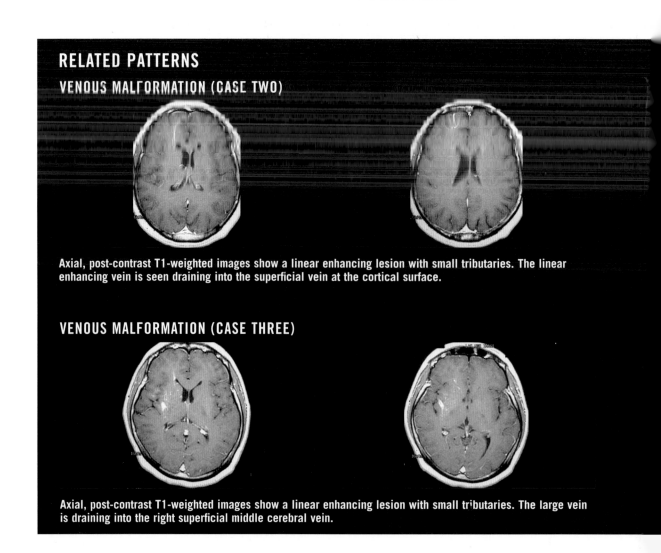

RELATED PATTERNS

VENOUS MALFORMATION (CASE TWO)

Axial, post-contrast T1-weighted images show a linear enhancing lesion with small tributaries. The linear enhancing vein is seen draining into the superficial vein at the cortical surface.

VENOUS MALFORMATION (CASE THREE)

Axial, post-contrast T1-weighted images show a linear enhancing lesion with small tributaries. The large vein is draining into the right superficial middle cerebral vein.

VENOUS MALFORMATION (CASE THREE) (continued)

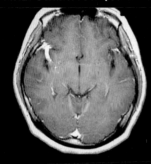

Axial, post-contrast T1-weighted images show a linear enhancing lesion with small tributaries. The large vein is draining into the right superficial middle cerebral vein.

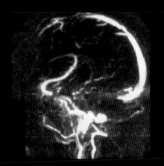

Magnetic resonance venogram demonstrates the venous malformation.

DIFFERENTIAL DIAGNOSIS

At a Glance:

* *Venous Malformation Associated with*
  Cavernous Hemangioma

VENOUS MALFORMATION ASSOCIATED WITH CAVERNOUS HEMANGIOMA

There is a frequent association between cavernous hemangioma and developmental venous malformation. When hemorrhage occurs, it is usually due to the cavernous angioma.

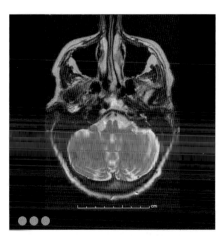

B1. Axial T2-weighted images show a hyperintense lesion with surrounding hypointensity.

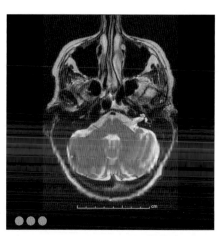

B2. Axial T2-weighted images show a hyperintense lesion with surrounding hypointensity.

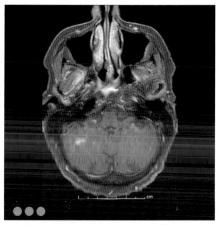

B3. Axial and coronal, post-contrast, T1-weighted images show a linear enhancing lesion with small tributaries adjacent to the round hyperintense lesion with peripheral hypointense rim.

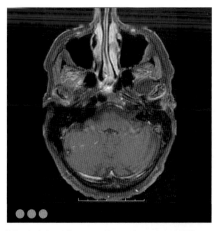

B4. Axial and coronal, post-contrast, T1-weighted images show a linear enhancing lesion with small tributaries adjacent to the round hyperintense lesion with peripheral hypointense rim.

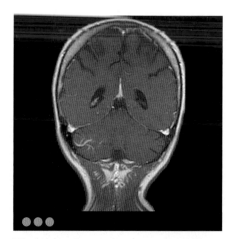

B5. Axial and coronal, post-contrast, T1-weighted images show a linear enhancing lesion with small tributaries adjacent to the round hyperintense lesion with peripheral hypointense rim.

AMYLOID ANGIOPATHY

Amyloid angiopathy results from deposition of amyloid in the media and adventitia of small and medium sized arteries of the superficial layer of the cerebral cortex and leptomeninges, with sparing of the deep gray matters. Amyloid deposition increases with age. Hemorrhages are usually lobar, involving frontal and parietal lobes. Subarachnoid and subdural hemorrhages have also been reported. There is a tendency for recurrent or multiple hemorrhages. MRI may exhibit variable signal intensity areas, consistent with hemorrhage at different stages.

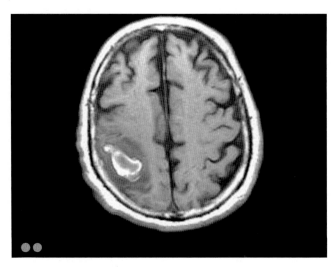

A. Axial T1-weighted image shows a hyperintense area of hemorrhage with surrounding hypointense edema in the right parietal lobe.

RELATED PATTERNS

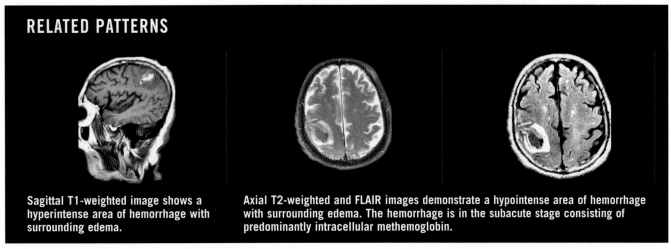

Sagittal T1-weighted image shows a hyperintense area of hemorrhage with surrounding edema.

Axial T2-weighted and FLAIR images demonstrate a hypointense area of hemorrhage with surrounding edema. The hemorrhage is in the subacute stage consisting of predominantly intracellular methemoglobin.

DIFFERENTIAL DIAGNOSIS

At a Glance:

- *Arteriovenous Malformation Rupture*
- *Cavernous Angioma*
- *Hemorrhagic Infarct due to Superior Sagittal Sinus Thrombosis*

- *Hemorrhagic Neoplasm (Primary or Metastatic)*
- *Hemorrhagic Metastatic Melanoma*
- *Toxoplasmosis*
- *Aneurysm Rupture* (not pictured)
- *Moya-Moya Syndrome* (not pictured)
- *Vasculitis* (not pictured)

ARTERIOVENOUS MALFORMATION RUPTURE

They are usually solitary, but occasionally they may be multiple (2%). These lesions are congenital and at 25% of patients have symptoms in childhood. Approximately 80-90% of arteriovenous malformations are supratentorial. AVMs are seen in approximately 0.10% of the general population and 3% in patients with cerebral hemorrhage. Flow-related aneurysm accounts for a major cause of intracranial hemorrhage in patients with AVM or AVF.

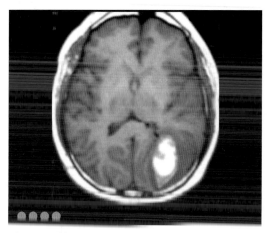

B1. Axial T1-weighted image shows a hyperintense lesion in the left parietooccipital region.

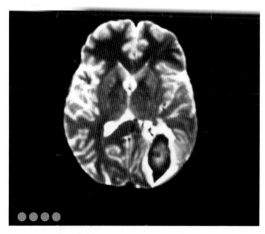

B2. Axial T2-weighted image shows a predominantly hypointense lesion in the left parietooccipital region.

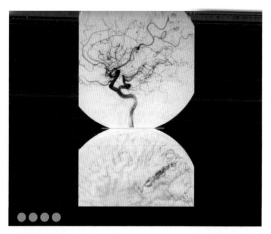

B3. A cerebral angiogram reveals an arteriovenous malformation in the left parietooccipital region. Incidentally seen in this patient is the presence of a trigeminal artery. The persistent trigeminal artery is the most cephalically located and frequently occurring persistent carotid-vertebrobasilar anastomosis. Its incidence is reported to be 0.1–0.6% in large angiographic series. There is an increased incidence of intracranial aneurysm in patients with persistent trigeminal artery.

CAVERNOUS ANGIOMA

Cavernous angiomas are the most common type of vascular malformations. There is a tendency for multiplicity and a familial predisposition. They may be discovered incidently or present with seizures or neurological symptoms, particularly if they are associated with hemorrhage. MR is the imaging modality of choice for cavernous angioma. The angioma is a round, well-circumscribed area that has mixed signal intensity due to the presence of various blood products. It may present as a hyperintense lesion on T1-weighted images because of the presence of methemoglobin in the cavernoma. It has been described as "popcorn-like" in appearance. There is a circumscribed ring of hemosiderin that is dark and has a blooming effect on T2-weighted images and particularly on T2*-weighted gradient-echo images. Contrast enhancement is usually present on MRI. The differentiation of a cavernous hemangioma from a hemorrhagic tumor may be challenging, but the evolution of hemorrhage in a tumor contrasts with the static appearance of the angioma. A complete hemosiderin ring and lack of mass effect and edema favor a cavernous angioma. If the angioma has an acute hemorrhage, it is more difficult to differentiate a hemorrhagic tumor; with time, however, it will evolve to the typical appearance of an angioma. They are seen intraparenchymally or extradurally.

CAVERNOUS ANGIOMA (CASE ONE)

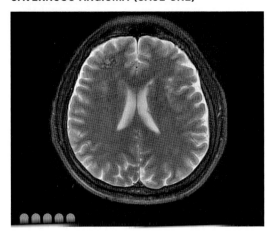

C1. Axial T2-weighted and FLAIR images show a low signal intensity rim surrounding a mixed, hyperintense lesion.

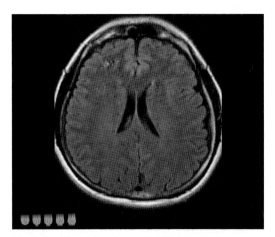

C2. Axial T2-weighted and FLAIR images show a low signal intensity rim surrounding a mixed, hyperintense lesion.

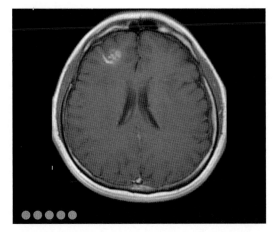

C3. Axial, post-contrast T1-weighted image shows a predominantly hyperintense lesion with some mixed hypointensity.

CAVERNOUS ANGIOMA (CASE TWO)

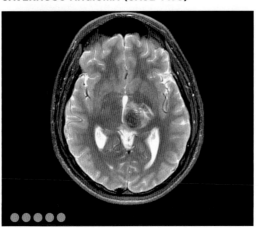

D1. Axial T2-weighted images show a lesion of mixed signal intensity with predominant hypointensity seen medially and hyperintensity seen laterally in the region of left thalamus and midbrain.

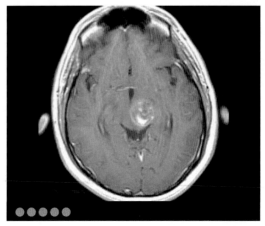

D2. Axial and coronal, post-contrast T1-weighted images show partial enhancement of the lesion.

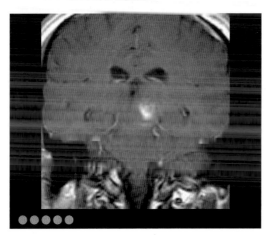

D3. Axial and coronal, post-contrast T1-weighted images show partial enhancement of the lesion.

HEMORRHAGIC INFARCT DUE TO SUPERIOR SAGITTAL SINUS THROMBOSIS

Cerebral venous thrombosis (CVT) is a rare disease, more cases are recognized recently due to modern imaging techniques. CVT causes venous infarcts in about 50% of cases. They are frequently hemorrhagic in nature. On the basis of clinical observation, however, this brain damage seems to be largely reversible and differs from arterial stroke.

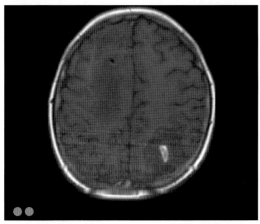

E1. Axial T1-weighted image shows a hyperintense area with surrounding hypointensity in the left parietal white matter, consistent with hemorrhagic infarct. Another hypointense area is seen in the right frontal white matter, consistent with white matter infarct.

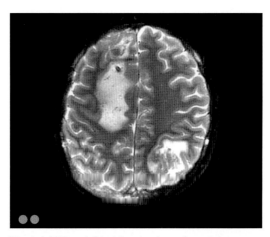

E2. Axial T2-weighted image shows hyperintense areas in the left parietal and right frontal region.

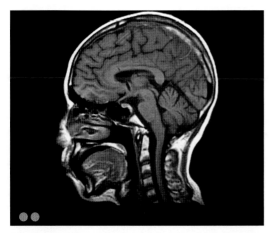

E3. Sagittal T1-weighted image shows hyperintensity along the superior sagittal sinus, consistent with thrombosis.

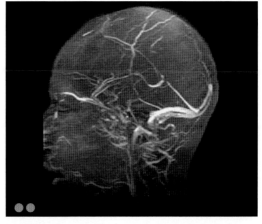

E4. MR venogram demonstrates sagittal sinus thrombosis.

HEMORRHAGIC NEOPLASM (PRIMARY OR METASTATIC)

Hemorrhage is common in the high-grade gliomas and certain highly vascular metastases. The diagnosis of a neoplastic source of hemorrhage may be difficult in the subacute phase. It is difficult to appreciate the contrast enhancement against the hyperintense methemoglobin seen on T1-weighted images. In such cases, CT with and without contrast may assist in the diagnosis by demonstrating enhancing component of the neoplasm. When a hematoma results from a primary or metastatic tumor, fluid--fluid levels may be seen. When followed sequentially, intratumoral hemorrhage may appear to evolve more slowly than parenchymal hematoma.

HEMORRHAGIC GLIOBLASTOMA MULTIFORME

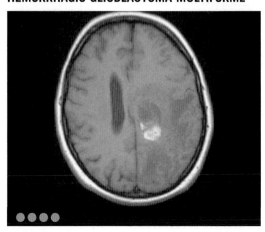

F1. Axial T1-weighted image shows a mass lesion in the left frontoparietal region. The anterior portion of the mass shows isointensity and the posterior portion of the mass shows hyperintensity, consistent with hemorrhage.

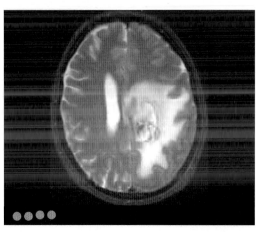

F2. Axial T2-weighted image shows a heterogeneous mass in the left frontoparietal region with surrounding edema.

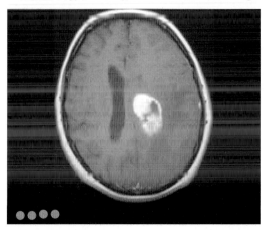

F3. Axial, post-contrast T1-weighted image demonstrates enhancement of the isointense portion of the mass.

HEMORRHAGIC METASTATIC ADENOCARCINOMA OF THE LUNG

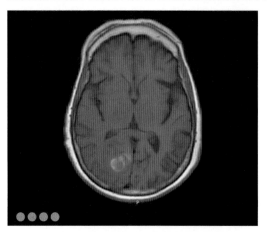

G1. Axial T1-weighted image shows a hyperintense lesion in the right occipital region, consistent with a hemorrhagic lesion.

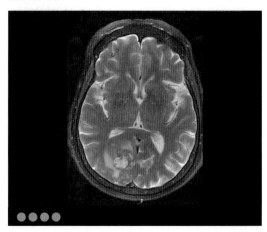

G2. Axial T2-weighted image reveals hyperintense lesion with surrounding edema in the right occipital region.

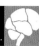

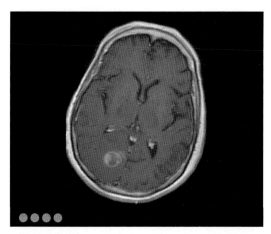

G3. Axial, post-contrast T1-weighted image shows some enhancement of the lesion.

HEMORRHAGIC METASTATIC MELANOMA

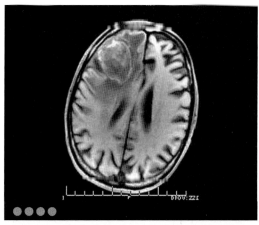

H1. Axial T1-weighted image shows a mixed intensity mass with focal, peripheral hyperintensity, consistent with hemorrhage in the right frontal region with surrounding edema.

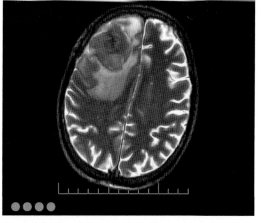

H2. Axial T2-weighted and FLAIR images reveal a large hypointense mass in the right frontal region with surrounding edema.

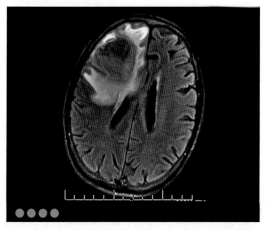

H3. Axial T2-weighted and FLAIR images reveal a large hypointense mass in the right frontal region with surrounding edema.

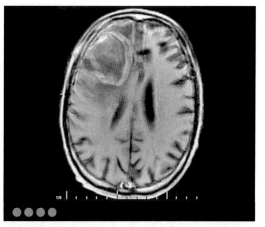

H4. Axial, post-contrast T1-weighted image shows an irregular ring-like enhancing mass.

TOXOPLASMOSIS

Toxoplasmosis lesions are hypointense on T1-weighted images and hyperintense on T2-weighted images. Toxoplasmosis demonstrates ring-like enhancement more frequently than lymphoma after administration of gadolinium.

T2-weighted and FLAIR images are useful for detection of multiple lesions. Although multiple lesions may occur in either condition, presence of thin-walled, multiple lesions favor toxoplasmosis. Occasionally, toxoplasmosis lesions may exhibit hyperintensity on T1-weighted images due to hemorrhage or calcification following treatment.

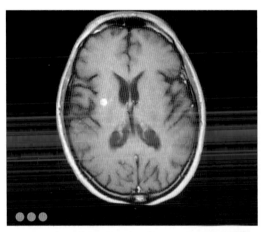

I1. Axial T1-weighted image shows a focal hyperintensity in the right basal ganglia due to hemorrhage in a lesion of toxoplasmosis.

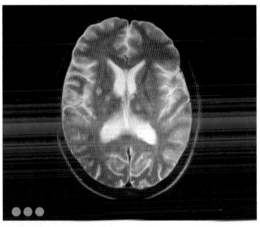

I2. Axial T2-weighted image reveals a focal hyperintensity in the right basal ganglia.

364

SAGITTAL SINUS THROMBOSIS AND AVF

A number of predisposing factors have been implicated in the development of venous sinus thrombosis. Trauma, infection, tumors, dehydration, hypercoagulable states such as pregnancy, oral contraceptives and nephrotic syndrome are common causes. Unusual causes include Behcet disease, acquired immunodeficiency syndrome, ulcerative colitis, chemotherapy (particularly with asparginase and cytarabine), and lupus. In addition, dural sinus thrombosis has also been associated with congenital heart disease, antiphospholipid syndrome, and protein S deficiency. Local infection, such as mastoiditis or cellulitis, can lead to venous sinus thrombosis. Approximately 20–25% of cases of dural sinus thrombosis are idiopathic. An association of venous sinus thrombosis and dural arteriovenous fistula has been described. Cerebral venous thrombosis often presents with hemorrhagic infarction in areas atypical for arterial vascular distribution. Magnetic resonance venography (MRV) in conjunction with conventional MRI can accurately diagnose cerebral venous thrombosis.

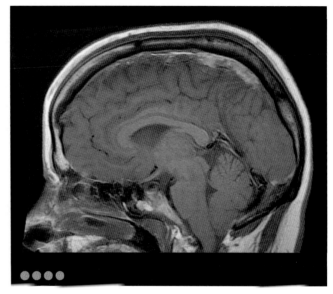

A. Sagittal T1-weighted image shows hyperintensity in the proximal superior sagittal sinus instead of the usual flow void.

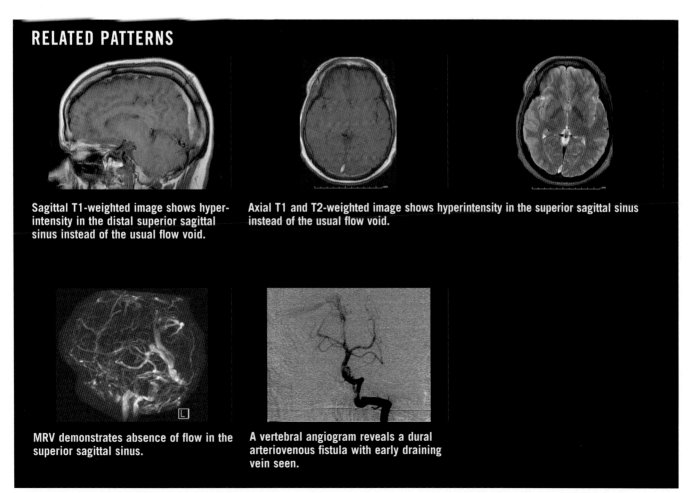

RELATED PATTERNS

Sagittal T1-weighted image shows hyperintensity in the distal superior sagittal sinus instead of the usual flow void.

Axial T1 and T2-weighted image shows hyperintensity in the superior sagittal sinus instead of the usual flow void.

MRV demonstrates absence of flow in the superior sagittal sinus.

A vertebral angiogram reveals a dural arteriovenous fistula with early draining vein seen.

RELATED PATTERNS (continued)
SAGITTAL SINUS THROMBOSIS (CASE TWO)

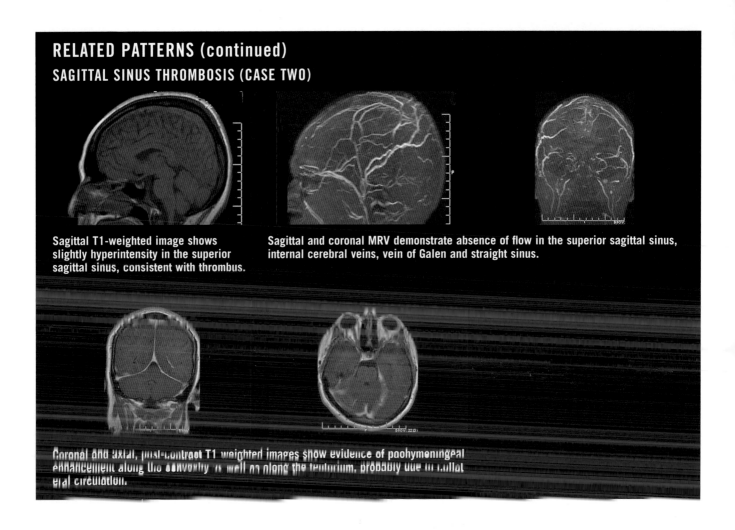

Sagittal T1-weighted image shows slightly hyperintensity in the superior sagittal sinus, consistent with thrombus.

Sagittal and coronal MRV demonstrate absence of flow in the superior sagittal sinus, internal cerebral veins, vein of Galen and straight sinus.

Coronal and axial, post-contrast T1 weighted images show evidence of pachymeningeal enhancement along the convexity as well as along the tentorium, probably due to collateral circulation.

DIFFERENTIAL DIAGNOSIS

At a Glance:

- *Straight Sinus Thrombosis*
- *Transverse Sinus Thrombosis*

STRAIGHT SINUS THROMBOSIS

Thrombosis of the deep cerebral veins such as the basal vein of Rosenthal, the internal cerebral veins and straight sinus can result in bilateral thalamic infarction, which could be hemorrhagic.

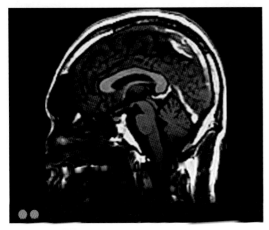

B1. Sagittal T1-weighted image shows hyperintensity in the straight sinus, vein of Galen as well as in the superior sagittal sinus, consistent with venous thrombosis.

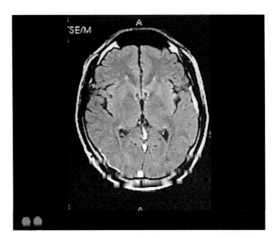

B2. Axial T2-weighted FLAIR image shows hyperintensity in the straight sinus, consistent with venous thrombosis. Slight hyperintensity is seen in the posterior aspect of the thalamus bilaterally due to early venous infarction.

TRANSVERSE SINUS THROMBOSIS

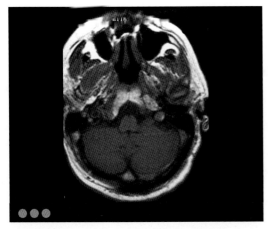

C1. Axial T1-weighted images show focal hyperintensity in the region of left transverse sinus.

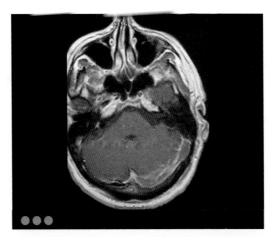

C2. Axial T1-weighted images show focal hyperintensity in the region of left transverse sinus.

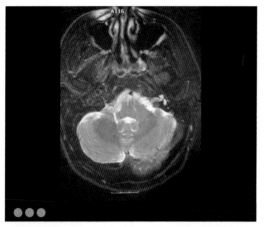

C3. Axial T2-weighted images show focal hypointensity in the region of left transverse sinus.

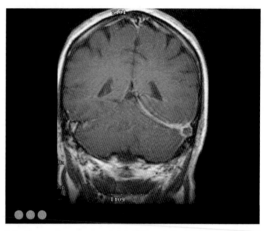

C4. Coronal, post-contrast T1-weighted image shows a filling defect in the left transverse sinus.

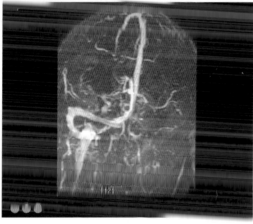

C5. Coronal MRV reveals absence of flow in the left transverse sinus.

THROMBOSIS OF THE SUPERIOR SAGITTAL SINUS, INTERNAL CEREBRAL VEIN, AND STRAIGHT SINUS

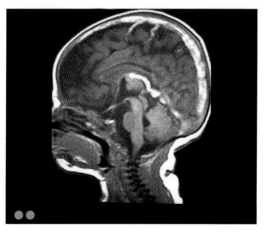

D1. Sagittal and axial T1-weighted image shows hyperintensity in the superior sagittal sinus, internal cerebral veins, vein of Galen and straight sinus.

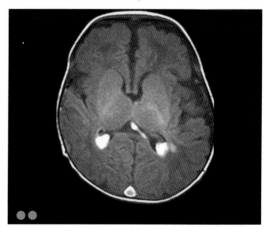

D2. Sagittal and axial T1-weighted image shows hyperintensity in the superior sagittal sinus, internal cerebral veins, vein of Galen and straight sinus.

Chapter 8

Lesions in the Cortical Gray Matter, White Matter, and Deep Gray Matter

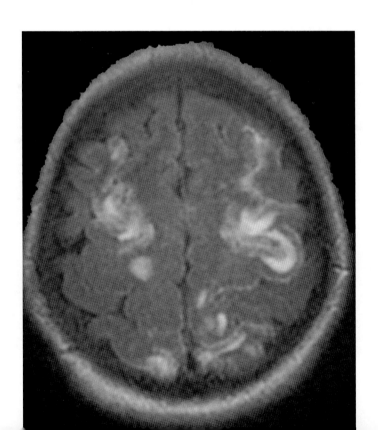

SYSTEMIC LUPUS ERYTHEMATOSUS (SLE)

Systemic lupus erythematosus may present with a wide variety of MR appearances. Multiple small foci of T2 hyperintensity are seen in the subcortical and deep hemispheric white matter. These lesions usually do not enhance with contrast and may represent old inflammatory foci or small white matter infarcts secondary to vasculitis. Another pattern is the presence of large areas of cortical and subcortical edema shown as T2 hyperintensity on MRI. Superficial contrast enhancement may be demonstrated.

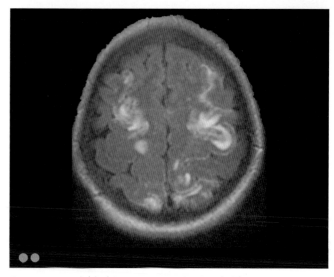

A, Axial T2-weighted image shows gyriform hyperintensity in frontal and parietal lobes bilaterally.

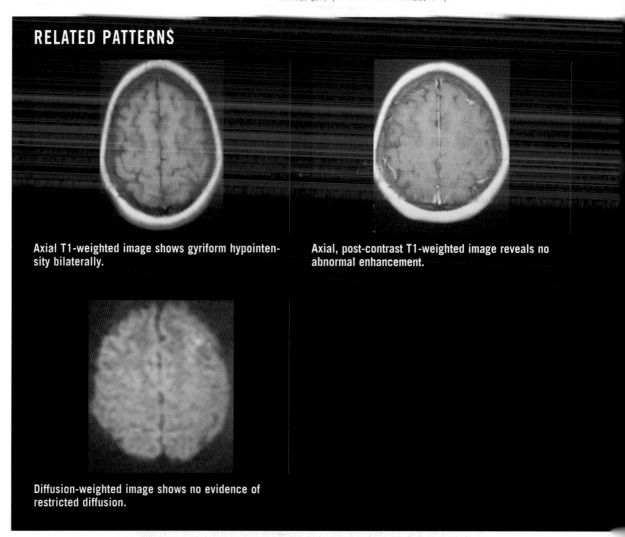

RELATED PATTERNS

Axial T1-weighted image shows gyriform hypointensity bilaterally.

Axial, post-contrast T1-weighted image reveals no abnormal enhancement.

Diffusion-weighted image shows no evidence of restricted diffusion.

INFARCT DUE TO LUPUS VASCULITIS

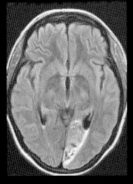
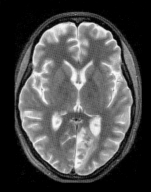

Axial T2-weighted and FLAIR images show gyriform hyperintensity in the left occipital region due to an old infarct in a patient with lupus.

LUPUS VASCULITIS

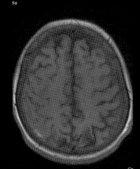
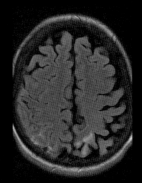

Axial T1-weighted image shows focal edema in the right parietal region with a hyperintense area seen, consistent with hemorrhage.

Axial T2 FLAIR image reveals gyriform hyperintensity in both parietal regions. Effacement of the cortical sulci is seen on the right side due to edema.

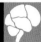

DIFFERENTIAL DIAGNOSIS

At a Glance:

- *Cerebral Contusion*
- *Cerebritis and Subdural Empyema*
- *Creutzfeldt Jakob Disease*
- *Embolic Infarct Post Cardiac Surgery*
- *Herpes Encephalitis*
- *Posterior Reversible Eencephalopathy*
- *Subacute Infarction*
- *Tuberous Sclerosis*
- *Vasculitis*
- *Wegner's Granulomatosis*
- *Hypoxic, Anoxic Injury* (not pictured)
- *Sarcoidosis* (not pictured)

CEREBRAL CONTUSION

Contusion of the brain presents bruises of the brain parenchyma with petechial hemorrhage. It tends to occur in the areas where the inner surface of the skull is rough, namely the temporal fossa and inferior frontal fossa. T2-weighted images and FLAIR images are useful to detect the edema following contusion. Cerebral contusion combines mechanical insults to brain tissue with an imbalance between cerebral blood flow and metabolism, excitotoxicity, edema formation, and inflammatory and apoptotic processes. The unpredictability of each patient's pathophysiology although common to trauma requires monitoring of the injured brain in order to tailor the treatment according to the specific status of the patient.

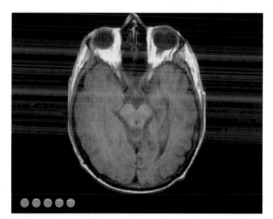

B1. Axial T1-weighted image shows hypointensity in the right temporal region.

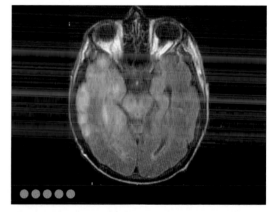

B2. Axial FLAIR image reveals gyriform hyperintensity in the right temporal region.

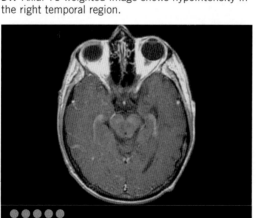

B3. Axial, post-contrast T1-weighted images demonstrate gyriform contrast enhancement in the right temporal region.

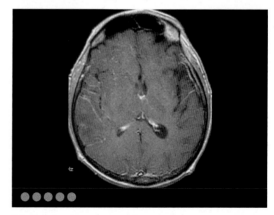

B4. Axial, post-contrast T1-weighted images demonstrate gyriform contrast enhancement in the right temporal region.

CEREBRITIS AND SUBDURAL EMPYEMA

Subdural empyema accounts for about 13% to 20% of all cases of intracranial infection. Subdural empyema is a collection of pus between the dura and the leptomeninges, which often occurs as a complication of meningitis, paranasal sinusitis, otitis media, osteomyelitis, or a penetrating wound of the skull. Frontal sinusitis is the most common cause of subdural empyema. Infective organisms probably enter the subdural space in a retrograde fashion through a dural sinus or through bridging veins. Complications of subdural empyema include venous thrombosis and infarction. Subjacent cerebritis may be seen, which presents as gyriform hyperintensity on T2 weighted images.

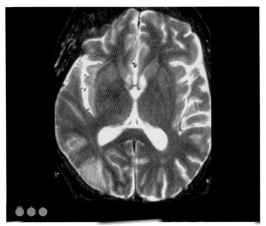

C1 Axial T2 weighted and FLAIR images show gyriform hyperintensity in the right parietal region, consistent with cerebritis. Linear hyperintensity along the falx posteriorly is also seen.

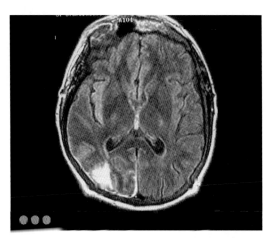

C2. Axial T2 weighted and FLAIR images show gyriform hyperintensity in the right parietal region, consistent with cerebritis. Linear hyperintensity along the falx posteriorly is also seen. Slight hyperintensity is seen involving the right insular cortex.

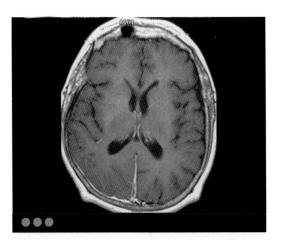

C3. Axial, post-contrast T1-weighted images demonstrate a parafalcine subdural empyema with right parietal pachymeningeal enhancement.

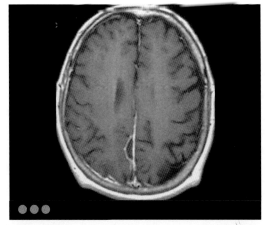

C4. Axial, post-contrast T1-weighted images demonstrate a parafalcine subdural empyema with right parietal pachymeningeal enhancement.

CREUTZFELDT JAKOB DISEASE

This fatal disease of the CNS was first described by Creutzfeldt in 1920 and by Jakob in 1921. Similar to kuru and scrapie, **Creutzfeldt Jakob disease (CJD)** is thought to be caused by an "unconventional virus" known as a prion. Prions are small proteinaceous infectious particles that differ from standard viruses, in that they contain little or no nucleic acid and do not evoke an immune response during infection. Creutzfeldt-Jakob disease is a rare, degenerative brain disease that causes progressive demen-

tia and, eventually, death. Prompt diagnosis is essential to prevent human-to-human transmission. Progressive brain atrophy and areas of high signal intensity in the cerebral cortex and basal ganglia are well-known features of Creutzfeldt-Jakob disease demonstrated on T2-weighted MR images. However, in the early stage of disease, abnormalities may not be seen on T2-weighted MR images. Diffusion-weighted imaging may be a useful modality for the early diagnosis of Creutzfeldt-Jakob disease. Areas of restricted diffusion are seen in the cerebral cortex, basal ganglia and thalamus.

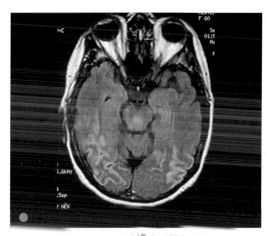

D1. Axial T2 weighted FLAIR image shows gyriform hyperintensity in the temporoccipital region bilaterally. Note the focal hyperintensity in the midbrain.

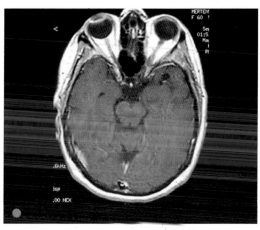

D2. Axial, post contrast T1 weighted image reveals no abnormal contrast enhancement. Note a dural based, extra-axial enhancing mass in the left posterior temporal region is probably a meningioma.

EMBOLIC INFARCT IN A PATIENT STATUS POST CARDIAC SURGERY

Current literature indicates a stroke rate of approximately 3.6% in patients who had cardiac surgery. The majority of

the patients were identified within the first 3 postoperative days. Stroke after cardiac surgery is a devastating complication. **Embolic infarction** causes multiple areas of abnormal signal intensity with evidence of restricted diffusion on MRI.

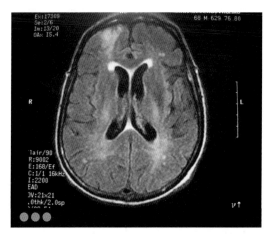

E1. Axial T2-weighted FLAIR images show several areas of gyriform hyperintensity, consistent with embolic infarctions. In addition, periventricular and subcortical white matter hyperintense areas are also seen.

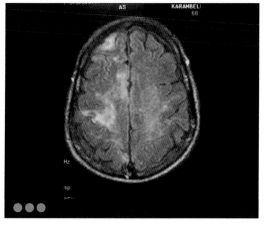

E2. Axial T2-weighted FLAIR images show several areas of gyriform hyperintensity, consistent with embolic infarctions. In addition, periventricular and subcortical white matter hyperintense areas are also seen.

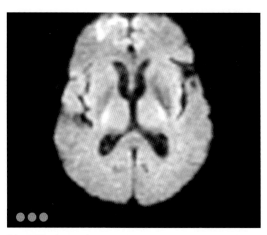

E3. Diffusion-weighted images show evidence of restricted diffusion corresponding to T2 abnormal signal intensity areas.

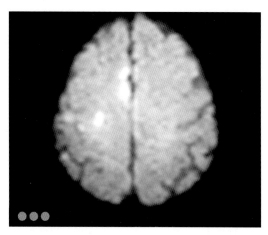

E4. Diffusion-weighted images show evidence of restricted diffusion corresponding to T2 abnormal signal intensity areas.

HERPES ENCEPHALITIS

Herpes encephalitis has a bimodal age distribution, with the first peak occurring in patients younger than 20 years and a second peak in those older than 50 years. It occurs as a superficial gray matter disease, and a breakdown of blood brain barrier produces gyral pattern of contrast enhancement. Herpes encephalitis often begins in the medial temporal lobes and in the cingulated gyrus of the medial frontal and parietal lobes.

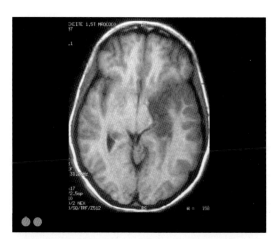

F1. Axial T1-weighted image shows hypointense lesion involving the cortex of the left temporal lobe, more medially.

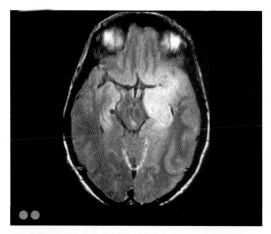

F2. Axial T2-weighted image shows hyperintense lesions involving both temporal lobes, more on the left side.

POSTERIOR REVERSIBLE ENCEPHALOPATHY

As the name indicates, this is a reversible condition with abnormal hyperintensity seen in the cortex and subcortical white matter in parietoccipital regions bilaterally on T2-weighted images. The abnormal signal can extend into temporal, frontal lobes, pons, and cerebellum. Enhancement may or may not be seen. Diffusion imaging characteristically does not show restricted diffusion unless there is superimposed infarction. There are a diverse group of etiologies including preeclampsia and eclampsia, hypertension, cyclosporine, Cisplatinum, SLE, cryoglobulinemia, hemolytic uremic syndrome, etc.

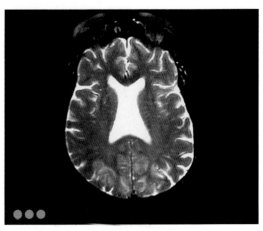

G1. Axial T2-weighted and FLAIR images show gyriform T2 hyperintensity in the parietoccipital region bilaterally.

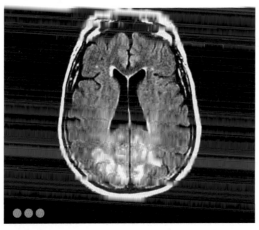

G2. Axial T2-weighted and FLAIR images show gyriform T2 hyperintensity in the parietoccipital region bilaterally.

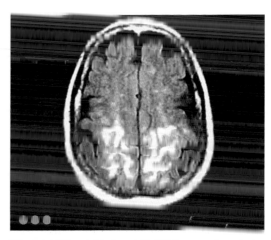

G3. Axial T2-weighted and FLAIR images show gyriform T2 hyperintensity in the parietoccipital region bilaterally.

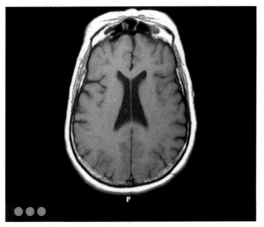

G4. Axial T1-weighted image does not show significant abnormality.

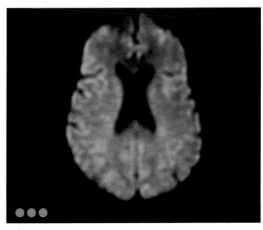

G5. Diffusion-weighted image shows no evidence of restricted diffusion.

SUBACUTE INFARCTION

Cerebral infarction is the third leading cause of death behind heart disease and cancer and is the number one cause of all disability in the United States. Thromboembolic disease is the most prevalent cause. Most patients present with neurologic deficits; however, the clinical findings are often nonspecific. The specificity of diagnosis is markedly improved with MR imaging with diffusion-weighted images. The early detection of cerebral infarction is important for identifying patients who may undergo tar-

geted treatments such as thrombolysis or thrombectomy. Acute infarction can be identified using diffusion-weighted imaging as early as 2 hours after the onset. Restricted diffusion presents as hyperintensity on diffusion-weighted images and hypointensity on ADC map. Subacute infarction (7–21 days) usually presents as areas of low T1 and high T2 signal intensity in a gyriform pattern. The ADC map findings may reverse and become bright, reflecting T2 shine through on the DWI due to vasogenic edema. Edema and associated mass effect slowly resolve.

SUBACUTE INFARCTION (CASE ONE)

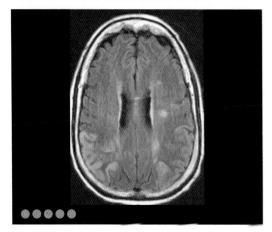

H1. Axial FLAIR image shows gyriform hyperintensity in both temporoparietal regions.

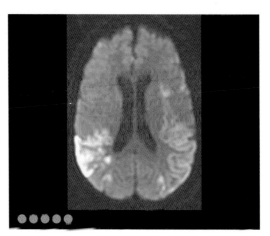

H2. Diffusion-weighted image shows restricted diffusion bilaterally, more on the right side.

SUBACUTE INFARCTION (CASE TWO)

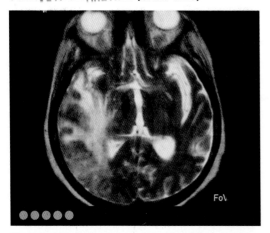

I1. Axial T2-weighted image shows gyriform hyperintensity in the right temporal region. Intermixed areas of hypointensity are due to hemorrhage within the infarct.

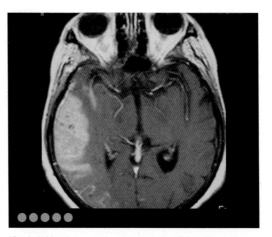

I2. Axial and coronal, post-contrast T1-weighted image demonstrates gyriform contrast enhancement.

377

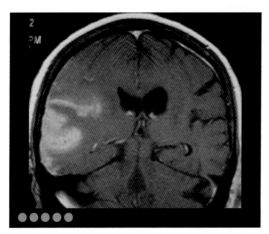

I3. Axial and coronal, post-contrast T1-weighted image demonstrates gyriform contrast enhancement.

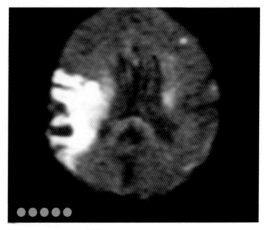

I4. Diffusion-weighted image and ADC map show restricted diffusion in the right temporal lobe, consistent with acute/subacute infarction.

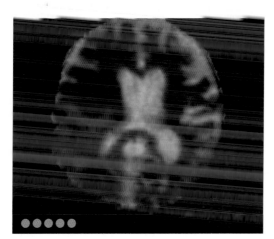

I5. Diffusion-weighted image and ADC map show restricted diffusion in the right temporal lobe, consistent with acute/subacute infarction.

TUBEROUS SCLEROSIS

Tuberous sclerosis is an autosomal dominant disease with classic triad of epilepsy, mental retardation, and adenoma sabeceum. Other features include ocular harmatomas, bilateral renal angiolipomas and cysts, cardiac rhabdomyomas, shagreen patch, and hypopigmented macules.

Characteristic subependymal nodules are seen in 95% of the patients. Cortical tubers may be seen on MRI in 95% of patients. Most show a smooth, expanded outer cortical surface. MRI signal intensity of the outer component is isointense to gray matter on all sequences. The inner core is isointense to hypointense on T1-weighted images and is hyperintense on T2-weighted images.

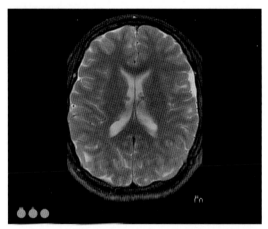

J1. Axial T2-weighted and FLAIR images show gyriform hyperintensity in both hemisphere. These actually represent subcortical tubers. In addition, multiple small subependymal tubers are seen.

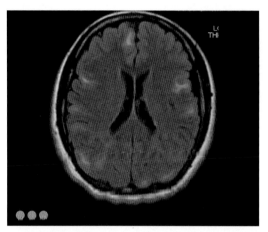

J2. Axial T2-weighted and FLAIR images show gyriform hyperintensity in both hemisphere. These actually represent subcortical tubers. In addition, multiple small subependymal tubers are seen.

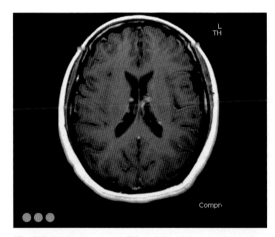

J3. Axial, post-contrast T1-weighted image demonstrates enhancement of the subependymal tubers.

379

VASCULITIS

Primary central nervous system vasculitis (PCNSV) is a rare form of vascular inflammatory disease involving the brain and spinal cord that is poorly understood. PCNSV diagnosis is established based on positive CNS tissue histopathology. Cerebral angiography may be negative in some cases although intracranial vascular stenosis can be demonstrated in some of the cases. Although no specific pattern for this entity exists on MR imaging, multiple infarcts of various ages in more than one vascular territory should raise the suspicion. MR angiography may be used to detect vascular stenosis in major intracranial vessels. CT angiography is now widely used and may replace conventional angiography as the primary imaging modality. The most frequent clinical presentations include hemiparesis, cerebral ischemia, headache and altered cognition. Patients with MR findings of T2 hyperintensity involving the white matter and cortical gray matter tend to show significantly worse modified Rankin disability scores compared to the other patients.

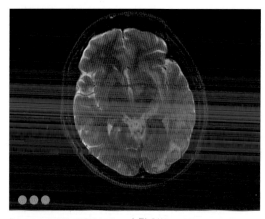

K1. Axial T2-weighted and FLAIR images demonstrate gyriform hyperintensity involving the left parietooccipital region as well as in the left basal ganglia, external capsule, and thalamus

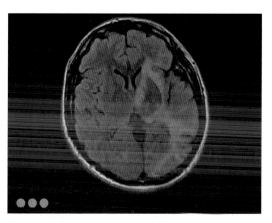

K2. Axial T2-weighted and FLAIR images demonstrate gyriform hyperintensity involving the left parietooccipital region as well as in the left basal ganglia, external capsule, and thalamus

WEGNER'S GRANULOMATOSIS

Wegener's granulomatosis is an uncommon multisystemic disorder of unknown etiology. Histopathologically, it is a necrotizing granulomatous vasculitis. Most commonly this involves the respiratory tract, with pulmonary involvement occurring at some stage of the disease in almost all patients. However, many other organ systems can also be affected including the kidneys, orbits, and central nervous system. Leptomeningeal or pachymeningeal disease is seen with adjacent gyriform hyperintensity seen on T2-weighted images.

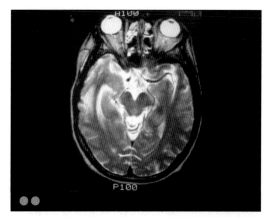

L1. Axial T2-weighted image shows gyriform hyperintensity in the right temporal lobe. Abnormal T2 hyperintense tissue is seen in both retroglobal region as well as in the right temporal subcutaneous soft tissue.

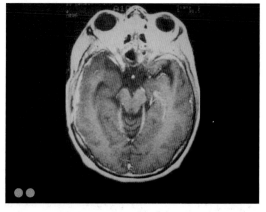

L2. Axial, post-contrast T1-weighted image reveals thick pachymeningeal enhancement in the right temporal region as well as in the left anterior temporal region. Note the presence of abnormal contrast enhancement in both retroglobal region and right temporal subcutaneous soft tissue.

MULTIPLE SCLEROSIS

Multiple sclerosis is a demyelinating disease that is characterized by multiple inflammatory plaques of demyelination involving the white matter of the central nervous system. Most common among northern Europeans or people of northern European extraction. Females are affected more frequently than males with a ratio of 3:2. MRI scan shows T1-hypointense and T2-hyperintense lesions with or without contrast enhancement.

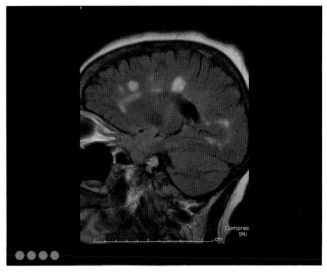

A. Sagittal, T2-weighted FLAIR image shows multiple hyperintense lesions in the periventricular white matter.

RELATED PATTERNS

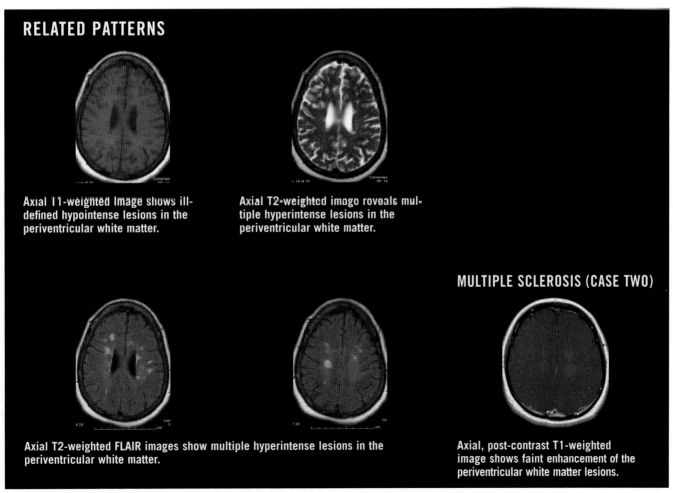

Axial T1-weighted image shows ill-defined hypointense lesions in the periventricular white matter.

Axial T2-weighted image reveals multiple hyperintense lesions in the periventricular white matter.

MULTIPLE SCLEROSIS (CASE TWO)

Axial T2-weighted FLAIR images show multiple hyperintense lesions in the periventricular white matter.

Axial, post-contrast T1-weighted image shows faint enhancement of the periventricular white matter lesions.

RELATED PATTERNS (continued)

MULTIPLE SCLEROSIS (CASE TWO) (continued)

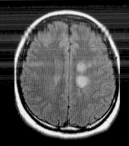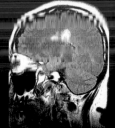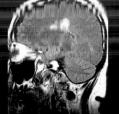

Axial and sagittal T2-weighted FLAIR images demonstrate several white matter lesions bilaterally.

MULTIPLE SCLEROSIS (CASE THREE)

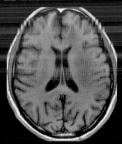

Axial T1-weighted image shows periventricular hypointense areas with a large one seen in the left corona radiata.

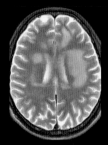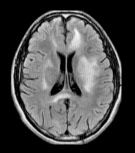

Axial T2-weighted and FLAIR images show bilateral periventricular hyperintense areas with a large one seen on the left side.

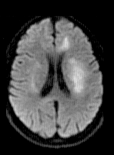

Diffusion-weighted image shows some of the MS plaques exhibit restricted diffusion.

MULTIPLE SCLEROSIS (CASE THREE) (continued)

MULTIPLE SCLEROSIS (CASE FOUR)

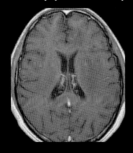

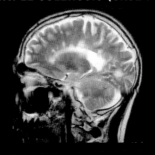

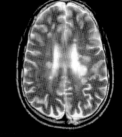

Axial, post-contrast T1-weighted image shows no abnormal enhancing lesion.

Sagittal, axial T2-weighted and FLAIR images demonstrate multiple, periventricular hyperintense lesions. Some of the lesions are perpendicular to the ventricular wall.

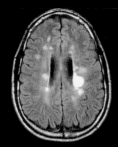

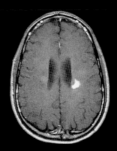

Sagittal, axial T2-weighted and FLAIR images demonstrate multiple, periventricular hyperintense lesions. Some of the lesions are perpendicular to the ventricular wall.

Axial, post-contrast T1-weighted image shows an enhancing lesion along the left lateral ventricle.

DIFFERENTIAL DIAGNOSIS

At a Glance:

- *Acute Disseminated Encephalomyelitis*
- *Chronic White Matter Ischemic Changes*
- *Human Immune Deficiency Virus Encephalitis*
- *Meningoencephalitis*
- *Progressive Multifocal Leukoencephalopathy*
- *Syphilis*
- *Vasculitis*
- *Dysmyelinating Disease* (not pictured)
- *Metachromatic Leukodystrophy* (not pictured)
- *Post Chemotherapy Changes* (not pictured)
- *Post Radiation Changes* (not pictured)

ACUTE DISSEMINATED ENCEPHALOMYELITIS

Acute disseminated encephalomyelitis is a monophasic demyelinating disease. There is usually a preceding viral infection, or vaccination. The etiology is supposed to be an allergic or autoimmune (cell-mediated immune response against myelin basic protein). These lesions may be multiple or large, usually exhibiting low signal intensity on T1-weighted images and high signal intensity on T2-weighted images. Contrast enhancement may be seen.

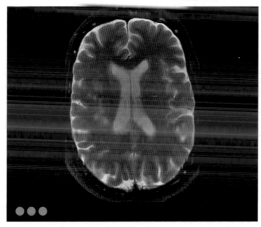

B1. Axial T2-weighted and FLAIR images show multiple periventricular white matter lesions.

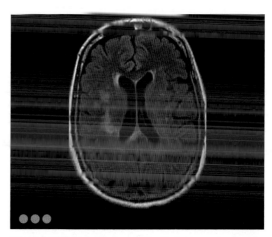

B2. Axial T2-weighted and FLAIR images show multiple periventricular white matter lesions.

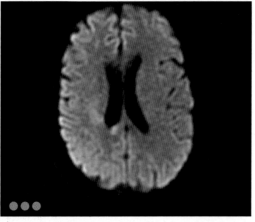

B3. Diffusion-weighted image shows some of the lesions with restricted diffusion.

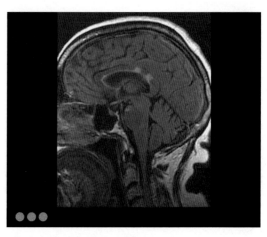

B4. Sagittal T2-weighted FLAIR image demonstrates lesions involving the corpus callosum.

CHRONIC WHITE MATTER ISCHEMIC CHANGES

With advancing age, the subcortical and periventricular white matter becomes susceptible to various assortment of tissue alterations that cannot be easily categorized in terms of traditionally defined neuropathologic disease. These changes appear as hyperintense areas involving the periventricular and subcortical white matter on T2-weighted MR imaging, and better demonstrated on FLAIR imaging. These findings are more commonly seen in patients with chronic hypertension and other microvascular arteriosclerotic risk factors. The majority of the tissue alterations are of low histopathologic grade, which include dilated perivascular (Virchow-Robin) spaces, mild demyelination, gliosis, and diffuse regions neuropil vacuolation. Associated clinical abnormalities are minimal and, when present, are usually confined to deficits of attention, mental processing speed, and psychomotor control.

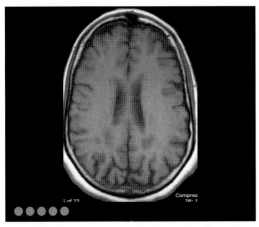

C1. Axial T1-weighted image shows ill defined hypointense areas in the periventricular white matter bilaterally.

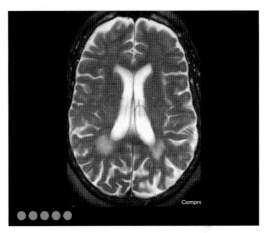

C2. Axial T2-weighted and FLAIR images show bilateral hyperintense lesions in the periventricular as well as in the subcortical white matter.

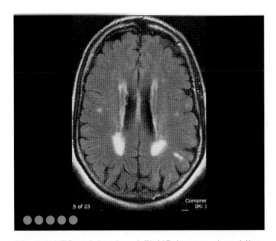

C3. Axial T2-weighted and FLAIR images show bilateral hyperintense lesions in the periventricular as well as in the subcortical white matter.

HUMAN IMMUNE DEFICIENCY VIRUS ENCEPHALITIS

Neurologic manifestations associated with human immune deficiency virus in the absence of opportunistic infection or neoplasm include encephalopathy, myelopathy, peripheral neuropathy, and myopathy. Approximately one third of AIDS autopsies show evidence of viral encephalopathy. CT shows low-density white matter lesions and atrophy. MRI shows periventricular white matter lesions diffusely or in a patchy pattern. Contrast enhancement is usually not seen.

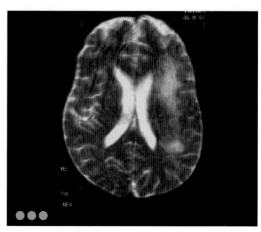

D. Axial T2-weighted images show white matter hyperintense lesions bilaterally.

MENINGOENCEPHALITIS

Meningoencephalitis is a term used to include infection/inflammation of the meninges and brain. Meningoencephalitis can be due to bacterial, viral, fungal or parasitic infections. They can be secondary to hematogenous spread of systemic infection or direct extension from sinusitis or mastoiditis through venous pathways.

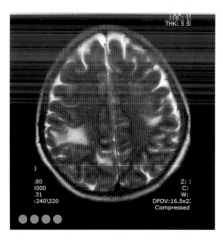

E1. Axial T2-weighted and FLAIR images show hyperintense lesions in the white matter bilaterally.

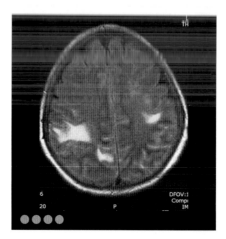

E2. Axial T2-weighted and FLAIR images show hyperintense lesions in the white matter bilaterally.

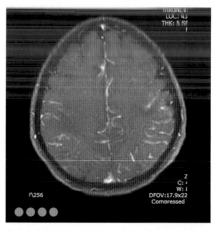

E3. Axial, post-contrast T1-weighted image shows diffuse leptomeningeal enhancement and some gyriform enhancement.

PROGRESSIVE MULTIFOCAL LEUKOENCEPHALOPATHY

Progressive multifocal leukoencephalopathy (PML) is a demyelinating disease caused by JC virus. The JC virus infects the oligodendrocytes, causing cytolytic destruction with resultant demyelination. In patients with HIV and sub-cortical white matter lesions, PML is more likely than other HIV-related infections. Clinically, the disease is a progressive one with death commonly occurring within 9 months after the onset of clinical symptoms. MRI shows hypointense lesions on T1 weighted images and hyperintense lesions on T2 weighted images involving the white matter, in the parietoccipital and frontal locations. Posterior fossa lesions are also seen. PML can involve the myelinated fibers in the deep gray matter. PML may be difficult to differentiate from HIV-related demyelination. White matter lesions in HIV-related encephalopathy are more diffuse and periventricular, whereas those in PML are more often multifocal, with a greater tendency for subcortical location.

PROGRESSIVE MULTIFOCAL LEUKOENCEPHALOPATHY (CASE ONE)

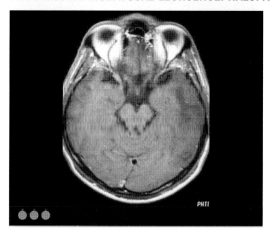

F1. Axial T1-weighted image shows hypointensity in the left temporal region.

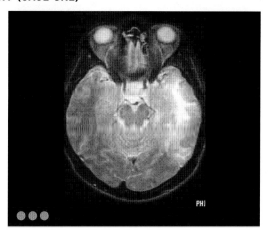

F2. Axial fat-suppressed T2-weighted images demonstrate hyperintense lesions in the white matter of temporal, parietal region.

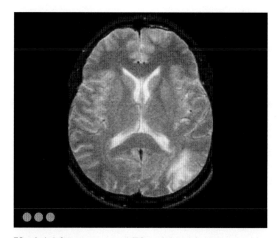

F3. Axial fat-suppressed T2-weighted images demonstrate hyperintense lesions in the white matter of temporal, parietal region.

PROGRESSIVE MULTIFOCAL LEUKOENCEPHALOPATHY (CASE TWO)

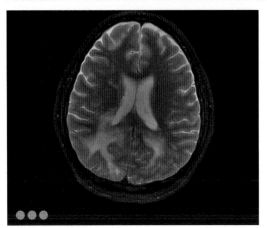

Q1. Axial T2-weighted and FLAIR images reveal bilateral periventricular white matter hyperintense lesions.

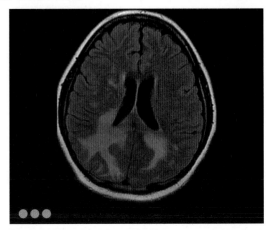

Q2. Axial T2-weighted and FLAIR images reveal bilateral periventricular white matter hyperintense lesions.

SYPHILIS

Syphilitic infection of the nervous system is the most chronic, insidious meningeal inflammatory process. Invasion of the CNS occurs early in the course of untreated syphilis. Neurosyphilis is diagnosed by a positive CSF VDRL test. The pathogenesis of neurosyphilis is similar to that in the rest of the body. Imaging findings in patients with neurosyphilis include ischemic lesions in meningovascular syphilis, intracerebral gummata, and syphilitic meningitis. Hydrocephalus and cranial nerve involvement, particularly the optic and vestibulocochlear nerves, has been reported. A gumma is a well-circumscribed mass of leptomeningeal granulation tissue. It results from a cell-mediated immune response to *T pallidum*. Gummas usually are extra-axial lesions and dura based. The cortex is often involved secondary to invasion and direct extension.

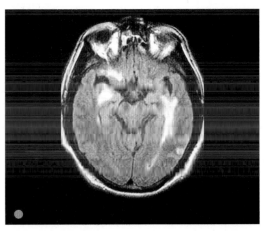

H1. Axial T2-weighted FLAIR images demonstrate bilateral hyperintense lesions in the periventricular as well as subcortical white matter.

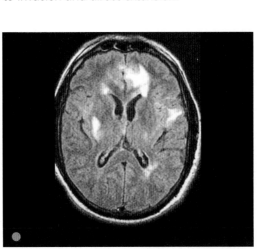

H2. Axial T2 weighted FLAIR image demonstrates bilateral, parasagittal, cortical and subcortical hyperintense lesions.

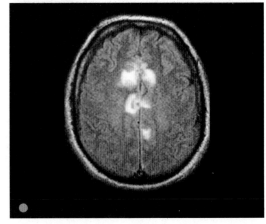

H3. Axial T2-weighted FLAIR images demonstrate bilateral hyperintense lesions in the periventricular as well as subcortical white matter.

VASCULITIS

Primary central nervous system vasculitis (PCNSV) is a rare form of vascular inflammatory disease involving the brain and spinal cord that is poorly understood. PCNSV diagnosis is established based on positive CNS tissue histopathology. PCNSV can be divided into two main diagnostic categories: large-medium vessel disease and small vessel disease. The diagnosis of large-medium disease can be made based on magnetic resonance angiography, computed tomographic angiography and digital subtraction angiography with findings of vascular stenosis in the CNS, without evidence of underlying systemic inflammatory disease. Lesions typically conform to the territory defined by a particular arterial distribution. Small vessel disease affects vessels smaller than those seen by neuro-angiography. Therefore, by definition, this condition has negative angiography findings. Lesions can be multifocal and bilateral and tend not to conform to a distinct vascular distribution. The diagnosis is confirmed by brain biopsy findings.

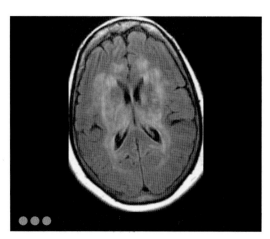

I1. Axial T2-weighted and FLAIR images show confluent white matter hyperintense lesions bilaterally.

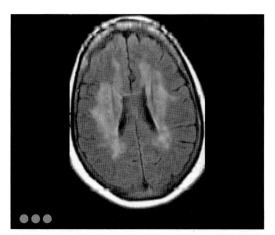

I2. Axial T2-weighted and FLAIR images show confluent white matter hyperintense lesions bilaterally.

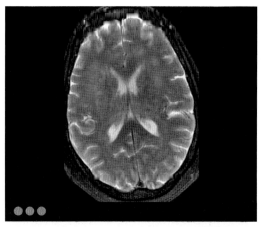

I3. Axial T2-weighted and FLAIR images show confluent white matter hyperintense lesions bilaterally.

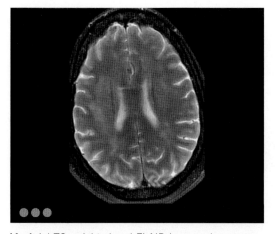

I4. Axial T2-weighted and FLAIR images show confluent white matter hyperintense lesions bilaterally.

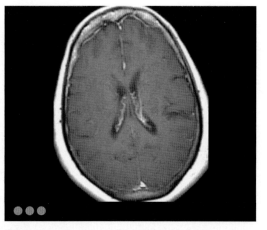

I5. Axial, post-contrast T1-weighted image reveals no abnormal contrast enhancement.

WILSON'S DISEASE

The brain lesions are usually bilateral and often symmetrical, involving the putamen, caudate nucleus, globus pallidus, claustrum, thalamus, cortical/subcortical regions, mesencephalon, pons, vermis, and dentate nucleus. The lesions of cerebral Wilson disease usually appear hyperintense on T2-weighted MR images. These changes seen on MRI have been attributed to cellular damage caused by accumulation of copper, chronic ischemia, vasculopathy, or demyelination.

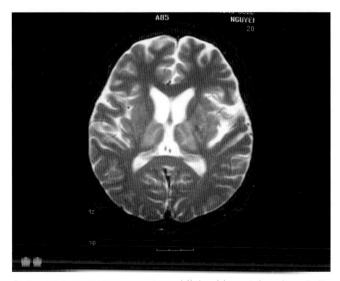

A. Axial T2-weighted image shows bilateral hyperintensity in both thalami, and basal ganglia

RELATED PATTERNS

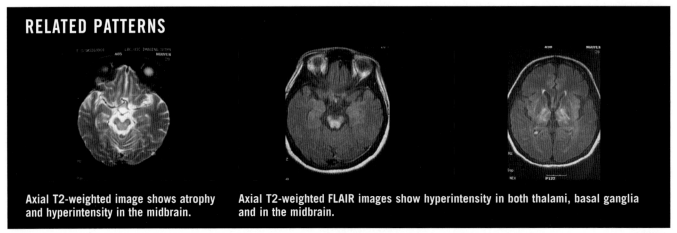

Axial T2-weighted image shows atrophy and hyperintensity in the midbrain.

Axial T2-weighted FLAIR images show hyperintensity in both thalami, basal ganglia and in the midbrain.

DIFFERENTIAL DIAGNOSIS

At a Glance:

- *Acute*
- *Fungal Infection*
- *Osmotic Myelinolysis*
- *Vasculitis*
- *Encephalitis* (not pictured)
- *Hypoxia* (not pictured)
- *Hypoglycemia* (not pictured)
- *Methanol* (not pictured)
- *Chronic*
- *Huntinglon's Disease*
- *Leigh's Disease*
- *Melas Syndrome*
- *Et Crible Multiple Dilated Perivascular Spaces in Basal Ganglia*
- *Cockayne's Syndrome* (not pictured)
- *Creutzfelt-Jacob Disease* (not pictured)
- *Kearns-Sayre Syndrome* (not pictured)
- *Neurofibromatosis* (not pictured)
- *Pelizaeus-Merzbacher Disease* (not pictured)

ACUTE

FUNGAL INFECTION

Fungal infection may involve intracranial blood vessels, leptomeninges, and brain parenchyma. Intracranial infection is frequently secondary to pulmonary disease. Prior to the era of immunosuppressive therapy in organ transplant patients and the increase in HIV infection, fungal infection of the CNS was rare. Other conditions that predispose patients to fungal infection include diabetes, pregnancy, and malignancy. Depending on the genera, fungi may exist as single cells (yeast) or in a branched appearance (hyphal form). The yeast and hyphal forms may coalesce and form mycelia. The fungi of yeast forms tend to spread hematogenously to the meningeal microcirculation, with resultant leptomeningitis attributable to their smaller size, the larger hyphal form more commonly involves the brain parenchyma, with resultant cerebritis or encephalitis. The genera that are present predominantly as yeast forms include *Blastomyces, Candida, Coccidioides, Cryptococcus, Histoplasma, Paracoccidioides,* and *Torulopsis.* Hyphal forms include *Aspergillus, Mucor* and other agents of mucormycosis, and *Pseudoallescheria.* CNS fungal infection displays neuroimaging features similar to those seen with tuberculosis. MRI characteristically demonstrate dilated Virchow-Robin space with T2 hyperintensity seen in both basal ganglia in patients with Cryptococcus. On contrast-enhanced MR images, enhancement within the Virchow-Robin space may be seen. However, similar findings may be seen in coccidioidomycosis and candidiasis.

FUNGAL INFECTION (CANDIDIASIS)

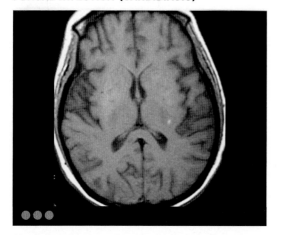

B1. Axial T1-weighted image shows hypointensity with focal hyperintensity in both basal ganglia.

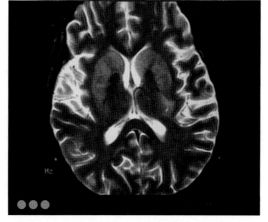

B2. Axial T2-weighted and FLAIR images demonstrate hyperintensity in both basal ganglia.

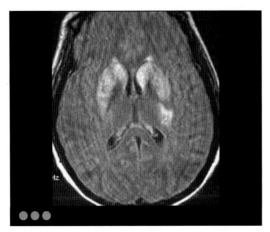

B3. Axial T2-weighted and FLAIR images demonstrate hyperintensity in both basal ganglia.

B4. Axial, post-contrast T1-weighted image shows intense enhancement in both basal ganglia

FUNGAL INFECTION (CRYPTOCOCCUS)

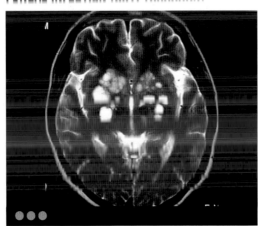

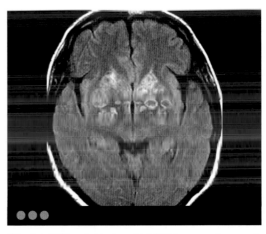

C1. Axial T2-weighted and FLAIR images show multiple hyperintense lesions in both basal ganglia, consistent with dilated perivascular spaces with gelatinous pseudocysts.

C2. Axial T2-weighted and FLAIR images show multiple hyperintense lesions in both basal ganglia, consistent with dilated perivascular spaces with gelatinous pseudocysts.

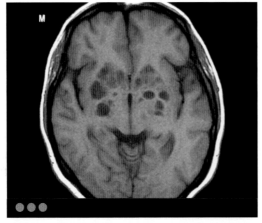

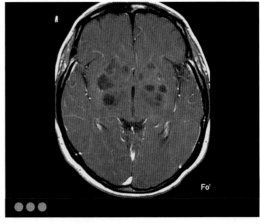

C3. Axial T1-weighted pre- and post-contrast images show multiple cystic lesions in the basal ganglia with no definite enhancement.

C4. Axial T1-weighted pre- and post-contrast images show multiple cystic lesions in the basal ganglia with no definite enhancement.

OSMOTIC MYELINOLYSIS

Central pontine myelinolysis (CPM) is symmetric, noninflammatory demyelination within the central basis pontis. In at least 10% of patients with CPM, demyelination also occurs in extrapontine regions, including the mid brain, thalamus, basal nuclei, and cerebellum. Prolonged hyponatremia followed by rapid correction probably results in cellular edema. Osmotic myelinolysis is a more appropriate term for demyelination occurring in extrapontine regions after the correction of hyponatremia.

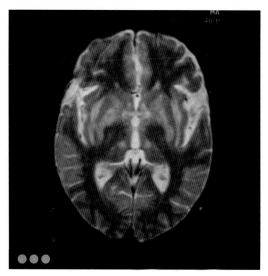

D. Axial T2-weighted image shows bilateral hyperintensity in both thalami and basal ganglia.

VASCULITIS

Primary vasculitis of the central nervous system includes giant cell arteritis, primary angiitis of the CNS, Takayasu's disease, periarteritis nodosa, Kawasaki disease, Churg-Strauss syndrome, Wegener's granulomatosis. Secondary vasculitis may be due to collagen vascular diseases, Behcet's disease, other systemic conditions and the use of illicit drugs. The diagnosis may be suggested on MR angiography, CT angiography or conventional angiography, but is confirmed by brain biopsy findings.

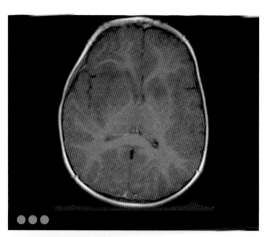

E1. Axial T1-weighted image shows bilateral hypointensity in both basal ganglia.

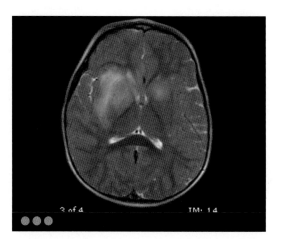

E2. Axial T2-weighted and FLAIR images demonstrate hyperintensity involving both basal ganglia, more on the right side.

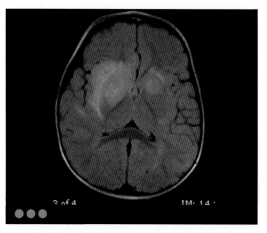

E3. Axial T2-weighted and FLAIR images demonstrate hyperintensity involving both basal ganglia, more on the right side.

393

CHRONIC
HUNTINGTON'S DISEASE

Huntington's disease is a neurodegenerative disorder characterized by progressive choreoathetosis, psychological behavioral changes, and subcortical dementia. It is an autosomal dominant disease with a defective gene locus on chromosome 4. MRI demonstrates bilateral basal ganglia T2 hyperintensity in early stage of the disease. In later stage of the disease, there is diffuse cortical atrophy as well as atrophy of the caudate and, less frequently, of the putamen.

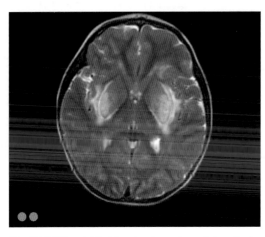

F1. Axial T2-weighted image shows hyperintensity in both basal ganglia.

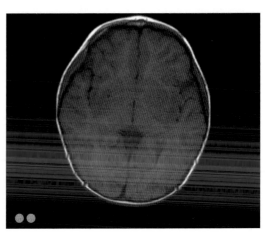

F2. Axial T1-weighted image reveals hypointensity in both basal ganglia.

LEIGH'S DISEASE

Leigh's disease is a mitochondrial encephalomyopathy and is a hereditary disease transmitted as an autosomal recessive disorder. The disease is present earlier in infancy with motor and intellectual regression. On MRI abnormal signal intensity areas are detected in basal ganglia, thalamus, brainstem, cerebellar white matter, cerebellar cortex, cerebral white matter. Marked progressive atrophy is seen.

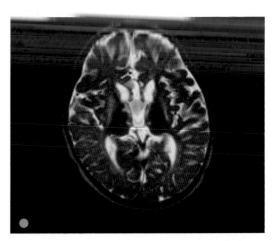

G. Axial T2-weighted image reveals bilateral hyperintensity in the basal ganglia, thalami with cerebral volume loss.

MELAS SYNDROME

MELAS consists of mitochondrial myopathy, encephalopathy, lactic acidosis and stroke. It is not single disorder, but group of systemic abnormalities. It involves CNS, skeletal muscle, eye, cardiac muscle, kidneys, and GI system. Common presentations include stroke, strokelike events, nausea, vomiting, encephalopathy, seizures, short stature, headaches, muscle weakness, exercise intolerance, neurosensory hearing loss, diabetes, and myopathy.

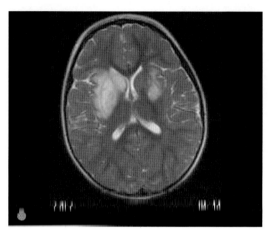

H1 Axial T2-weighted and FLAIR images demonstrate hyperintensity in bilateral basal ganglia, more on the right side.

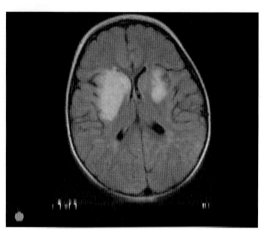

H2 Axial T2-weighted and FLAIR images demonstrate hyperintensity in bilateral basal ganglia, more on the right side.

ET CRIBLE-MULTIPLE DILATED PERIVASCULAR SPACES IN BASAL GANGLIA

There is an increased incidence of perivascular spaces (Virchow Robin space), often greater than 2 mm in diameter, in elderly people. Increased frequency of perivascular space dilatation can be seen in healthy subjects with advancing age or hypertension. Associated small lacunar infarcts and focal lesions of the white matter can be seen in these patients.

Two mechanisms are considered potentially responsible for age related dilatation of perivascular space. The first concept suggests that the ventricles and subarachnoid space dilate with age, with consequent dilatation of perivascular spaces as the anatomic continuation of these structures. The second mechanism is based on presumption atherosclerotic changes common in elderly patients. Blood vessels become wider and more tortuous, which can explain increased amount of perivascular interstitium containing vacuoles and eventual dilatation of perivascular spaces.

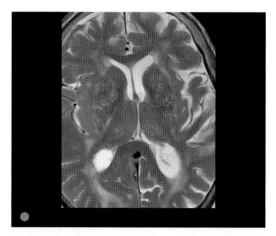

I1. Axial T2 weighted image shows multiple, dilated perivascular spaces in both basal ganglia. In addition periventricular white ischemic changes are seen bilaterally.

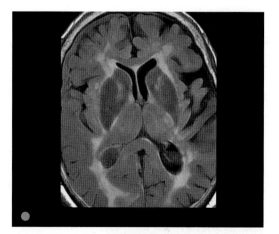

I2. Axial T2 weighted FLAIR image shows multiple, dilated perivascular spaces in both basal ganglia. In addition, periventricular white matter ischemic changes are seen bilaterally.

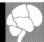

NEURODEGENERATION WITH BRAIN IRON ACCUMULATION (HALLERVORDEN–SPATZ DISEASE)

Rare autosomal recessive disorder characterized by the hallmarks of progressive extrapyramidal dysfunction and eventual loss of ambulation. Onset is most commonly in late childhood or early adolescence. The classic presentation is in the late part of the first decade or early part of the second decade, when the individual is aged 7–15 years, but cases with adult onset have been described.

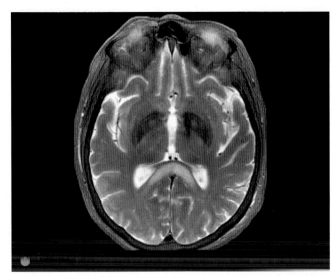

A. Axial T2-weighted image shows hypointensity in both basal ganglia with a small central hyperintensity. Hyperintensity is seen involving the splenium of the corpus callosum

RELATED PATTERN

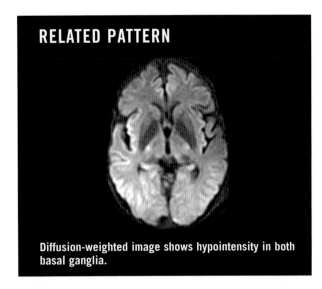

Diffusion-weighted image shows hypointensity in both basal ganglia.

DIFFERENTIAL DIAGNOSIS

At a Glance:

- *Parkinson's Disease*
- *Wilson's Disease*
- *Multiple Sclerosis* (not pictured)

PARKINSON'S DISEASE

Parkinson's disease (PD) is a progressive movement disorder marked by tremors, rigidity, slow movements (bradykinesia), and posture instability. It occurs when neurons in substantia nigra begin to die or become impaired for unknown reasons. Normally, these neurons produce dopamine, which is a chemical messenger responsible for transmitting signals between the substantia nigra and the corpus striatum, to produce smooth, purposeful muscle activity. Loss of dopamine causes the nerve cells of the striatum to fire out of control, leaving patients unable to control their movements in a normal manner. PD was first noted by British physician James Parkinson in the early 1800s

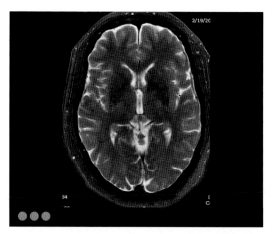

B1. Axial T2-weighted image shows hypointensity in both globus pallidi and putamen due to iron deposition.

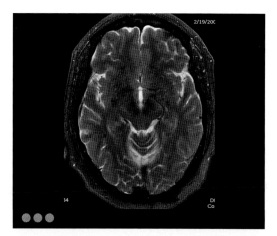

B2. Axial T2-weighted image shows volume loss in the pars compacta of the substantia nigra. (The tissue between the low signal red nucleus and low signal pars radiculata of substantia nigra.)

WILSON'S DISEASE

The brain lesions of **Wilson's disease** are usually bilateral and often symmetrical, involving the putamen, caudate nucleus, globus pallidus, claustrum, thalamus, cortical/ subcortical regions, mesencephalon, pons, vermis, and dentate nucleus. Initial imaging findings are hyperintensity on T2-weighted images with restricted diffusion seen on diffusion-weighted images, but later on hypointensity may be seen on T2-weighted images with increased diffusion.

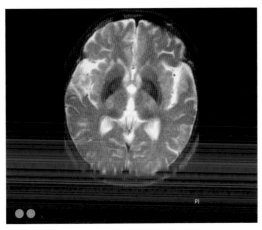

C1. Axial and coronal T2-weighted images demonstrate hypointnesity in both basal ganglia.

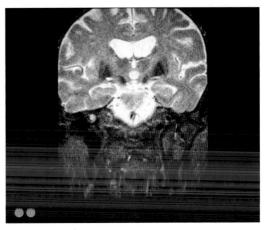

C2. Axial and coronal T2-weighted images demonstrate hypointnesity in both basal ganglia.

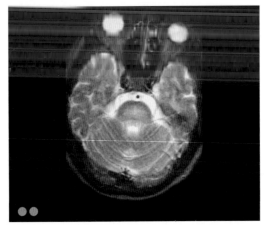

C3. Axial T2-weighted image shows hyperintensity in the pons.

HEPATIC ENCEPHALOPATHY

In patients with hepatic encephalopathy, hyperintensity is seen in globus pallidus, putamina, and midbrain on T1-weighted images. Deposition of manganese, which bypasses the detoxification in the liver presumed to be the source of hyperintnesity in the globus pallidus.

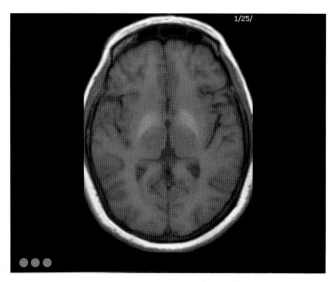

A. Axial T1-weighted image shows hyperintensity in both basal ganglia, predominantly in globus pallidi.

RELATED PATTERNS

HEPATIC ENCEPHALOPATHY (CASE TWO)

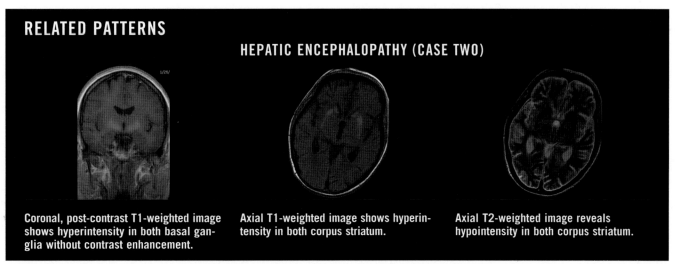

Coronal, post-contrast T1-weighted image shows hyperintensity in both basal ganglia without contrast enhancement.

Axial T1-weighted image shows hyperintensity in both corpus striatum.

Axial T2-weighted image reveals hypointensity in both corpus striatum.

DIFFERENTIAL DIAGNOSIS

At a Glance:

- *Basal Ganglia Calcification*
- *Parenteral Nutrition*
- *Neurofibromatosis* (not pictured)
- *Nonketotic Hyperglycemia* (not pictured)
- *Wilson's Disease* (not pictured)

BASAL GANGLIA CALCIFICATION

Basal ganglia calcification can be due to a number of disorders including hypoparathyroidism, pseudohypoparathyroidism, pseudopseudohypoparathyroidism, hyperparathyroidism, Fahr's disease, Cockayne syndrome, Down syndrome, anoxia, carbon monoxide poisoning, mineralizing microangiopathy, radiation therapy, neurofibromatosis, etc. **T1** hyperintensity is seen in basal ganglia calcification due to the hydration layer around the calcium. The most common cause of basal gnaglia calcification is physiological calcification due to aging.

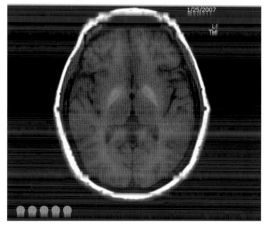

B. Axial T1 weighted image shows hyperintensity in both bsal ganglia in a patient with bilateral basal ganglia physiological calcification due to aging.

PARENTERAL NUTRITION

Hyperalimentation is a procedure in which nutrients and vitamins are given to a person in liquid form through an intravenous catheter placed in vena cava. It is only given to someone who cannot get nutrients from food. T1 hyperintense lesion in patients with **parenteral nutrition** is probably also due to manganese. The signal abnormality is reversible when peroral alimentation is resumed.

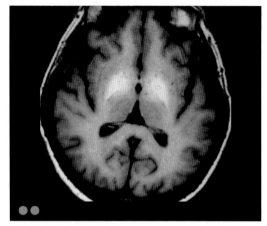

C1. Axial T1-weighted image shows hyperintensity in both basal ganglia.

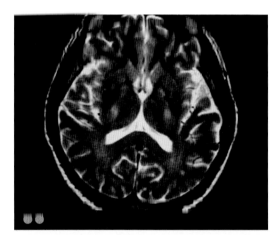

C2. Axial T2-weighted image shows hypointensity with small areas of hyperintensity in both basal ganglia.

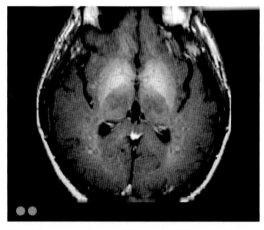

C3. Axial, post-contrast T1-weighted image demonstrates no definite enhancement.

THALAMIC HEMORRHAGE

Intracranial hemorrhage is the pathological accumulation of blood within the cranial vault. It may occur within brain parenchyma or the surrounding meningeal spaces. Intracerebral hemorrhage (ICH) can occur in any part of the cerebrum and cerebellum. Intracerebral hemorrhage accounts for 8–13% of all strokes and results from a wide spectrum of disorders, including hypertensive hemorrhage, trauma, bleeding into a neoplasm, vasculitis, rupture of an AVM, etc. Intracerebral hemorrhage and surrounding edema may compress adjacent brain tissue or cause herniation, leading to neurological dysfunction.

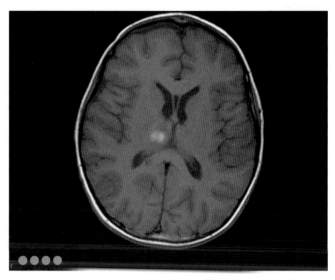

A. Axial T1-weighted image shows a focal hyperintense lesion in the right thalamus, consistent with hemorrhage in a patient with head trauma.

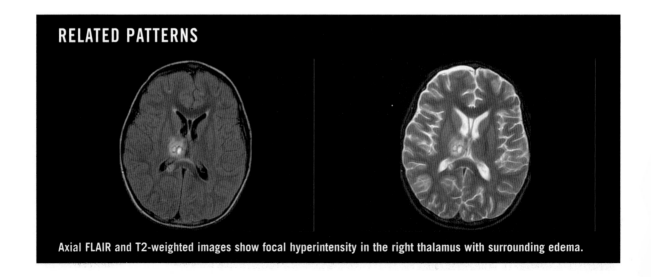

RELATED PATTERNS

Axial FLAIR and T2-weighted images show focal hyperintensity in the right thalamus with surrounding edema.

DIFFERENTIAL DIAGNOSIS

At a Glance:

- *Bilateral Thalamic Infarcts*
- *Creutzfeldt–Jakob Disease*
- *Metastatic Disease*
- *Thalamic Neoplasm*
- *Vasculitis*
- *Bilateral Thalamic Infarcts due to Straight Sinus Thrombosis* (not pictured)

BILATERAL THALAMIC INFARCTS

A rare variation of the arterial blood supply in the thalamic and midbrain region is the artery of Percheron, which is a solitary arterial trunk that arises from the one of the proxi-mal posterior cerebral arteries and supplies the parame-dian thalami and rostral midbrain bilaterally. Occlusion of this artery can cause **bilateral thalamic infarction** as well as midbrain infarction.

BILATERAL THALAMIC INFARCTS (CASE ONE)

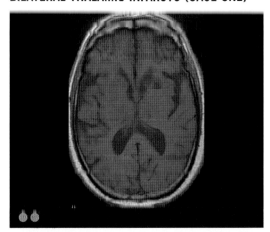

B1. Axial T1-weighted image shows ill-defined hypoint-nesity in both thalami. In addition, an old infarct of the left head of caudate nucleus is seen.

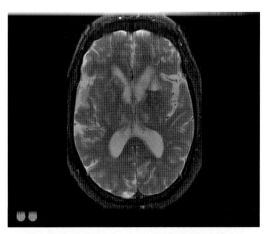

B2. Axial T2-weighted and FLAIR images demonstrate bilateral thalamic, left head of caudate old infarcts. A right temporal infarct is also seen. White matter ischemic changes are also seen.

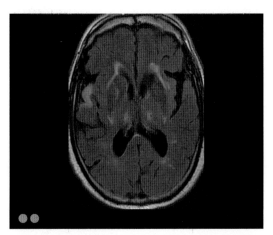

B3. Axial T2-weighted and FLAIR images demonstrate bilateral thalamic, left head of caudate old infarcts. A right temporal infarct is also seen. White matter ischemic changes are also seen.

403

BILATERAL THALAMIC INFARCTS (CASE TWO)

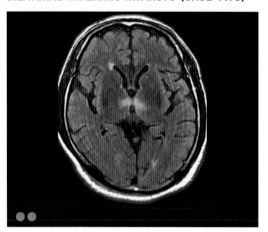

C1. Axial T2-weighted FLAIR image shows small hyperintense areas in the medial aspect of both thalami.

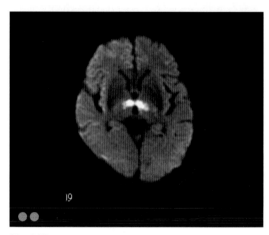

C2. Diffusion-weighted image and ADC map demonstrate restricted diffusion in the corresponding areas, consistent with acute infarction.

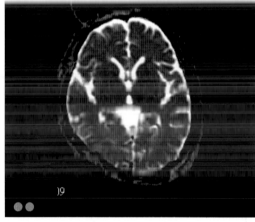

C3. Diffusion-weighted image and ADC map demonstrate restricted diffusion in the corresponding areas, consistent with acute infarction.

CREUTZFELDT–JAKOB DISEASE

Creutzfeldt–Jakob disease (CJD) is a human spongiform encephalopathy that results from an infection by a prion. The mode of transmission has been traced to inoculations by injections of human growth hormone, transplantation of corneas, and implantation of cerebral electrodes. In addition, butchers and meat handlers are at greater risk of contracting the disease. A new variant of Creutzfeldt–Jakob disease is due to bovine spongiform encephalopathy (so-called mad cow disease).

The infective prion is a proteinaceous particle that contains little or no nucleic acid. The disease occurs in adults in their late 50s. However, the new variant of the disease can affect all age groups. Dementia with rapid progression to stupor is seen clinically. CT and MRI studies are useful to document the rapid progression of atrophy. Cortical gray matter involvement without cerebral atrophy may represent an early phase of the disease. Hyperintensity may be seen in corpus striata, thalami bilaterally on T2-weighted images or FLAIR images, and on diffusion-weighted images, which may reflect areas of gliosis and microvacuolization pathologically. Later on, hyperintensity may be in basal ganglia, thalami, and white matter bilaterally on T2-weighted images and FLAIR images. In contrast to CJD where bilateral involvement of the corpus striata and thalami are seen on the imaging studies, the bovine spongiform encephalopathy characteristically demonstrate bilateral thalamic pulvinar hyperintensity on T2-weighted and FLAIR images.

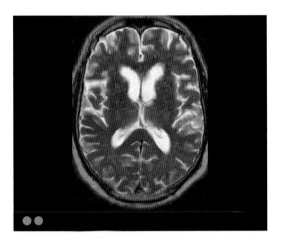

D1. Axial T2-weighted and FLAIR images show hyperintense lesion in both thalami.

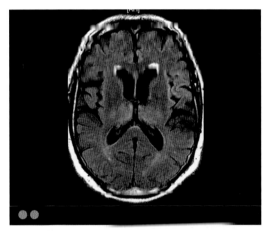

D2. Axial T2-weighted and FLAIR images show hyperintense lesion in both thalami.

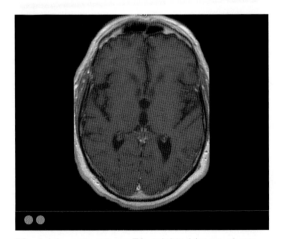

D3. Axial, post-contrast T1-weighted image shows no abnormal contrast enhancement.

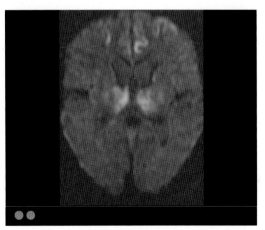

D4. Diffusion-weighted image shows restricted diffusion in both thalami.

METASTATIC DISEASE

Metastatic tumors are among the most common mass lesions in the brain. The incidence of brain metastasis is thought to be 120,000–140,000 per year. This disease accounts for 20% of cancer deaths annually, a rate that can be traced to an increase in the median survival of patients with cancer because of advanced therapies, increased availability of modern imaging techniques for early detection of cancer, and vigilant clinical surveillance protocols for monitoring recurrence. Furthermore, the use of chemotherapeutic agents in the treatment of systemic disease may transiently weaken the blood-brain barrier and allow systemic disease to be seeded in the CNS, resulting in increased incidence of brain metastasis.

METASTATIC LESION

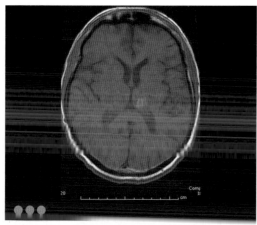

E1, Axial T1-weighted image shows a focal hyperintense lesion in the left thalamus.

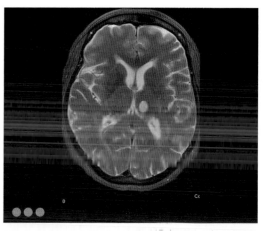

E2, Axial T2-weighted and FLAIR images show a hyperintense mass in the left.

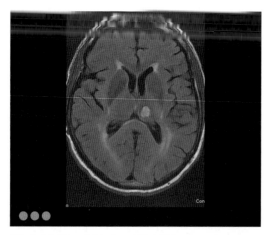

E3. Axial T2-weighted and FLAIR images show a hyperintense mass in the left.

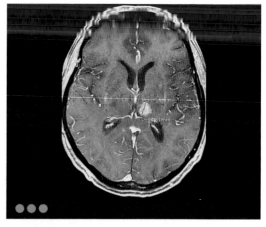

E4. Axial, post-contrast T1-weighted image demonstrates an enhancing mass in the left thalamus.

THALAMIC NEOPLASM

Thalamic tumors are typical deep brain tumors. Thalamic tumors account for approximately 1% of all intracranial neoplasms. They are seen predominantly in children and young adults. The majority of the cases in the thalamus consist of low-grade astrocytomas, followed by primitive neuroectodermal tumors, ganglion cell tumors, oligodendrogliomas, lymphomas, and germ cell neoplasms.

THALAMIC ASTROCYTOMA

Low-grade astrocytomas are a heterogeneous group of intrinsic central nervous system neoplasms that share certain similarities in their clinical presentation, radiologic appearance, prognosis, and treatment. The World Health Organization (WHO) classification is based on the appearance of certain pathological features including atypia, mitoses, endothelial proliferation, and necrosis. These pathological characteristics reflect the malignant potential of the tumor in terms of invasion and growth rate. Tumors without any of these features are grade I, and those with one of these features (usually atypia) are considered grade II. Tumors with 2 criteria and tumors with 3 or 4 criteria are WHO grades III and IV, respectively. Thus, the low-grade astrocytomas are grades I and II according to the WHO classification. There is a subset of astrocytomas, due to their distinctive pathology, cannot be evaluated by the usual four featured grading system. These tumors may have endothelial proliferation and marked atypia on hisopathology. However, they are slow growing and well circumscribed tumors. They include juvenile pilocytic astrocytoma (JPA), pleomorphic xanthoastrocytoma (PXA), and subependymal giant-cell astrocytoma (SGCA).

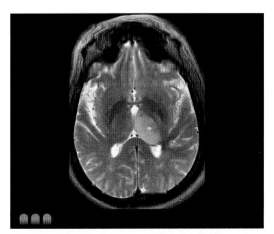

F1. Axial T2-weighted and FLAIR images show a hyperintense mass lesion in the left thalamus.

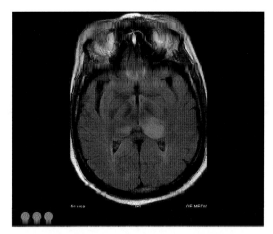

F2. Axial T2-weighted and FLAIR images show a hyperintense mass lesion in the left thalamus.

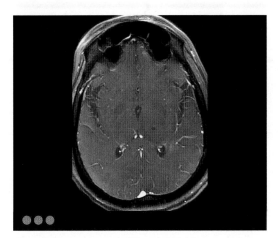

F3. Axial, post-contrast T1-weighted image demonstrates no abnormal enhancement.

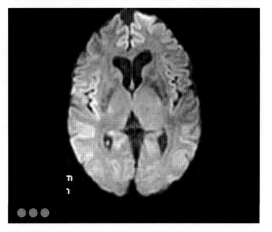

F4. Diffusion-weighted image shows no evidence of restricted diffusion, indicating it is a low-grade astrocytoma.

THALAMIC PNET

Supratentorial primitive neuroectodermal tumors (PNET) are relatively rare, representing approximately one tenth the frequency of medulloblastoma, and 3 to 7% of pediatric CNS tumors. They are diagnosed at a younger median age than medulloblastomas; more than 65% of supratentorial PNETs are reported in patients younger than 5 years of age with no significant sex predominance. Furthermore, supratentorial PNETs can present as congenital tumors. Although supratentorial PNET is generally considered almost exclusively a pediatric tumor, rarely they can be seen in adults. A supratentorial PNET most commonly arises in the cerebrum, and basal ganglia and thalamus are less frequently involved.

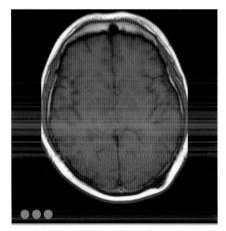

G1 Axial T1-weighted image shows a mixed hypointense to isointense lesion in the right thalamus.

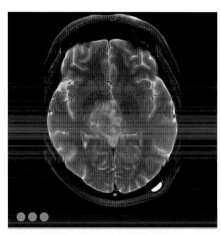

G2 Axial T2-weighted and FLAIR images show a slightly heterogeneous mass in the right thalamus with surrounding edema.

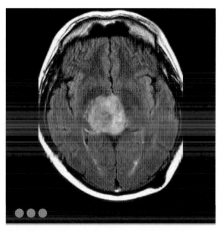

G3. Axial T2-weighted and FLAIR images show a slightly heterogeneous mass in the right thalamus with surrounding edema.

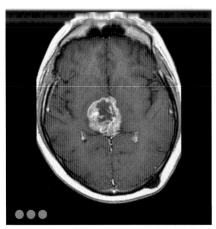

G4. Axial and coronal, post-contrast T1-weighted images show an enhancing mass in the right thalamus with a central necrotic area.

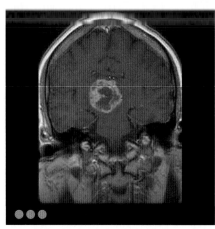

G5. Axial and coronal, post-contrast T1-weighted images show an enhancing mass in the right thalamus with a central necrotic area.

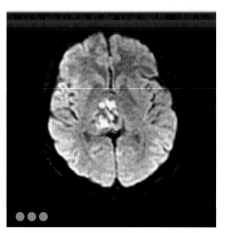

G6. Diffusion-weighted image shows restricted diffusion in the right thalamic mass.

VASCULITIS

Primary vasculitis of the central nervous system includes giant cell arteritis, primary angiitis of the CNS, Takayasu's disease, periarteritis nodosa, Kawasaki disease, Churg-Strauss syndrome, Wegener's granulomatosis. Secondary vasculitis may be due to collagen vascular diseases, Behcet's disease, other systemic conditions and the use of illicit drugs. The diagnosis may be suggested on neuro-angiography, but is confirmed by brain biopsy findings.

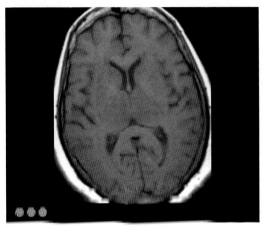

H1. Axial T1-weighted image shows slightly hypointense lesions in both thalami.

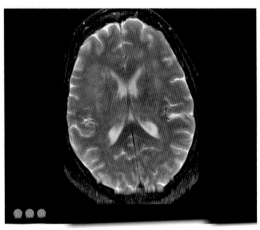

H2. Axial T2-weighted and FLAIR images reveal hyperintensity in both thalami as well as in the periventricular white matter.

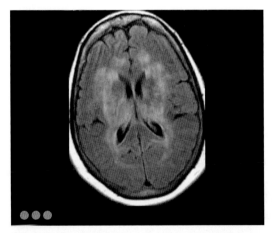

H3. Axial T2-weighted and FLAIR images reveal hyperintensity in both thalami as well as in the periventricular white matter.

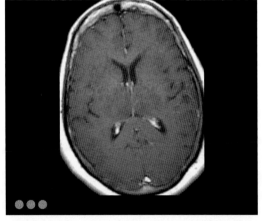

H4. Axial, post-contrast T1-weighted image demonstrates no abnormal contrast enhancement.

AMYOTROPHIC LATERAL SCLEROSIS

Amyotrophic lateral sclerosis (ALS) is a disease of unknown cause characterized by slowly progressive degeneration of upper motor neurons and lower motor neurons. Hyperreflexia and spasticity are due to upper motor neuron disease. They result from degeneration of the corticospinal tract. Weakness, atrophy, and fasciculations are a direct consequence of muscle denervation due to lower motor neuron disease. ALS is eventually fatal because of respiratory muscle weakness. On magnetic resonance imaging, hyperintensity is seen along the corticospinal tract on T2-weighted images and abnormal iron deposition can be seen in the motor cortex.

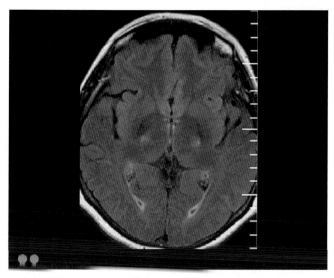

A. Axial T2-weighted FLAIR image shows T2 hyperintense lesions in the posterior limb of internal capsules bilaterally.

RELATED PATTERNS

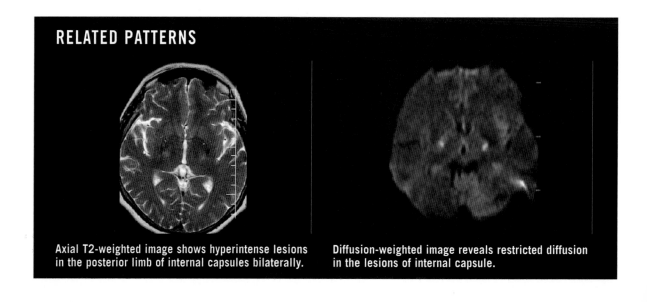

Axial T2-weighted image shows hyperintense lesions in the posterior limb of internal capsules bilaterally.

Diffusion-weighted image reveals restricted diffusion in the lesions of internal capsule.

DIFFERENTIAL DIAGNOSIS

At a Glance:

- *Behcet's Syndrome*
- *Infarct*
- *Osmotic Myelinolysis (Extrapontine Myelinolysis)*
- *Wallerian Degeneration*
- *Multiple Sclerosis* (not pictured)
- *Normal Variant* (not pictured)

BEHCET'S SYNDROME

Behcet's syndrome is a multisystemic inflammatory disorder, characterized as a triad of symptoms that include recurring crops of mouth ulcers, genital ulcers, and uveitis and with relapsing courses. In the central nervous system during the acute phase of Behcet's disease, MR imaging shows hyperintense lesions, usually involving the brainstem, basal ganglia, and cerebral hemisphere on T2-weighted sequences. The lesions usually demonstrate contrast enhancement.

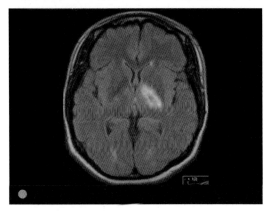

B1. Axial T2-weighted FLAIR image shows hyperintensity involving the left posterior limb of internal capsule with extension into the basal ganglia, thalamus, and midbrain

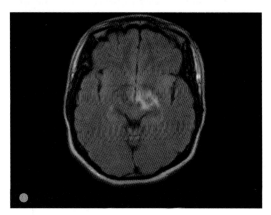

B2. Axial T2-weighted FLAIR image shows hyperintensity involving the left posterior limb of internal capsule with extension into the basal ganglia, thalamus, and midbrain.

INFARCT

Small infarcts of the internal capsule are called lacunes. Lacunes are usually caused by occlusion of a single deep penetrating artery. These deep penetrating arteries are small, nonbranching end arteries (usually smaller than 500 μm in diameter). They arise directly from much larger arteries, such as the middle cerebral artery, anterior choroidal artery, anterior cerebral artery, posterior cerebral artery, posterior communicating artery, and so on. Their small size and proximal position predispose them to the development of microatheroma and lipohyalinosis, which cause the occlusion of these vessels. Embolic phenomenon is also a possible etiology in the occlusion of these penetrating arteries.

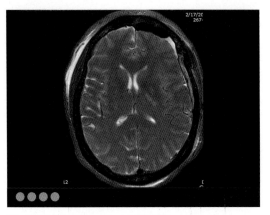

C1. Axial T2-weighted and FLAIR images show a focal hyperintense lesion involving the posterior limb of the left internal capsule.

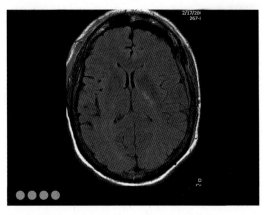

C2. Axial T2-weighted and FLAIR images show a focal hyperintense lesion involving the posterior limb of the left internal capsule.

411

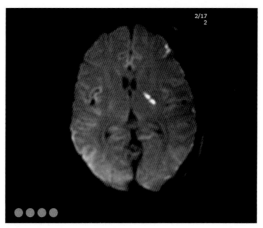

C3. Diffusion-weighted image and ADC map image demonstrate restricted diffusion due to infarct involving the posterior limb of the left internal capsule.

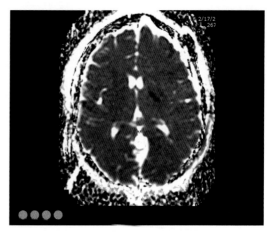

C4. Diffusion-weighted image and ADC map image demonstrate restricted diffusion due to infarct involving the posterior limb of the left internal capsule.

OSMOTIC MYELINOLYSIS (EXTRAPONTINE MYELINOLYSIS)

Central pontine myelinolysis is a noninflammatory demyelination within the central basis pontis that is frequently symmetrical. In approximately 10% of patients with central pontine myelinolysis, demyelination also occurs in extrapontine regions, including the mid brain, thalamus, basal ganglia, and cerebellum. They are usually seen in patients with prolonged hyponatremia followed by rapid sodium correction. During the period of hyponatremia, the concentration of intracellular charged protein moieties is altered. Reversal of hyponatremai cannot induce a rapid correction of electrolyte balance. The term osmotic myelinolysis is more appropriate than central pontine myelinolysis for demyellination occurring in extrapontine regions after the correction of hyponatremia.

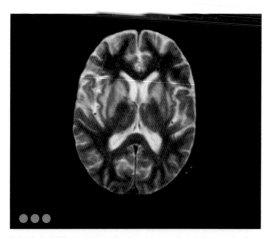

D1. Axial T2-weighted image shows hyperintensity in basal ganglia, external capsules, and posterior limb of internal capsules bilaterally as well as in the cerebral peduncles of the midbrain in a patient with rapidly corrected hyponatremia.

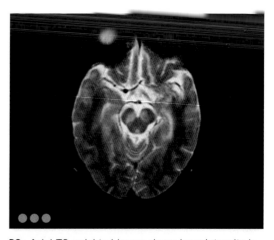

D2. Axial T2-weighted image shows hyperintensity in basal ganglia, external capsules, and posterior limb of internal capsules bilaterally as well as in the cerebral peduncles of the midbrain in a patient with rapidly corrected hyponatremia.

WALLERIAN DEGENERATION

Wallerian degeneration is the process of progressive demyelination and disintegration of the distal axonal segment following the damage to the neuron. The cause of Wallerian degeneration consists of cerebral infarction, hemorrhage, trauma, necrosis, and focal demyelination. MRI provides excellent visualization of intergraded (Wallerian) degeneration in brain. In the early stage of the disease, diffusion abnormality may be seen along the corticospinal tract. In the later stage of the disease process, focal atrophy and abnormal hyperintensity on T2-weighted images may be seen along the corticospinal tract.

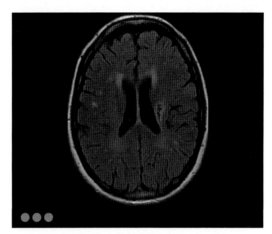

E1. Axial T2-weighted FLAIR image shows an old infarct involving the left corona radiata with mixed signal intensity.

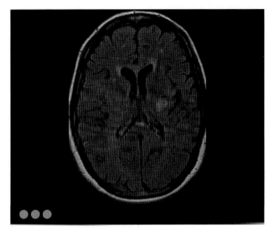

E2. Axial T2-weighted FLAIR images show hyperintensity along the left internal capsule, consistent with Wallerian degeneration.

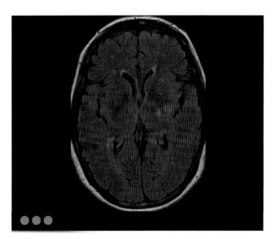

E3. Axial T2-weighted FLAIR images show hyperintensity along the left internal capsule, consistent with Wallerian degeneration.

413

OLIVOCEREBELLOPONTINE DEGENERATION (OPCD)

The olivocerebellopontine degenerations are progressive neurodegenerative conditions. Sporadic forms involve abnormalities of alpha-synuclein, but that does not fully explain the abnormality. Many specific genes have been identified for the genetic forms. However, all the clinical findings cannot be explained by the genetic abnormalities. The pons is atrophic, especially in the area of the basis pontis. Degeneration of the cerebellum is seen, especially in the cerebellar white matter. Loss of Purkinje cells is common. Major neuronal loss occurs in the inferior olivary, arcuate, and pontine nuclei. There is well preservation of the dentate nuclei. The middle cerebellar peduncles are usually atrophic, possibly secondary to degeneration of the basal pontine gray matter. The substantia nigra of the midbrain also shows evidence of tissue loss.

A group of inherited and sporadic disorders is presented clinically with symptoms of progressive ataxia and anatomically with atrophy of the cerebellum, pons, and inferior olivary nuclei. The familial form has an earlier onset (second decade) and may feature spinal cord atrophy. The sporadic form tends to present in the fifth or sixth decade, and is considered a clinical subtype of multisystem atrophy

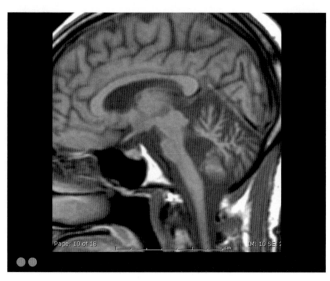

A. Sagittal T1-weighted image shows volume loss involving the cerebellum and brainstem, especially pons.

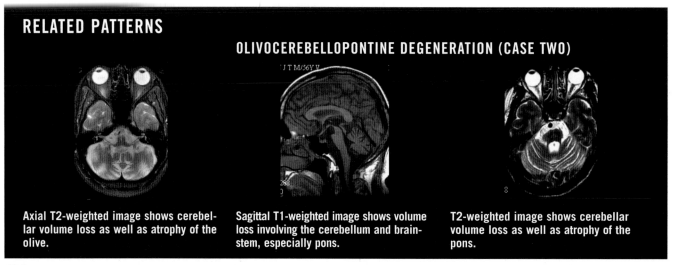

RELATED PATTERNS

OLIVOCEREBELLOPONTINE DEGENERATION (CASE TWO)

Axial T2-weighted image shows cerebellar volume loss as well as atrophy of the olive.

Sagittal T1-weighted image shows volume loss involving the cerebellum and brainstem, especially pons.

T2-weighted image shows cerebellar volume loss as well as atrophy of the pons.

DIFFERENTIAL DIAGNOSIS

At a Glance:

- *Paraneoplastic Syndrome*
- *Seizure and Phenytoin*
- *Chronic Alcohol Abuse* (not pictured)
- *Trauma* (not pictured)

PARANEOPLASTIC SYNDROME

Paraneoplastic cerebellar degenerations are disorders of the cerebellum, which are associated with certain neoplasms, particularly small cell lung carcinoma, ovarian cancer, uterine cancer, or breast cancer. These syndromes affect 1–3% of all cancer patients. They arise when tumors express proteins that are normally found only in neurons, and it is believed that the immune system, in its attempt to kill the tumor, also damages the cerebellum. Only about 1% of all persons thought to have a paraneoplastic syndrome turn out to have antibodies to neurons or Purkinje cells.

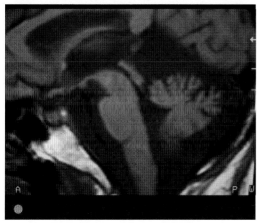

B1. Sagittal T1-weighted and axial T1- and T2-weighted images demonstrate cerebellar volume loss in a patient with lung cancer.

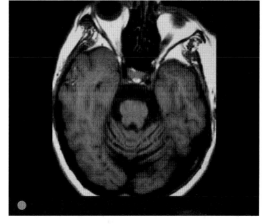

B2. Sagittal T1-weighted and axial T1- and T2-weighted images demonstrate cerebellar volume loss in a patient with lung cancer.

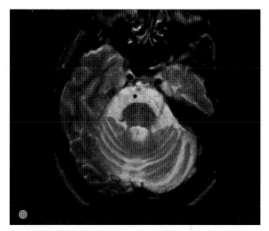

B3. Sagittal T1-weighted and axial T1- and T2-weighted images demonstrate cerebellar volume loss in a patient with lung cancer.

SEIZURE AND PHENYTOIN

Chronic Phenytoin overdose has been implicated to cause cerebellar atrophy. Experimental studies have also shown loss of Purkinje cells and other evidence of cerebellar damage in animals given Phenytoin. However, some authors argue that seizure itself can cause hypoxic injury to the cerebellum with resultant atrophy.

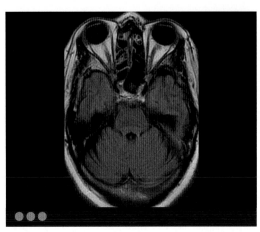

G.1 Axial T1- and T2-weighted images show cerebellar volume loss due to long-term seizure treatment with Phenytoin administration.

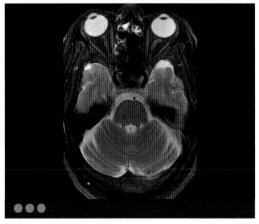

G.2 Axial T1- and T2-weighted images show cerebellar volume loss due to long-term seizure treatment with Phenytoin administration.

SECTION II

SPINE

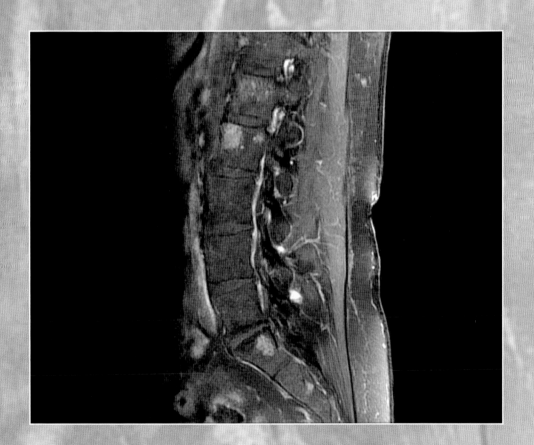

Chapter 9

Spinal Disease

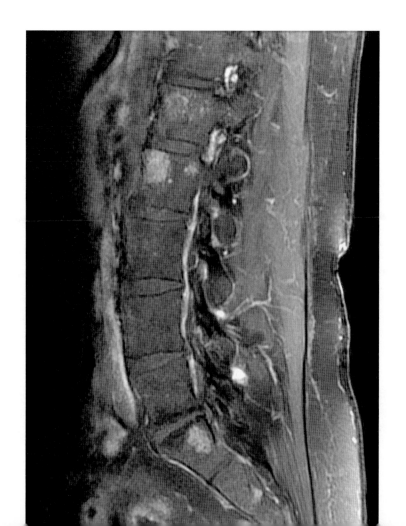

SARCOIDOSIS

Sarcoidosis is a multisystem disease of unknown origin, occurring predominantly in young adults. In the United States, sarcoidosis affects African Americans more often than Caucasian. Black Americans are more likely to be affected for a short period of time but with more severe symptoms, including neurosarcoidosis. Black women are affected more than black men whereas there is no such gender preference in white people. While involvement of virtually every tissue and organ has been described, the usual sites are lymph nodes, liver, spleen, lungs, skin, and the uveo-parotid region. Diagnosis is supported by clinical and radiological manifestations and histological features consisting of widespread, noncaseating epithelioid cell granuloma. The precise incidence of bone marrow involvement is not known, but bone lesions are identified in 1–13% of patients during the course of the disease. Bone lesions often involve small bones of the hands and feet. Vertebral lesions are rarely reported, located mainly at the dorsolumbar junction. Radiologically, the vertebral lesion appeared lytic in most of the cases and occasionally, they can be sclerotic or mixed.

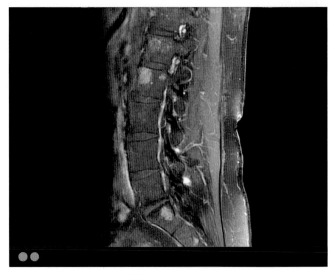

A. Sagittal, post-contrast T1-weighted, fat-suppressed image shows multiple enhancing lesions within the marrow cavity of the spine.

RELATED PATTERNS

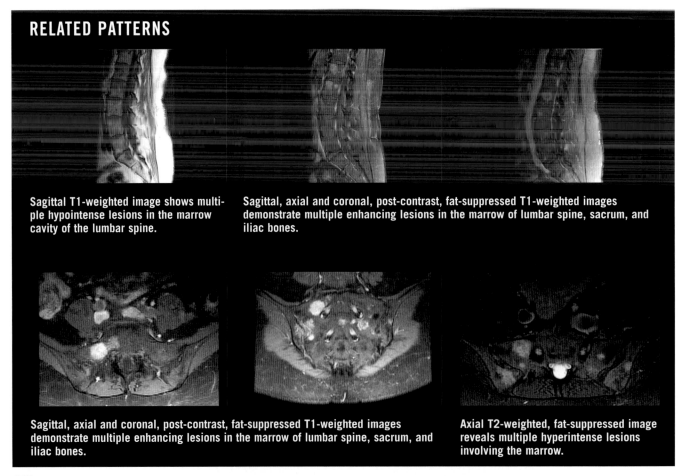

Sagittal T1-weighted image shows multiple hypointense lesions in the marrow cavity of the lumbar spine.

Sagittal, axial and coronal, post-contrast, fat-suppressed T1-weighted images demonstrate multiple enhancing lesions in the marrow of lumbar spine, sacrum, and iliac bones.

Sagittal, axial and coronal, post-contrast, fat-suppressed T1-weighted images demonstrate multiple enhancing lesions in the marrow of lumbar spine, sacrum, and iliac bones.

Axial T2-weighted, fat-suppressed image reveals multiple hyperintense lesions involving the marrow.

At a Glance:

- *Anemia (Sickle Cell Anemia)*
- *Coccidiomycosis*
- *Enostosis*
- *Metastatic Disease*
- *Myeloma*
- *Renal Osteodystrophy with Brown Tumor*

ANEMIA (SICKLE CELL ANEMIA)

Sickle cell anemia and its variants are genetic disorders of mutant hemoglobins (Hb). The most common form found in North America is homozygous HbS disease. The major consequence of this sickle shape of the red blood cells is that they become much less deformable; therefore, they obstruct the microcirculation, causing tissue hypoxia. Bone infarction and less frequently osteomyelitis can occur.

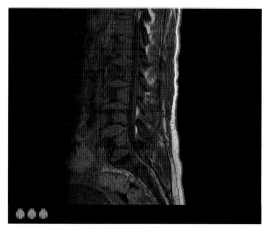

B1. Sagittal T1-weighted image shows hypointensity in the bone marrow with loss of fatty marrow. Loss of height of vertebral bodies is also seen.

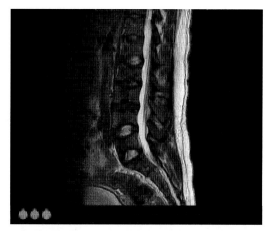

B2. Sagittal T2-weighted images demonstrate hypointensity within the bone marrow with loss of height of the vertebral bodies seen.

COCCIDIOMYCOSIS

Coccidioidomycosis is endemic in San Joaquin Valley of Central California. Most exposed patients are actually asymptomatic. Disseminated coccidioidomycosis is rare. The symptoms of disseminated coccidioidomycosis usually develop insidiously, which causes frequent delays in diagnosis. Extrapulmonary dissemination of coccidioidmycosis is relatively prevalent in Mexican Americans and Filipino Americans, pregnant women, and immunocompromised patients. MR imaging is used frequently to evaluate patients in whom infectious or neoplastic processes in the spine are clinically suspected. Coccidioidomycosis spondylitis can have a variable appearance on MR imaging. Despite the preservation of disk height on plain radiographs, disk space involvement is shown by abnormal signal intensity or enhancement. MR is superior to other imaging modalities in demonstrating bone marrow abnormality. Heterogeneous signal intensity is seen in the vertebral body marrow. Extraosseous soft tissue involvement is typical and usually extensive. Epidural disease, spread of infection beneath the longitudinal ligaments, and paraspinal disease are commonly seen, resulting in cord compression and nerve root impingement.

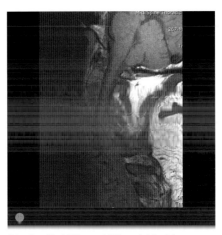

C1. Sagittal T1- and T2-weighted images show compression fractures of C7 and T2 vertebral bodies. There is an epidural mass lesion with cord compression as well as paraspinal mass seen.

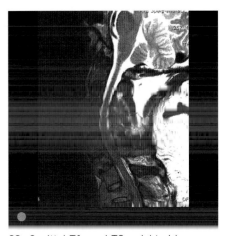

C2. Sagittal T1- and T2-weighted images show compression fractures of C7 and T2 vertebral bodies. There is an epidural mass lesion with cord compression as well as paraspinal mass seen.

ENOSTOSIS

An enostosis (bone island) is a focus of mature compact (cortical) bone within the cancellous bone (spongiosa). It is a benign lesion and probably congenital or developmental in origin. It probably occurs as a result in failure of resorption during endochondral ossification. An enostosis is usually an incidental finding and typically asymptomatic. There is a preference for the pelvis, femur, and other long bones, although it can occur anywhere in the skeleton, including the spine.

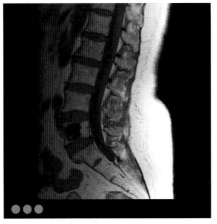

D1. Sagittal T1-weighted image shows a multi-lobulated, hypointense lesion in the L5 vertebral body.

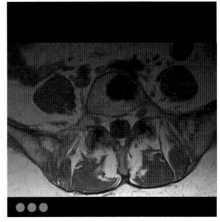

D2. Axial T1-weighted image shows a multi-lobulated, hypointense lesion in the L5 vertebral body.

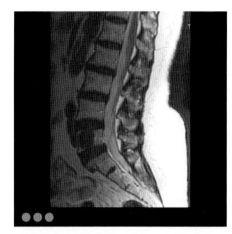

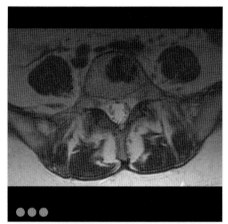

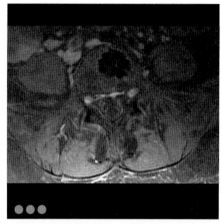

D3. Sagittal T2-weighted image demonstrates a multi-lobulated, hypointense lesion in the L5 vertebral body.

D4. Axial T2-weighted image demonstrates a multi-lobulated, hypointense lesion in the L5 vertebral body.

D5. Axial, post-contrast, fat-suppressed T1-weighted image shows no abnormal enhancement in the hypointense lesion.

METASTATIC DISEASE

The spine is a common site of spread of metastatic disease, which results in pathologic compression fractures and paraspinal masses. Spinal cord compression is a serious consequence and requires immediate treatment. With conventional MR imaging, it is often difficult to discriminate whether the cause of acute vertebral compression fracture is osteoporosis or metastasis. Recently, it has been advocated to use diffusion weighted imaging to differentiate benign from pathological compression fractures of the vertebral bodies.

METASTATIC DISEASE (CASE ONE)

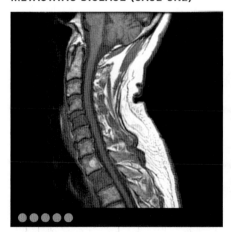

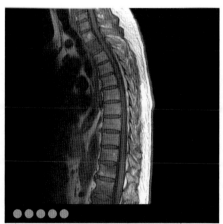

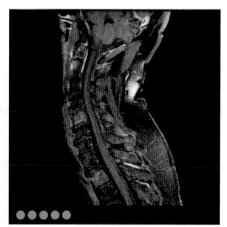

E1. Sagittal T1-weighted image shows multiple hypointense lesions involving multiple vertebral bodies.

E2. Sagittal T1-weighted image shows multiple hypointense lesions involving multiple vertebral bodies.

E3. Sagittal post-contrast T1-weighted fat-suppressed image shows multiple enhancing lesions involving vertebral bodies.

METASTATIC DISEASE (CASE TWO)

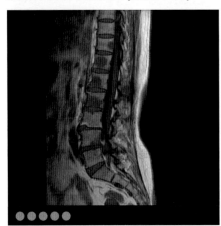

F1. Sagittal T1-weighted image shows multiple hypointense lesions involving multiple vertebral bodies

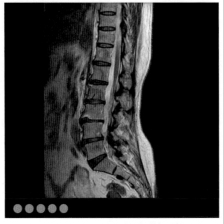

F2. Sagittal T2 and fat-suppressed T2 images reveal multiple hyperintense lesions involving thoracic and lumbar bodies

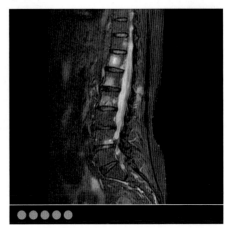

F3. Sagittal T2 and fat-suppressed T2 images reveal multiple hyperintense lesions involving thoracic and lumbar bodies.

METASTATIC DISEASE (CASE THREE)

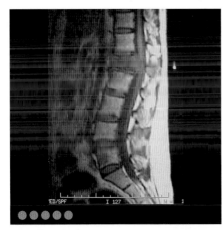

G1. Sagittal T1-weighted image shows hypointense lesions involving L1 and L5 vertebral bodies. L1 vertebral body pathological compression fracture with spinal canal compromise is seen.

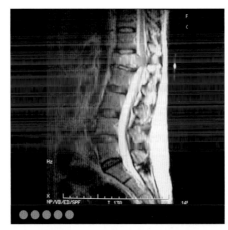

G2. Sagittal T2 and fat-suppressed images reveal different intensity hyperintense lesions in L1 and L5 vertebral bodies.

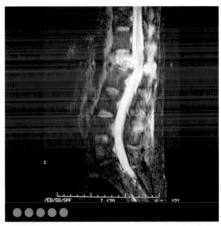

G3. Sagittal T2 and fat-suppressed images reveal different intensity hyperintense lesions in L1 and L5 vertebral bodies.

MYELOMA

Multiple myeloma is a malignant B-cell neoplasm that involves the skeleton in approximately 80% of the patients. It has an average age of onset at 60 years and its 5-years survival is nearly 45%. The disease can be very aggressive and debilitating. MRI and FDG-PET in combination with low-dose CT are the imaging modalities of choice in diagnosing multiple myeloma.

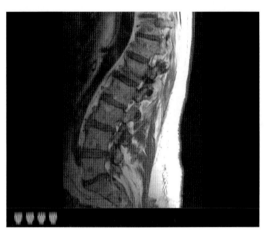

H1. Sagittal T1-weighted image shows multiple hypointense areas within the bone marrow of lumbar spine.

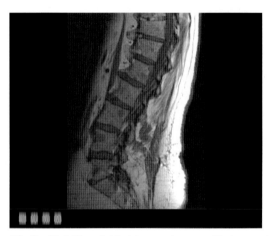

H2. Sagittal T1-weighted image shows multiple hypointense areas within the bone marrow of lumbar spine.

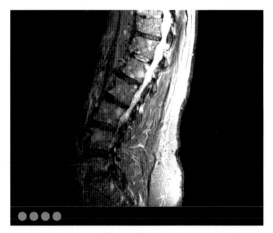

H3. Sagittal T2-weighted image demonstrates multiple hyperintense lesions within the bone marrow of lumbar spine.

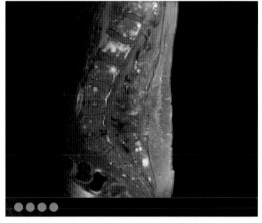

H4. Sagittal post-contrast, fat-suppressed T1-weighted image shows multiple enhancing lesions within the lumbar spine.

RENAL OSTEODYSTROPHY WITH BROWN TUMOR

Brown tumor is an extreme form of osteitis fibrosa cystica, which is caused by hyperparathyroidism and is the most common manifestation of renal osteodystrophy. Brown tumors are less common with secondary hyperparathy-roidism than they are with primary hyperparathyroidism. However, as the life expectancy of patients with chronic renal disease is increased, the incidence of Brown tumors has increased proportionally in patients with renal osteody-strophy. Brown tumors may occur in the spine and form expansile masses.

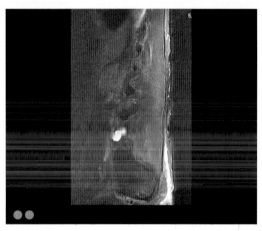

I1. Sagittal T2 weighted image demonstrates a hyper-intense lesion involving the left pedicle of L5 due to Brown tumor in a patient with renal osteodystrophy.

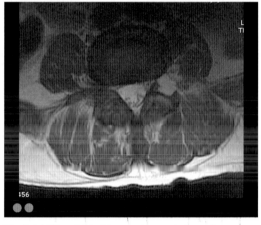

I2. Axial T2-weighted image demonstrates a hyperin-tense lesion involving the left pedicle of L5 due to Brown tumor in a patient with renal osteodystrophy.

OSSIFICATION OF THE POSTERIOR LONGITUDINAL LIGAMENT (OPLL)

Ossification of the posterior longitudinal ligament (OPLL) is most prevalent in Asian population with most reports from the Japanese literature and has a genetic linkage. Most individuals with this condition are asymptomatic and only a minority of them develop radiculopathy. Lesions of the posterior longitudinal ligament may include hypertrophy, calcification, and ossification. Hypertrophy may occur as a primary entity or secondary to disc protrusions. OPLL usually involves the cervical spine. Occasionally, it may be seen in the thoracic or lumbar region. OPLL is usually seen in the fifth to seventh decades with predominance in males. Posterior longitudinal ligament consists of two layers, superficial and deep. They are attached to the vertebral bodies and annulus of the discs by fibrous tissue. The ossification of posterior longitudinal ligament initially occurs in its superficial layer. In some, the herniated or bulging disc material may deform the deep layer of the PLL leading to reactive fibrous proliferation and inflammatory cellular changes. Proliferating small vessels may be seen in the ligament leading to contrast enhancement. The ossified mass consists mainly of lamellar bone with areas of calcified cartilage in between. It expands in thickness and width beyond its anatomical boundaries and is firmly attached to the posterior margin of the vertebral bodies and annulus of the discs.

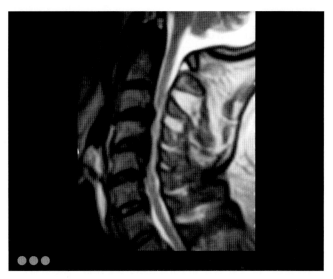

A. Sagittal T2-weighted image shows hypointense tissue at the anterior aspect of the bony spinal canal extending from C3-C4 through C6-C7 levels with compression of the cord consistent with ossification of the posterior longitudinal ligament.

RELATED PATTERNS

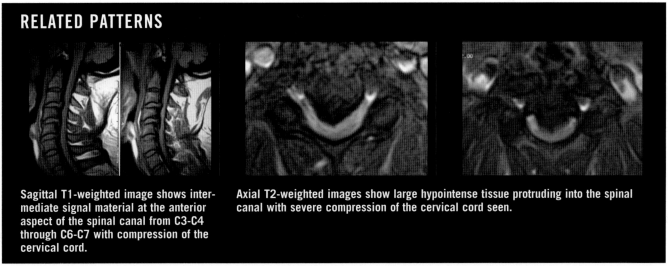

Sagittal T1-weighted image shows intermediate signal material at the anterior aspect of the spinal canal from C3-C4 through C6-C7 with compression of the cervical cord.

Axial T2-weighted images show large hypointense tissue protruding into the spinal canal with severe compression of the cervical cord seen.

DIFFERENTIAL DIAGNOSIS

At a Glance:

- *Ossification of Ligament of Flavum*
- *Congenitally Short Pedicles*
- *Degenerative Disease*

OSSIFICATION OF LIGAMENT OF FLAVUM

Ossification of the ligamentum flavum (OLF) is uncommon and their incidence in the thoracic, lumbar and cervical spine is approximately 38.6% and 26.5% and 0.9%, respectively. OLF frequently occurs at the thoracic and thoracolumbar regions below the level of C6-7, as ossification starts at the densely adherent ligament-osseous junction (enthesis). Due to increased craniocaudal thickness of the ligament of flavum in combination with a narrower thoracic canal diameter, OLF is usually detected early in the thoracic spine due to clinical symptoms related to cord compression.

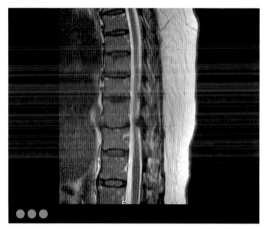

B1. Sagittal T2-weighted image shows calcification of the ligament of flavum involving one of the thoracic levels on the right side causing mild spinal stenosis.

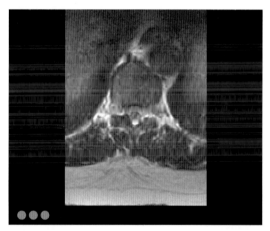

B2. Axial T2-weighted image shows calcification of the ligament of flavum involving one of the thoracic levels on the right side causing mild spinal stenosis.

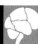

CONGENITALLY SHORT PEDICLES

Congenitally short pedicles can result in spinal stenosis with the onset of degenerative hypertrophic changes of the spine. They are seen more frequently in the cervical or lumbar spine. Cervical or lumbar spine stenosis most com-monly affects the middle-aged and elderly population. Nar-rowed spinal canals may be a result of congenitally short pedicles, thickened lamina and facets, or excessive scoli-otic or lordotic curves. With the onset of degenerative dis-ease of the spine, the condition becomes worse and patients may be symptomatic.

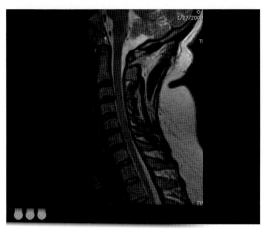

C1 Sagittal T2-weighted image demonstrates spinal canal stenosis extending from C3 through C6 due to congenitally short pedicles.

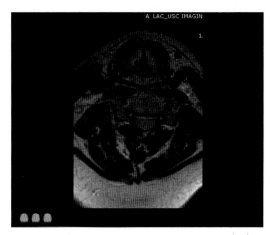

C2. Axial T2-weighted image demonstrates spinal canal stenosis extending from C3 through C6 due to congenitally short pedicles.

DEGENERATIVE DISEASE

Degenerative or arthritic changes of the spine can involve the intervertebral discs, ligaments and facet joints sur-rounding the spinal canal. These changes include carti-laginous hypertrophy of the articulations surrounding the canal, intervertebral disc bulges or herniation, hypertrophy of the ligamentum flavum and bony osteophyte formation.

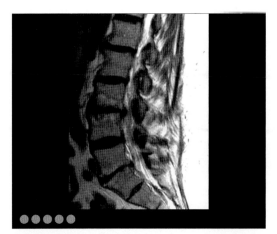

D1. Sagittal T2-weighted image of the lumbar spine demonstrates degenerative changes of the lumbar spine with disc space narrowing and osteophyte formation at L3-L4 and L5-S1 levels with mild spinal stenosis. In addition, mild retrolisthesis of L3 over L4 is seen.

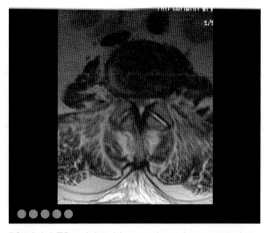

D2. Axial T2-weighted image shows bony osteophyte formation, ligament of flavum hypertrophy with resultant mild spinal stenosis.

Anatomically, the superior articular process of the vertebral body below prevents the inferior articular process of the body above to move forward. When spondylolysis is present, a loss of the stability offered by the locking mechanism of the articular processes of the vertebrae that allow the superior vertebrae to slide forward over the inferior vertebrae. The etiologies of spondylolisthesis can be classified as congenital (dysplastic), spondylolytic (isthmic), degenerative (facet joints), or traumatic.

SPONDYLOLISTHESIS DUE TO SPONDYLOLYSIS

The spondylolytic (isthmic) type is due to the presence of defects in pars interarticularis and is the most common cause of spondylolisthesis. A defect at this point functionally separates the vertebral body, pedicle, and superior articular process from the inferior articular process, lamina, and spinous process. Thus, the defects separate the vertebra into two components. The portion of the vertebra posterior to the defect remains fixed, and the anterior portions are potentially allowed to slip forward relative to the posterior structures and the spine below. Therefore, the bony spinal canal is widened at the level of spondylolisthesis. Bilateral pars defects are needed to allow for significant slippage to happen. Unilateral pars defect may result in a mild rotational type of slippage. In young athletes, trauma can cause an acute fracture through a normal pars interarticularis and result in spondylolisthesis.

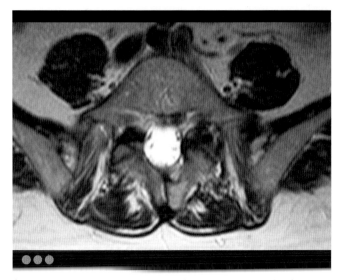

A. Axial T2-weighted image shows bilateral pars interarticularis defects. Note the defects are seen anterior to the facet joints. The bony spinal canal is widened.

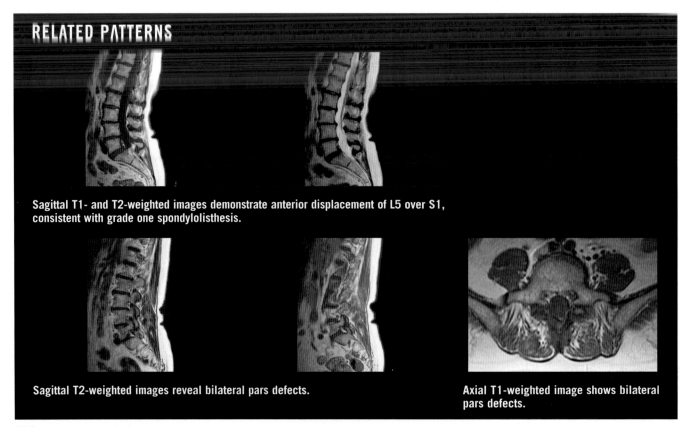

Sagittal T1- and T2-weighted images demonstrate anterior displacement of L5 over S1, consistent with grade one spondylolisthesis.

Sagittal T2-weighted images reveal bilateral pars defects.

Axial T1-weighted image shows bilateral pars defects.

DIFFERENTIAL DIAGNOSIS

At a Glance:

- *Spondylolisthesis due to Degenerative Changes of the Facet Joints*

- *Spondylolisthesis due to Congenital Defects* (not pictured)

SPONDYLOLISTHESIS DUE TO DEGENERATIVE CHANGES OF THE FACET JOINTS

In the degenerative type of spondylolisthesis, there is no pars interarticularis defect present. Long-standing intersegmental instability leads to degenerative spondylolisthesis. This may arise from other problems, such as disc degeneration or spondylolytic spondylolisthesis. Surgical laminectomy is another cause. Arthritic changes develop in the facet joints. Eburnation and erosive changes occur, which may lead to abnormal vertical alignment of the articular surfaces allowing the inferior articular facet of the vertebral body above to slip forward in relation to the superior articular facet of the body below. Other factors include abnormalities of the ligaments and intervertebral disc. A constellation of these factors combined can cause spondylolisthesis. Usually, the degree of spondylolisthesis is not severe in this group. The L4-L5 vertebral space is affected 6–10 times more commonly than at other levels. There is always associated spinal canal stenosis.

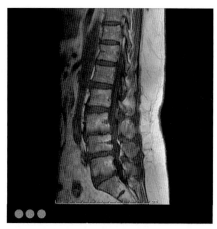

B1. Sagittal T1 weighted image shows anterior displacement of L3 over L4, consistent with grade one spondylolisthesis. Note the bony spinal canal shows stenosis at L3-4.

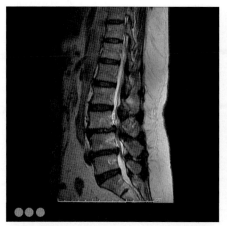

B2. Sagittal T2 weighted image shows anterior displacement of L3 over L4, consistent with grade one spondylolisthesis. Note the bony spinal canal shows stenosis at L3-4.

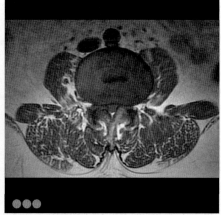

B3. Axial T1 weighted image demonstrates degenerative changes of the facet joints at L3-4 and spinal canal stenosis.

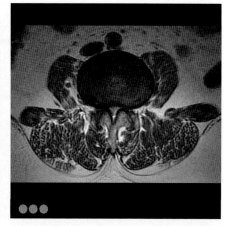

B4. Axial T2 weighted image demonstrates degenerative changes of the facet joints at L3-4 and spinal canal stenosis. Note the inferior facet of L3 is seen in front of superior facet of L4.

431

SPONDYLITIS

Early detection of infectious spondylitis is a challenge. Early MR findings include abnormal signal involving only one vertebral body, one body and one disc space, or two bodies without intervening disc. It is a challenge to differentiate early infectious spondylitis from spondylosis. Correlation with clinical findings is essential. Contrast enhancement is a good indicator for response to treatment. Diminishing contrast enhancement in the adjacent soft tissue and vertebral bodies suggest favorable response to treatment.

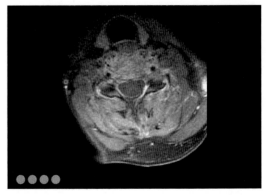

A. Axial post-contrast T1-weighted, fat-suppressed image shows abnormal enhancement in the disc, paraspinal tissue and muscles as well as epidural tissue.

RELATED PATTERNS

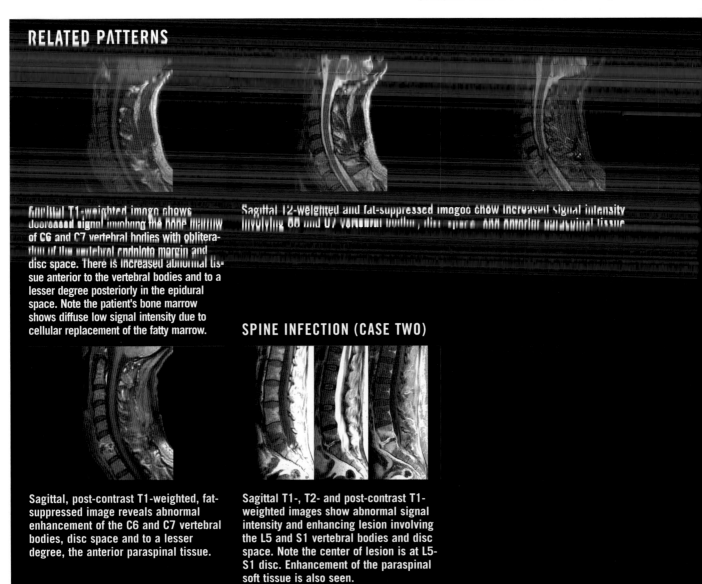

Sagittal T1-weighted image shows decreased signal involving the bone marrow of C6 and C7 vertebral bodies with obliteration of the vertebral endplate margin and disc space. There is increased abnormal tissue anterior to the vertebral bodies and to a lesser degree posteriorly in the epidural space. Note the patient's bone marrow shows diffuse low signal intensity due to cellular replacement of the fatty marrow.

Sagittal T2-weighted and fat-suppressed images show increased signal intensity involving C6 and C7 vertebral bodies, disc space and anterior paraspinal tissue.

Sagittal, post-contrast T1-weighted, fat-suppressed image reveals abnormal enhancement of the C6 and C7 vertebral bodies, disc space and to a lesser degree, the anterior paraspinal tissue.

SPINE INFECTION (CASE TWO)

Sagittal T1-, T2- and post-contrast T1-weighted images show abnormal signal intensity and enhancing lesion involving the L5 and S1 vertebral bodies and disc space. Note the center of lesion is at L5-S1 disc. Enhancement of the paraspinal soft tissue is also seen.

SPINE INFECTION (CASE THREE)

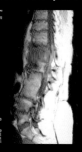

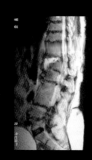

Sagittal T1-weighted image shows decreased signal involving the bone marrow of T12 and L1 vertebral bodies with obliteration of the vertebral endplate margin and disc space. Slight kyphotic deformity is seen. The narrowing L2-L3 disc space is due to previous infection.

Sagittal T2-weighted image demonstrates abnormal hyperintense fluid collection at T12-L1 level with abnormal vertebral bodies and disc space.

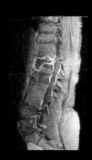

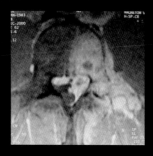

Sagittal and axial, post-contrast T1-weighted images reveal abnormal enhancement around the fluid collection, soft tissue, and vertebral bodies consistent with pus collection at T12-L1 level.

DIFFERENTIAL DIAGNOSIS

At a Glance:

- *Spondylosis*
- *Tuberculous Spondylitis*

SPONDYLOSIS

Spondylosis is due to degenerative changes of the disc, resulting in disc space narrowing and changes in the adjacent vertebral endplates. Initially, the portion of vertebral bodies adjacent to endplates may show decreased signal intensity on T1-weighted images and increased signal intensity on T2-weighted images. Narrowing of the disc space is seen with dehydration of the nucleus pulposus, resulting in decreased signal intensity on T2-weighted images. This is followed by fatty changes in the portion of the vertebral bodies next to the involved endplates, which exhibit hyperintensity on both T1-weighted and T2-weighted images. The disc space generally shows decreased intensity, but occasionally slight hyperintensity may be seen. Finally, sclerotic changes in the portion of the vertebral bodies adjacent to the disc space will present as hypointensity on both T1- and T2-weighted images. Contrast enhancement of the portion of vertebral bodies adjacent to the disc space may be seen, but the disc space does not exhibit any enhancement. It is challenging attempting to differentiate spondylosis from infectious spondylitis. A number of imaging findings may be seen. Absence of paraspinal soft tissue abnormality favors spondylosis but clinical correlation and follow-up examination is required.

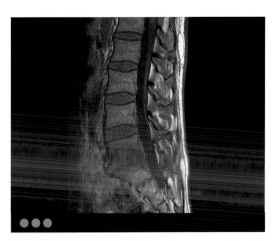

B1. Sagittal T1-weighted image shows narrowing of the disc space at L5-S1 level. Abnormal, hypointensity is seen involving the lower portion of L5 and upper portion of S1 vertebral bodies.

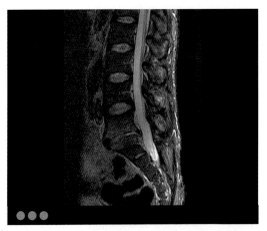

B2. Sagittal T2-weighted image reveals hyperintensity in the lower portion of L5 and upper portion of S1 as well as in the narrowed L5-S1 disc space.

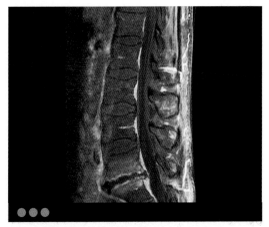

B3. Sagittal, contrast-enhanced T1-weighted, fat-suppressed image shows abnormal contrast enhancement involving the lower endplate of L5 and upper endplate of S1. The disc space is spared and there is no abnormal enhancement of the surrounding soft tissue.

434

TUBERCULOUS SPONDYLITIS

Differentiation of tuberculous spondylitis from pyogenic spondylitis can be a difficult task clinically and radiologically. Relative preservation of disc in patients with tuberculous spondylitis is thought to be due to the lack of proteolytic enzymes in the tuberculous mycobacterium. A well-defined abnormal signal intensity involving the paraspinal soft tissue, subligamentous spread of infection to involve more than three vertebral levels, presence of paraspinal or intraosseous abscesses with thin and smooth wall are all signs in favor of tuberculous spondylitis. Tuberculous spondylitis tends to involve thoracic spine with resultant kyphotic deformity.

TUBERCULOUS SPONDYLITIS (CASE ONE)

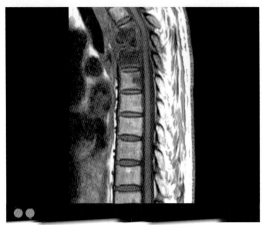

C1. Sagittal T1-weighted image shows abnormal decreased signal involving three adjacent vertebral bodies with pathological compression fractures. Gibbus deformity is seen with increased kyphosis.

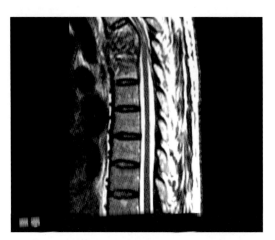

C2. Sagittal T2-weighted and fat-suppressed images reveal abnormal signal intensity involving three adjacent vertebral bodies with pathological compression fractures.

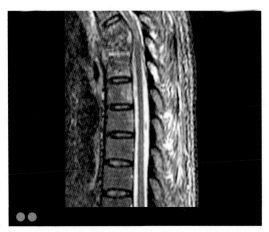

C3. Sagittal T2-weighted and fat-suppressed image reveals abnormal signal intensity involving three adjacent vertebral bodies with pathological compression fractures. Note the abnormal high signal within the cord due to compression.

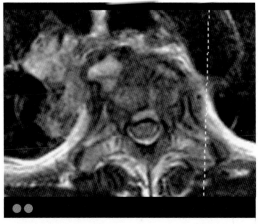

C4. Axial T2-weighted image shows pathological fracture of one of the vertebral bodies and abnormal paraspinal soft tissue.

TUBERCULOUS SPONDYLITIS (CASE TWO)

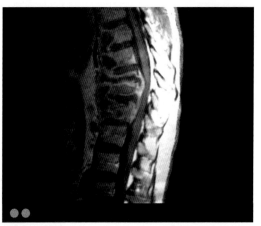

D1. Sagittal, post-contrast T1-weighted images demonstrate large, multiloculated paraspinal abscesses involving several vertebral bodies and disc spaces. Note the presence of epidural abscess compressing on the spinal cord.

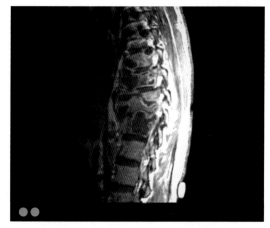

D2. Sagittal, post-contrast T1-weighted images demonstrate large, multiloculated paraspinal abscesses involving several vertebral bodies and disc spaces. Note the presence of epidural abscess compressing on the spinal cord.

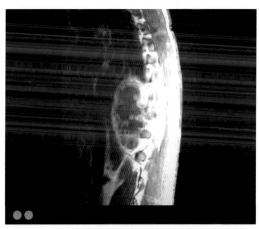

D3. Sagittal, post-contrast T1-weighted images demonstrate large, multiloculated paraspinal abscesses involving several vertebral bodies and disc spaces. Note the presence of epidural abscess compressing on the spinal cord.

TUBERCULOUS SPONDYLITIS (CASE THREE)

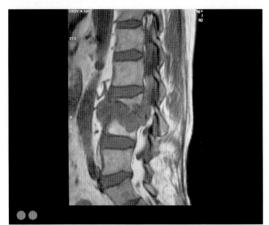

E1. Sagittal T1- and T2-weighted image shows abnormal hypointense signal lesion involving L2 and L3 vertebral bodies and loss of disc space. Compression of the thecal sac is seen by the epidural abscess.

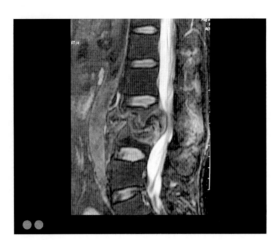

E2. Sagittal T1- and T2-weighted image shows abnormal hypointense signal lesion involving L2 and L3 vertebral bodies and loss of disc space. Compression of the thecal sac is seen by the epidural abscess.

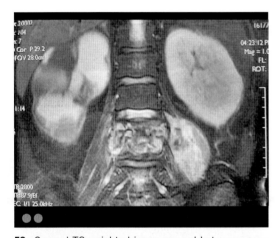

E3. Coronal T2-weighted images reveal heterogeneous hyperintense lesion involving L2 and L3 vertebral bodies and disc space. A left paraspinal abscess is seen.

GIANT CELL TUMOR

Giant cell tumors are rare primary bone tumors and represent about 4% of all primary bone tumors. Generally, these tumors are expansile, osteolytic lesions but soft tissue mass without bony change can be seen. These tumors are often very vascular, containing osteoclast-like multinucleated giant cells. Most of the giant cell tumors of the spine occur in the sacrum, followed in order of decreasing frequency by the thoracic, cervical, and lumbar segments. Spinal lesions are more frequently found in women and affect patients in their second to fourth decades of life.

A sacral giant cell tumor commonly involves both sides of the midline, and an extension across the sacroiliac joint is frequently seen.

The MR images of a giant cell tumor often show heterogeneously low-to-intermediate signal intensity on both T1- and T2-weighted images.

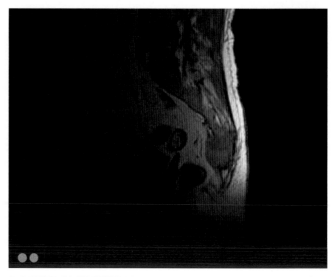

A. Sagittal T1-weighted image shows a hypointense mass involving the lower sacrum with bone destruction.

RELATED PATTERNS

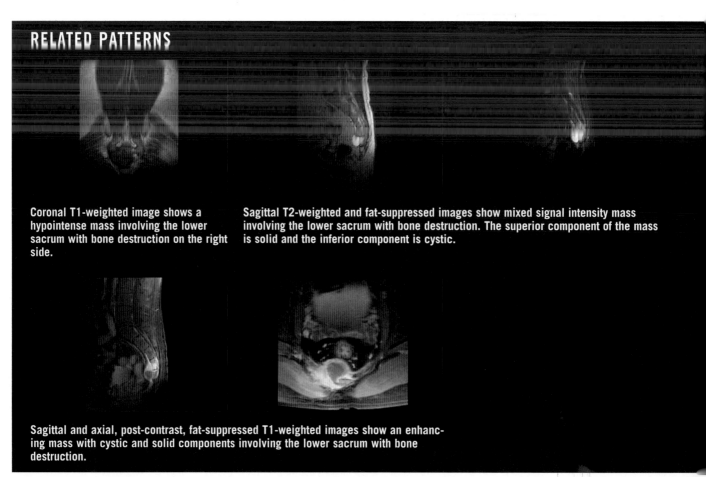

Coronal T1-weighted image shows a hypointense mass involving the lower sacrum with bone destruction on the right side.

Sagittal T2-weighted and fat-suppressed images show mixed signal intensity mass involving the lower sacrum with bone destruction. The superior component of the mass is solid and the inferior component is cystic.

Sagittal and axial, post-contrast, fat-suppressed T1-weighted images show an enhancing mass with cystic and solid components involving the lower sacrum with bone destruction.

GIANT CELL TUMOR (CASE TWO)

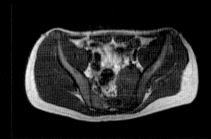

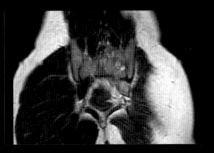

Axial T1-weighted image shows a hypointense mass involving the sacrum with bone destruction on the left side.

Coronal T2-weighted and fat-suppressed images show mixed signal intensity mass involving the sacrum with bone destruction.

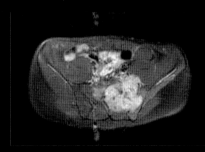

Axial post-contrast, fat-suppressed T1-weighted image demonstrates a slightly heterogeneously enhancing mass with cystic components.

DIFFERENTIAL DIAGNOSIS

At a Glance:

Benign Lesions Involving the Sacrum

- *Hemangioma*
- *Neurofibroma*
- *Schwannoma*
- *Aneurysm Bone Cyst* (not pictured)
- *Osteoblastoma* (not pictured)
- *Osteochondroma* (not pictured)
- *Radiation Osteonecrosis* (not pictured)

Malignant Lesions of the Sacrum

- *Lymphoma*
- *Metastasis*
- *Multiple Myeloma*
- *Angiosarcoma* (not pictured)
- *Chondrosarcoma* (not pictured)
- *Ewing's Sarcoma* (not pictured)
- *Osteosarcoma* (not pictured)

Congenital Lesions Involving the Sacrum

- *Lipomyelomeningocele*
- *Sacral Agenesis*
- *Spinal Dysraphism and Tethered Cord*

HEMANGIOMA

Hemangioma is the most common primary tumor of the spine, and it is frequently seen on the magnetic resonance imaging of the spine as an incidental finding. However, it is rarely seen in the sacrum. It contains fat and exhibits fatty signal on both T1- and T2-weighted images

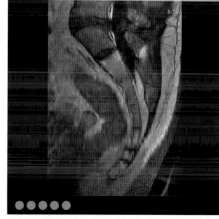

B1. Sagittal and axial T1-weighted images show a hyperintense lesion involving the S2.

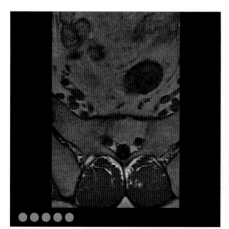

B2. Sagittal and axial T1-weighted images show a hyperintense lesion involving the S2.

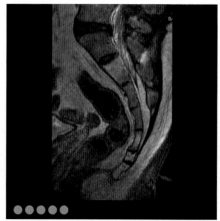

B3. Sagittal and axial T2-weighted images show a hyperintense lesion involving the S2.

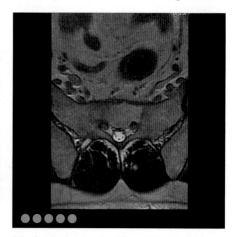

B4. Sagittal and axial T2-weighted images show a hyperintense lesion involving the S2.

440

NEUROFIBROMA

Neurofibromas are benign fibroblastic neoplasms of penipheral nerves and they are slow growing and non-invasive. Their histologic appearance consists of various mixture of myxoid and fibrous tissue. The bulk of the tumor volume consists of intercellular collagen fibrils in a nonorganized myxoid matrix. They present as a fusiform lesion with neural fibers dispersed within the lesion. They rarely calcify, and frequently have a bilobed "dumbbell" appearance. On MR imaging, neurofibromas tend to be isointense on T1-weighted images and show marked hyperintensity on T2-weighted images. The signal intensity of neurofibromas may be inhomogeneous and largely depend on the relative amounts of fibrous and myxoid material within the tumor.

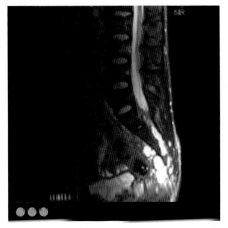

C1. Sagittal T2-weighted image shows multiple, lobulated, hyperintense lesions in the region of sacrum.

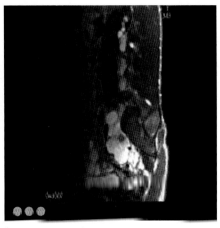

C2. Sagittal, post-contrast, fat-suppressed T1-weighted image reveals multiple enhancing masses in the region of sacrum and along the lumbar neuroforamina.

SCHWANNOMA

Schwannomas may arise from sacral nerve root sheath. They are usually seen as an intradural extramedullary mass and therefore are not true sacral neoplasms. They may be large and dumbbell shaped with extradural components that may erode and enlarge the sacral neural foramina. Occasionally bone destruction may be seen.

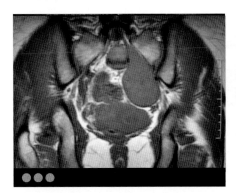

D1. Coronal T1-weighted image shows an ovoid mass lesion arising from the region of left S1 nerve root.

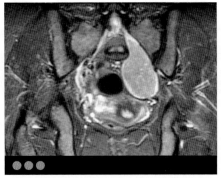

D2. Coronal, post-contrast T1-weighted image demonstrates a homogeneously enhancing mass adjacent to left S1 sacral foramen.

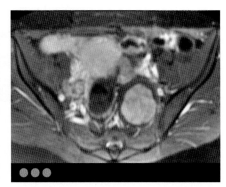

D3. Axial, post-contrast T1-weighted image demonstrates a homogeneously enhancing mass adjacent to left S1 sacral foramen.

CHORDOMA

Chordoma is the most common tumor involving the sacrum, representing 40% of all primary sacral neoplasms. 50% of all **chordomas** involve the sacrum; within the sacrum, the S4 and S5 levels are the most commonly involved. On MR imaging, **chordomas** exhibit low signal intensity on T1-weighted and very high signal intensity on T2-weighted images. Intense contrast enhancement is seen.

CHORDOMA (CASE ONE)

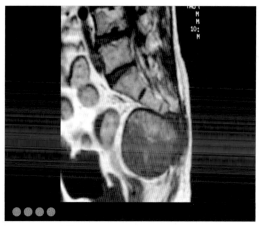

E1. Sagittal T1 weighted image shows a hypointense mass in the pre-sacral region.

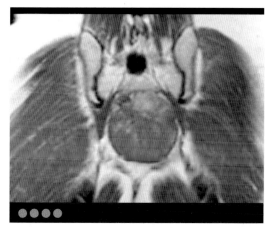

E2. Coronal T1-weighted image shows a hypointense mass in the pre-sacral region.

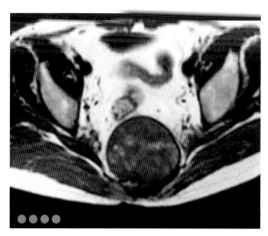

E3. Axial T1-weighted image shows a hypointense mass in the pre-sacral region.

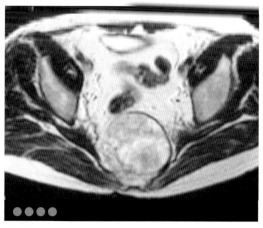

E4. Axial T2-weighted image demonstrates a hyperintense pre-sacral mass.

CHORDOMA (CASE TWO)

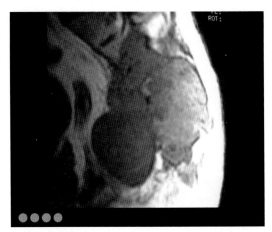

F1. Sagittal T1-weighted image shows a large multilobulated, hypointense mass with bony destruction involving the sacrum.

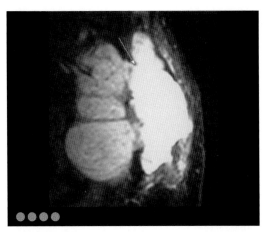

F2. Sagittal T1-weighted image shows a large multilobulated, hypointense mass with bony destruction involving the sacrum.

LYMPHOMA

Primary lymphoma of bone is a rare lesion but is the third most common primary malignant neoplasm of the sacrum.

It may appear as either an aggressive lesion causing distinct bone destruction or as the osseous structures that may show permeation, with a large associated soft tissue mass seen.

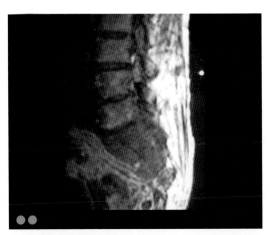

G1. Sagittal T1-weighted image reveals a hypointense, pre-sacral mass with involvement of the bony sacrum.

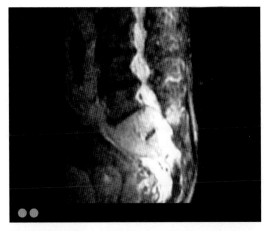

G2. Sagittal T2-weighted image reveals a hyperintense mass, pre-sacral mass with involvement of the bony sacrum.

METASTASIS

The spine including sacrum is a common site for metastatic disease. The more common primary tumors to metastasize to the spine are lung and breast carcinoma, followed by prostatic carcinoma. Any malignancy has the potential to metastasize to bone, and thus sacrum. Bony involvement results in epidural and paraspinal masses, which could cause nerve root compression.

METASTASIS (CASE ONE)

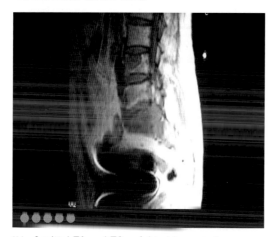

H1. Sagittal T1 and T2 weighted images show hypointense lesions involving the sacrum and L4 vertebral body.

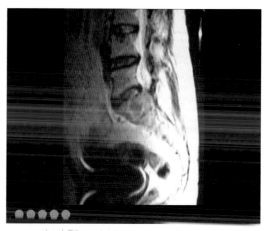

H2. Sagittal T1 and T2-weighted images show hypointense lesions involving the sacrum and L4 vertebral body.

METASTASIS (CASE TWO)

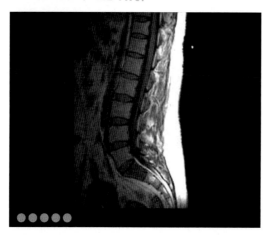

I1. Sagittal T1-weighted image shows a large hypointense lesion involving the left side of sacrum.

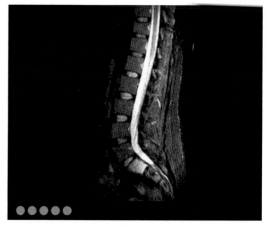

I2. Sagittal T2-weighted, fat-suppressed image shows a hyperintense lesion involving the sacrum.

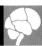

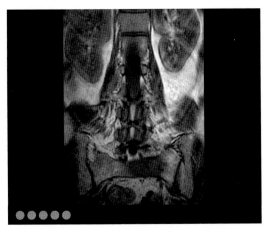

I3. Coronal T1-weighted image shows a large hypointense lesion involving the left side of sacrum.

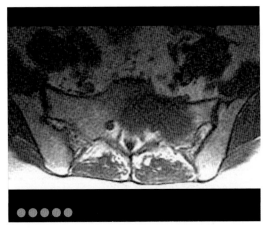

I4. Axial T1-weighted image shows a hypointense lesion involving the sacrum.

MULTIPLE MYELOMA

Multiple myeloma is the second most common primary malignant neoplasm of the sacrum following chordoma. It is most frequently seen in the sixth and seventh decades, with a male to female ratio of 2:1. **Multiple myeloma** is seen in the sacrum and other bones as multiple round "punched-out" lytic lesions. The earlier solitary form, plasmacytoma, can be more difficult to diagnose because it has a less distinctive lytic appearance. An associated soft tissue mass may be seen.

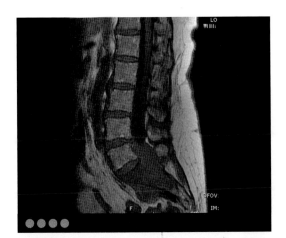

J1. Sagittal T1-weighted image shows a hypointense mass lesion in the sacral region with bone destruction involving the sacrum and extension of the mass into the sacral spinal canal.

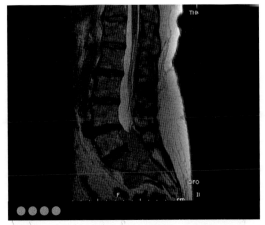

J2. Sagittal T2-weighted image shows an iso- to hypointense mass lesion in the sacral region with bone destruction involving the sacrum and extension of the mass into the sacral spinal canal.

445

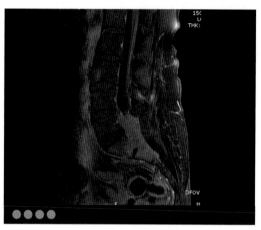

J3. Sagittal, post-contrast T1-weighted image shows an enhancing mass lesion in the sacral region with bone destruction involving the sacrum and extension of the mass into the sacral spinal canal.

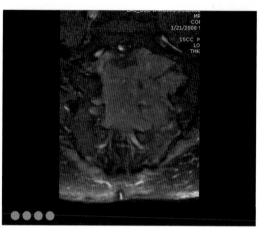

J4. Axial, post-contrast T1-weighted image shows an enhancing mass lesion in the sacral region with bone destruction involving the sacrum and extension of the mass into the sacral spinal canal.

LIPOMYELOMENINGOCELE

When a lipoma extends from the subcutaneous tissues to the dorsal aspect of the cord, tethering the cord inferiorly, it is called a **lipomyelomeningocele**. This is due to a premature separation of the cutaneous ectoderm during the process of neurulation that allows mesenchyme to enter the unclosed neural tube and differentiate into fat

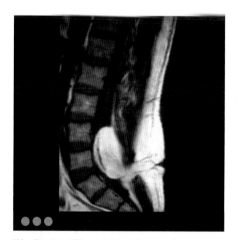

K1. Sagittal T1-weighted image shows spinal dysraphism with a dermal sinus tract. A hyperintense, lipomatous lesion is seen extending from the intradural space to subcutaneous region.

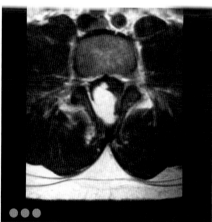

K2. Axial T1-weighted image shows spinal dysraphism with a dermal sinus tract. A hyperintense, lipomatous lesion is seen extending from the intradural space to subcutaneous region.

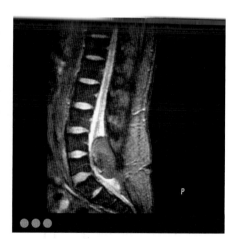

K3. Sagittal T2-weighted, fat-suppressed image shows spinal dysraphism with a dermal sinus tract. A hypointense, lipomatous lesion is seen extending from the intradural space to subcutaneous region.

SACRAL AGENESIS

Sacral agenesis is a rare congenital deformity of the sacrum, which is characterized by absence of the variable portion of the caudal portion of the spine. It occurs in approximately 1 in 25,000 livebirths. Renshaw classified patients with **sacral agenesis** according to the amount of sacrum remaining and the characteristics of the articulation between the spine and the pelvis. The classification types are as follows:

Type I—Unilateral sacral agenesis, partial or total.

Type II—Bilateral symmetrical sacral defects, a normal or hypoplastic sacral vertebra, and a stable articulation between the ilia and the first sacral vertebra.

Type III—Variable degree of lumbar and complete **sacral agenesis,** with the presence of articulation between the ilia and the lowest vertebra.

Type IV—Variable degree of lumbar and complete **sacral agenesis,** with the caudal endplate of the lowest vertebra resting above either fused ilia or an iliac amphiarthrosis.

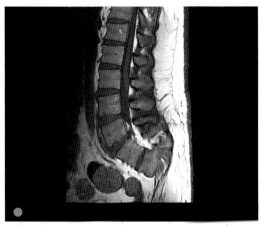

L1. Sagittal T1- and T2-weighted images show hypogenesis of the sacrum with low-lying cord.

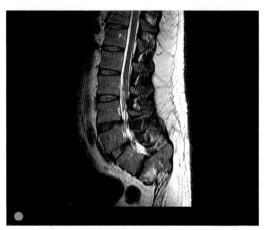

L2. Sagittal T1- and T2-weighted images show hypogenesis of the sacrum with low-lying cord.

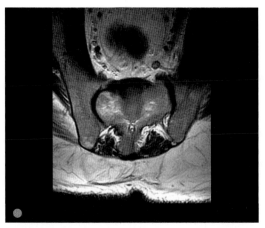

L3. Axial T2-weighted image shows hypogenesis of the sacrum and absence of the sacral neural foramina.

SPINAL DYSRAPHISM AND TETHERED CORD

Spinal dysraphism, or neural tube defect (NTD), is a broad term consisting of a heterogeneous group of congenital spinal anomalies, which result from defective closure of the neural tube early in fetal life. **Spinal dysraphism** in its open form includes myelocele, meningocele, and myelomeningocele. These open forms are often associated with hydrocephalus and Chiari malformation type II.

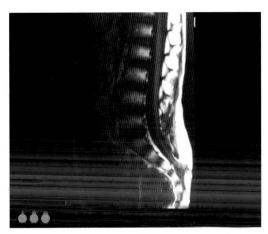

M1. Sagittal T1- and T2-weighted images demonstrate spinal dysraphism involving the sacrum associated with tethered cord.

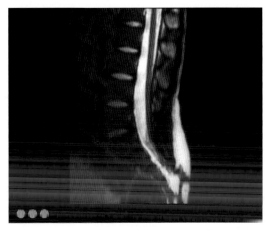

M2. Sagittal T1- and T2-weighted images demonstrate spinal dysraphism involving the sacrum associated with tethered cord.

Chapter 10

Extradural Lesions

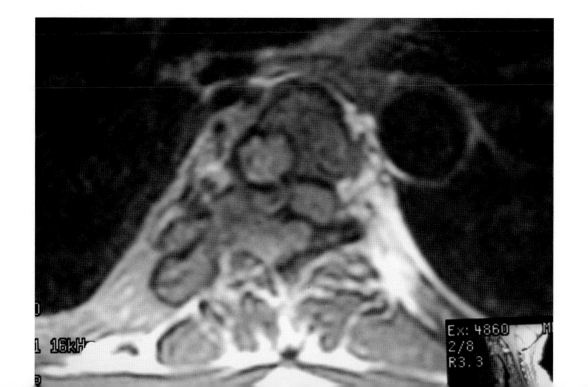

OSTEOBLASTOMA

The most common location for osteoblastoma is in the vertebral arch, mainly in the transverse and spinous processes. About 50% of the cases have vertebral body involvement. They are seen in young adults in the second and third decade. Patient usually complains of dull localized pain.

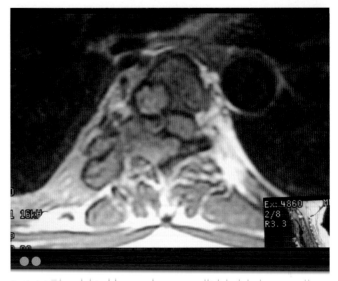

A. Axial T1-weighted image shows a multi-lobulated mass with low signal that involving the right transverse process, right side of the body, and posterior elements.

RELATED PATTERNS

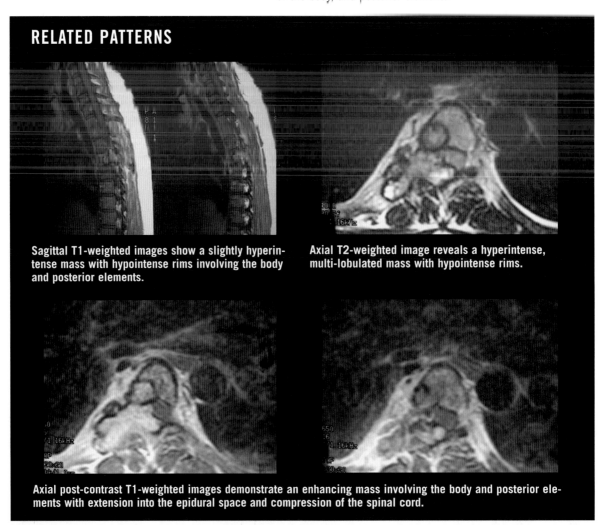

Sagittal T1-weighted images show a slightly hyperintense mass with hypointense rims involving the body and posterior elements.

Axial T2-weighted image reveals a hyperintense, multi-lobulated mass with hypointense rims.

Axial post-contrast T1-weighted images demonstrate an enhancing mass involving the body and posterior elements with extension into the epidural space and compression of the spinal cord.

DIFFERENTIAL DIAGNOSIS

At a Glance:

- *Aneurysmal Bone Cyst*
- *Chondrosarcoma*
- *Chordoma*
- *Ewing's Sarcoma*
- *Giant Cell Tumor*
- *Hemangioma*
- *Multiple Myeloma*
- *Hemangioblastoma* (not pictured)
- *Osteoid Osteoma* (not pictured)
- *Osteochondroma* (not pictured)
- *Osteogenic Sarcoma* (not pictured)

ANEURYSMAL BONE CYST

Aneurysmal bone cyst (ABC) is a benign bone lesion and commonly affects young adolescents. It usually grows rapidly with hypervascularity. The majority of the **ABC** is seen before the age of 30. MRI can show multiple cystic areas with fluid—fluid levels due to sedimentation of the blood byproducts.

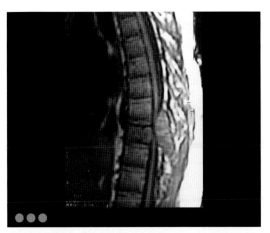

B1. Sagittal T1-weighted image shows a mixed, hypointense lesion involving one of the lumbar vertebral bodies and posterior elements.

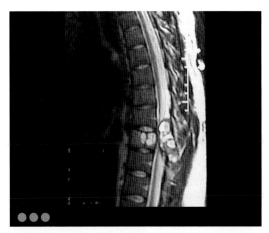

B2. Sagittal T2-weighted image shows expansile cystic, hyperintense lesions involving the vertebral body and posterior elements.

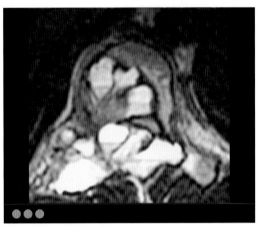

B3. Axial T2-weighted image shows expansile cystic, hyperintense lesions involving the vertebral body and posterior elements.

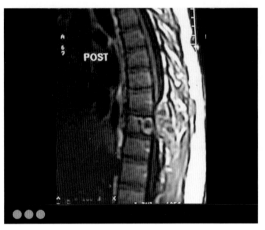

B4. Sagittal, post-contrast T1-weighted image shows a multicystic enhancing lesion involving the vertebral body and posterior elements.

CHONDROSARCOMA

Chondrosarcoma is the third most common primary malignancy of bone after myeloma and osteosarcoma, affecting primarily the shoulder girdles and pelvis. It is extremely rare in the spine. The incidence of **chondrosarcoma** of the spine is reported to be 12% of all malignant spinal neoplasms and 4–10% of all **chondrosarcomas**. **Chondrosarcomas** of the spine are locally aggressive tumors with limited potential for metastasis. Metastases have a tendency to involve the lungs and usually appear late in the course of the disease.

CHONDROSARCOMA (CASE ONE)

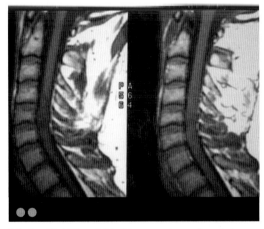

C1. Sagittal T1-weighted images show a hypointense, extradural mass at the level of C5 on the left side.

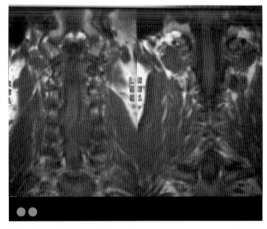

C2. Coronal T1-weighted images show a hypointense, extradural mass at the level of C5 on the left side.

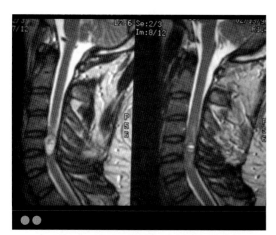

C3. Sagittal T2-weighted images demonstrate a hyperintense mass in the extradural space on the left side extending into the neuroforamen at C4-C5 level. There is compression and displacement of the cervical cord seen.

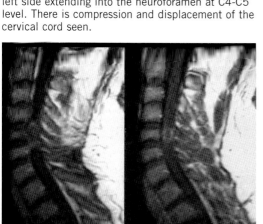

C5. Sagittal, post-contrast T1-weighted images show faint enhancement of the mass with a peripheral ring.

CHONDROSARCOMA (CASE TWO)

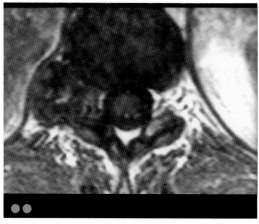

D. Axial T1-weighted image shows a predominantly hypointense mass involving the right side of body and pedicle.

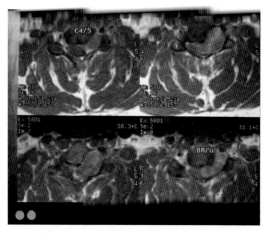

C4. Axial T2-weighted images demonstrate a hyperintense mass in the extradural space on the left side extending into the neuroforamen at C4-C5 level. There is compression and displacement of the cervical cord seen.

C6. Axial, post-contrast T1-weighted images show faint enhancement of the mass with a peripheral ring.

CHORDOMA

Chordomas are slow-growing, locally invasive malignant tumors derived from remnants of the notochord. Sacro-coccygeal involvement is seen in 50% of the cases and vertebral involvement is seen in 15% of the cases. In the spine, there is a tendency for chordoma to involve the C2 vertebral body. They usually present with bone destruction with a soft tissue mass. Intervertebral disc may or may not be involved. **Chordomas** usually have low signal intensity on T1-weighted images and high signal intensity on T2-weighted images. Contrast enhancement is seen.

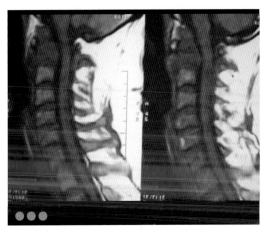

E1. Sagittal T1-weighted image shows a hypointense mass involving C2 vertebral body with epidural and prevertebral components

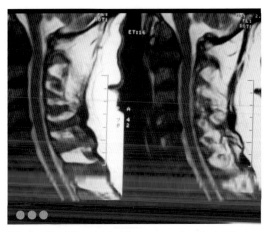

E2. Sagittal T2-weighted image reveals a hypointense mass involving C2 vertebral body with epidural and prevertebral components.

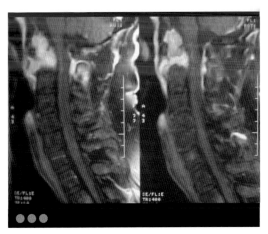

E3. Sagittal, post-contrast T1-weighted and fat-suppressed images demonstrate an enhancing mass involving C2 vertebral body extending into epidural space posteriorly and prevertebral space anteriorly.

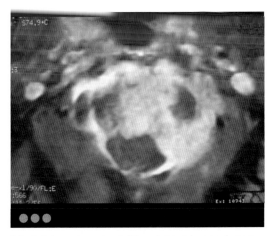

E4. Axial, post-contrast T1-weighted image demonstrates an enhancing mass involving the body and posterior elements of C2 with poorly defined margin.

EWING'S SARCOMA

Ewing's sarcoma present as ill-defined, permeative destruction of the vertebral bodies associated with paraspinal mass. Collapse of the vertebral body may be seen. Primary **Ewing's sarcoma** of the spine is extremely rare; most spinal **Ewing's sarcomas** are metastatic in nature.

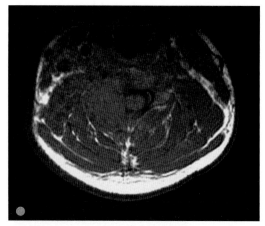

F1. Axial T1-weighted image shows an isointense mass lesion with bone destruction involving the right side of the vertebral body and posterior elements.

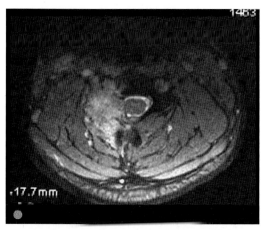

F2. Axial T2-weighted, fat-suppressed image shows a hyperintense mass lesion with bone destruction involving the right side of the vertebral body and posterior elements.

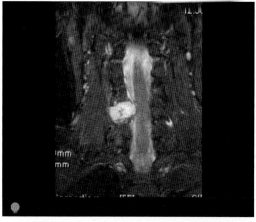

F3. Coronal T2-weighted, fat-suppressed image shows a hyperintense mass lesion with bone destruction involving the right side of the vertebral body and posterior elements.

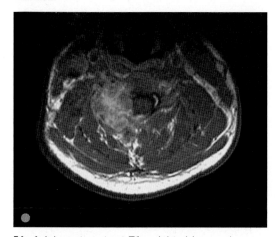

F4. Axial, post-contrast T1-weighted image shows an enhancing mass lesion with bone destruction involving the right side of the vertebral body and posterior elements.

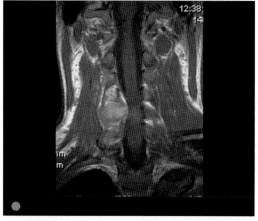

F5. Coronal, post-contrast T1-weighted image shows an enhancing mass lesion with bone destruction involving the right side of the vertebral body and posterior elements.

455

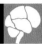

GIANT CELL TUMOR

Giant cell tumor of the bone is a relatively uncommon benign tumor that is pathologically characterized by the presence of multinucleated giant cells. In most patients, **giant cell tumors** have an indolent course, but they can recur locally. The majority of **giant cell tumors** occur in the

long bones, and almost all are located at the articular end of the bone. They may involve the spine with predominance in the sacrum. Sacral tumors may be so extensive that they involve the entire sacrum. Rarely, the tumor may extend across the sacroiliac joint to involve the adjacent ilium or may extend across the L5-S1 disc to involve the posterior elements of the L5 vertebral body.

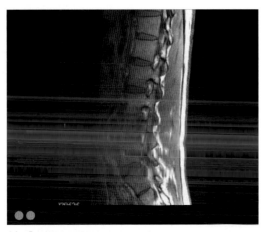

G1. Sagittal T1-weighted image shows a hypointense expansile lytic lesion involving L4 vertebral body with prevertebral components.

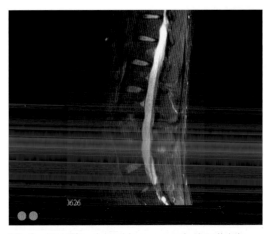

G2. Sagittal T2-weighted image reveals the slightly hyperintense lesion involving L4 vertebral body.

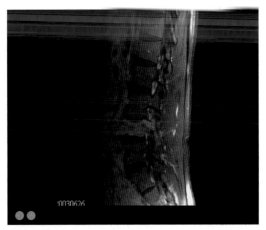

G3. Sagittal post-contrast T1-weighted image demonstrates an enhancing lesion involving L4 vertebral body with paravertebral soft tissue mass.

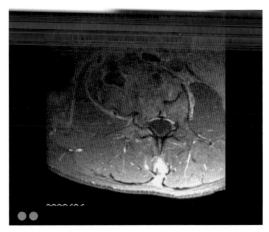

G4. Axial post-contrast T1-weighted image demonstrates an enhancing lesion involving L4 vertebral body with paravertebral soft tissue mass.

HEMANGIOMA

Hemangiomas are commonly seen on spine imaging. On MRI, they usually present as hyperintense lesions with well-defined margin on both T1- and T2-weighted images. They are usually incidental findings without clinical significance. Occasionally, they can be destructive lesions with vascular soft tissue mass.

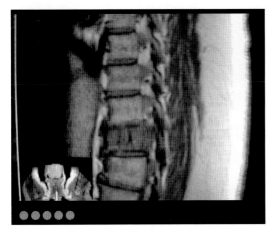

H1. Sagittal T1-weighted image shows a mass with striated appearance involving the entire vertebral body in the lower thoracic spine.

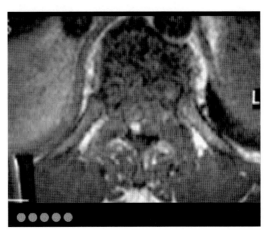

H2. Axial T1-weighted image shows a mass with striated appearance involving vertebral body with extension into the epidural space.

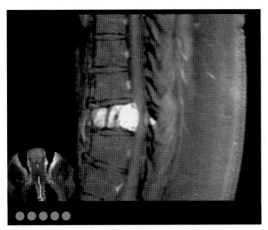

H3. Sagittal, post-contrast, T1-weighted and fat-suppressed image demonstrates an intensely enhancing lesion involving the entire vertebral body.

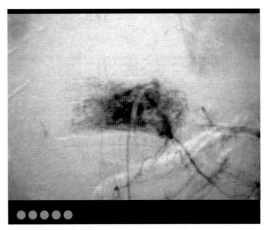

H4. A digital subtraction angiography shows extreme vascularity of the mass lesion.

457

MULTIPLE MYELOMA

Multiple myeloma is the most common malignant primary neoplasm of the skeletal system. It is a disease involving malignant plasma cells. The etiology of the disease is the monoclonal proliferation of B cells, which results in an increase of a single immunoglobulin and its fragments in serum and urine. Axial skeleton is the predominant site of involvement, which includes the vertebral column, ribs, skull, pelvis, and femur. Patients can present with multiple lytic lesions or diffuse demineralization at the time of diagnosis.

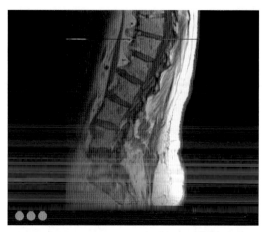

I1. Sagittal T1-weighted image shows multiple hypointense lesions involving vertebral bodies as well as posterior elements.

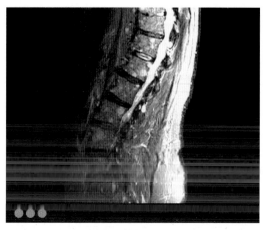

I2. Sagittal T2-weighted image shows multiple hyperintense lesions involving the spine.

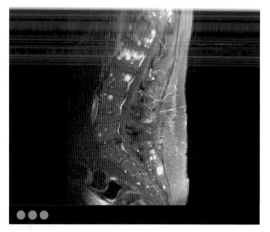

I3. Sagittal, post-contrast T1-weighted, fat-suppressed image reveals multiple enhancing lesions involving the spine.

LYMPHOMA

Lymphomas are extradural masses associated with marrow replacement in the vertebral bodies. Pure extradural masses are usually spread from retroperitoneal lymph nodes.

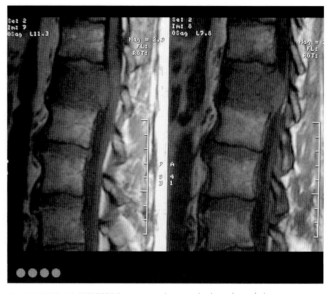

A. Sagittal T1-weighted images demonstrate a hypointense mass involving the vertebral body of L2 with an epidural component extending into the spinal canal, compressing the spinal cord.

RELATED PATTERNS

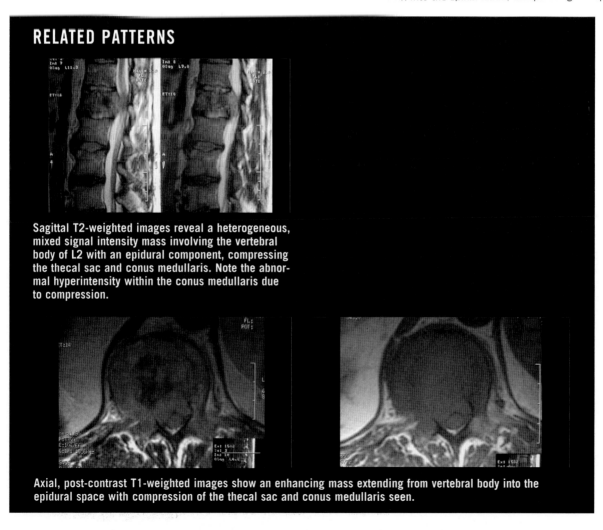

Sagittal T2-weighted images reveal a heterogeneous, mixed signal intensity mass involving the vertebral body of L2 with an epidural component, compressing the thecal sac and conus medullaris. Note the abnormal hyperintensity within the conus medullaris due to compression.

Axial, post-contrast T1-weighted images show an enhancing mass extending from vertebral body into the epidural space with compression of the thecal sac and conus medullaris seen.

RELATED PATTERNS (continued)
LYMPHOMA (CASE TWO)

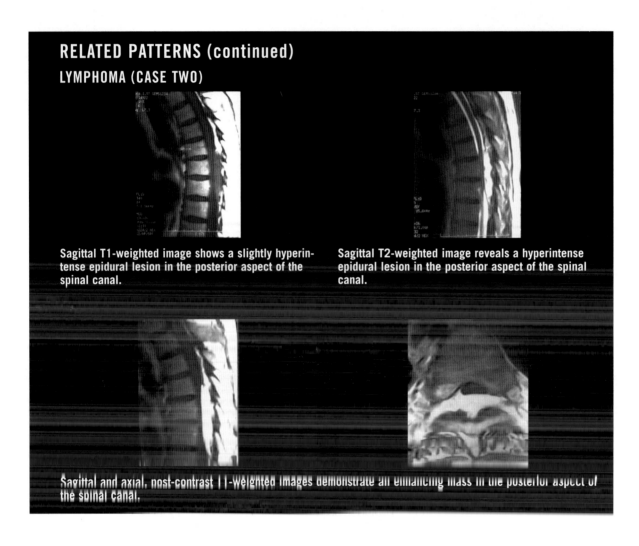

Sagittal T1-weighted image shows a slightly hyperintense epidural lesion in the posterior aspect of the spinal canal.

Sagittal T2-weighted image reveals a hyperintense epidural lesion in the posterior aspect of the spinal canal.

Sagittal and axial, post-contrast T1-weighted images demonstrate an enhancing mass in the posterior aspect of the spinal canal.

DIFFERENTIAL DIAGNOSIS

At a Glance:

- Extradural Hemangioma
- Ganglioneuroma
- Leukemia
- Metastatic Disease
- Neuroblastoma (not pictured)
- Sarcoma (not pictured)

EXTRADURAL HEMANGIOMA

Spinal cavernous hemangiomas are common lesions involving the vertebral bodies. Purely epidural soft tissue lesions are extremely rare. These lesions are hypointense on T1-weighted images and hyperintense on T2-weighted images. Following intravenous injection of contrast material, intense enhancement is seen.

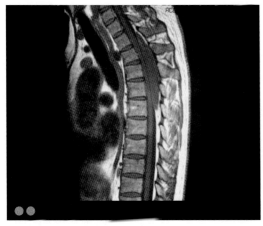

B1. Sagittal T1-weighted image shows an isointense, epidural mass in the posterior aspect of the spinal canal.

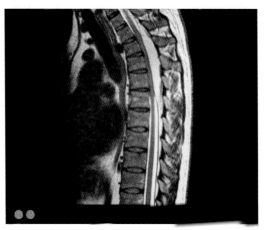

B2. Sagittal T2-weighted image reveals a hyperintense lesion.

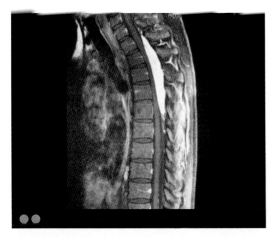

B3. Sagittal, post-contrast T1-weighted image shows an enhancing, epidural mass in the posterior aspect of the bony spinal canal with compression of the thoracic cord.

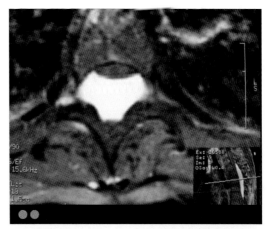

B4. Axial, post-contrast T1-weighted image shows an enhancing, epidural mass in the posterior aspect of the bony spinal canal with compression of the thoracic cord.

GANGLIONEUROMA

Ganglioneuromas are rare, benign, fully differentiated tumors that contain mature Schwann cells, ganglion cells, fibrous tissue, and nerve fibers. These lesions can grow almost anywhere along the paravertebral sympathetic ganglia and sometimes in the adrenal medulla. Along with neuroblastomas, **ganglioneuromas** and ganglioneuroblastomas are collectively known as neuroblastic tumors. Some **ganglioneuromas** may secrete catecholamines. Ganglioneuromas appear homogeneous on MRI and have relatively low signal intensity on T1-weighted images and intermediate-to-high signal intensity on T2-weighted images. Contrast enhancement may be early or in a delayed fashion.

GANGLIONEUROMA (CASE ONE)

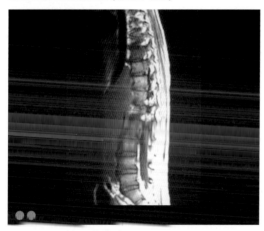

C1 Sagittal T1-weighted image demonstrates a large, hypointense, anterior paravertebral mass

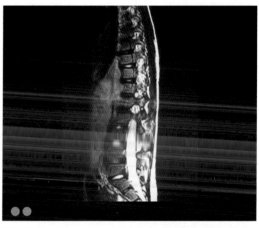

C2. Sagittal T2-weighted image demonstrates a large, hyperintense, anterior paravertebral mass

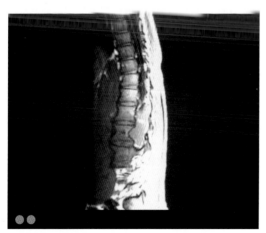

C3. Sagittal post-contrast T1-weighted image demonstrates a large, enhancing paravertebral mass with extension into the epidural space on the right side. Compression of the thoracic cord is seen.

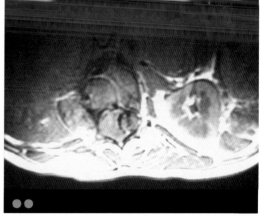

C4. Axial post-contrast T1-weighted image demonstrates a large, enhancing paravertebral mass with extension into the epidural space on the right side. Compression of the thoracic cord is seen.

GANGLIONEUROMA (CASE TWO)

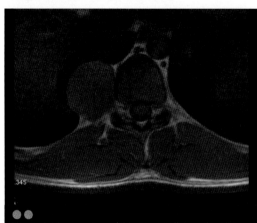

D1. Axial T1-weighted image shows a hypointense lesion in the right paraspinal region.

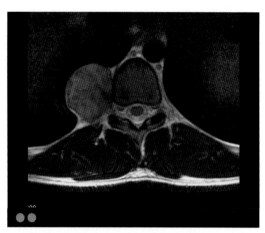

D2. Axial T2-weighted image shows a slightly hyperintense lesion in the right paraspinal region.

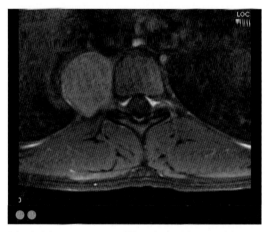

D3. Axial, post-contrast T1-weighted image shows an ovoid, enhancing mass lesion in the right paraspinal region.

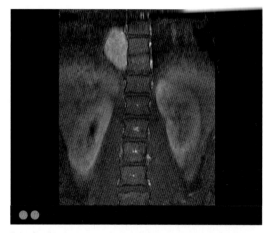

D4. Sagittal, post-contrast T1-weighted image shows an ovoid, enhancing mass lesion in the right paraspinal region.

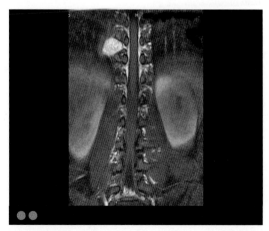

D5. Sagittal, post-contrast T1-weighted image shows an ovoid, enhancing mass lesion in the right paraspinal region.

LEUKEMIA

Leukemias account for about 2% of all cancers. It is the most common form of cancer in children. However, leukemias affect nine times as many adults as children. 50% of all leukemia patients are over 60 years. The incidence of acute and chronic leukemias is about equal. On MR imaging, leukemia may involve the bone marrow diffusely and/or present as an epidural mass.

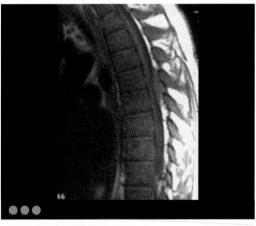

E1. Sagittal T1-weighted image shows an isointense, posterior epidural mass with compression of the thoracic cord. Note the diffuse hypointensity of all the vertebral bodies due to leukemic infiltration.

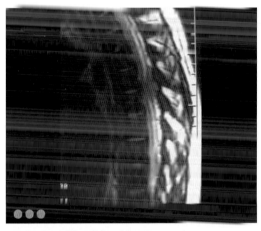

E2. Sagittal T2-weighted image reveals a hypointense, posterior epidural mass compressing the thoracic cord. Note the diffuse hypointensity of the vertebral bodies due to leukemic infiltration. A right paraspinal mass is seen on the axial image.

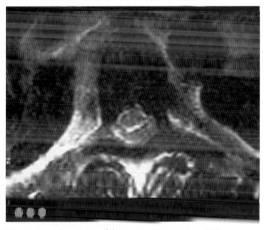

E3. Axial T2-weighted image reveals a hypointense, posterior epidural mass compressing the thoracic cord. Note the diffuse hypointensity of the vertebral bodies due to leukemic infiltration. A right paraspinal mass is seen on the axial image.

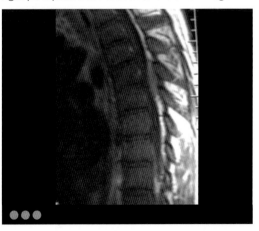

E4. Sagittal, post-contrast T1-weighted image demonstrates an enhancing posterior epidural mass with compression of the cord. Note the right paraspinal mass as well as retroperitoneal mass.

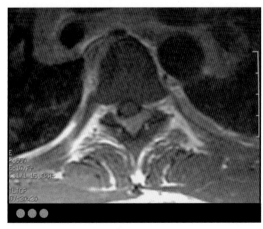

E5. Axial, post-contrast T1-weighted image demonstrates an enhancing posterior epidural mass with compression of the cord. Note the right paraspinal mass as well as retroperitoneal mass.

METASTATIC DISEASE

Spinal **metastatic disease** most commonly involves the vertebral bodies, followed by pedicles and neural arch. They are most frequently seen in the thoracic spine, followed by lumbar spine.

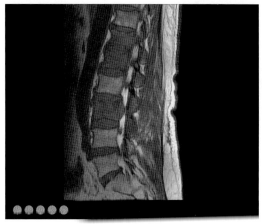

F1. Sagittal T1-weighted image shows hypointensity involving vertebral bodies of T12, L1 and L3, consistent with metastatic disease. Slight posterior extension of the metastatic disease into the spinal canal is seen at L3 level.

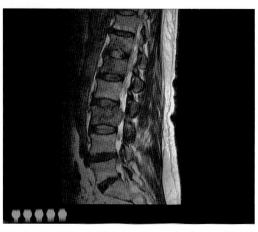

F2. Sagittal T2-weighted image reveals abnormal hyperintensity involving these vertebral bodies.

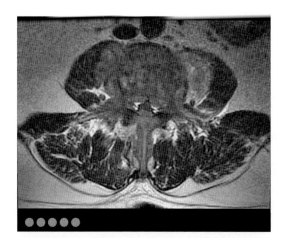

F3. Axial, post-contrast T1-weighted image shows abnormal enhancement of the metastatic disease with epidural component. Note the sagittal image is fat-suppressed.

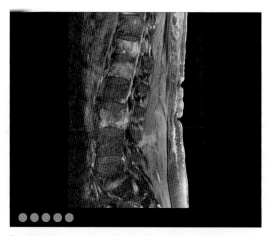

F4. Sagittal, post-contrast T1-weighted image shows abnormal enhancement of the metastatic disease with epidural component. Note the sagittal image is fat-suppressed.

SYNOVIAL CYST

According to the classification described by Nabors et al. for spinal meningeal cysts, extramedullary cysts of the spinal canal can be divided into three main groups. The first group, meningeal cysts, can be further classified into subgroups as type 1, extradural meningeal cysts that contain no neural tissue; type 2, extradural meningeal cysts that contain neural tissue (perineurial cyst or Tarlov's cyst); and type 3, intradural meningeal cysts. The second main group, non-meningeal epidural cysts, includes non-neoplastic lesions such as synovial cysts, as well as neoplastic lesions such as dermoids, cystic schwannomas, and cystic metastatic lesions. In addition, cyst-like lesions may result from trauma, hemorrhage, and inflammation. The third group of spinal cysts is neurenteric cysts.

Synovial cyst is an example of a non-neoplastic non-meningeal epidural cyst. It belongs to the second group of spinal extramedullary cysts according to Nabors' classification.

Synovial cysts may be contiguous with the synovium or they may be juxtaarticular without synovial attachment. Some 75% occur at the L4-L5 level, most of the remainder in L3-L4 and L5-S1. Cysts are always seen adjacent to

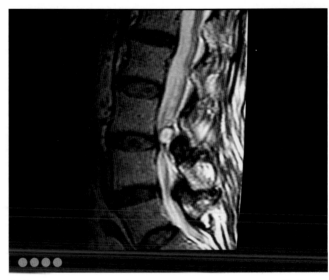

A. Sagittal T2-weighted image shows a hyperintense, cystic lesion with a hypointense rim at L3-L4 level.

degenerative facet joints. The diagnosis of a synovial cyst can be made by CT or MRI by demonstrating an epidural cystic mass adjacent to degenerated facet joint.

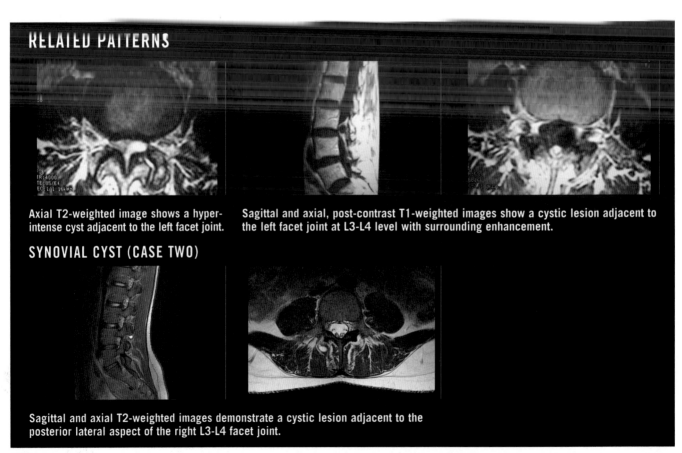

RELATED PATTERNS

Axial T2-weighted image shows a hyperintense cyst adjacent to the left facet joint.

Sagittal and axial, post-contrast T1-weighted images show a cystic lesion adjacent to the left facet joint at L3-L4 level with surrounding enhancement.

SYNOVIAL CYST (CASE TWO)

Sagittal and axial T2-weighted images demonstrate a cystic lesion adjacent to the posterior lateral aspect of the right L3-L4 facet joint.

DIFFERENTIAL DIAGNOSIS

At a Glance:

- *Cystic Schwannoma*
- *Dermoid Cyst*
- *Echinococcal Cyst*
- *Epidural Abscess*
- *Epidural Cyst*
- *Epidural Hematoma*
- *Tarlov's Cyst*

CYSTIC SCHWANNOMA

According to Nabors' classification, **cystic schwannoma** belongs to the second main group of extramedullary spinal cysts, the non-meningeal epidural cysts. Schwannomas are benign, slow-growing, solitary and well encapsulated masses that arise from Schwann cells without incorporating nerve root. Rarely, malignant transformation of schwannoma may occur. Extracranial Schwannomas may present in any part of the body as mass lesions. The spinal and sympathetic nerves are often involved. When a fusiform, cystic mass with a tail extending into the neuroforamen is seen, the diagnosis of Cystic Schwannoma should be considered.

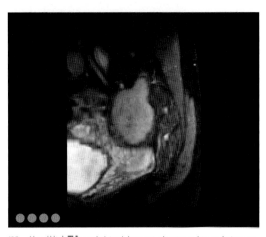

B1. Sagittal T2-weighted image shows a hyperintense cystic lesion arising from the sacral foramen.

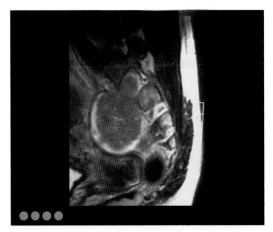

B2. Sagittal, post-contrast, fat-suppressed T1-weighted image shows a ring-like enhancing, cystic lesion arising from the sacral foramen.

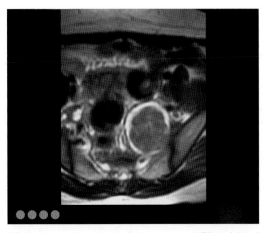

B3. Axial, post-contrast, fat-suppressed T1-weighted image shows a ring-like enhancing, cystic lesion arising from the sacral foramen.

DERMOID CYST

According to Nabors' classification, **dermoid cyst** belongs to the second main group of extramedullary spinal cysts, the non-meningeal epidural cysts.

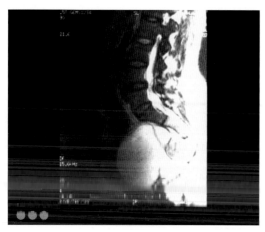

C1. Sagittal T2-weighted image reveals a large pre-sacral, hyperintense cystic lesion.

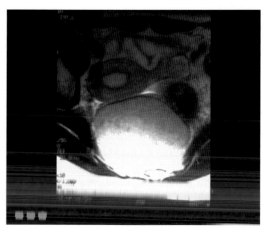

C2. Axial T2-weighted image reveals a large pre-sacral, hyperintense cystic lesion.

ECHINOCOCAL CYST

Primary hydatid cysts of the spine are rare and account for approximately 1% of all cases of hydatid disease. Echinococcus granulosus is most often responsible for liver and lung hydatidosis. Primary spinal hydatid cyst is extremely rare. Spinal hydatid cysts are usually situated in the dorsal region and generate medullary or radicular symptoms depending on their location. Magnetic resonance imaging (MRI) is the imaging modality of choice.

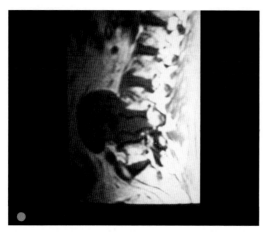

D1. Sagittal T1-weighted image shows lobulated cystic lesion involving the vertebral body and prevertebral space.

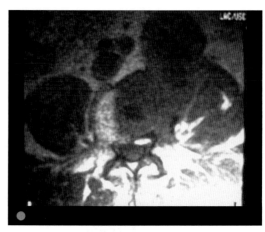

D2. Axial T1-weighted image shows lobulated cystic lesion involving the vertebral body and prevertebral space.

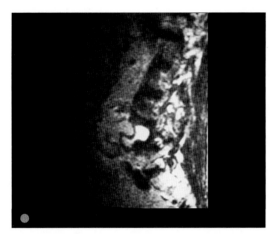

D3. Sagittal T2-weighted image reveals the cystic mass to be of mixed hyperintensity.

EPIDURAL ABSCESS

The posterior spinal epidural space consists of fat and blood vessels including the venous plexus. The anterior epidural space is a potential space with dura attached to the posterior vertebral bodies, the posterior longitudinal ligament. Infections in the epidural space can spread over several vertebral levels. **Epidural abscesses** tend to occur more frequently in the larger posterior epidural space. Most spinal **epidural abscesses** are seen in the thoracic region.

A spinal **epidural abscess** may be seen in patients with spondylitis or spondylodiscitis (vertebral infections) and after back surgery or other invasive procedures involving the spine. Immunocompromised patients and drug abusers are also at an increased risk of spinal **epidural abscess**. **Epidural abscess** is a rare disorder. Nine out of ten cases are located in the spine. The most common causative agent is *Staphylococcus aureus*.

EPIDURAL ABSCESS (CASE ONE)

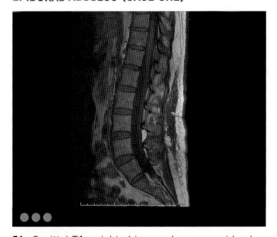

E1. Sagittal T1-weighted image shows an epidural collection posteriorly at T11-T12 level.

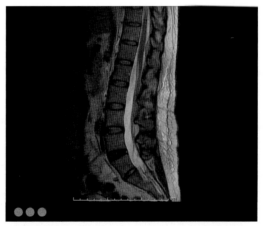

E2. Sagittal T2-weighted image reveals an epidural collection which is slightly hypointense as compared to CSF.

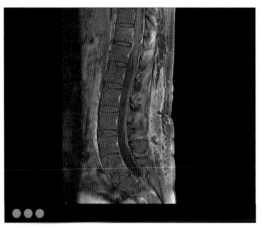

E3. Sagittal, post-contrast, fat-suppressed T1-weighted image demonstrates an epidural collection at posterior aspect of T11-T12 level. Note the extensive, abnormal enhancement of the paraspinal, subcutaneous soft tissue in the thoracolumbar region.

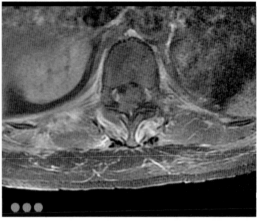

E4. Axial, post-contrast, fat-suppressed T1-weighted image demonstrates an epidural collection at posterior aspect of T11-T12 level. Note the extensive, abnormal enhancement of the paraspinal, subcutaneous soft tissue in the thoracolumbar region.

EPIDURAL ABSCESS (CASE TWO)

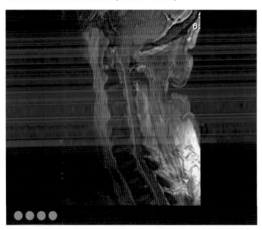

F1. Sagittal, post-contrast, fat-suppressed T1-weighted image demonstrates an anterior epidural collection with enhancing membrane extending from C1 through C6. In addition, abnormal soft tissue enhancement is seen in the prevertebral soft tissue.

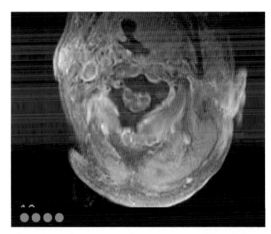

F2. Axial, post-contrast, fat-suppressed T1-weighted image demonstrates an anterior epidural collection with enhancing membrane extending from C1 through C6.

EPIDURAL ABSCESS (CASE THREE)

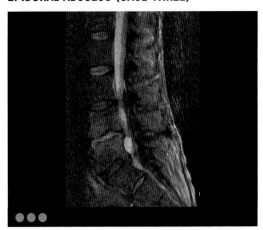

G1. Sagittal T2-weighted, fat-suppressed image shows abnormal hyperintensity involving the L4-L5 disc as well as the adjacent vertebral bodies, consistent with spondylodiscitis. In addition, a hyperintense fluid collection is seen posterior to L5 in the ventral aspect of the spinal canal

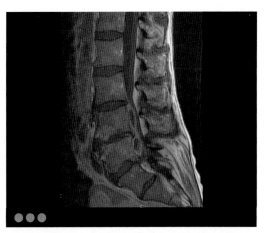

G2. Sagittal, post-contrast image shows abnormal enhancement of intervertebral disc as well as adjacent vertebral bodies at L4-L5 level. In addition epidural abscesses are seen.

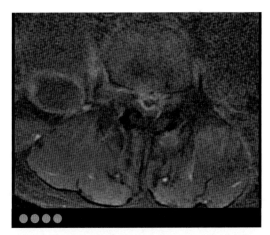

G3. Axial, post-contrast, fat-suppressed image shows abnormal enhancement of epidural abscesses in the ventral aspect of the spinal canal. In addition, a right paraspinal abscess is seen.

471

EPIDURAL CYST

According to Nabors' classification, Group 1, type 1 (extradural meningeal cysts that contain no neural tissue) cysts can be subdivided into extradural arachnoid cysts (type 1A) and sacral meningoceles (type 1B). Type 1A cysts probably arise from the herniation of the arachnoid through congenital or acquired dural defects. These cysts usually arise in the mid-to-lower thoracic spine. Type 1A lesions most commonly project dorsally and may partially protrude into the adjacent neural foramen.

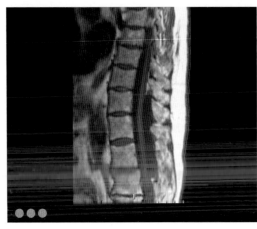

H1. Sagittal T1- and T2-weighted images show an epidural cyst posterior to the thecal sac in the lower thoracic region.

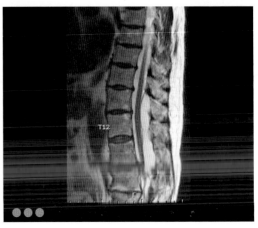

H2. Sagittal T1- and T2-weighted images show an epidural cyst posterior to the thecal sac in the lower thoracic region.

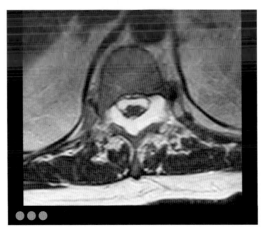

H3. Axial T2-weighted image shows the presence of epidural cyst dorsal to the thecal sac with partial extension into the neuroforamina.

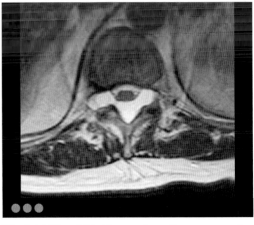

H4. Axial T2-weighted image shows the presence of epidural cyst dorsal to the thecal sac with partial extension into the neuroforamina.

EPIDURAL HEMATOMA

Spinal **epidural hematomas** have been reported to be associated with approximately 1–8% of spinal fractures. Because of the large amount of sizable veins in the epidural space, their disruption is an enticing etiology. CT can show non-specific epidural masses. MRI shows an **epidural hematoma** that may vary in signal intensity depending on the age of the hematoma and the relative proportion of the hemoglobin breakdown products present.

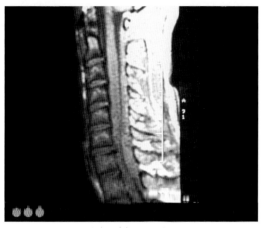

I1. Sagittal T1-weighted image shows an isointense mass at the posterior aspect of the spinal canal with compression of the cervical cord.

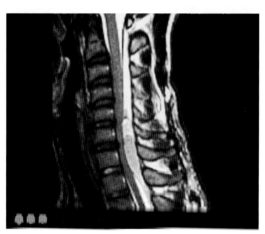

I2. Sagittal T2-weighted image reveals mixed signal intensity, predominantly hyperintense lesion at the posterior aspect of the spinal canal.

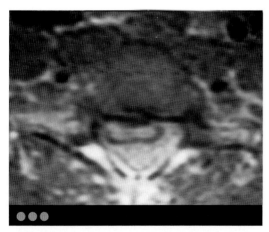

I3. Axial T2-weighted image shows a hyperintense lesion at the posterior aspect of the spinal canal with displacement of the cord anteriorly.

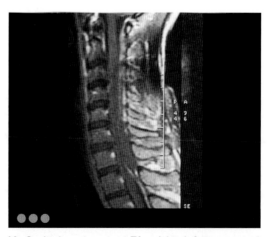

I4. Sagittal, post-contrast T1-weighted, fat-suppressed image shows no enhancement of the mass. Enhancement of the dura is seen, separating the mass from the cord.

TARLOV'S CYST

Tarlov's cyst belongs to Nabors' classification, Group 1, type 2 spinal extramedullary cysts. It is an outpouching of the perineurial space on the extradural portion of the posterior sacral or coccygeal nerve roots at the junction of the root of the ganglion.

Most cases are asymptomatic, but the cyst can impinge on the adjacent nerve roots causing low back pain or other neurological findings.

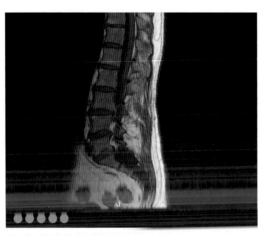

J1. Sagittal T1-weighted image shows cystic lesions expanding the bony spinal canal.

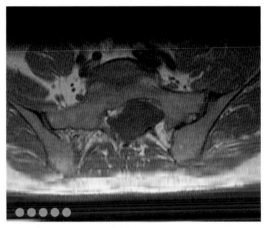

J2. Axial T1 and T2-weighted images show cystic lesions expanding the spinal canal as well as the sacral neural foramenina.

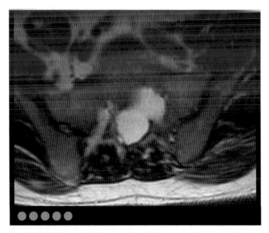

J3. Axial T1 and T2-weighted images show cystic lesions expanding the spinal canal as well as the sacral neural foramenina.

HERNIATED DISC

Lumbar disc herniation is the most common type of disc herniation. Thoracic disc herniation is the least common type. MR in the lumbar area demonstrates displacement of the anterior epidural and foraminal fat by **herniated disc** material, which may also obscure the nerve roots. Little epidural fat is present in the cervical region, thus cervical herniations are not usually outlined by displaced fat but by subtle soft tissue enchroachment upon the spinal canal.

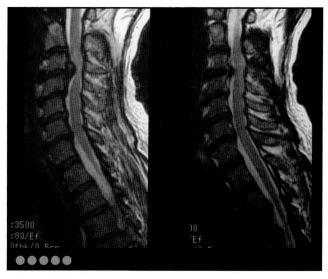

A. Sagittal T2-weighted image shows an extruded disc at C3-C4 level. Note the vertical dimension of the extruded fragment is greater than the width of disc space.

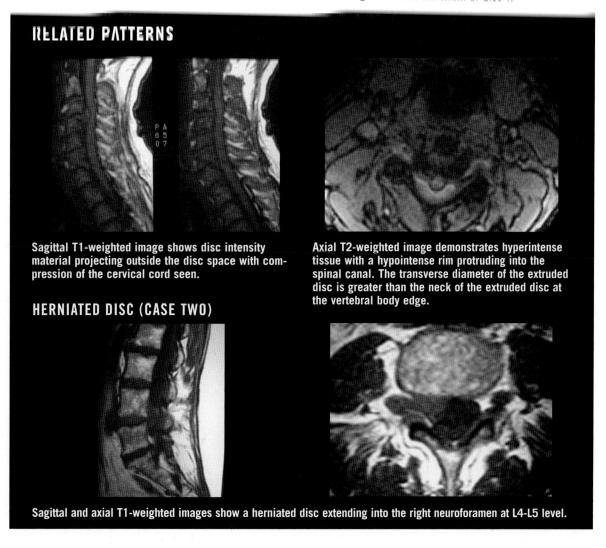

RELATED PATTERNS

Sagittal T1-weighted image shows disc intensity material projecting outside the disc space with compression of the cervical cord seen.

Axial T2-weighted image demonstrates hyperintense tissue with a hypointense rim protruding into the spinal canal. The transverse diameter of the extruded disc is greater than the neck of the extruded disc at the vertebral body edge.

HERNIATED DISC (CASE TWO)

Sagittal and axial T1-weighted images show a herniated disc extending into the right neuroforamen at L4-L5 level.

475

RELATED PATTERNS (continued)

HERNIATED DISC (CASE TWO) (continued)

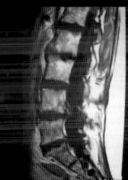
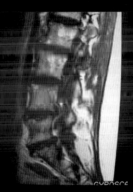

Sagittal, post-contrast T1-weighted images demonstrate enhancement of the epidural vein surrounding the herniated disc fragment.

THORACIC DISC (FREE FRAGMENT)

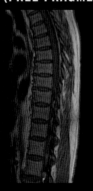
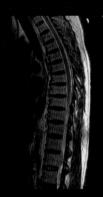

Sagittal T1- and T2-weighted images show an intermediate signal intensity disc material posterior to T12 vertebral body.

THORACIC DISC (FREE FRAGMENT) (Continued)

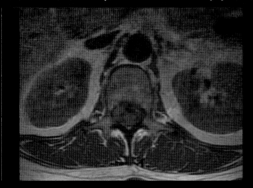
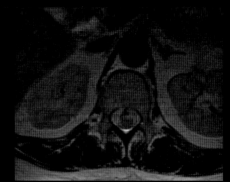

Axial T1- and T2-weighted images show an intermediate signal intensity disc material posterior to T12 vertebral body on the right anterior aspect of the spinal canal with slight compression of the thecal sac.

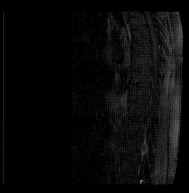
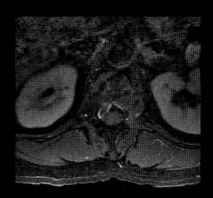

Sagittal and axial, post-contrast, fat-suppressed T1-weighted images demonstrate enhancing scar tissue surrounding the free disc fragment.

477

BONY FRACTURE/DISLOCATION

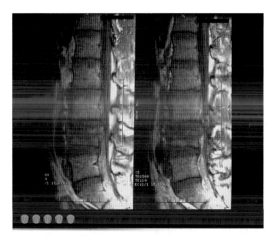

B1. Sagittal T1-weighted images show a burst fracture of L4 vertebral body with posterior protrusion of the bony fragments into the spinal canal. The fractured vertebral body shows mixed hypo- to isointensity.

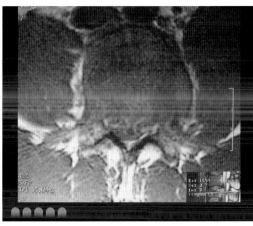

B2. Axial T1-weighted image shows a burst fracture of L4 vertebral body with posterior protrusion of the bony fragments into the spinal canal. The fractured vertebral body shows mixed hypo- to isointensity.

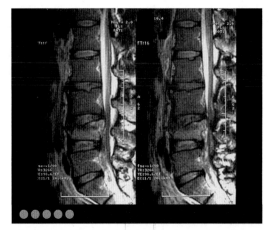

B3. Sagittal T2-weighted images show a burst fracture of L4 vertebral body with posterior protrusion of the bony fragments into the spinal canal.

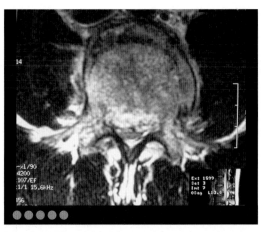

B4. Axial T2-weighted image shows a burst fracture of L4 vertebral body with posterior protrusion of the bony fragments into the spinal canal.

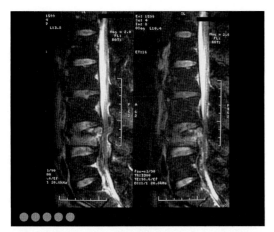

B5. Sagittal T2-weighted, fat-suppressed images show a burst fracture of L4 vertebral body with posterior protrusion of the bony fragments into the spinal canal. Note the hyperintense edema seen in the fractured vertebral body indicating an acute fracture.

EOSINOPHILIC GRANULOMA

Eosinophilic granuloma is not a common pathological condition in the spine. When it involves the spine, it is most commonly seen in the thoracic spine and frequently present as vertebra plana (loss of height of a single vertebra). Occasionally multiple lesions may be seen.

EOSINOPHILIC GRANULOMA (CASE ONE)

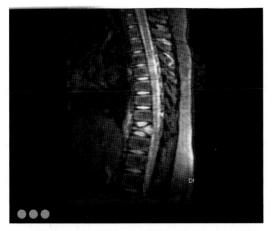

C1. Sagittal T2-weighted image shows loss of height of one of the thoracic vertebral bodies with epidural and paraspinal masses.

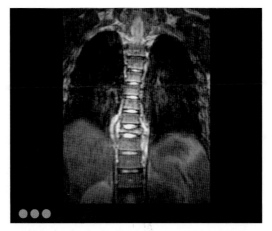

C2. Coronal T2-weighted image shows loss of height of one of the thoracic vertebral bodies with epidural and paraspinal masses.

479

EOSINOPHILIC GRANULOMA (CASE TWO)

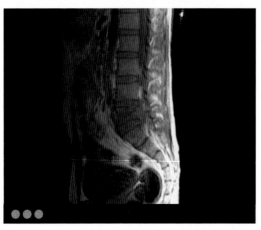

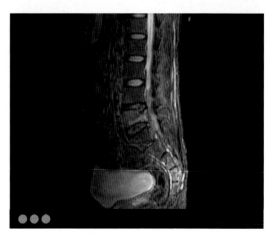

D1. Sagittal T1-weighted image shows loss of height of L5 vertebral body with epidural mass. Mild retropulsion into the spinal canal is seen.

D2. Sagittal T2-weighted and fat-suppressed images show hyperintense lesion involving the L5 vertebral body.

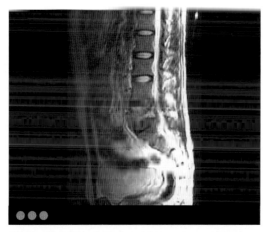

D3. Sagittal T2-weighted and fat-suppressed images show hyperintense lesion involving the L5 vertebral body.

EPIDURAL LIPOMATOSIS

Epidural lipomatosis can occur due to obesity, steroid use, or Cushing's syndrome. The fatty tissue presents as hyperintense mass on T1-weighted images. Cord compression may be seen.

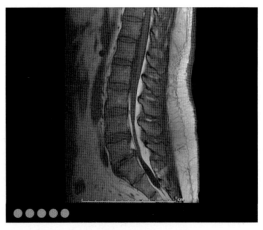

E. Sagittal T1-weighted image shows epidural, hyperintense fat in the distal lumbar spinal canal with compression of the thecal sac.

EXTRAMEDUALLARY HEMATOPOIESIS

Extramodullary hematopoiesis can occur anywhere in the body. It can present as paraspinal masses.

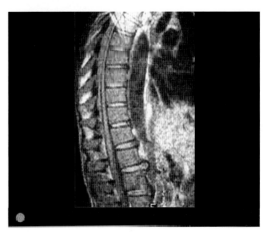

F1. Sagittal T1-weighted image shows an isointense, epidural lesion in the posterior aspect of the spinal canal.

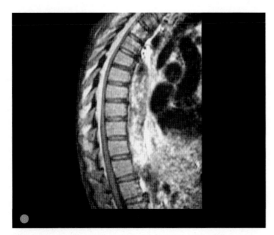

F2. Sagittal, post-contrast T1-weighted image demonstrates enhancing epidural lesions in the posterior aspect of the spinal canal on sagittal image and in the paraspinal region bilaterally on the coronal image.

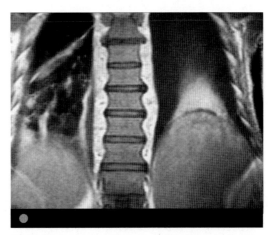

F3. Coronal, post-contrast T1-weighted image demonstrates enhancing epidural lesions in the posterior aspect of the spinal canal on sagittal image and in the paraspinal region bilaterally on the coronal image.

481

OPLL

Ossification of the posterior longitudinal ligament (OPLL) begins with hypervascular fibrosis and hypertrophy of the posterior longitudinal ligament, followed by cartilaginous proliferation, and lamellar bone formation. OPLL are seen in the cervical spine in about 70% of the cases, with the remaining 30% equally divided between thoracic and lumbar spine.

MRI can demonstrate the hypointense calcified posterior longitudinal ligament as well as the presence of cord contusion, which is seen as a focal hyperintense area in the cord.

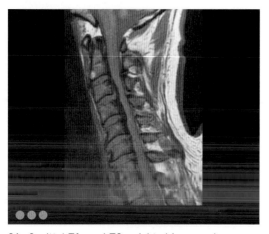

G1. Sagittal T1- and T2-weighted images show hypointense lesion at the anterior aspect of the spinal canal with cord compression extending from C3 through C5

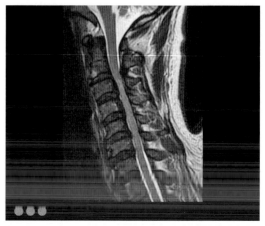

G2. Sagittal T1- and T2-weighted images show hypointense lesion at the anterior aspect of the spinal canal with cord compression extending from C3 through C5.

TUMORAL CALCINOSIS

Tumoral Calcinosis is a rare disorder characterized by soft tissue calcification deposition, typically in a periarticular distribution most commonly seen in the regions of the hip, shoulder, and elbow. Spinal involvement is rare.

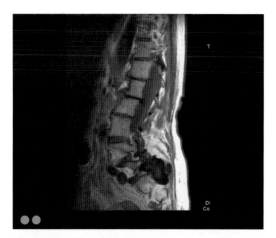

H1. Sagittal T1-weighted image shows a hypointense lesion adjacent to left lamina and facet joint extending from L5 through S2.

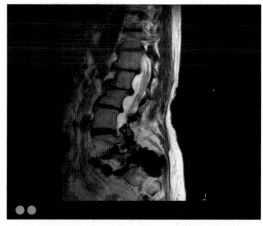

H2. Sagittal T2-weighted image reveals a hypointense lesion adjacent to left lamina and facet joint.

Chapter 11

Intradural Extramedullary Lesions

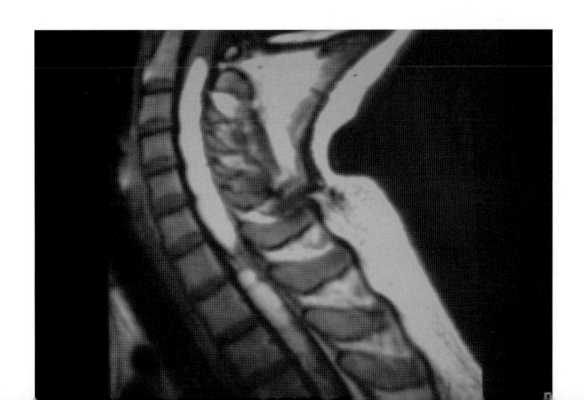

LIPOMA

Intradural lipomas are rare congenital tumors consisting of approximately 4% of spinal lipomas. They are usually associated with spinal dysraphysm such as spina bifida, lipomeningocele. Intradural lipomas without spinal dysraphysm are very rare. Intradural lipomas can be intradural, subpial or juxtamedullary in location. They are seen in young adults in second and third decades of life with no sex predilection. Upper thoracic and cervical spine are most commonly affected regions. The lesion is elongated in shape and may involve several segments. MRI is the imaging modality of choice. The fat component of the lesion is seen as a hyperintense mass on T1 weighted image and the fat signal is suppressed by using the fat-suppression technique. MRI can also localize the lipoma and delineates its relationship with the adjacent structures.

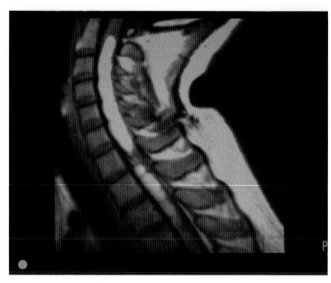

A Sagittal T1-weighted image shows a hyperintense mass in the subpial location of the the cervical cord.

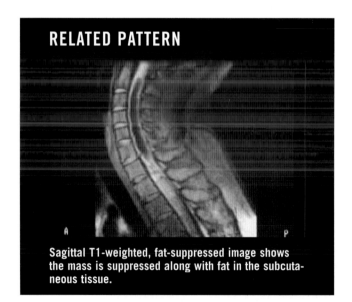

RELATED PATTERN

Sagittal T1-weighted, fat-suppressed image shows the mass is suppressed along with fat in the subcutaneous tissue.

DIFFERENTIAL DIAGNOSIS

At a Glance:

• *Dermoid*

• *Fibrolipoma of the Filum Terminale*

• *Teratoma*

DERMOID

Dermoids in the spinal canal may cause back or leg pain due to focal mass effect. Headache and meningitis may occur if an associated dermal sinus tract becomes infected. Dermal sinuses, dermoid tumors, or epidermoid tumors are frequently seen in association with vertebral abnormalities, such as diastematomyelia, hemivertebra, and scoliosis.

Approximately 60% of both epidermoids and **dermoids** are extramedullary in location.

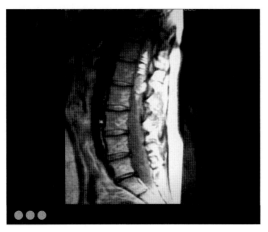

A. Sagittal T1-weighted image shows a hyperintense, intradural lesion with irregular contour extending from T12 to L2.

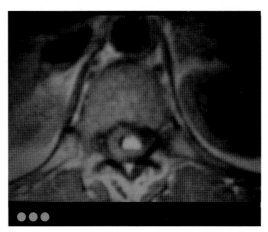

B. Axial T1-weighted image reveals a hyperintense, intradural lesion. A rim of hypointensity on the right side is due to calcification.

FIBROLIPOMA OF THE FILUM TERMINALE

Small amounts of fat in the filum terminale can be identified on MRI as an area of linear hyperintensity on T1 weighted images. They are usually asymptomatic in kids and may be termed "fibrolipomas." The occurrence of incidental fat within the filum terminale in the normal, asymptomatic adult population has been estimated to be approximately 5%.

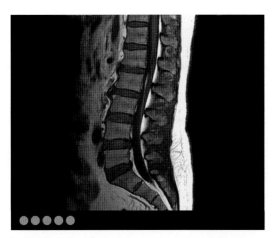

C. Sagittal T1-weighted image shows hyperintense, fatty signal intensity along the filum terminale.

TERATOMA

Spinal **teratomas** are rare masses and may be intra- or extradural in location. Fat and calcification may be seen within the lesion.

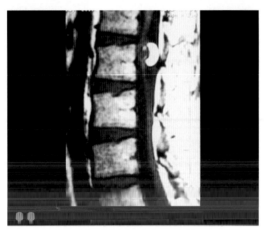

D1. Sagittal T1-weighted image shows a hyperintense, intradural lesion displacing the cauda equina anteriorly.

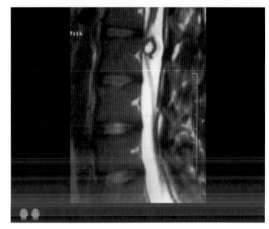

D2. Sagittal T2-weighted image shows a hyperintense lesion with similar signal intenisty as CSF. A broken ring of hypointensity is due to calcification within the lesion.

ARTERIOVENOUS FISTULA

Intradural, extramedullary vascular malformations are of the type I (dural AV fistula), type III (juvenile type of AVMs), and type IV (intradural, extramedullary AVFs) varieties. Type III vascular malformations are large and located in both intramedullary and extramedullary compartments. Type IV vascular malformations are AVFs, in which typically the anterior spinal artery feeds directly into a draining vein on the anterior surface of the cord without an interposed nidus of vessels. Type I vascular malformations are AVFs in which arteries located on the cord surface or within root sleeves feed directly into perimedullary veins and may eventually produce cord edema secondary to perimedullary venous hypertension. This is the most common variety of spinal AVMs. Type II spinal AVMs are true intramedullary arteriovenous malformations with a nidus and early draining vein.

DURAL AV FISTULA (TYPE I)

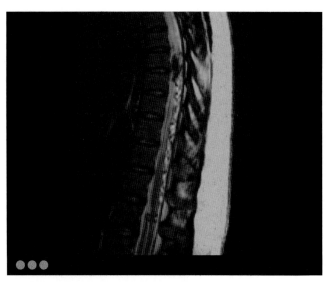

A. Sagittal T2-weighted image reveals multiple serpiginous flow void areas along the spinal cord. A focal hypointensity in the upper portion of the cord is probably due to old hemorrhage. Hyperintense edema is seen involving a long segment of the cord

RELATED PATTERNS

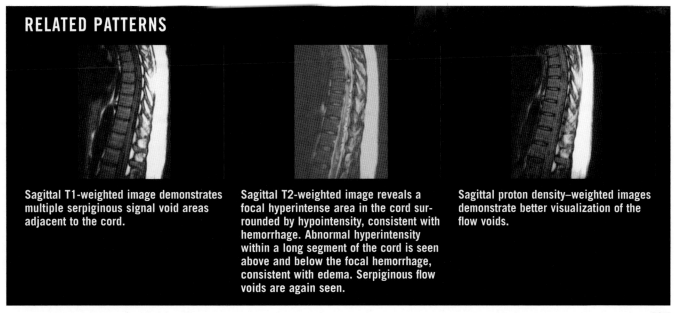

Sagittal T1-weighted image demonstrates multiple serpiginous signal void areas adjacent to the cord.

Sagittal T2-weighted image reveals a focal hyperintense area in the cord surrounded by hypointensity, consistent with hemorrhage. Abnormal hyperintensity within a long segment of the cord is seen above and below the focal hemorrhage, consistent with edema. Serpiginous flow voids are again seen.

Sagittal proton density–weighted images demonstrate better visualization of the flow voids.

DIFFERENTIAL DIAGNOSIS

At a Glance:

- *Intradural, Extramedullary AVF (Type IV)*
- *Juvenile Type of AVM (Type III)*
- *Intramedullary Spinal AVM (Type II)* (not pictured)

INTRADURAL, EXTRAMEDULLARY AVF (TYPE IV)

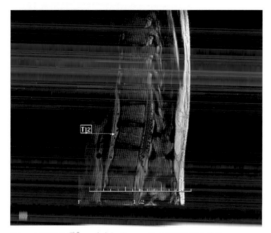

B1. Sagittal T2-weighted image shows serpiginous flow voids on the surface of the cord.

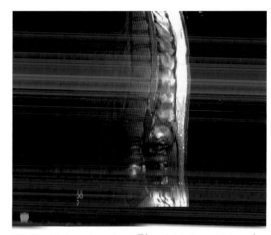

B2. Sagittal, post contrast T1-weighted image reveals enhancement of the serpiginous flow void areas seen on T2-weighted image.

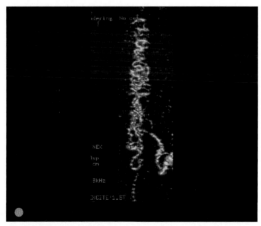

B3. MRA of the spine demonstrates serpiginous vessels in the region of conus medullaris. The feeding radicular artery is seen and it provides useful information for performing spinal angiogram.

JUVENILE TYPE OF AVM (TYPE III)

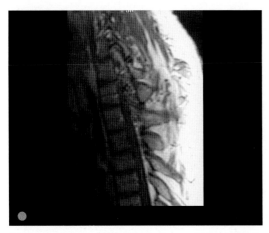

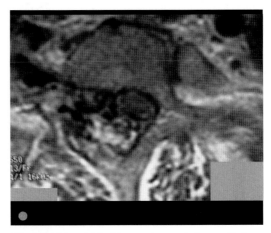

C1. Sagittal T1-weighted image demonstrates multiple flow voids in the intradural as well as in the extradural space.

C2. Axial T1-weighted image demonstrates multiple flow voids in the intradural as well as in the extradural space.

ARACHNOID CYST

Arachnoid cyst may be extradural or intradural extramedullary in location. Combined intradural/extradural location is also seen. The majority of the arachnoid cysts occur in the thoracic spine. They are defined as diverticula of the sub-arachnoid space, usually with a communication through a relatively narrow neck. Focal widening of the spinal canal may be seen with displacement of the spinal cord.

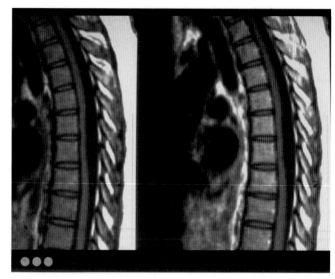

A. Sagittal T1-weighted images demonstrate a CSF signal intensity lesion at the dorsal aspect of the spinal canal with compression of the spinal cord.

RELATED PATTERNS

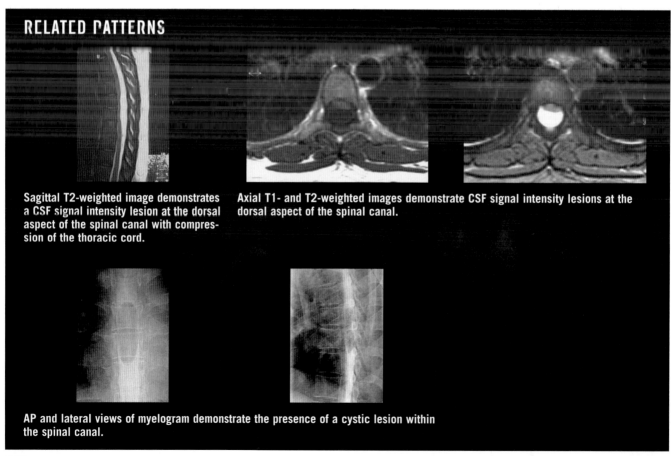

Sagittal T2-weighted image demonstrates a CSF signal intensity lesion at the dorsal aspect of the spinal canal with compression of the thoracic cord.

Axial T1- and T2-weighted images demonstrate CSF signal intensity lesions at the dorsal aspect of the spinal canal.

AP and lateral views of myelogram demonstrate the presence of a cystic lesion within the spinal canal.

ARACHNOID CYST (CASE TWO)

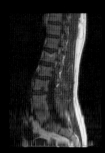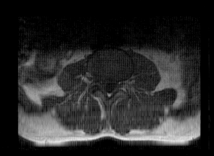

Sagittal and axial T1-weighted images show an intradural cystic lesion in the distal thecal sac with displacement of the nerve roots seen anteriorly.

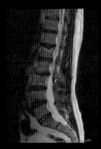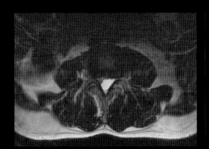

Sagittal and axial T2-weighted images show an intradural cystic lesion in the distal thecal sac with displacement of the nerve roots seen anteriorly.

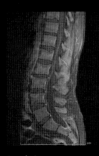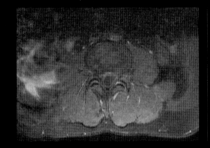

Sagittal and axial, post-contrast, fat-suppressed T1-weighted images show an intradural cystic lesion in the distal thecal sac with displacement of the nerve roots seen anteriorly. No enhancement of the cystic lesion is seen.

491

BRONCHOGENIC CYST

Bronchogenic cysts are rare benign congenital cysts that result from abnormal budding of the developing tracheo-bronchial tree. Bronchogenic cysts are lined by respiratory epithelium with bronchial glands, smooth muscle, and cartilage. Bronchogenic cysts are frequently seen in the mediastinum; they are rarely seen in the spine.

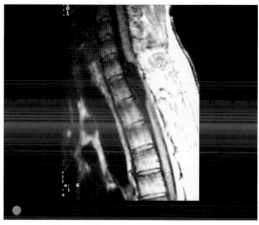

B. Sagittal T1 weighted image shows a cystic lesion anterior to the cord in the intradural location.

CYSTICERCOSIS

Although neurocysticercosis is a common parasitic disease, spinal cysticercosis is rare when compared to intracranial cysticercosis. Cysticercosis cysts probably gain access into the spinal canal by way of gravity. Intraventricular cysticercosis cysts can exit the foramen of Magendie or Luschka and migrate through the subarachnoid space into the spinal canal. Intramedullary cysticercosis cysts involving the spinal cord is probably due to hematogenous spread.

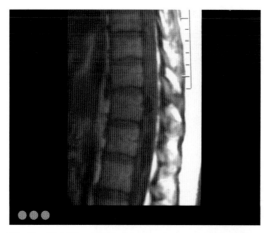

C1. Sagittal T1- weighted image demonstrates multiple intradural cysts in the spinal canal, compressing on the thoracic cord.

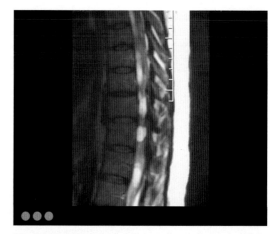

C2. Sagittal T2-weighted image demonstrates multiple intradural cysts in the spinal canal, compressing on the thoracic cord.

EPIDERMOID CYST

Epidermoid cysts in the spine are rare and composed of a connective tissue capsule lined by stratified squamous epithelium. The cavity of an **Epidermoid cyst** is filled with white keratinized debris shed from the epithelial lining. Most

spinal **epidermoid cysts** involve the thoracic and lumbar spine. Most spinal **epidermoid cysts** are located intradurally and the majority are intramedullary in location. Even when they are extramedullary, they are often firmly attached to the cord or cauda equina. They can occur congenitally or as an acquired lesion, such as from prior lumbar puncture.

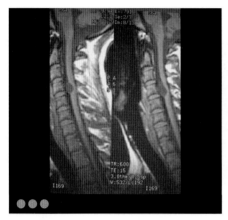

D1. Sagittal T1-weighted image shows an intradural, extramedullary cystic lesion compressing and displacing the cord posteriorly.

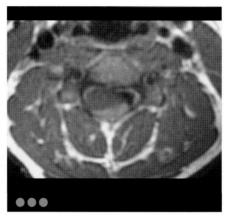

D2. Axial T1 weighted image shows an intradural, extramedullary cystic lesion compressing and displacing the cord posteriorly.

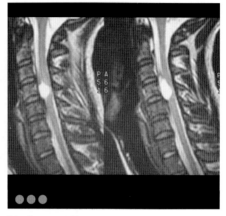

D3. Sagittal T2-weighted image shows an intradural, extramedullary cystic lesion compressing and displacing the cord posteriorly.

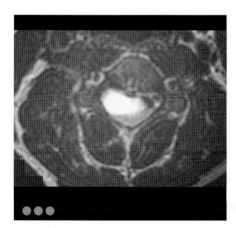

D4. Axial T2-weighted image shows an intradural, extramedullary cystic lesion compressing and displacing the cord posteriorly.

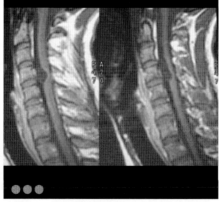

D5. Sagittal, post-contrast T1-weighted image shows an intradural, extramedullary cystic lesion compressing and displacing the cord posteriorly. No enhancement of the cystic mass is seen.

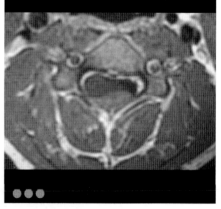

D6. Axial, post-contrast T1-weighted image shows an intradural, extramedullary cystic lesion compressing and displacing the cord posteriorly. No enhancement of the cystic mass is seen.

NEUROENTERIC CYST

Neuroenteric cysts are rare foregut duplication cysts. Foregut duplication cysts can be classified pathologically into three different types: (1) enteric duplications and cysts (lined by intestinal epithelium), (2) bronchogenic cysts (lined by respiratory epithelium), (3) **neuroenteric cysts** (associated with vertebral anomalies or have a connection with the nervous system). **Neuroenteric cysts** are commonly seen in the thoracic cavity, but they can also present as a cystic lesion in the spinal canal, especially in the lower cervical and upper thoracic region. According to Nabors' classification, it belongs to Group 3 of spinal meningeal cysts.

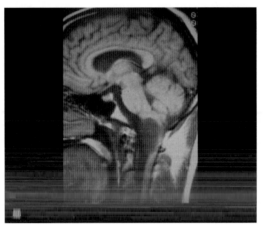

E1. Sagittal T1-weighted image shows a cystic lesion at the right anterior aspect of the spinal canal with marked compression of the cord.

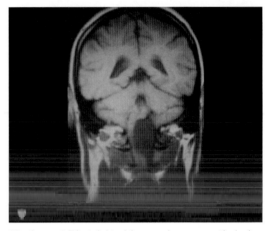

E2. Coronal T1-weighted image shows a cystic lesion at the right anterior aspect of the spinal canal with marked compression of the cord.

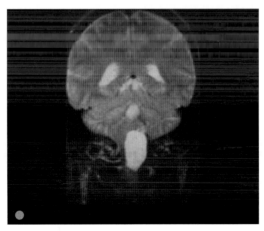

E3. Coronal T2-weighted image reveals a cystic lesion at the right anterior aspect of the spinal canal with marked compression of the cord.

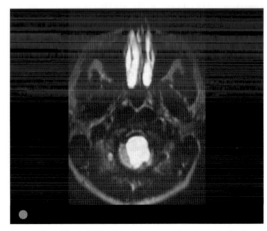

E4. Axial T2-weighted image reveals a cystic lesion at the right anterior aspect of the spinal canal with marked compression of the cord.

SUBDURAL FLUID COLLECTION

Subdural collection of cerebrospinal fluid (CSF) is produced when there is leakage of CSF through the dural defect created during lumbar puncture. This occurs only in neonates and children because this population has less well developed connective tissue in the subdural space to tamponade the defect. These collections usually resolve spontaneously over time.

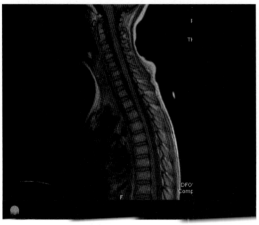

F1. Sagittal T1 weighted image of the thoracic spine shows increased subarachnoid space posterior to the cord.

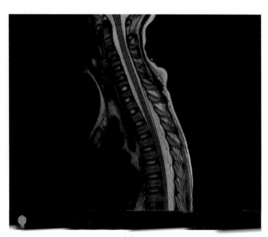

F2. Sagittal T2 weighted image demonstraton the presence of a subdural fluid collection caudal to C7 level.

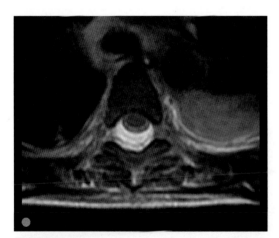

F3. Axial T2 weighted image shows a subdural fluid collection posterior to the cord.

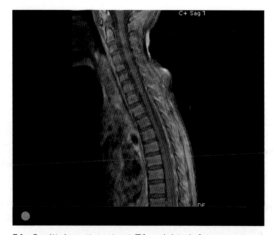

F4. Sagittal, post-contrast T1 weighted, fat-suppressed image shows no abnormal enhancement.

GUILLAIN-BARRE SYNDROME

Guillain-Barre syndrome is an autoimmune disorder that can affect anybody. Usually, the patient had preceding respiratory or gastrointestinal infection. Occasionally, surgery or vaccination will trigger the syndrome. In patients with Guillen-Barre syndrome, the immune system starts to destroy the myelin sheath that surrounds the axons of many peripheral nerves, or even the axons themselves.

Enhancement of the nerve roots along cauda equina can be seen in patients with Guillain-Barre syndrome.

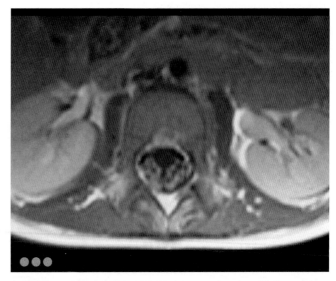

A. Axial, post-contrast T1-weighted image shows multiple nodular enhancements in the spinal canal due to enhancement of the thickened nerve roots

RELATED PATTERNS

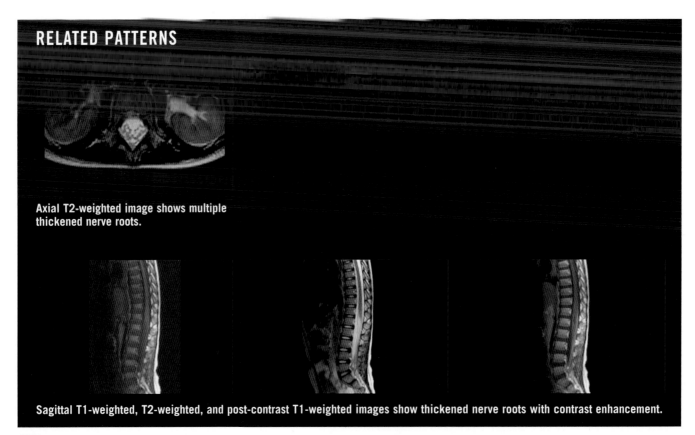

Axial T2-weighted image shows multiple thickened nerve roots.

Sagittal T1-weighted, T2-weighted, and post-contrast T1-weighted images show thickened nerve roots with contrast enhancement.

DIFFERENTIAL DIAGNOSIS

At a Glance:

- *Arachnoiditis (Due to Cysticercosis)*
- *HIV Arachnoiditis*
- *Metastatic Seeding from Intracranial Tumor*
- *Metastatic Disease (Metastatic Melanoma)*
- *Neurofibromatosis*
- *Sarcoidosis*
- *Tuberculosis*
- *CMV Polyradiculopathy* (not pictured)
- *Inflammatory Nerve Roots (Due to Compression)* (not pictured)
- *Lymphoma* (not pictured)

ARACHNOIDITIS (DUE TO CYSTICERCOSIS)

Arachnoiditis is a general term for arachnoidal inflammation associated with arachnoidal adhesions. The arachnoidal adhesion results in the adherence of the nerve roots, variable degree of obliteration of subarachnoid space, intradural cyst formation, and intramedullary cavity formation. Among the reported causes of **arachnoiditis** are infection, trauma, SAH, surgery, lumbar puncture, intraspinal neoplasm, tuberculosis, sarcoidosis, intrathecal injection, and idiopathic.

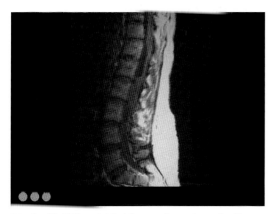

B1. Sagittal T1-weighted image shows irregular tissue in the distal thecal sac. A cystic lesion is seen anterior to the conus medullaris, displacing it posteriorly.

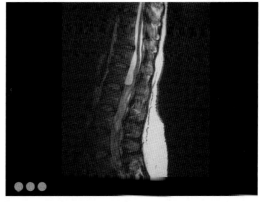

B2. Sagittal T2-weighted image shows irregular, heterogeneous tissue in the distal thecal sac. A cystic lesion is seen anterior to the conus medullaris, displacing it posteriorly.

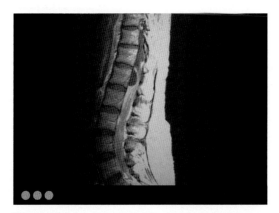

B3. Sagittal, post-contrast T1-weighted images demonstrate irregular, heterogeneously enhancing tissue in the distal thecal sac. A cystic lesion is seen anterior to the conus medullaris, displacing it posteriorly.

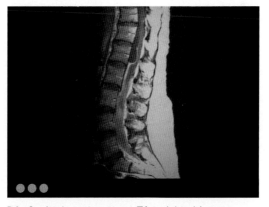

B4. Sagittal, post-contrast T1-weighted images demonstrate irregular, heterogeneously enhancing tissue in the distal thecal sac. A cystic lesion is seen anterior to the conus medullaris, displacing it posteriorly.

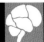

HIV ARACHNOIDITIS

Arachnoiditis is a broad term used to describe inflammation of the meninges and subarachnoid space in the spinal canal. A wide variety of etiologies exist, including infectious, inflammatory, and neoplastic processes. Infectious etiologies include bacterial, viral, fungal, and parasitic agents. Due to the increase in immunocompromised patients, there is an increase in the incidence of spinal infection as well as neoplasm.

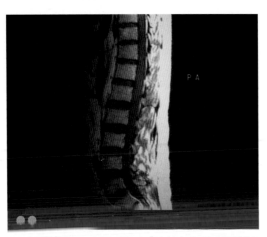

C1. Sagittal T1 weighted image shows abnormal signal in the distal thecal sac extending to the level of conus.

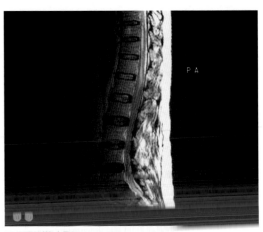

C2. Sagittal T2 weighted image shows heterogeneous, abnormal signal in the distal thecal sac extending to the level of conus.

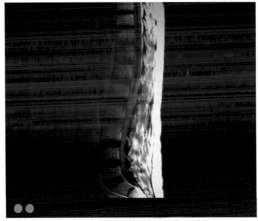

C3. Sagittal, post-contrast T1-weighted image shows abnormal enhancement in the distal thecal sac extending to the level of conus. In this case, the enhancement pattern is more diffuse, but enhancing nerve roots can be identified distally.

METASTATIC SEEDING FROM INTRACRANIAL TUMOR

Leptomeningeal metastases usually occur from either seeding of the CSF from CNS neoplasms or from hematogenous spread from systemic tumors. The lumbosacral region is involved in 75% of the cases. In the cervical and thoracic regions, involvement is usually posterior in location probably because the CSF flow dynamics involve flow away from the brain primarily dorsal to the cord. The usual sources of origin for metastatic seeding are PNET (medulloblastoma) (48%), glioblastomas multiforme (14%), ependymomas (12%), oligodendroglioma (12%), astrocytoma (7%), and retinoblastoma (5%).

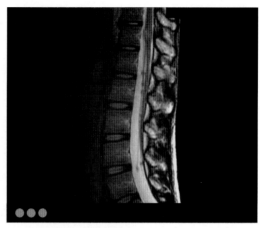

D1. Sagittal T2-weighted image shows small intradural lesions in contrast to the CSF.

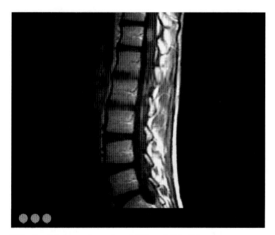

D2. Sagittal, post-contrast T1-weighted images demonstrate multiple enhancing, intradural, nodular lesions.

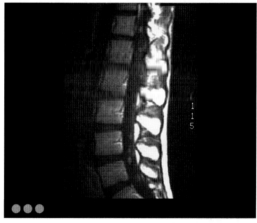

D3. Sagittal, post-contrast T1-weighted images demonstrate multiple enhancing, intradural, nodular lesions.

METASTATIC DISEASE (METASTATIC MELANOMA)

Leptomeningeal metastases usually occur from either seeding of the CSF from CNS neoplasms or from hematogenous spread from systemic tumors. The two most common systemic sources of **metastatic disease** are carcinomas of the breast and lung, followed by melanoma, lymphoma, leukemia, and carcinoma of the GI tract and GU tract, and head and neck region.

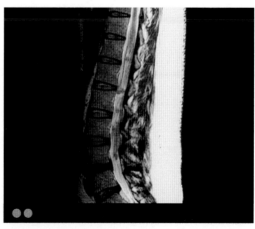

E1. Sagittal T2-weighted image shows multiple nodular lesions in the intradural space.

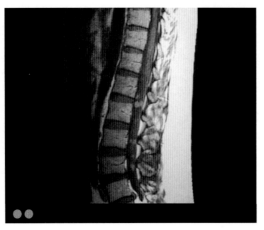

E2. Sagittal post-contrast T1-weighted image shows multiple enhancing nodular lesions within the thecal sac.

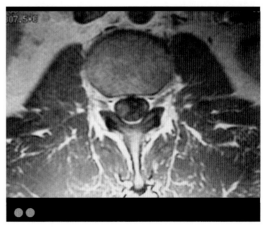

E3. Axial post-contrast T1-weighted image shows multiple enhancing nodular lesions within the thecal sac.

NEUROFIBROMATOSIS

Neurofibromatosis type 1 (NF1), the most common neuro-cutaneous syndrome, is estimated to occur in approximately one of every 3300 infants. Clinical diagnosis is made according to the diagnostic criteria established by the National Institutes of Health Consensus Development Conference. Manifestations of **neurofibromatosis** are diverse and can arise from almost any system in the body. In the spine, lesions that can be detected on MR imaging are dysplasia of the dura, including lateral meningoceles and dural ectasia, and spinal tumors, most of which are nerve sheath tumors. The neurofibroma is the hallmark lesion of NF1 and develops from peripheral nerves. They can occur intradu-rally and extradurally.

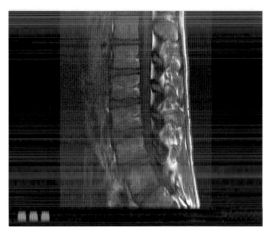

F1. Sagittal T1-weighted image shows thickened nerve roots in the lumbar region, seen within the thecal sac as well as in the neuroforamen.

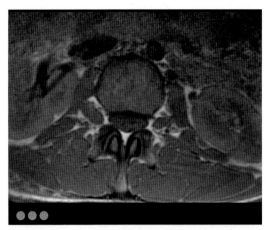

F2. Axial T1-weighted image shows thickened nerve roots in the lumbar region, seen within the thecal sac as well as in the neuroforamen.

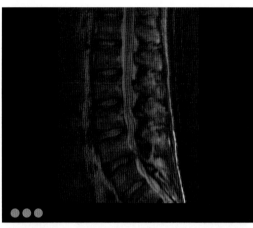

F3. Sagittal T2-weighted image shows thickened nerve roots in the lumbar region.

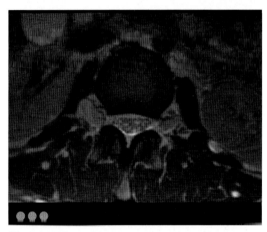

F4. Axial T2-weighted image shows thickened nerve roots in the lumbar region. Neurofibromas are seen in both neural foramina.

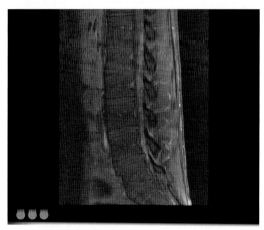

F5. Sagittal post-contrast T1-weighted image demonstrates multinodular enhancement of the nerve roots, consistent with multiple neurofibromas.

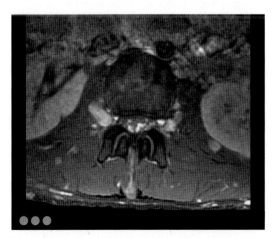

F6. Axial post-contrast T1-weighted image demonstrates multinodular enhancement of the nerve roots, consistent with multiple neurofibromas. Bilateral foraminal neurofibromas are seen.

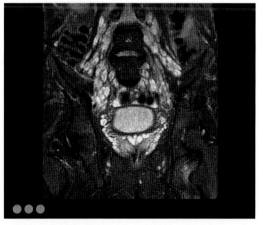

F7. Coronal T2-weighted fat-suppressed image shows multiple neurofibromas involving the lumbosacral plexus.

SARCOIDOSIS

Sarcoidosis is a systemic granulomatous disease of unknown etiology that has been shown to affect nearly every organ system. Typical intradural manifestations include leptomeningeal enhancement, enhancing spinal cord mass, nerve root "clumping," and enhancing nerve root.

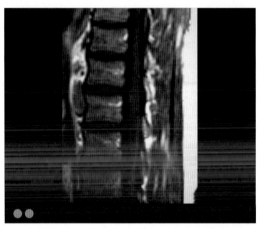

G1. Sagittal T1 weighted image shows thickening of the nerve roots.

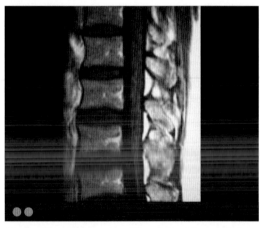

G2. Sagittal, post-contrast T1 weighted image shows nodular enhancement of the thickened nerve roots.

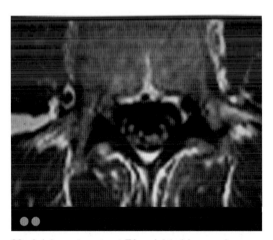

G3. Axial, post-contrast T1-weighted image shows multiple nodular enhancing lesions along the nerve roots.

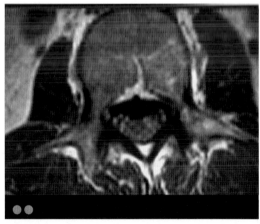

G4. Axial, post-contrast T1-weighted image shows multiple nodular enhancing lesions along the nerve roots.

TUBERCULOSIS

Tuberculosis of the spine is the most common form of skeletal tuberculosis. The common presentations of the spinal tuberculosis are tubercular spondylitis, followed by intradural tuberculosis or tubercular arachnoiditis and tubercular myelitis in decreasing frequency. Involvement of the spinal cord in the absence of skeletal lesion is uncommon. Isolated intradural tuberculosis is predominantly seen in thoracic spine and presents as gradually progressive weakness in the lower limbs, sometimes associated with urinary symptoms. Spinal tubercular arachnoiditis is rare. It may occur primarily or secondary to intracranial or vertebral infection. Unlike other types of arachnoiditis, it frequently involves the spinal cord and the nerve roots in addition to the meninges.

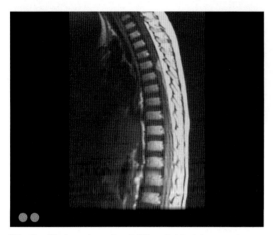

H1. Sagittal post-contrast T1-weighted image shows nodular enhancing lesion at the dorsal aspect of the spinal canal as well as enhancement of the thickened nerve roots.

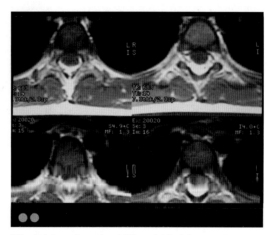

H2. Axial post-contrast T1-weighted image shows nodular enhancing lesion at the dorsal aspect of the spinal canal as well as enhancement of the thickened nerve roots.

MENINGIOMA

Meningiomas comprise 25–45% of intraspinal tumors. Meningiomas typically present between the ages of 40 and 60 years and demonstrate an 80% female preponderance. Approximately 80% of the spinal meningiomas occur in the thoracic region, 15% are cervical, 3% are lumbar, and 2% are located at foramen magnum. Thoracic meningiomas tend to be located posterior or lateral to the cord whereas cervical meningiomas tend to be located anterior to the cord. Typically, meningiomas are broad, dura-based mass with isointensity on both T1- and T2- weighted images. Homogeneous contrast enhancement is seen.

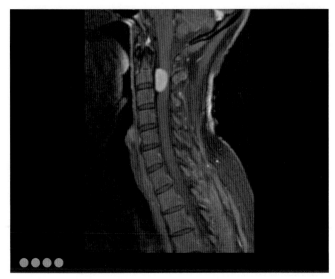

A. Sagittal, post-contrast T1 weighted and fat-suppressed image shows an enhancing intradural, extramedullary mass at C1-C2 level with broad-based attachment to the dura anteriorly.

RELATED PATTERNS

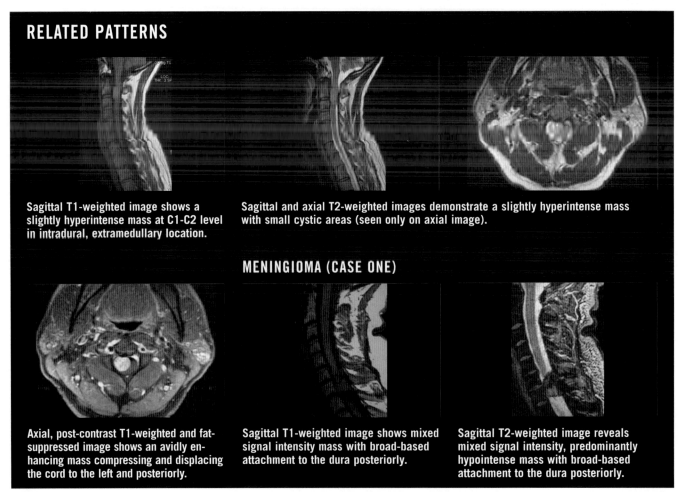

Sagittal T1-weighted image shows a slightly hyperintense mass at C1-C2 level in intradural, extramedullary location.

Sagittal and axial T2-weighted images demonstrate a slightly hyperintense mass with small cystic areas (seen only on axial image).

MENINGIOMA (CASE ONE)

Axial, post-contrast T1-weighted and fat-suppressed image shows an avidly enhancing mass compressing and displacing the cord to the left and posteriorly.

Sagittal T1-weighted image shows mixed signal intensity mass with broad-based attachment to the dura posteriorly.

Sagittal T2-weighted image reveals mixed signal intensity, predominantly hypointense mass with broad-based attachment to the dura posteriorly.

MENINGIOMA (CASE TWO) (continued)

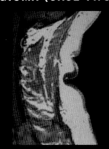 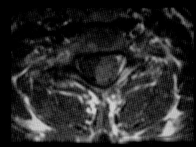 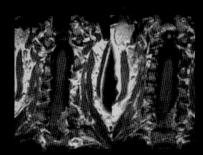

Sagittal, axial, and coronal, post-contrast T1 weighted images demonstrate an enhancing mass with broad-based attachment to the dura posteriorly and on the left side. There is compression and displacement of the cord to the right side seen.

MENINGIOMA (CASE THREE)

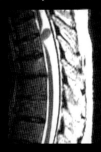 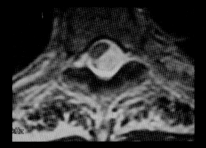

Sagittal and axial T2-weighted images show a slightly hyperintense mass in the intradural, extramedullary location displacing the cord anteriorly and to the right side.

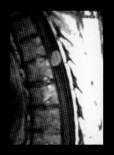 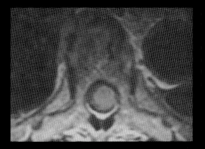

Sagittal and axial, post-contrast T1-weighted images show an intensely enhancing mass in the intradural, extramedullary location displacing the cord anteriorly and to the right side.

RELATED PATTERNS (continued)

MENINGIOMA (CASE FOUR)

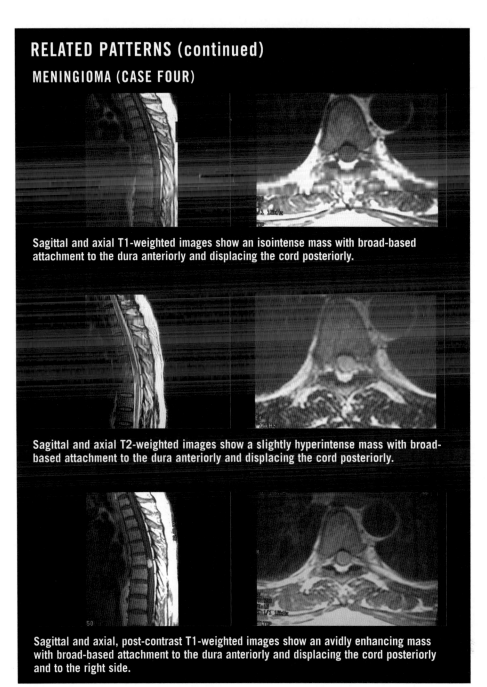

Sagittal and axial T1-weighted images show an isointense mass with broad-based attachment to the dura anteriorly and displacing the cord posteriorly.

Sagittal and axial T2-weighted images show a slightly hyperintense mass with broad-based attachment to the dura anteriorly and displacing the cord posteriorly.

Sagittal and axial, post-contrast T1-weighted images show an avidly enhancing mass with broad-based attachment to the dura anteriorly and displacing the cord posteriorly and to the right side.

DIFFERENTIAL DIAGNOSIS

At a Glance:

- *Carney's Complex*
- *Filum Terminale Ependymoma*
- *Schistosomiasis*
- *Schwannoma*

CARNEY'S COMPLEX

Patients with **Carney complex** exhibit spotty pigmentation of the skin, cardiac myxomas, and extracardiac myxomas (in breast, testis, thyroid, brain, or adrenal gland). Non-myxomatous tumors, such as pituitary adenoma, psammomatous melanotic schwannoma, and Sertoli cell tumors of the testis, also may be observed. Patients can exhibit a spectrum of endocrine overactivity, including Cushing syndrome and thyroid and pituitary dysfunction.

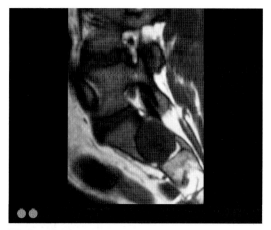

B1. Sagittal T1-weighted image shows a hypointense mass at the left S1 neural foramen with enlargement of the foramen seen.

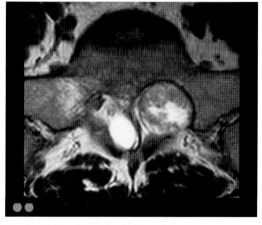

B2. Axial T2-weighted image reveals a heterogeneous, predominantly hyperintense mass at the left S1 neural foramen.

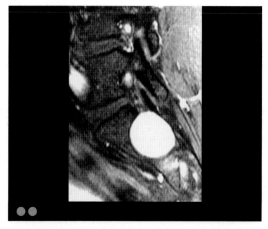

B3. Sagittal, post-contrast T1-weighted image demonstrates a homogeneously enhancing mass.

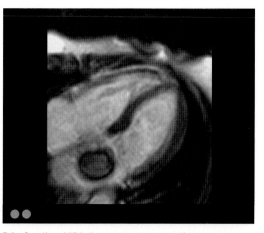

B4. Cardiac MRI demonstrates a cardiac myxoma.

FILUM TERMINALE EPENDYMOMA

Scloff and associates reported finding intradural extramedullary ependymomas (3.4%) and astrocytomas (2.7%) among 301 intraspinal gliomas. These were felt to be secondary to the presence of heterotopic glial tissue. **Filum terminale ependymomas** are actually exophytic growth of intramedullary (filum) ependymomas.

FILUM TERMINALE EPENDYMOMA (CASE ONE)

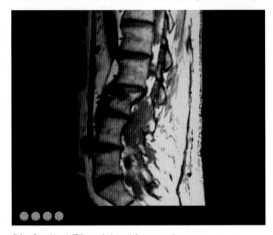

C1. Sagittal T1-weighted image shows a heterogeneous, predominantly hypointense mass in the lower lumbar spinal canal.

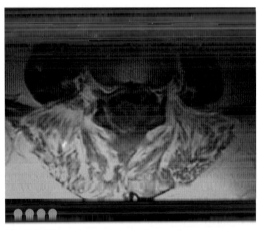

C2. Axial T1-weighted image shows a heterogeneous, predominantly hypointense mass in the lower lumbar spinal canal.

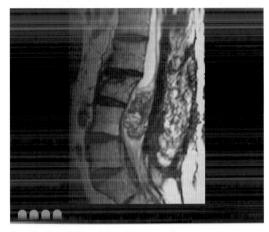

C3. Sagittal T2-weighted image shows a heterogeneous, mixed iso- to hyperintense mass at L3-L4 level.

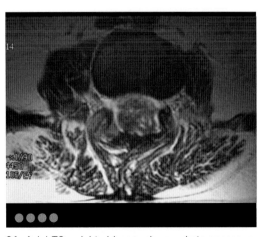

C4. Axial T2-weighted image shows a heterogeneous, mixed iso- to hyperintense mass at L3-L4 level.

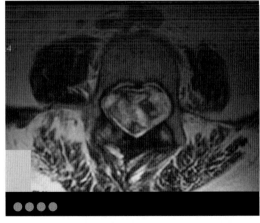

C5. Axial T2-weighted image shows a heterogeneous, mixed iso- to hyperintense mass at L3-L4 level.

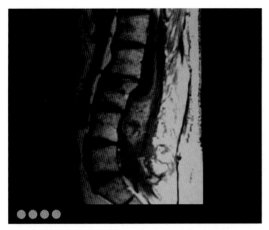

C6. Sagittal post-contrast T1-weighted image demonstrates a heterogeneously enhancing mass.

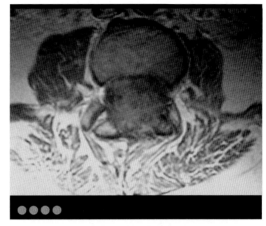

C7. Axial post-contrast T1-weighted image demonstrates a heterogeneously enhancing mass.

FILUM TERMINALE EPENDYMOMA (CASE TWO)

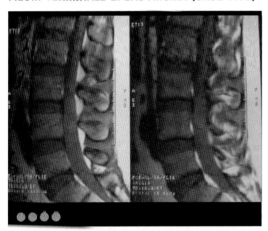

D1. Sagittal T1-weighted images show a slightly hyperintense mass at L3-L4 level. Note the slightly hyperintense CSF distal to the mass is due to lack of pulsation secondary to obstruction by the mass.

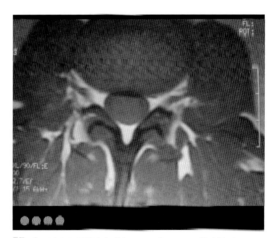

D2. Axial T1 weighted image shows a slightly hyperintense mass intradurally.

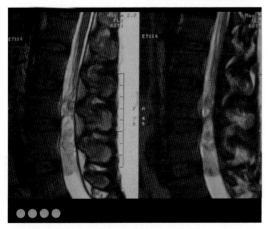

D3. Sagittal T2-weighted image shows a heterogeneously hyperintense mass.

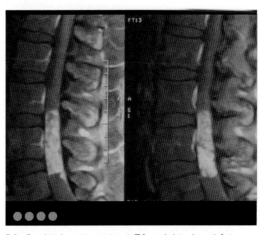

D4. Sagittal post-contrast T1-weighted and fat-suppressed image demonstrates avid enhancement of the mass.

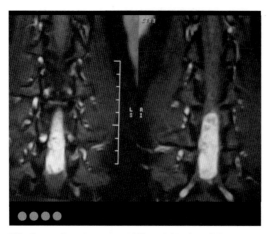

D5. Coronal post-contrast T1-weighted and fat-suppressed image demonstrates avid enhancement of the mass.

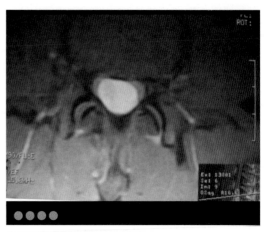

D6. Axial post-contrast T1-weighted and fat-suppressed image demonstrates avid enhancement of the mass.

SCHISTOSOMIASIS

Human **schistosomiasis** is principally caused by one of the 6 species of parasitic worms. Schistosome eggs are usually excreted from the infected individuals into the environment, but approximately 50% of the eggs can embolize to other parts of the body, leading to a host immune reaction and granuloma formation. Granulomas may be seen in the intradural space of the spinal canal.

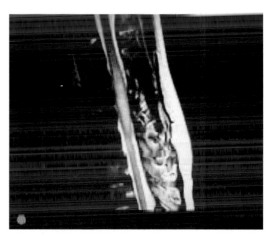

E1. Sagittal T2-weighted image shows abnormal hyperintensity within the cord.

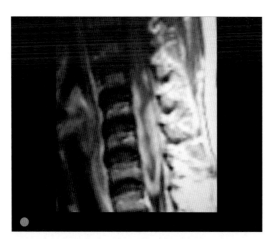

E2. Sagittal post-contrast T1-weighted image demonstrates intradural, extramedullary enhancing lesions surrounding the cord.

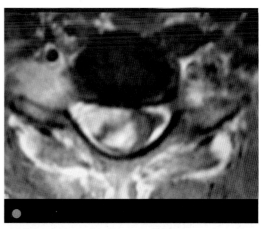

E3. Axial, post-contrast T1 weighted image shows an enhancing mass in the intradural, extramedullary space as well as epidural, paraspinal region on the right side with compression of the cord.

SCHWANNOMA

Nerve sheath tumors consist of **schwannomas** and neurofibromas. Nerve sheath tumors have been reported to comprise 15–30% of primary spinal tumors. Nerve sheath tumors usually involve the dorsal nerve roots and may be located anywhere in the spine. The most common site is the thoracic spine (43%), followed by lumbar spine (34%). Approximately 70% are intradural, extramedullary, about 15% each are extradural and combined intradural/extradural, and less than 1% intramedullary in location. They are usually hypo to isointense to cord on T1-weighted images and hyperintense on T2-weighted images. Homogeneous, intense contrast enhancement is seen. Sometimes, **schwannomas** can be cystic and exhibit ring-like contrast enhancement.

CERVICAL SCHWANNOMA

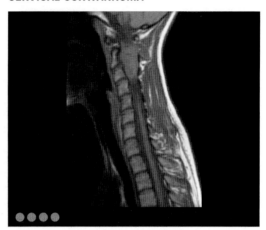

F1. Sagittal T1-weighted image shows a large isointense mass at C2-C3 level.

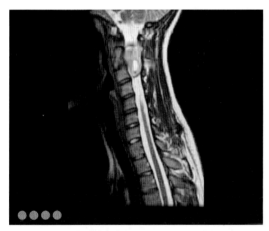

F2. Sagittal T2-weighted image reveals a slightly hyperintense mass with cystic areas at C2-C3 level with widening of the right neuroforamen.

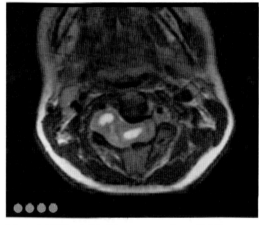

F3. Axial T2-weighted image reveals a slightly hyperintense mass with cystic areas at C2-C3 level with widening of the right neuroforamen.

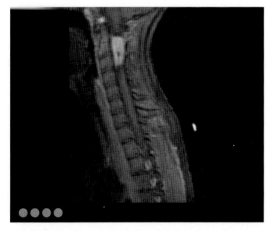

F4. Sagittal post-contrast T1-weighted, fat-suppressed image demonstrates an avidly enhancing mass with cystic changes.

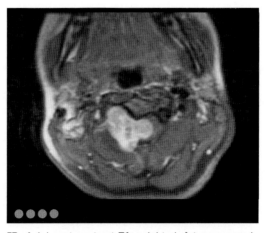

F5. Axial post-contrast T1-weighted, fat-suppressed image demonstrates an avidly enhancing mass with cystic changes.

511

THORACIC SCHWANNOMA

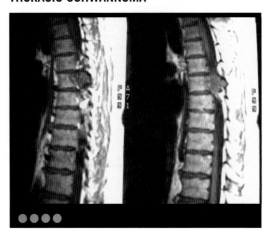

G1. Sagittal T1-weighted images show an isointense, extramedullary mass with intradural and extradural components extending across a thoracic neuroforamen on the left side with compression of the thoracic cord seen.

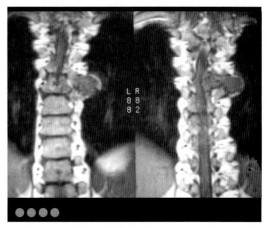

G2. Coronal T1-weighted images show an isointense, extramedullary mass with intradural and extradural components extending across a thoracic neuroforamen on the left side with compression of the thoracic cord seen.

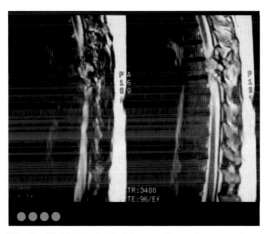

G3. Sagittal T2-weighted image shows the mass to be hyperintense.

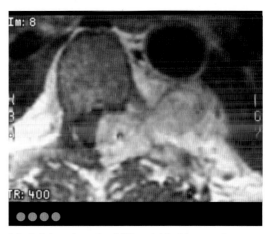

G4. Axial post-contrast T1-weighted image shows an enhancing, lobulated mass extending across the neuroforamen on the left side with extramedullary, intradural, and extradural components.

THORACOLUMBAR SCHWANNOMA

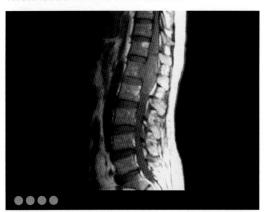

H1. Sagittal T1-weighted image demonstrates an isointense, lobulated mass extending from T12 to L2 in the intradural, extramedullary location. Note the scalloping of the posterior margin of L1 vertebral body.

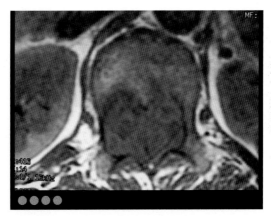

H2. Axial T1-weighted image demonstrates an isointense, lobulated mass extending from T12 to L2 in the intradural, extramedullary location. Note the scalloping of the posterior margin of L1 vertebral body.

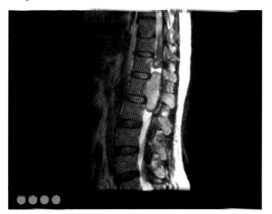

H3. Sagittal T2-weighted image shows the lobulated mass to be predominantly hyperintense with a hypointense peripheral rim seen.

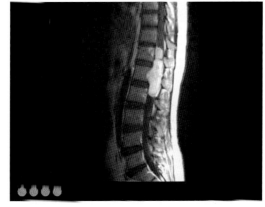

H4. Sagittal post-contrast T1-weighted image demonstrates an enhancing, lobulated mass in the intradural, extramedullary location with scalloping of the vertebral body of L1 and remodeling of the spinal canal.

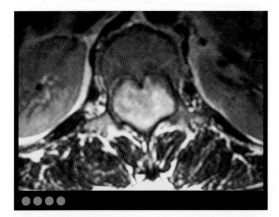

H5. Axial post-contrast T1-weighted image demonstrates an enhancing, lobulated mass in the intradural, extramedullary location with scalloping of the vertebral body of L1 and remodeling of the spinal canal.

CYSTIC SCHWANNOMA

Sometimes, schwannomas can be cystic and exhibit ring-like contrast enhancement. When a cystic lesion involving the spine is seen, schwannoma should be considered in the differential diagnosis.

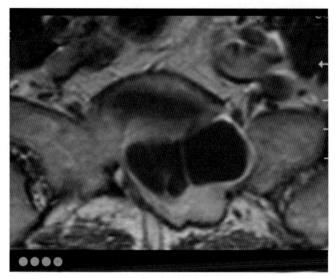

A Axial, post contrast T1 weighted image shows a large cystic mass with enhancing rims bilaterally and a solid component located posteriorly in the sacral region.

RELATED PATTERNS

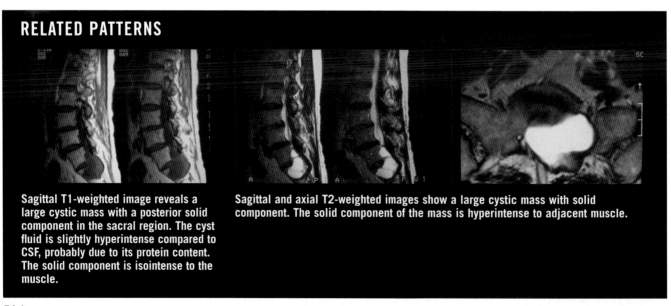

Sagittal T1-weighted image reveals a large cystic mass with a posterior solid component in the sacral region. The cyst fluid is slightly hyperintense compared to CSF, probably due to its protein content. The solid component is isointense to the muscle.

Sagittal and axial T2-weighted images show a large cystic mass with solid component. The solid component of the mass is hyperintense to adjacent muscle.

DIFFERENTIAL DIAGNOSIS

At a Glance:

- *Cysticercosis*
- *Ependymoma*
- *Echinococcus* (not pictured)
- *Metastasis* (not pictured)

CYSTICERCOSIS

Spinal cysticercosis is rare and consists of 1% of all cases of neurocysticercosis. Spinal cysticercosis can be intradural, extramedullary or intramedullary in location. Intradural, extramedullary cysticercosis can occur secondary to intracranial disease or through retrograde flow of the larvae within venous blood in the vertebral plexus. However, it is very rare to see intradural, extramedullary cysticercosis without intracranial disease. MRI with contrast is the imaging modality of choice in the evaluation of spinal cysticercosis.

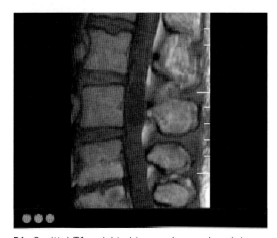

B1. Sagittal T1-weighted image shows a hypointense cystic lesion in the lumbar region.

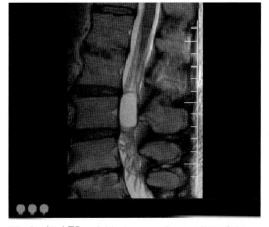

B2. Sagittal T2-weighted image shows a hyperintense cystic lesion in the lumbar region.

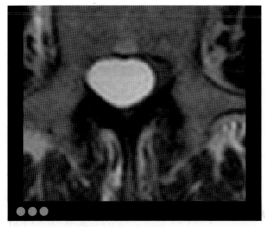

B3. Axial T2-weighted image shows a hyperintense cystic lesion in the lumbar region.

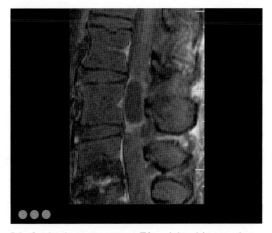

B4. Sagittal, post-contrast T1-weighted image shows a ring-like enhancing cystic lesion in the lumbar region.

EPENDYMOMA

Ependymomas are glial tumors that arise from ependymal cells lining the ventricular wall within the central nervous system. The World Health Organization (WHO) classification scheme for these tumors includes 4 categories: (1) ependymoma (with cellular, papillary, and clear cell variants), (2) anaplastic ependymoma, (3) myxopapillary ependymoma, and (4) subependymoma. Intracranial ependymomas present as intraventricular or intraparenchymal masses, while spinal ependymomas present as intramedullary masses arising from the central canal or exophytic masses arising from the conus medullaris, cauda equine and filum terminale. The majority (60%) of the intracranial ependymomas occur infratentorially and arise from the roof of the fourth ventricle in children, whereas supratentorial ependymomas are seen predominantly in adolescents and adults. Interestingly, spinal ependymomas are usually seen in adults as well.

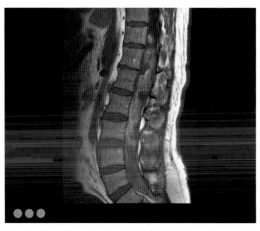

C1. Sagittal T1-weighted image shows a heterogeneous mass with multiple cystic areas. Widening of the bony spinal canal with scalloping of the posterior vertebral margin of L1 and L2 is seen.

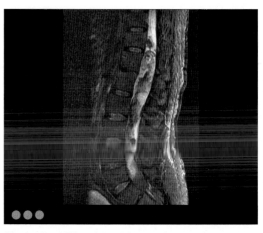

C2. Sagittal T2-weighted image shows a heterogeneous mass with multiple cystic areas.

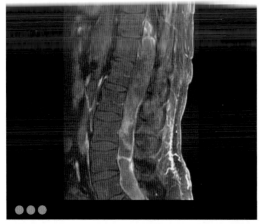

C3. Sagittal, post-contrast, fat-suppressed T1-weighted image shows a heterogeneous mass with multiple cystic areas.

EPIDERMOID

Approximately 60% of epidermoids are extramedullary in location. Epidermoids are usually isointense to CSF on both T1- and T2-weighted images. Epidermoid in the lumbar spine may be secondary to previous lumbar puncture. It is postulated that epidermal cells may be implanted into the spinal canal during the puncture if a needle without stilette is used and epidermoid can develop years later following the lumbar puncture.

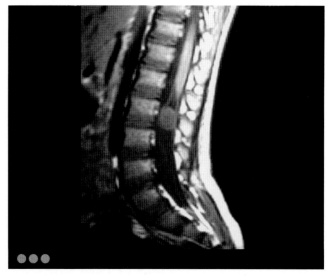

A. Sagittal T1-weighted image shows an intradural, extramedullary mass in the lumbar thecal sac. The mass is hypointense to cord and hyperintense to CSF.

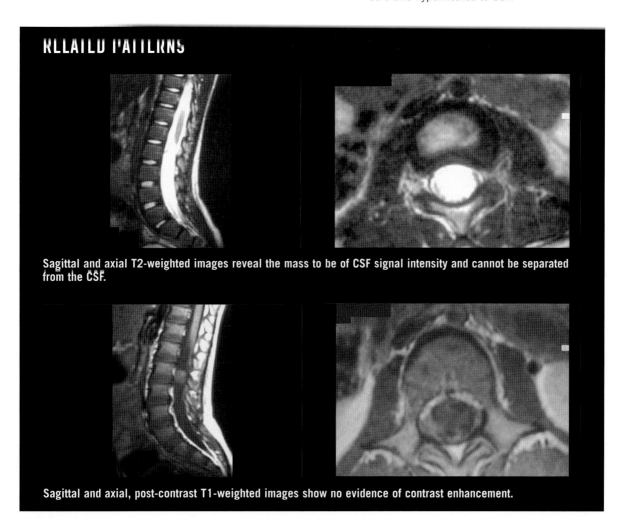

RELATED PATTERNS

Sagittal and axial T2-weighted images reveal the mass to be of CSF signal intensity and cannot be separated from the CSF.

Sagittal and axial, post-contrast T1-weighted images show no evidence of contrast enhancement.

517

LIPOMA

Spinal subpial lipoma is a rare entity and comprises only 0.9% of spinal cord tumors and 4% of spinal lipomas. It arises from premature dysjunction of the cutaneous ecto-derm during neural tube formation. Intradural lipomas can be intradural, subpial or juxtamedullary in location. They are seen in young adults in second and third decades of life with no sex predilection. Upper thoracic and cervical spine is affected most frequently.

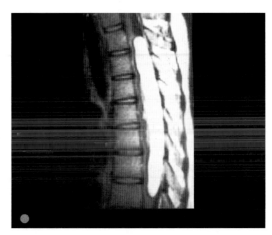

B. Sagittal T1-weighted image shows a large hyper-intense mass over the dorsal aspect of the spinal cord

SEQUESTERED INTRADURAL DISC

Intradural disc herniations frequently develop in patients with a history of chronic back pain as in our patient. The exact mechanism of intradural disc is not well understood. Adhesions are thought to be an important factor in the development of intradural disc. Lumbar intradural disc rupture must be considered in the differential diagnosis of mass lesions causing nerve root or cauda equina syn-dromes. The majority of them occurred at the L4-L5 levels and only occasionally seen at L5-S1. Peripheral enhance-ment around the non-enhancing free disc fragment is characteristically seen on contrast-enhanced MRI. A her-niated disc fragment will rarely be enhanced centrally, which is attributed to vascular granulation tissue infiltrating the disc fragment.

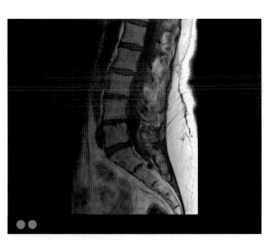

C1. Sagittal T1-weighted image shows an irregular, isointense mass intradurally with a left paracentral disc protrusion.

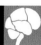

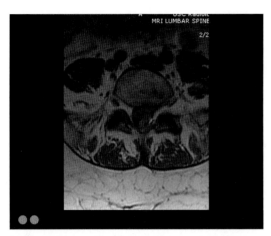

C2. Axial T1-weighted image shows an irregular, isointense mass intradurally with a left paracentral disc protrusion.

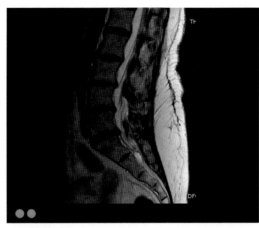

C3. Sagittal T2-weighted image shows an irregular, hypointense mass intradurally with a left paracentral disc protrusion.

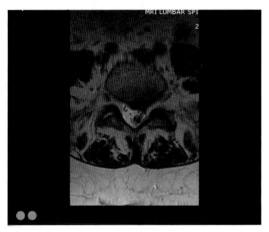

04. Axial T2 weighted image shows an irregular hypointense mass intradurally with a left paracentral disc protrusion.

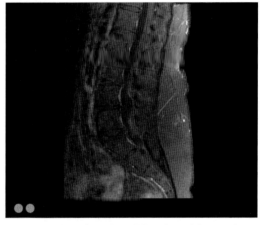

C5. Sagittal, post-contrast T1-weighted image shows a peripherally enhancing mass intradurally with a left paracentral disc protrusion.

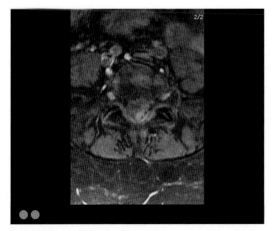

C6. Axial, post-contrast T1-weighted image shows a peripherally enhancing mass intradurally with a left paracentral disc protrusion.

Chapter 12

Intramedullary Lesions

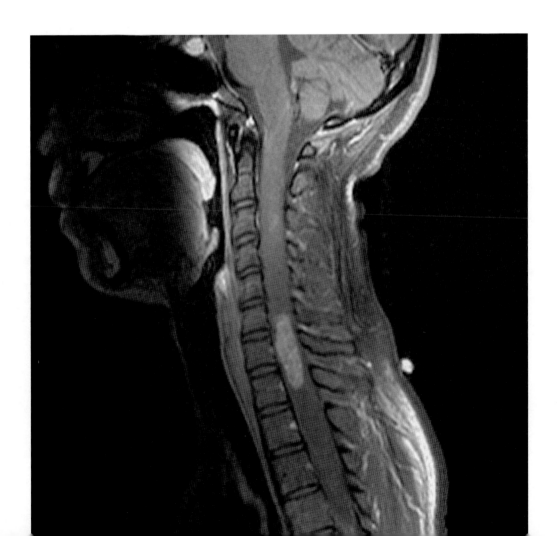

EPENDYMOMA

Ependymoma is the second most common spinal glioma of childhood and overall the most common spinal glioma. In a large series of 273 spinal intramedullary gliomas, Slooff and associates found 169 or 61.9% to represent ependymomas of the spinal cord and filum terminale. The vascular myxopapillary ependymoma is the predominant variant found in the regions of conus medullaris and filum terminale (95%). However, the epithelial, cellular, and papillary types are also seen in these sites. Ependymomas are an occasional source of subarachnoid hemorrhage. On MRI, ependymomas show focal enlargement of the cord or filum and are typically hypointense or isointense on T1-weighted images and hyperintense on T2-weighted images. Hemorrhage may be seen with a peripheral ring of hemosiderin and mixed signal intensity of various blood byproducts within the mass. Marked contrast enhancement is seen. Associated cystic changes or syringohydromyelia is common (50%).

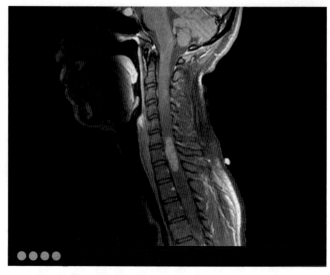

A. Sagittal, post-contrast T1-weighted image shows an intramedullary, enhancing mass extending from C6 through T1.

RELATED PATTERNS

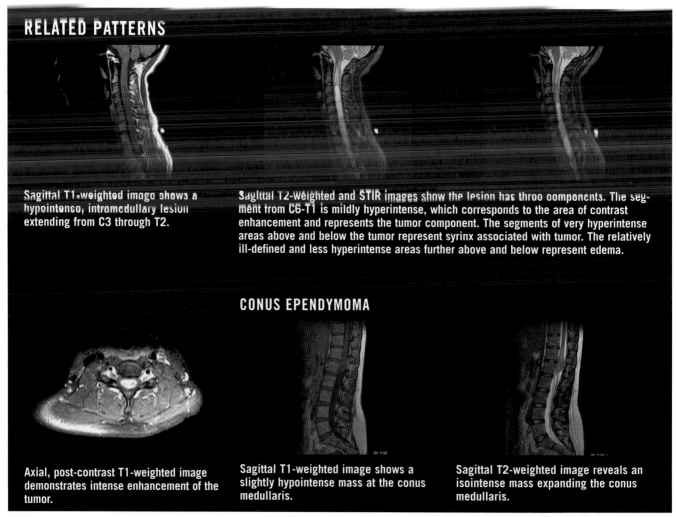

Sagittal T1-weighted image shows a hypointense, intramedullary lesion extending from C3 through T2.

Sagittal T2-weighted and STIR images show the lesion has three components. The segment from C6-T1 is mildly hyperintense, which corresponds to the area of contrast enhancement and represents the tumor component. The segments of very hyperintense areas above and below the tumor represent syrinx associated with tumor. The relatively ill-defined and less hyperintense areas further above and below represent edema.

CONUS EPENDYMOMA

Axial, post-contrast T1-weighted image demonstrates intense enhancement of the tumor.

Sagittal T1-weighted image shows a slightly hypointense mass at the conus medullaris.

Sagittal T2-weighted image reveals an isointense mass expanding the conus medullaris.

CONUS EPENDYMOMA (continued)

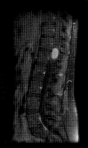
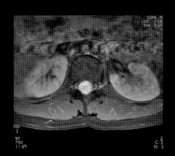

Sagittal and axial, post-contrast T1-weighted, fat-suppressed images demonstrate an intensely enhancing mass at conus medullaris.

THORACIC EPENDYMOMA

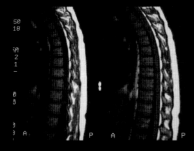
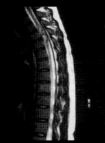

Sagittal T1-weighted image shows slight expansion of the cord at T3-T4 level.

Sagittal T2-weighted image reveals a hyperintense lesion with adjacent hypointensity, probably due to hemorrhage.

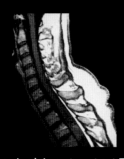
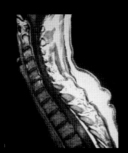
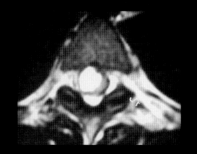

Sagittal and axial, post-contrast T1-weighted images demonstrate an enhancing mass at T3-T4 level.

DIFFERENTIAL DIAGNOSIS

At a Glance:

- *Astrocytoma*
- *Cavernous Hemangioma*
- *Cysticercosis*
- *Hemangioblastoma*
- *Metastasis*
- *Multiple Sclerosis*
- *Radiation Myelitis*
- *Sarcoid*
- *Tuberculosis*
- *Acute Disseminated Encephalomyelitis* (not pictured)
- *Ganglioglioma* (not pictured)
- *Oligodendroglioma* (not pictured)
- *Subacute Necrotizing Myelopathy* (not pictured)

ASTROCYTOMA

Astrocytomas account for approximately 25–30% of intramedullary gliomas overall but account for 50–60% of these tumors in the pediatric group. Spinal **astrocytomas** are more common in adults. Over 80% of spinal **astrocytomas** are located in the cervical and upper thoracic spine. Long segments of cord may be involved. MRI shows cord expansion with inhomogeneous enhancement that is less intense than ependymoma.

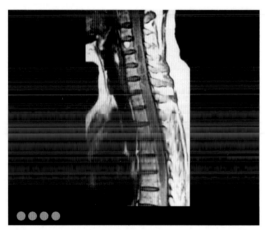

B1. Sagittal T1 weighted image shows expansion of the cervical and upper thoracic cord with multiseptated cystic areas seen within the cord.

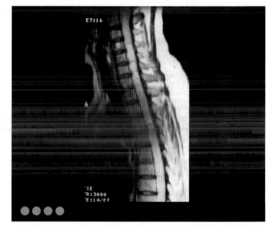

B2. Sagittal T2-weighted image reveals expansion of the cord with diffuse hyperintensity.

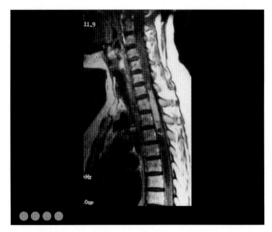

B3. Sagittal, post-contrast T1-weighted image demonstrates an enhancing mass within the cord extending from C7 through T3 with cystic cavity (syrinx) above and below the enhancing mass.

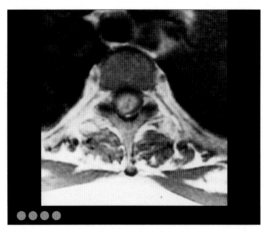

B4. Axial, post-contrast T1-weighted image demonstrates an enhancing mass within the cord extending from C7 through T3 with cystic cavity (syrinx) above and below the enhancing mass.

CAVERNOUS HEMANGIOMA

Intramedullary cavernous angioma of spinal cord is very rare. They are seen slightly more frequently in females. The size of cavernous angiomas may vary from few millimeters to several centimeters. These lesions may evolve over time and increase their size slowly due to recurrent chronic hemorrhage. Slowly, progressive course of the hemangioma may be due to local pressure effects on the adjoining spinal cord and or repeated episodes of bleeding. Acute symptoms are probably caused by relatively large, acute hemorrhages. Clinical onset of symptoms is in the 3rd to 6th decade of life with progressive paraparesis, sensory loss, frequently associated pain. Some lesions are found incidentally on MRI without any clinical symptoms.

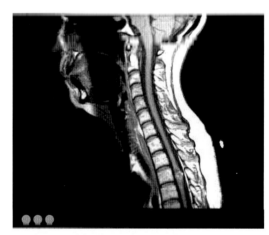

C1. Sagittal T1-weighted image shows a heterogeneous mass with predominant hyperintensity.

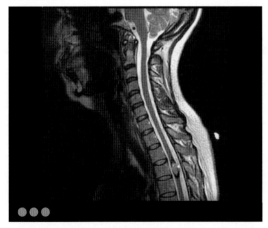

C2. Sagittal T2-weighted image shows a hyperintense lesion with a hypointense rim.

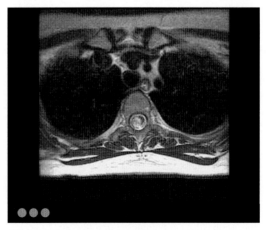

C3. Axial T2-weighted image shows a hyperintense lesion with a hypointense rim.

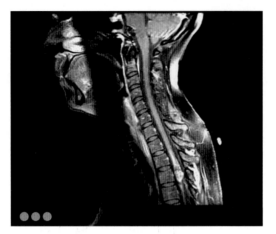

C4. Sagittal post-contrast T1-weighted image demonstrates an enhancing mass within the cervical cord.

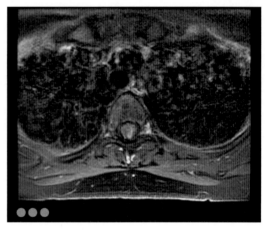

C5. Axial post-contrast T1-weighted image demonstrates an enhancing mass within the cervical cord.

CYSTICERCOSIS

Spinal involvement of cysticercosis occurs in only 0.7–5.85% of patients afflicted with the disease, and the low incidence of spinal involvement is believed to be related to the fact that the blood flow to the brain is approximately 100-fold greater than to the spine, since the disease is spread hematogenously.

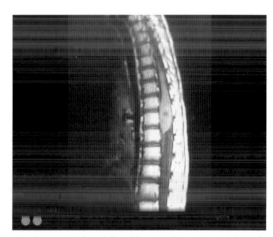

D1. Sagittal T1-weighted image shows expansion of the cord at the level of conus.

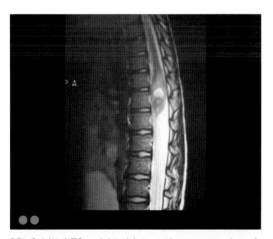

D2. Sagittal T2-weighted image shows expansion of the conus with a hypointense, ring-like lesion and adjacent edema.

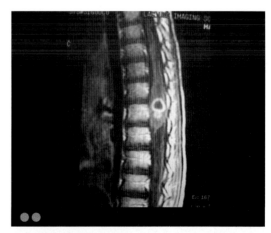

D3. Sagittal, post-contrast T1-weighted image reveals a ring-like enhancing lesion at the conus medullaris.

HEMANGIOBLASTOMA

Hemangioblastomas represent approximately 3% of spinal intramedullary tumors. Approximately 13% of the **hemangioblastomas** are within the spinal canal. Approximately 60% are intramedullary, 11% both intramedullary and intradural extramedullary, 21% intradural extramedullary, and 8% extradural in location. On MRI, mixed signal intensity is seen on T1-weighted images and high signal intensity is seen on T2-weighted images. Contrast-enhanced MRI shows enhancement of the entire solid tumor or tumor nodule of the cystic tumor.

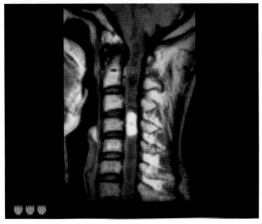

I1. Sagittal, post-contrast T1 weighted image shows an intensely enhancing mass within the cord at C4 level with septated cystic areas (syrinx) above and below the mass.

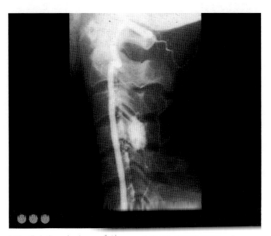

I2. A lateral view of the vertebral angiogram shows an intense vascular tumor stain early on.

METASTASIS

Intramedullary metastases are rare lesions and represent only 4–8.5% of central nervous system metastases. An important feature of intramedullary metastases is the rapid progression of neurological deficits which necessitates immediate treatment. Since primary neoplasms of the cord tend to have a gradual onset, metastatic disease must be suspected when a patient has an acute onset of clinical symptoms and MRI shows an intramedullary mass lesion.

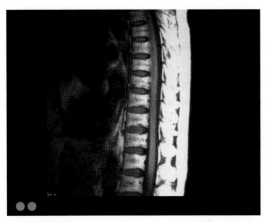

F1. Sagittal T1-weighted image shows slightly enlarged cord.

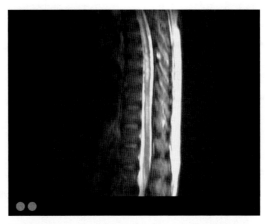

F2. Sagittal T2-weighted image reveals slightly enlarged cord with abnormal T2 hyperintensity seen extensively.

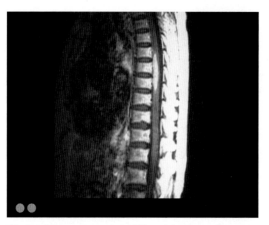

F3. Sagittal, post-contrast T1-weighted image shows intense contrast enhancement of the intramedullary metastatic disease.

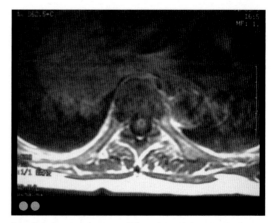

F4. Axial, post-contrast T1-weighted image shows intense contrast enhancement of the intramedullary metastatic disease.

MULTIPLE SCLEROSIS

Multiple sclerosis (MS) in the most common demyelinating disease of the spinal cord. Less than 10% of the patients have cord involvement only. CT is noncontributory. MRI shows plaques with the cord similar to those in the brain.

The typical MRI findings of spinal **MS** are vertically elongated regions of hyperintensity involving the lateral or posterior aspect of the cord on T2-weighted images. Sometimes contrast enhancement is seen. Expansion of the cord may be seen, mimicking an intramedullary neoplasm.

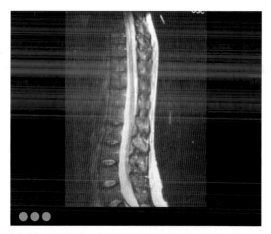

G1. Sagittal T2-weighted image shows abnormal hyperintensity within the cord.

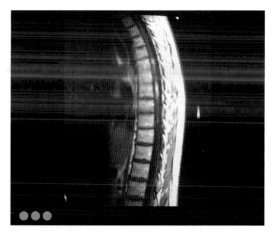

G2. Sagittal, post-contrast T1-weighted image demonstrates multiple areas of contrast enhancement within the cord.

RADIATION MYELITIS

Radiation myelitis is usually a self-limited disorder that produces symptoms starting a few weeks or months after radiation therapy. The involved area is within the treatment port. However, a progressive myelopathy may commence several months to years following therapy and progress to permanent paralysis. MRI may demonstrate a normal or expanded cord with T1-hypointensity and T2-hyperintnesity. Contrast enhancement is usually present. The vertebral bodies included in the radiation ports demonstrate marked T1-hyperintensity due to fatty replacement of the irradiated marrow. Cord atrophy may be seen later in the disease process.

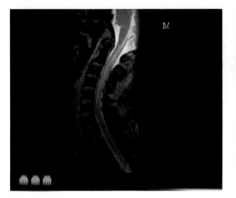

I1. Sagittal T2-weighted image shows expansion of the cord with diffuse hyperintensity.

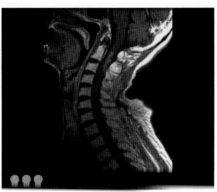

I2. Sagittal, post contrast T1-weighted Image demonstrates an enhancing intramedullary lesion in the cervical cord.

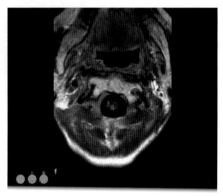

I3. Axial, post contrast T1-weighted image demonstrates an enhancing intramedullary lesion in the cervical cord.

SARCOID

Sarcoidosis is a multi-organ disease that is characterized by idiopathic non-caseating granulomatous disease. In the cervical and upper thoracic spine, sarcoidosis is generally seen in the intramedullary location. In the lumbar spine, it tends to be located in extramedullary, intradural location. MR findings include focal or diffuse cord expansion with isointensity seen on T1 weighted images, hyperintensity on T2 weighted images. Focal or leptomeningeal contrast enhancement is seen on post-contrast images.

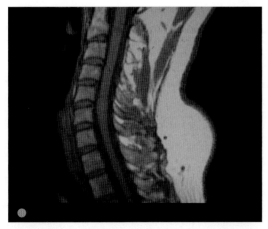

I1. Sagittal T1-weighted image shows focal expansion of the cord at C5-C6 level.

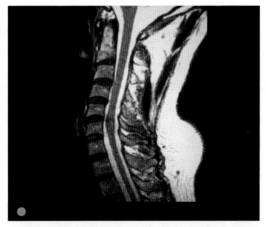

I2. Sagittal T2-weighted image shows a focal mixed signal intensity lesion with cord expansion.

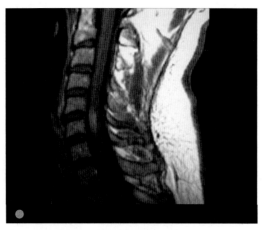

I3. Sagittal, post-contrast T1-weighted image demonstrates an enhancing intramedullary lesion.

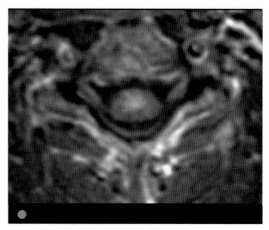

I4. Axial, post-contrast T1-weighted image demonstrates an enhancing intramedullary lesion.

TUBERCULOSIS

Intramedullary spinal tuberculoma is rare, and its diagnosis is often difficult. Tuberculoma is an evolving granuloma involving the nervous system. In the initial phase of tuberculoma formation, one finds chronic granulomatous inflammation with formation of giant cells, which homogeneously enhances with contrast due to break down of blood-brain barrier. Subsequently, collagen is deposited along the capsule of the tuberculoma and its contents is transformed into caseous material. The homogenous, nodular enhancing lesion becomes a ring-like enhancing lesion at this stage. Following treatment, the lesion regresses in size and eventually disappears, with an residual area of gliosis, which probably is seen as an area of hypointensity on T2 weighted MRI.

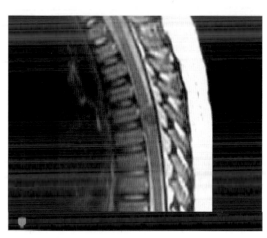

J1. Sagittal T2-weighted image shows a hypointense lesion in the thoracic cord.

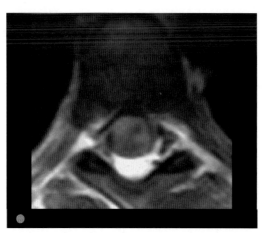

J3. Axial, post-contrast T1-weighted image demonstrates a thick ring-like enhancing lesion within the cord.

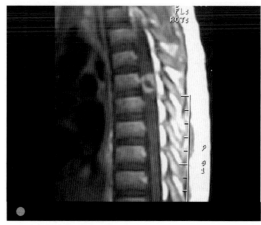

J2. Sagittal, post-contrast T1-weighted image demonstrates a thick ring-like enhancing lesion within the cord.

MULTIPLE SCLEROSIS

The spinal cord is frequently and often extensively involved in patients with multiple sclerosis. T2-hyperintense lesions are seen in the cord similar to plaques involving the brain. Enhancing plaques of multiple sclerosis in the spinal cord are not uncommon. Most enhancing lesions were homogeneous, nodular, and relatively small. Patchy and ring enhancement are unusual.

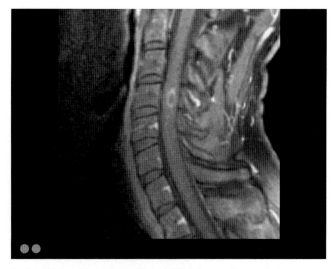

A. Sagittal, post-contrast T1 weighted image demonstrates a ring-like enhancing lesion in the cervical cord at C4.

RELATED PATTERNS

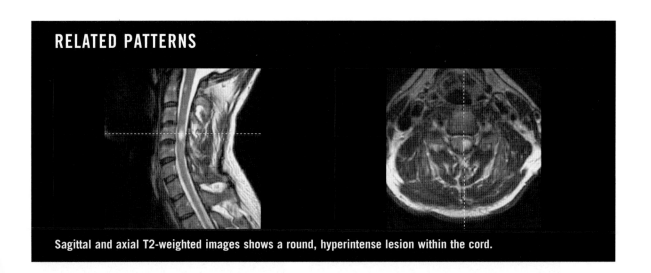

Sagittal and axial T2-weighted images shows a round, hyperintense lesion within the cord.

DIFFERENTIAL DIAGNOSIS

At a Glance:

- *Cysticercosis*
- *Metastasis*
- *Tuberculosis*

CYSTICERCOSIS

Intramedullary **cysticercosis** is uncommon. They occur as a result of hematogenous spread of the larva of **cysticercosis.**

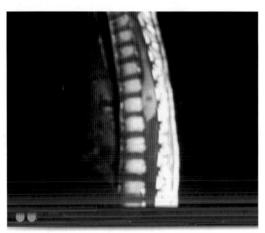

B1. Sagittal T1-weighted image shows focal expansion of the conus medullaris with a small cystic area within it.

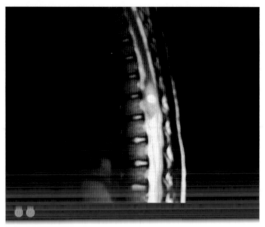

B2. Sagittal T2-weighted image shows focal expansion of the conus medullaris with a small cystic area within it. Some surrounding edema is seen.

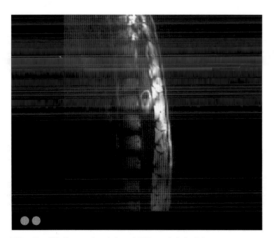

B3. Sagittal, post-contrast T1-weighted image shows focal expansion of the conus medullaris with two ring-like enhancing lesions within it.

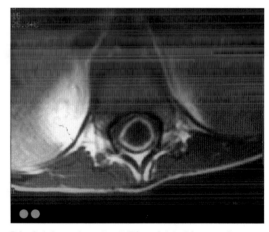

B4. Axial, post-contrast T1-weighted image shows focal expansion of the conus medullaris with two ring-like enhancing lesions within it.

METASTASIS

Intramedullary metastatic disease has been reported to be less than 3% in cancer patients at autopsy. Approximately 50% involve the thoracic cord and 35% involve the cervical cord. Lung cancer accounts for almost 66%, with the breasts being the second most common site. MRI shows variable cord expansion with marked contrast enhancement.

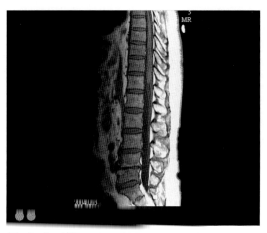

C1. Sagittal T1-weighted image shows focal enlargement of the conus medullaris.

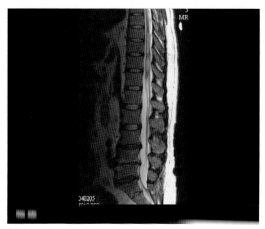

C2. Sagittal T2-weighted image shows focal enlargement of the conus with abnormal hyperintensity seen within it.

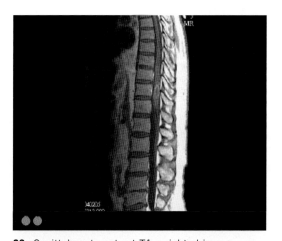

C3. Sagittal post-contrast T1-weighted image demonstrates a ring-like enhancing lesion in the conus medullaris.

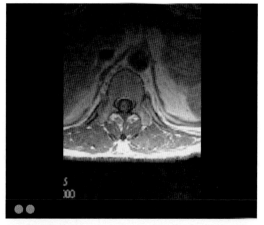

C4. Axial post-contrast T1-weighted image demonstrates a ring-like enhancing lesion in the conus medullaris.

TUBERCULOSIS

Intramedullary spinal tuberculoma is rare, and its diagnosis is often difficult. Tuberculoma is an evolving granuloma involving the nervous system. In the initial phase of tuberculoma formation, one finds chronic granulomatous inflammation with formation of giant cells, which homogeneously enhances with contrast due to break down of blood-brain barrier. Subsequently, collagen is deposited along the capsule of the tuberculoma and its contents is transformed into caseous material. The homogenous, nodular enhancing lesion becomes a ring-like enhancing lesion at this stage.

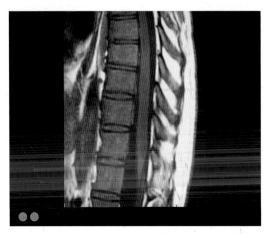

D1. Sagittal T1-weighted image shows focal expansion of the cord.

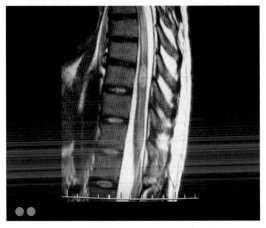

D2. Sagittal T2-weighted image shows focal expansion and an ovoid hyperintense lesion within the cord. Some hyperintense edema is seen above and below the lesions.

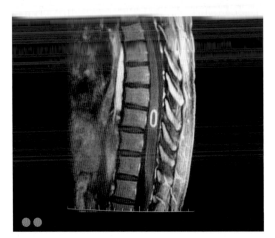

D3. Sagittal, post-contrast T1-weighted image shows focal expansion of the cord with a ring-like enhancing lesion.

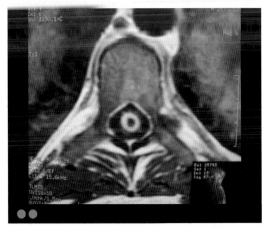

D4. Axial, post-contrast T1-weighted image shows focal expansion of the cord with a ring-like enhancing lesion.

MULTIPLE SCLEROSIS

Multiple sclerosis is the most common demyelinating disease of the spinal cord. Less than 10% of the patients have cord involvement only. CT is noncontributory. MRI shows plaques with the cord similar to those in the brain. The typical MRI findings of spinal MS are vertically elongated regions of hyperintensity involving the lateral or posterior aspect of the cord on T2-weighted images. Sometimes contrast enhancement is seen. Expansion of the cord may be seen, mimicking an intramedullary neoplasm.

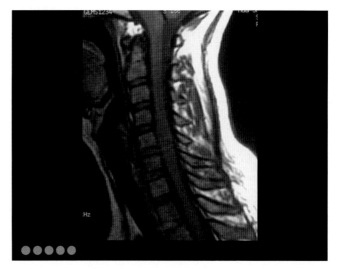

A. Sagittal T2-weighted image demonstrates abnormal hyperintense signal within the cord at C4-C6 levels.

RELATED PATTERNS

MULTIPLE SCLEROSIS (CASE TWO)

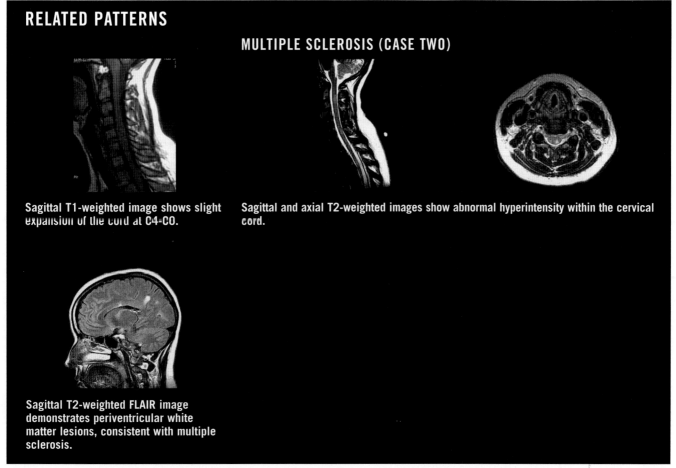

Sagittal T1-weighted image shows slight expansion of the cord at C4-C6.

Sagittal and axial T2-weighted images show abnormal hyperintensity within the cervical cord.

Sagittal T2-weighted FLAIR image demonstrates periventricular white matter lesions, consistent with multiple sclerosis.

DIFFERENTIAL DIAGNOSIS

At a Glance:

- *ADEM*
- *Aids Myelopathy*
- *Contusion*
- *Infarct*
- *Hematomyelia (Due to a Hemorrhagic Cavernoma)*
- *Sarcoidosis*
- *Subacute Combined Degeneration*
- *Transverse Myelitis*
- *Wallerian Degeneration*

ADEM

ADEM is usually a monophasic demyelinating disease, affecting children after a recent vaccination or viral infection. The imaging findings are similar to MS.

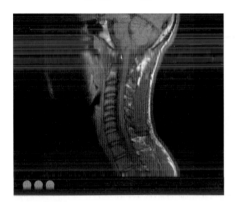 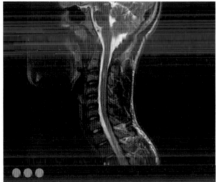 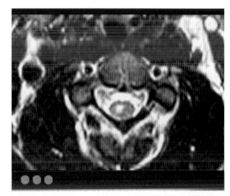

B1. Sagittal T1-weighted image is unremarkable.

B2. Sagittal T2-weighted image reveals focal hyperintense lesion within the cord.

B3. Axial T2 weighted image reveals focal hyperintense lesion within the cord.

AIDS MYELOPATHY

The diagnosis of AIDS-associated myelopathy is one of exclusion, based on clinical, laboratory, and imaging findings. MR imaging is important in the evaluation of myelopathy in HIV infected patients, and is essential in the exclusion of other extrinsic or intrinsic disease processes, such as primary or metastatic neoplasm, infectious processes. On MRI, there is usually no swelling of the cord, abnormal T2 hyperintensity is seen. Cord atrophy may be seen in the later stage of the disease. Usually, there is no contrast enhancement seen on the post contrast studies.

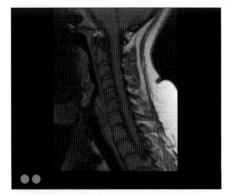 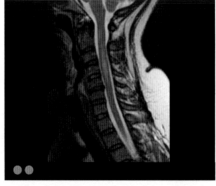 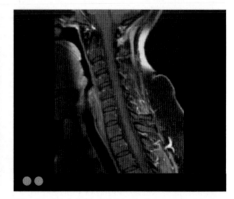

C1. Sagittal T1-weighted image shows mild focal enlargement of the cervical cord.

C2. Sagittal T2-weighted image reveals abnormal signal intensity within the cervical cord.

C3. Sagittal, T1 weighted, fat-suppressed post-contrast image shows no abnormal enhancement of the cord.

CONTUSION

MRI findings of cord injuries range from normal to edema to hemorrhage to transaction. The findings of blood and edema in the cord are analogous to those in the brain.

Kolkarni and coworkers have typed these categories as follows:

Type I—Hematomyelia, poor prognosis, with no recovery of function.

Type II—Edematous **contusion,** best recovery of function.

Type III—Hemorrhagic **contusion,** mixture of edema and blood, intermediate recovery of function.

CONTUSION (CASE ONE)

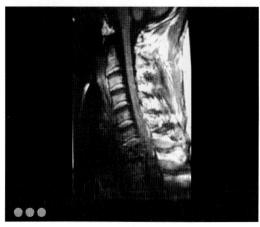

D1. Sagittal T1-weighted image shows a burst fracture of C7 with retropulsion of the bony fragments and compression of the cervical cord.

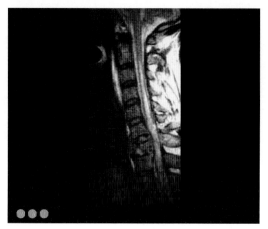

D2. Sagittal T2-weighted image reveals abnormal signal intensity within the cord extending from C2 through T1 due to contusion. Burst fracture of the C7 vertebral body is again seen.

CONTUSION (CASE TWO)

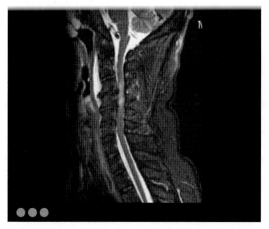

E. Sagittal T2-weighted image demonstrates hyperintense lesion within the cervical cord at C3 and C4 level. Note the presence of spinal stenosis due to degenerative changes of the cervical spine. There is a pre-vertebral hyperintense hematoma seen from C1 to C4.

537

INFARCT

Occlusive vascular lesions affecting the spinal cord are diagnostic challenges. An acute onset of symptoms is a clue to the diagnosis similar to intracranial infarct. The circulation to the spinal cord is characterized by the presence of rich anastomosis to the cord that result in relative rarity of spinal cord infarction in comparison to cerebral infarction. Most frequently affected location is the thoracic cord. Clinical presentation may be variable from paraplegia to mild weakness, etc.

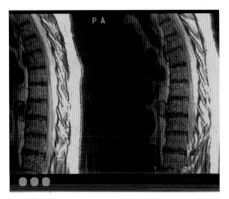
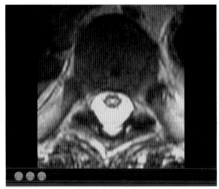
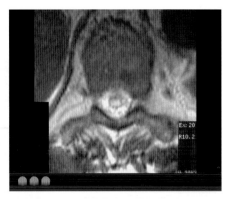

F1. Sagittal T2 weighted images demonstrate hyperintensity within the thoracic cord.

F2. Axial T2-weighted images demonstrate hyperintensity within the thoracic cord.

F3. Axial T2-weighted image demonstrating hyperintensity within the thoracic cord.

HEMATOMYELIA (DUE TO A HEMORRHAGIC CAVERNOMA)

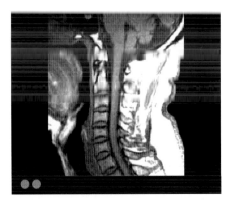
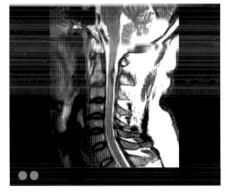
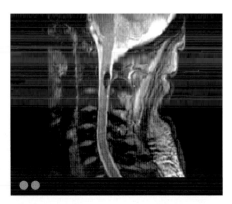

G1. Sagittal T1-weighted image shows patchy hyperintensity within the cervical cord at C2 level.

G2. Sagittal T2-weighted and T2 STIR images demonstrate a ring-like hypointensity with central hyperintensity and surrounding edema at C2 level.

G3. Sagittal T2-weighted and T2 STIR images demonstrate a ring-like hypointensity with central hyperintensity and surrounding edema at C2 level.

SARCOIDOSIS

In spine, **sarcoidosis** may involve either the bony vertebral column or the spinal cord. Typical spinal bony manifestations are lytic lesions with sclerotic borders that enhance on MRI. Typical intradural manifestations are leptomeningeal enhancement, enhancing spinal cord mass, nerve root "clumping," and enhancing nerve root.

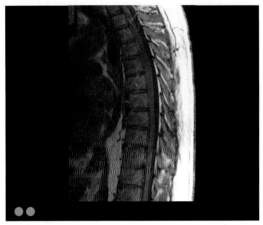

H1. Sagittal T1 weighted image shows slight focal cord expansion.

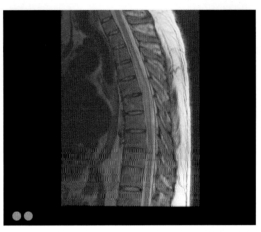

H2. Sagittal T2-weighted and T2-weighted, fat-suppressed images demonstrate hyperintensity within the thoracic cord with slight cord expansion.

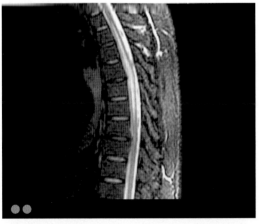

H3. Sagittal T2-weighted and T2-weighted, fat-suppressed images demonstrate hyperintensity within the thoracic cord with slight cord expansion.

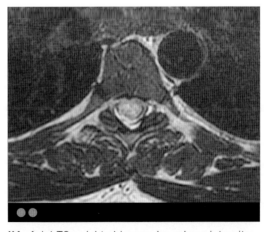

H4. Axial T2 weighted image shows hyperintensity in the thoracic cord.

SUBACUTE COMBINED DEGENERATION

Subacute combined degeneration is due to Vitamin B12 deficiency causing demyelination and vacuolation of the posterior and lateral columns. Pathologically, degeneration of myelin sheaths and axonal loss are seen. Symptoms include generalized weakness, paresthesias (tingling) involving hands and feet with loss of position and vibration, particularly in legs. The disease is progressive if not treated.

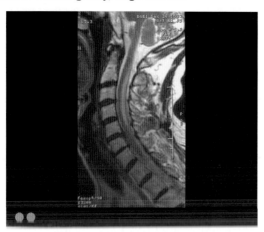

I1. Sagittal T2-weighted image shows abnormal hyperintensity in the posterior aspect of the thoracic cord in a patient with B12 deficiency.

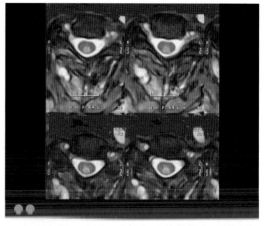

I2. Axial T2-weighted image shows abnormal hyperintensity in the posterior aspect of the thoracic cord in a patient with B12 deficiency.

TRANSVERSE MYELITIS

Transverse myelitis is an inflammatory condition of the spinal cord associated with rapidly progressive neurologic dysfunction. Diseases causing the condition include ADEM, MS, connective tissue disease, sarcoidosis, vascular malformations, vasculitides, and idiopathic forms. Authors believe there is a distinct entity termed idiopathic acute transverse myelitis. On MRI, there is hyperintense lesion extending over several segment of the cord on T2-weighted images. The contrast enhancement pattern is variable.

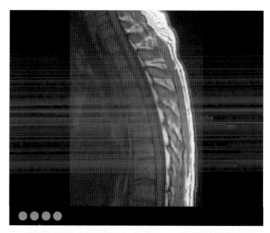

J1. Sagittal T1-weighted image is unremarkable.

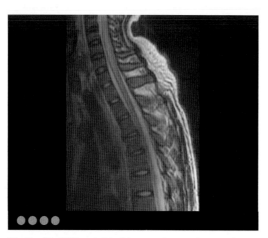

J2. Sagittal T2-weighted image shows abnormal hyperintensity within the cord.

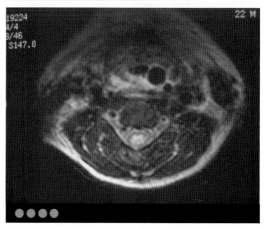

J3. Axial T2-weighted image shows abnormal hyperintensity within the cord.

WALLERIAN DEGENERATION

Wallerian degeneration refers to antegrade degeneration of axons and their accompanying myelin sheaths, and results from injury to the proximal portion of the axon or its cell body. It is progressive over a period of weeks to months, followed by an extended period of removal of the breakdown products of the myelinated axons. A focal cerebral infarct can cause secondary degeneration in fiber pathways remote from the primary infarct. Delayed disintegration of such a fiber tract is considered to be **Wallerian degeneration.**

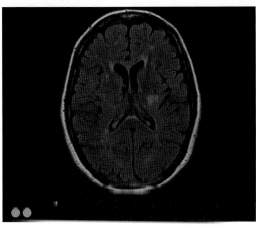

K1. Axial T2 weighted FLAIR image shows an infarct in the left basal ganglia and posterior limb of internal capsule.

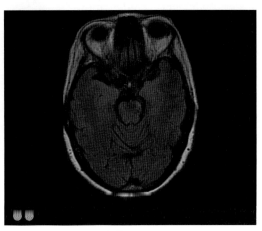

K2. Axial T2-weighted FLAIR image shows a hyperintense area in the left cerebral peduncle.

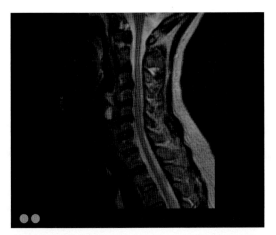

K3. Sagittal T2-weighted image shows hyperintensity in the right side of the spinal cord in the region of lateral corticospinal tract, consistent with Wallerian degeneration.

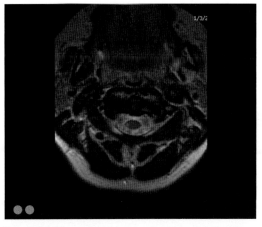

K4. Axial T2-weighted image shows hyperintensity in the right side of the spinal cord in the region of lateral corticospinal tract, consistent with Wallerian degeneration.

SYRINX

The term syringohydromyelia represents cystic cavitation of the cord. They may be congenital or acquired. The congenital form is usually associated with Chiari I malformations, and less frequently with Chiari II malformations or other congenital lesions such as spinal dysraphism, diastematomyelia. Acquired syringohydromyelia is usually related to trauma, spinal cord neoplasms, cord hemorrhage, ischemia, and arachnoiditis. MRI shows cystic cavity within the cord.

SYRINX WITH CHIARI I MALFORMATION

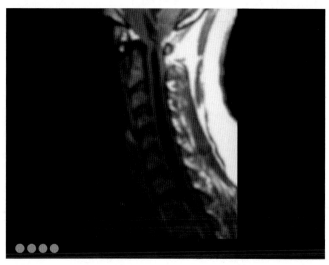

A Sagittal T1-weighted image demonstrates large cystic cavity within the cord extending from craniovertebral junction to the thoracic cord. Note the low-lying tonsil in this patient due to Chiari type I malformation.

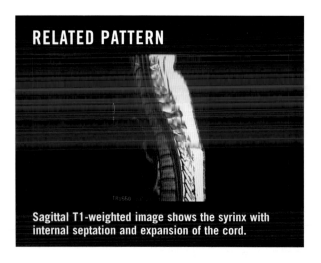

RELATED PATTERN

Sagittal T1-weighted image shows the syrinx with internal septation and expansion of the cord.

DIFFERENTIAL DIAGNOSIS

At a Glance:

* Syrinx and Spinal Dysraphism

* Syrinx Due to Cysticercosis

* Syrinx Due to Previous Surgery for Clipping Pica Aneurysm

* Syrinx with Ependymoma

* Syrinx (Idiopathic)

* Syrinx with Astrocytoma

* Syrinx Due to Trauma (not pictured)

SYRINX AND SPINAL DYSRAPHISM

Spinal dysraphism can be associated with **syrinx** due to the disruption of CSF flow in the spinal canal.

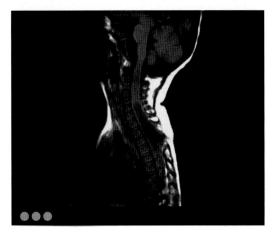

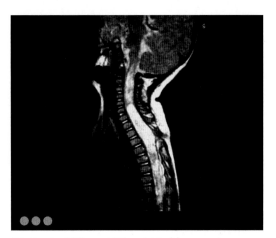

B1. Sagittal T1- and T2-weighted images show a cystic cavity within the cord in the cervicothoracic region with spinal dysraphism and tethered cord seen at T4-5 level. In this case, not only the spinal dysraphism contributed to the formation of syrinx but the tethered cord also was a factor in the disturbed CSF flow dynamics.

B2. Sagittal T1- and T2-weighted images show a cyst cavity within the cord in the cervicothoracic region with spinal dysraphism and tethered cord seen at T4-5 level. In this case, not only the spinal dysraphism contributed to the formation of syrinx but the tethered cord also was a factor in the disturbed CSF flow dynamics.

SYRINX DUE TO CYSTICERCOSIS

Cysticercosis occurs when human beings ingest ova by way of water or vegetables contaminated with feces from human who carries the adult worm of Taenia solim in gastrointestinal tract. Pigs are the intermediate hosts of Taenia solium. Pigs can also ingest water and food contaminated with human feces and develop cysticercosis. When human beings eat poorly cooked pork infected with the larva of cysticercosis, human beings become the permanent host and result in growth of the adult tapeworm. Cysticercosis may involve the muscle, brain, skin and eyes. Spinal involvement is rare. Subarachnoid disease in the spinal canal is more common than intramedullary disease. Syrinx may develop as a consequence of subarachnoid disease.

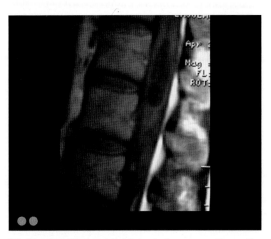

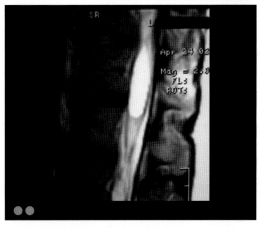

C1. Sagittal T1-weighted image shows a cystic cavity within the cord.

C2. Sagittal T2-weighted image shows a cystic cavity within the cord.

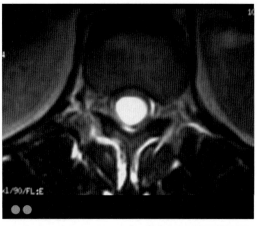

C3. Axial T2-weighted image shows a cystic cavity within the cord.

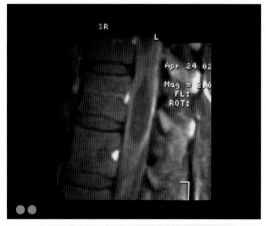

C4. Sagittal, post-contrast T1-weighted image shows a cystic cavity within the cord. No abnormal contrast enhancement is seen.

SYRINX DUE TO PREVIOUS SURGERY FOR CLIPPING PICA ANEURYSM

Alteration of the CSF flow dynamic at the craniovertebral junction due to previous surgery can cause syrinx formation.

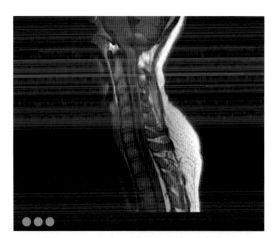

D1. Sagittal T1-weighted image shows a multi-septated cystic lesion within the cord extending from C1-T3. Note the metallic artifact at the craniovertebral junction is due to previous surgery for clipping PICA aneurysm.

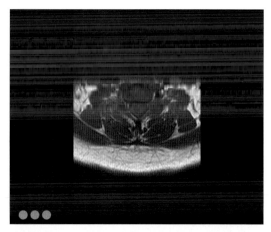

D2. Axial T1-weighted image shows a multi-septated cystic lesion within the cord extending from C1-T3. Note the metallic artifact at the craniovertebral junction is due to previous surgery for clipping PICA aneurysm.

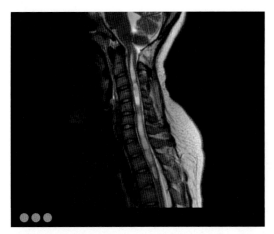

D3. Sagittal T2-weighted image shows a multiseptated cystic lesion within the cord extending from C1-T3. The artifact is more exaggerated on T2-weighted image.

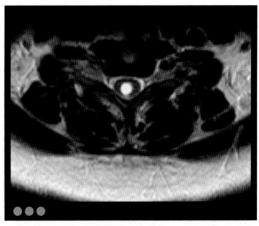

D4. Axial T2-weighted image shows a multiseptated cystic lesion within the cord extending from C1-T3. The artifact is more exaggerated on T2-weighted image.

SYRINX WITH EPENDYMOMA

Intramedullary spinal tumors consist of approximately 2–4% of all central nervous system neoplasms. The most common kinds of intramedullary tumors are ependymomas, followed by astrocytomas and hemangioblastomas. Ependymomas are the most common spinal cord tumor in adults and constitute 40–60% of all intramedullary spinal tumors, with the mean age of presentation being 35–40 years. In children, astrocytomas are the most common tumor type, accounting for around 60% of all intramedullary spinal tumors, and the mean age of presentation is 5–10 years. Interestingly, a syrinx may develop at a remote site from the primary tumor. However, in the majority of the cases, they are seen adjacent to the tumor.

The common intramedullary tumors associated with syringomyelia are **ependymomas** and hemangioblastomas. Dilatation of the central canal can occur in **ependymoma.** Cystic cavity may be created by fluid accumulation due to hemorrhage or fluid secreted by tumor cells. Cystic degeneration of the tumor may also occur.

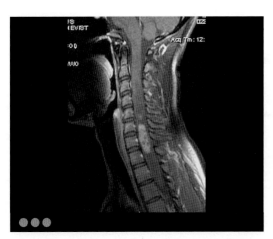

E1. Sagittal, post-contrast T1-weighted image shows an enhancing mass within the cord extending from C6 through T1.

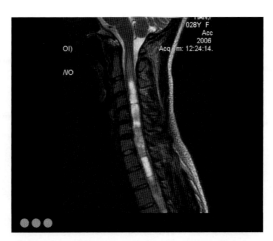

E2. Sagittal T2-weighted image shows the slightly hyperintense tumor with syrinx cavity seen above and below the mass.

SYRINX (IDIOPATHIC)

Syrinxes are rare entities. In about 50% of the patients with a syrinx, it is present at birth, and it gradually enlarges when they become teens or young adults. Frequently, patients who have a syrinx at birth also have congenital abnormalities of the brain and spine, such as Chiari type I malformation. Syrinxes that develop in adult life are usually due to injuries, infections or associated neoplasms. Idiopathic Syrinx means a syringomyelia is seen without an associated congenital anomaly of the brain or spine and no history of injury, no associated neoplasm.

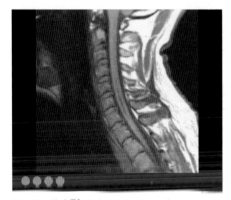

I1. Sagittal T1-weighted image shows a hypointense, cystic area within the cord extending from C5-C7.

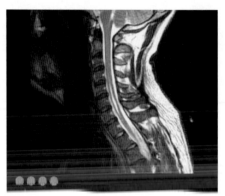

F2. Sagittal T2-weighted image shows a hyperintense, cystic area within the cord extending from C5-C7.

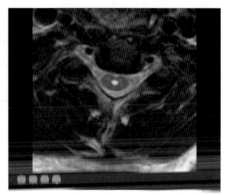

F3. Axial T2-weighted image shows a hyperintense, cystic area within the cord extending from C5-C7.

SYRINX WITH ASTROCYTOMA

Astrocytomas of the spinal cord arise from astrocytes in the spinal cord and occur in the pediatric as well as in adult populations. These tumors characteristically presents with focal cord expansion, often with cysts and a variable enhancement pattern. Associated syrinx may be seen. There are four types of macroglial cells in the central nervous system (CNS) including astrocytes, Schwann cells, oligodendrocytes, and ependymal cells. These cells all serve a variety of supportive functions. Astrocytomas arise from astrocytes, which is essential for structural and metabolic support in the CNS. Approximately 30% of pediatric and adult intramedullary spinal cord tumors are astrocytomas with the thoracic cord being the most common location, followed by cervical cord. Astrocytomas may be associated with tumor cyst or syrinx. Approximately 30% of spinal cord neoplasms may eventually produce a syrinx.

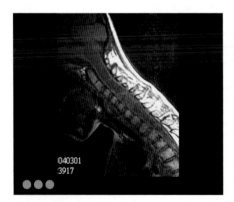

G1. Sagittal T1-weighted image shows a heterogeneously hypointense, cystic lesion within the cord involving the entire cervical spine.

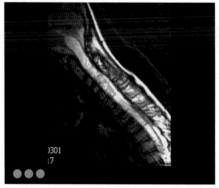

G2. Sagittal T2-weighted image reveals a hyperintense multicystic lesion within the entire cervical cord.

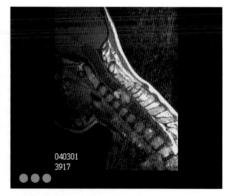

G3. Sagittal, post-contrast T1-weighted image demonstrates a heterogeneously enhancing lesion from C4 through C6 level. Note the presence of syrinx above and below the enhancing mass.

PART II

COMPUTED
TOMOGRAPHY

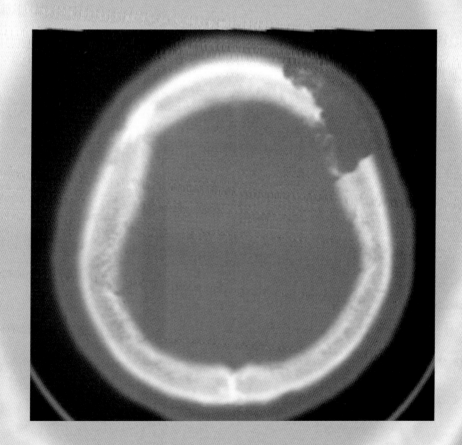

Chapter 13

Skull Defects and Lesions

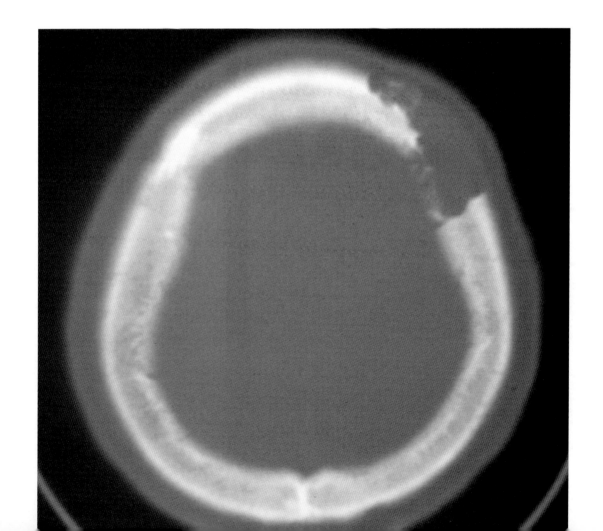

ANEURYSM BONE CYST

Aneurysm bone cyst involving the skull is rare and consists about 3–6% of all the aneurysm bone cysts. Aneurysm bone cyst has a lytic appearance composed of lobulated compartments containing blood. Fluid–blood level may be seen in these small compartments on magnetic resonance imaging. They usually present as a scalp mass, but occasionally may cause intracranial mass effect or intracranial hemorrhage.

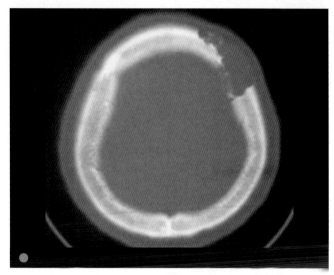

A, Axial CT shows a lytic lesion involving the bony calvarium with irregular margin along the inner table and broken outer table. This is a rare case of aneurysm bone cyst.

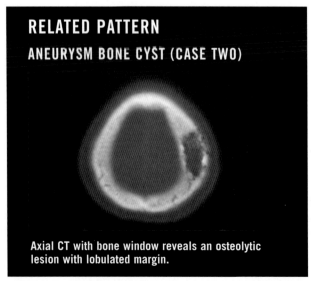

RELATED PATTERN

ANEURYSM BONE CYST (CASE TWO)

Axial CT with bone window reveals an osteolytic lesion with lobulated margin.

DIFFERENTIAL DIAGNOSIS

At a Glance:

- *Arachnoid Granulation (Normal Structure)*
- *Coccidiomycosis*
- *Encephalocele (Transethmoidal)*
- *Eosinophilic Granuloma (Langerhan's Cell Granulomatosis)*
- *Epidermoid*
- *Hemangioma*
- *Meningioma*
- *Metastatic Lesion*

- *Neurofibromatosis*
- *Osteomyelitis*
- *Plasmacytoma*
- *Venous Lake (Normal Structure)*
- *Encephalocele* (not pictured)
- *Fibrous Dysplasia* (not pictured)
- *Leptomeningeal Cyst* (not pictured)
- *Lymphoma* (not pictured)
- *Paget's Disease* (not pictured)
- *Osteoblastoma* (not pictured)

ARACHNOID GRANULATION (NORMAL STRUCTURE)

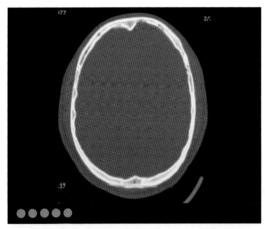

B. Axial CT shows remodelling of the inner table of skull due to pacchionian granulation.

ARACHNOID GRANULATION (CASE TWO)

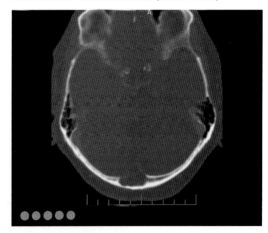

C. Axial CT shows a lytic lesion involving the inner table of the skull and diploic space in the region of transverse sinus.

COCCIDIOMYCOSIS

There are two types of coccidioidomycosis infection. Acute primary coccidioidomycosis causes mild infection of the lungs, which disappears spontaneously without treatment. It accounts for about half of the cases. The second form, severe, progressive coccidioidomycosis is an infection of the whole body, which could be fatal. It is more common among men and among blacks, Filipinos, and Native Americans. This form is more likely to occur in immuno-compromised patients, but can be seen in immunocom-petent patients. The infection may spread from the lungs to other organs, such as bones, joints, liver, spleen, and kidneys. The fungi can also iinvolve the brain and the meninges. Skull involvement is rare.

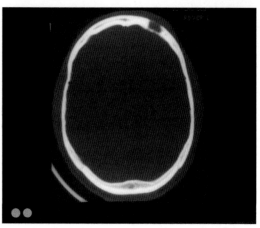

D. Axial CT shows a lytic lesion involving the skull in the left frontal region due to coccidiomycosis.

ENCEPHALOCELE (TRANSETHMOIDAL)

Basal **encephaloceles** are rare lesions including transethmoidal, sphenoethmoidal, transsphenoidal, and frontosphenoidal varieties. Due to their internal location, they are not generally externally visible. Transsphenoidal and transethmoidal encephaloceles are the most common types of basal **encephaloceles.** The former project through a defect in the floor of the sella and into the nasal cavity, whereas the latter project through cribriform plate defect into the nasal cavity.

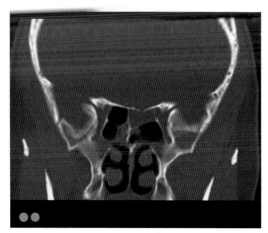

E1. Axial CT scan demonstrates the presence of a skull defect at the left cribriform plate with a soft tissue density seen in the ethmoid sinus representing encephalocele.

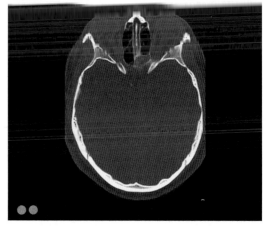

E2. Axial CT scan demonstrates the presence of a skull defect at the left cribriform plate with a soft tissue density seen in the ethmoid sinus representing encephalocele.

EOSINOPHILIC GRANULOMA (LANGERHAN'S CELL GRANULOMATOSIS)

Eosinophilic granuloma shows uneven destruction of the inner and outer table of the skull creating so-called "beveled edge" or "hole in a hole" appearance. The margin is usually not sclerotic.

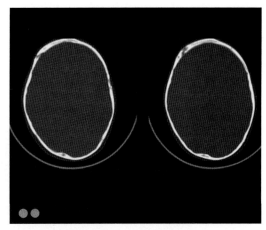

F. Axial CT shows a lytic lesion involving the skull in the right frontal region.

EPIDERMOID

Epidermoids are of developmental origin, derived from epithelial cell rests ectopically included in the bone during development. They may occur anywhere in the calvarium, with a preference for the frontal or occipital regions or in the temporal bone. They originate in the diploic space and enlarge in the both directions expanding and thinning both the inner and outer tables by continuous growth pressure. Sclerotic changes are seen at the edge of the lesions. The lesion may break through the thin tables and expand under the scalp or extradurally. A lesion in the midline location, especially over the torcula may involve the venous sinuses. The larger epidermoids are called giant epidermoids and they have a tendency to get infected.

EPIDERMOID (CASE ONE)

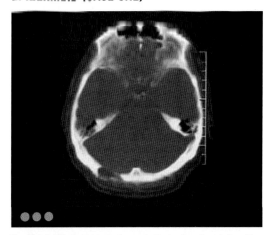

G. Axial CT demonstrates a lytic lesion involving the left occipital bone.

EPIDERMOID (CASE TWO)

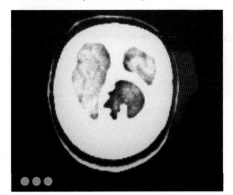

H1. Axial CT with soft tissue and bone window image shows an expansile lesion with central hypointensity and sclerotic margin involving the calvarium.

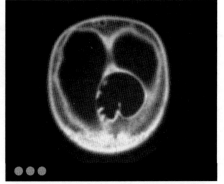

H2. Axial CT with soft tissue and bone window image shows an expansile lesion with central hypointensity and sclerotic margin involving the calvarium.

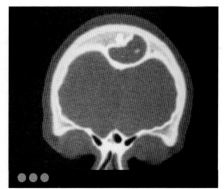

H3. Coronal CT shows an expansile lesion.

555

HEMANGIOMA

Hemangiomas constitute approximately 7% of all skull lesions. About two thirds of hemangiomas of skeletal system occur in the cranium or the spine. They arise from the vascular elements of the diploic space, mainly in the cranial vault and to a lesser extent in the roof of orbit or petrous temporal bone. They are slow growing and may reach a large size. They are painless and the presence of a swelling is the chief complaint. The skull is involved by erosion and their margins are usually not discernable.

HEMANGIOMA (CASE ONE)

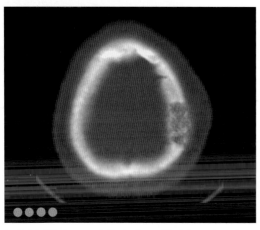

I. Axial CT shows a lytic lesion with internal septation.

HEMANGIOMA (CASE TWO)

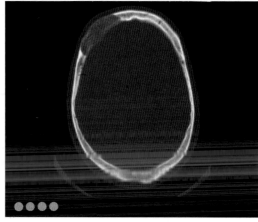

J. Axial CT shows an expansile lesion with internal septation with erosion of both the outer and inner table of the skull. Outer table is commonly involved, but inner table erosion is unusual, which could lead to the development of epidural or less likely subdural hematoma.

MENINGIOMA

Occasionally **meningioma** may show lytic changes. A tumor mass is seen on the soft tissue window and the mass enhances with contrast.

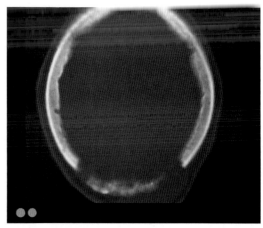

K. Axial CT shows a lytic defect due to a meningioma.

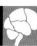

METASTATIC LESION

The primary sites for skull metastasis are usually from the breast, the lungs, the prostate, the thyroid, and the kidney. Although metastasis can affect any part of the skull, cranial vault is the common site. They are usually osteolytic lesions with the exception of prostate cancer. Occasionally in some cases of breast cancer, the skull metastasis may appear as a mixed lesions of osteolytic and osteoblastic changes. CT scan is positive in 85% of the cases. Extradural and scalp soft tissue extension exhibit as areas of contrast enhancement.

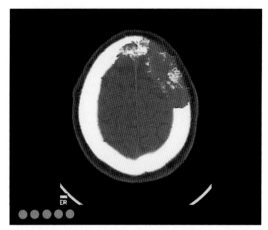

L. Axial CT show a lytic skull defect due to metastatic disease.

NEUROFIBROMATOSIS

Skull defects associated with **neurofibromatosis** can occur along the sagittal suture (single) or lambdoid suture (uni or bilateral).

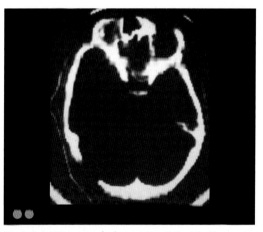

M. Axial CT demonstrates a lytic defect in the parietal region, which is due to dysplastic change secondary to neurofibromatosis.

OSTEOMYELITIS

Acute **osteomyelitis** is always a lytic process. As the disease progresses, small lucencies coalesce into larger areas. All three tables of the skull may be involved. Adjacent sinusitis, mastoiditis, or post-surgical changes may be seen on imaging studies.

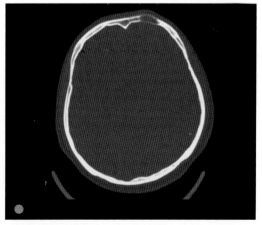

N. Axial CT shows a lytic skull defect in the right frontal bone secondary to osteomyelitis caused by frontal sinusitis.

557

PLASMACYTOMA

Classically, **plasmacytoma** appears as a rounded, well-circumscribed lucency a few millimeters in diameter, without reactive sclerosis.

PLASMACYTOMA (CASE ONE)

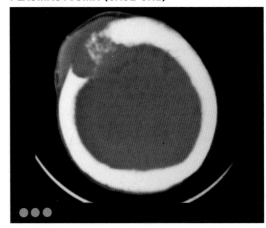

O. Axial CT shows a lytic skull defect in the right frontal region associated with a soft tissue mass due to plasmacytoma.

PLASMACYTOMA (CASE TWO)

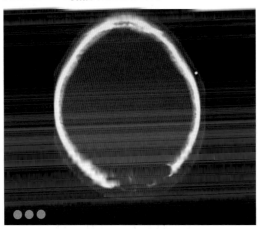

P1. Axial CT with bone window demonstrates a lytic skull defect in the parieto-occipital region.

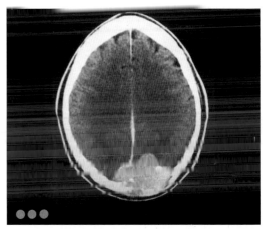

P2. Axial, post-contrast CT reveals an enhancing mass involving the calvarium and epidural space.

VENOUS LAKE (NORMAL STRUCTURE)

Venous lakes seen on skull are normal variants. They are well-defined lytic areas in the cranium, often with visible diploic veins going to them. Their location is within the diploic space. There is no bony expansion. The inner and outer tables are usually intact.

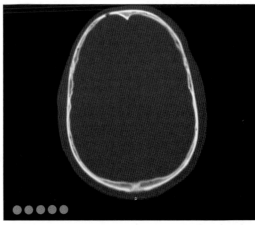

Q. Axial CT shows a small right frontal skull defect due to venous lake.

METASTATIC LESIONS

Primary sites are usually the breasts, lungs, prostate, kidneys, thyroid, and melanoma. Diploic space is involved before the inner or outer table of the skull. Because of its rich blood supply, the calvarium is more commonly involved than the skull base.

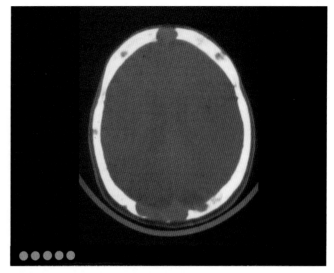

A. Axial CT with bone window demonstrates multiple lytic skull defects, consistent with metastatic disease.

DIFFERENTIAL DIAGNOSIS

At a Glance:

* Langerhan's Cell Histiocytosis
* Multiple Myeloma
* Hyperparathyroidism (not pictured)

* Osteomyelitis (not pictured)
* Pacchionian Granulation (Normal Structure) (not pictured)
* Parietal Foramina (not pictured)
* Radiation Necrosis (not pictured)
* Venous Lake (not pictured)

LANGERHAN'S CELL HISTIOCYTOSIS

In Langerhans's histiocytosis, the Langerhans' cells are admixed with a mixed population of acute and chronic inflammatory cells. Langerhans' histiocytosis is an all-inclusive term that covers the formerly known clinicopathologic entities of histiocytosis X that includes Lettere-Siwe disease, Hand-Schüller-Christan, disease, and eosinophilic granulomas. The disease typically involves children and young adults. The skull and femur are most commonly involved sites. The lesion may be solitary or multiple.

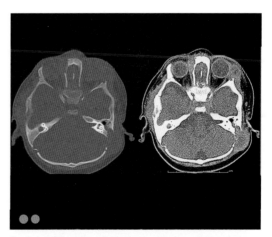

B. Axial CT with soft tissue and bone window images show multiple skull defects involving the right sphenoid, both occipital, and left temporal bones associated with soft tissue mass.

MULTIPLE MYELOMA

Multiple myeloma is the most common primary neoplasm of the skeletal system. Multiple myeloma is a malignancy of plasma cells. Radiologically, there are four distinct patterns, including (1) normal, (2) diffuse demineralization with no lytic lesion, (3) a solitary lytic lesion, and (4) diffuse, multiple lytic lesions.

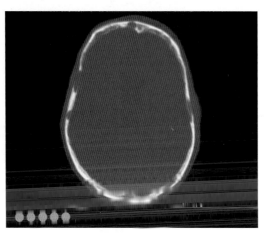

C1. Axial CT scan demonstrates multiple lytic skull defects with destruction of both the inner and outer table of the skull.

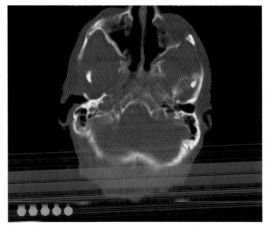

C2. Axial CT scan shows a lytic lesion involving the left mandibular condyle. Mandibular involvement is seen in a third of the cases and may help to differentiate myeloma from metastatic disease.

OSTEOMA

Osteomas of the skull may involve the outer or inner tables of the skull, more frequently involving the outer table. Osteomas appear as flat-based, well marginated domes of dense bone. They do not involve the diploic space. Osteomas are the common tumors of the paranasal sinuses, especially in the frontal and ethmoid sinuses. They are benign tumors of membranous bone consisting of dense, compact bone. Obstruction of a sinus ostium may lead to infection or formation of a mucocele. Multiple osteomas involving the maxilla and mandible are found in Gardner's syndrome (associated with CNS malignancy).

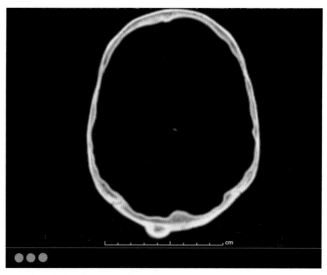

A. Axial CT shows a well-marginated bony growth from the outer table of the skull in the right occipital region. The diagnosis is an osteoma arising from the outer table of the calvarium.

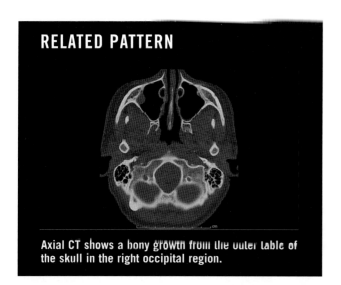

RELATED PATTERN

Axial CT shows a bony growth from the outer table of the skull in the right occipital region.

DIFFERENTIAL DIAGNOSIS

At a Glance:

• *Fibrous Dysplasia*

• *Meningioma*

• *Metastatic Lesion*

• *Paget's Disease* (not pictured)

• *Osteomyelitis* (not pictured)

FIBROUS DYSPLASIA

Skull abnormalities seen in **fibrous dysplasia** may be sclerotic or cystic. The more common sclerotic form consists of dense, expanded bone with loss of the diploic space and of trabecular pattern. The sclerotic form is seen when both the skull base and facial bone are involved along with the calvarium.

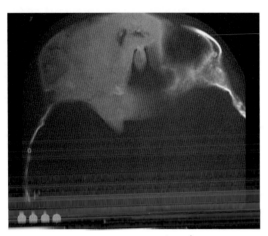

D1. Axial and coronal CT scans show focal thickening of the bony orbital roof on the right side due to fibrous dysplasia.

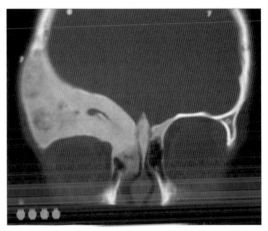

B2. Axial and coronal CT scans show focal thickening of the bony orbital roof on the right side due to fibrous dysplasia.

MENINGIOMA

The incidence of hyperostosis in meningiomas reported in literature is quite variable. It tends to occur more frequently in meningioma en plaque than globular ones and its incidence has been reported up to 49% of the cases. It is generally accepted that in most patients the hyperostosis represents a true infiltration of the bone by the tumor cells. Most of the cases of hyperostosis involve the frontal bone and the orbit. It should be noted that hyperostotic bone reaction is seen with osteoblastic metastases, meningiomas, fibro osseous lesions or previous radiotherapy.

MENINGIOMA (CASE ONE)

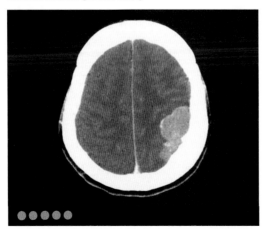

C. Axial, post-contrast CT image demonstrates a left parietal extra-axial mass with adjacent bony hyperostosis.

MENINGIOMA (CASE TWO)

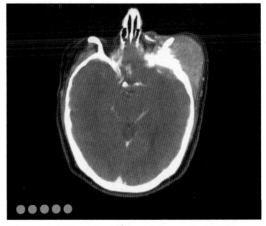

D1. Axial CT in soft tissue and bone window images show a left sphenoid meningioma with significant extracranial component and a small orbital component. Hyperostosis of the sphenoid and temporal bone is seen with spiculated appearance.

MENINGIOMA (CASE THREE)

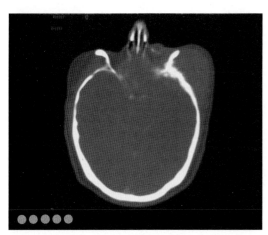

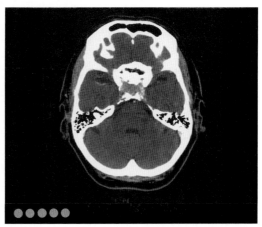

D2. Axial CT in soft tissue and bone window images show a left sphenoid meningioma with significant extracranial component and a small orbital component. Hyperostosis of the sphenoid and temporal bone is seen with spiculated appearance.

E. Axial CT with contrast demonstrates focal hyperostosis of the planum sphenoidale with an enhancing mass.

METASTATIC LESION

Sclerotic calvarial metastasis are most frequently due to breast cancer, followed by prostate and lung cancer. Most metastatic skull lesions are asymptomatic, although they can cause symptoms due compression of dural sinuses and cranial nerves. In case of solitary lesion, the metastasis need to be differentiated from primary skull tumors like osteoma, chondroma, chondrosarcoma, chordoma, etc. and tumor-like lesions like fibrous dysplasia, hyperostosis, etc. Patients with skull metastases tend to be elderly patients with shorter duration of symptoms as compared from those with primary bone lesions.

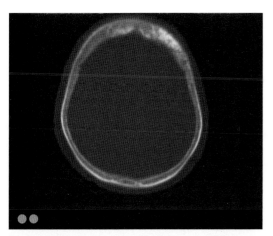

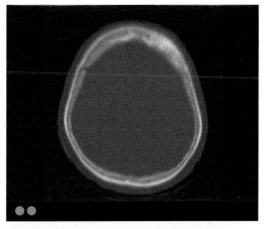

F1. Axial CT demonstrates focal mixed, predominantly hyperdense lesion in left frontal region.

F2. Axial CT demonstrates focal mixed, predominantly hyperdense lesion in left frontal region.

SHUNTED HYDROCEPHALUS

The thickening of the calvarium involves predominantly the diploic space. History of hydrocephalus with shunt placement is important.

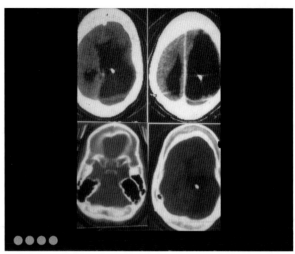

A. Axial CT shows diffuse calvarial thickening. In addition, there is ventricular dilation and a shunt tube seen in the left lateral ventricle. The diagnosis is skull thickening due to shunted hydrocephalus.

DIFFERENTIAL DIAGNOSIS

At a Glance:

- *Acromegaly*
- *Fibrous Dysplasia*
- *Seizure and Phenytoin*
- *Sickle Cell Anemia*
- *Thalassemia*

- *Fluorosis* (not pictured)
- *Mucolipidosis* (not pictured)
- *Myelofibrosis* (not pictured)
- *Osteomyelitis* (not pictured)
- *Osteopetrosis* (not pictured)
- *Paget's Disease* (not pictured)

ACROMEGALY

Acromegaly is due to the overproduction of growth hormone in adults. Growth hormone stimulates the growth of bones, muscles, and many internal organs. It is almost always caused by a benign pituitary adenoma. Certain rare tumors of the pancreas and lungs also can produce hormones that stimulate the pituitary to produce excessive amounts of growth hormone, with similar consequences. An x-ray or CT of the skull may show thickening of the bones and enlargement of the nasal sinuses. The sella turcica may be enlarged due to the pituitary tumor.

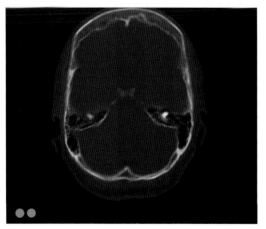

B1. Axial CT demonstrates diffuse calvarial thickening due to acromegaly.

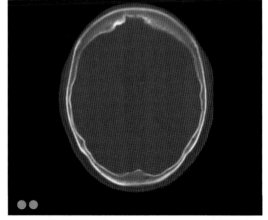

B2. Axial CT demonstrates diffuse calvarial thickening due to acromegaly.

FIBROUS DYSPLASIA

Fibrous dysplasia is a relatively common disorder of skeletal system. When it involves the facial bone and cranium, it produces a wide variety of clinical presentations. Plain film assessment of craniofacial fibrous dysplasia may be confusing due to varying appearances and complex, overlapping structures. The MRI appearances of fibrous dysplasia are often non-specific and may be confusing due to contrast enhancement. CT findings are more likely to lead to a specific diagnosisdue to its characteristic ground-glass appearance of woven bone.

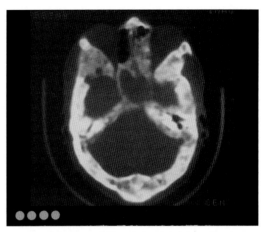

C. Axial CT shows diffuse calvarial thickening in a patient with fibrous dysplasia.

SEIZURE AND PHENYTOIN

Phenytoin is known to cause calvarial thickening. Phenytoin has been shown to stimulate osteoblast proliferation and differentiation via upregulation of transforming growth factor-β1 and bone morphogenetic proteins. The incidence of calvarial thickening is approximately 30% among patients with seizure disorder and receiving Phenytoin treatment.

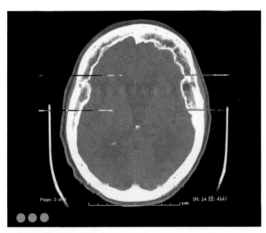

D1. Axial CT with bone window shows diffuse calvarial thickening in a patient taking dilantin for treatment of chronic seizure.

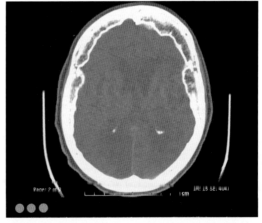

D2. Axial CT with bone window shows diffuse calvarial thickening in a patient taking dilantin for treatment of chronic seizure.

SICKLE CELL ANEMIA

Severe, chronic anemias (such as thalassemias and sickle cell anemia) can increase the bone marrow response to form red blood cells. This drive for erythropoiesis may cause hyperplasia of marrow and lead to widening of the diploic space. Trabeculae are oriented perpendicular to the inner table, giving a hair-on-end appearance.

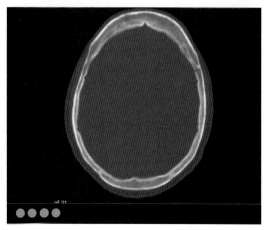

E. Axial CT demonstrates diffuse calvarial thickening in a patient with sickle cell anemia.

THALASSEMIA

Severe, chronic anemias (such as thalassemias and sickle cell anemia) can increase the bone marrow response to form red blood cells. This drive for erythropoiesis may cause hyperplasia of marrow and lead to widening of the diploic space. Trabeculae are oriented perpendicular to the inner table, giving a hair-on-end appearance.

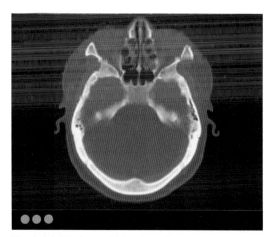

F1. Axial CT shows thickening of the skull in a patient with thalassemia.

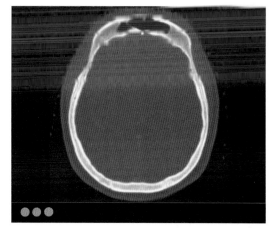

F2. Axial CT shows thickening of the skull in a patient with thalassemia.

DYKE-DAVIDOFF-MASON SYNDROME

The characteristic findings consist of unilateral calvarial thickening (especially of the diploic space), expansion of the ipsilateral ethmoid, frontal sinuses and mastoid, and asymmetry of the planum sphenoidale, anterior clinoid processes.

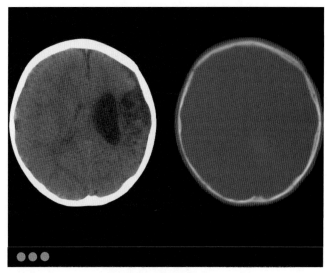

A. Axial CT with soft tissue and bone window demonstrates left cerebral hemiatrophy, dilated left lateral ventricle, volume loss in left hemisphere, and left calvarial thickening.

DIFFERENTIAL DIAGNOSIS

At a Glance:

- *Fibrous Dysplasia*
- *Sturge–Weber Syndrome*
- *Unilateral Megalencephaly* (not pictured)

FIBROUS DYSPLASIA

Skull abnormalities seen in **fibrous dysplasia** may be sclerotic or cystic. The more common sclerotic form consists of dense, expanded bone with loss of the diploic space and of trabecular pattern. The sclerotic form is seen when both the skull base and facial bone are involved along with the calvarium.

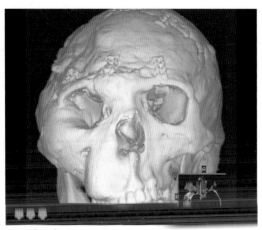

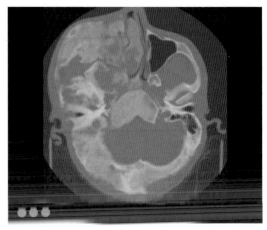

B1. 3D reformat shows unilateral calvarial thickening involving the skull as well as the skull base. Fibrous dysplasia is a disease of unknown etiology in which the osteoblasts fail to mature and differentiate. Skull and facial bone involvement occurs in 20–30% of these patients.

B2. Axial CT shows unilateral calvarial thickening involving the skull as well as the skull base. Fibrous dysplasia is a disease of unknown etiology in which the osteoblasts fail to mature and differentiate. Skull and facial bone involvement occurs in 20–30% of these patients.

STURGE–WEBER SYNDROME

Sturge–Weber syndrome is a congenital disorder caused by the persistence of the transitory primordial sinusoidal plexus stage of vessel development. It is usually sporadic in nature. The disease is characterized by a capillary and/or venous malformation that involves the face, choroid of the eye, and leptomeninges. The facial vascular malformation has a predilection for the distribution of the ophthalmic division of the fifth cranial nerve. In association with leptomeningeal vascular malformation, underlying cerebral hemiatrophy is often present. Unilateral skull thickening, associated with enlargement of paranasal sinuses and mastoids may be seen. The disease process is usually unilateral, but rarely may be bilateral. Clinically, they present with seizure and/or mental retardation.

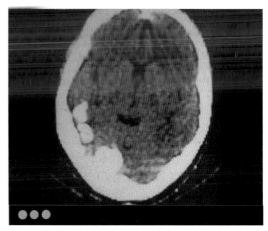

C. Axial CT image shows thickening of the calvarium on the right side with intracranial calcification seen in the right temporal, parietoccipital region.

Chapter 14

Meningeal and Sulcal Diseases

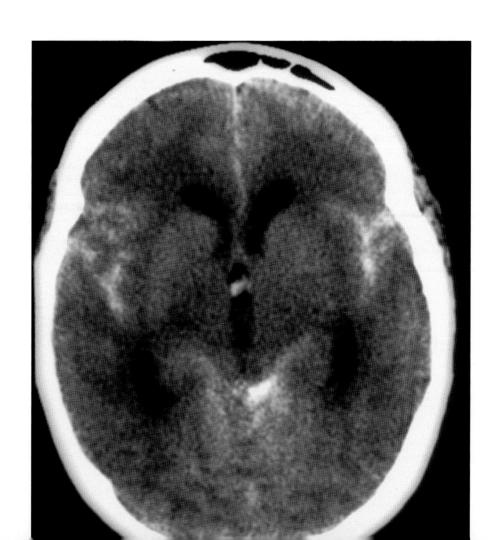

SUBARACHNOID HEMORRHAGE

Subarachnoid hemorrhage can occur in patients with ruptured intracranial aneurysm. The classic symptom is the sudden onset of severe, disabling headache. Neckache and neck stiffness follows. Focal neurologic deficit, obtundation, and coma may follow. Another cause of subarachnoid hemorrhage is head trauma. Subarachnoid hemorrhage stems primarily from laceration of the pial vessels or a small cortical injury with blood leakage into the subarachnoid space. Subarachnoid hemorrhage can occur around the perimesencephalic cistern and is not associated with an aneurysm.

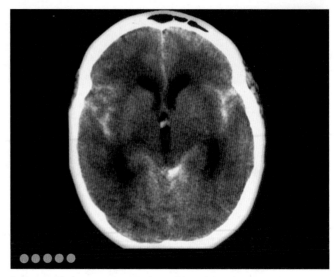

A. Axial CT shows hyperdensity in the sylvian fissure bilaterally, quadrigeminal cistern and superior vermian cistern consistent with subarachnoid hemorrhage.

RELATED PATTERNS

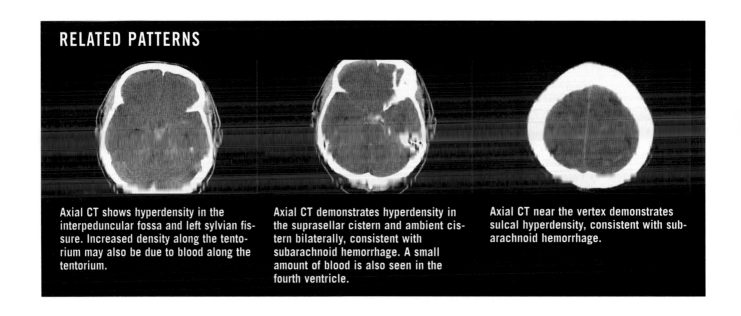

Axial CT shows hyperdensity in the interpeduncular fossa and left sylvian fissure. Increased density along the tentorium may also be due to blood along the tentorium.

Axial CT demonstrates hyperdensity in the suprasellar cistern and ambient cistern bilaterally, consistent with subarachnoid hemorrhage. A small amount of blood is also seen in the fourth ventricle.

Axial CT near the vertex demonstrates sulcal hyperdensity, consistent with subarachnoid hemorrhage.

DIFFERENTIAL DIAGNOSIS

At a Glance:

- *Coccidioidomycosis*
- *Subarachnoid Contrast*
- *Subarachnoid Pantopaque*

COCCIDIOIDOMYCOSIS

Coccidioidomycosis is a systemic infection caused by *Coccidiodes immitis*. The organism is endemic to the southwestern United States and northern Mexico. The majority of the patients are asymptomatic and only 4–5% of symptomatic patients may develop disseminated disease with associated morbidity and mortality, especially in immunocompromized patients. Central nervous system involvement is usually secondary to hematogenous dissemination from the pulmonary disease. Imaging findings of CNS **coccidioidomycosis** include meningitis and ependymitis with secondary hydrocephalus; solitary or multiple granulomas; vasculitis with ischemic infarction or rarely mycotic aneurysm.

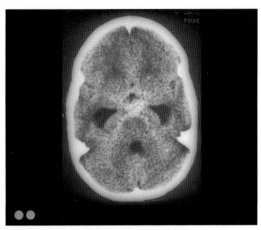

B. Axial CT without contrast shows hyperdense material in the suprasellar cistern, consistent with pus.

SUBARACHNOID CONTRAST

Subarachnoid contrast is usually introduced iatrogenically while performing a myelogram or cisternogram. Patient may suffer from seizure activity due to the cortical stimulation from the contrast. Since contrast material is of higher density than blood, it can readily be recognized on the CT scan.

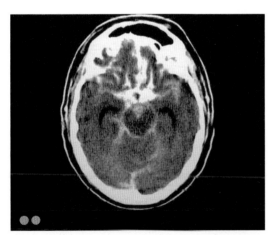

C1. Axial CT demonstrates hyperdensity in the suprasellar cistern, ambient cistern, and cerebral sulci. This patient had intrathecal contrast injection for a cisternogram.

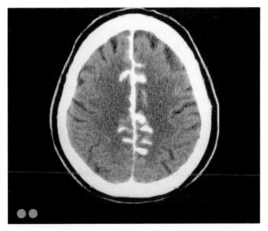

C2. Axial CT near the vertex region demonstrates hyperdensity in the cerebral sulci bilaterally in the same patient.

SUBARACHNOID PANTOPAQUE

Pantopaque is an oil-based contrast agent, which was used for myelography prior to the invention of water soluble, non-ionic contrast agent. It can stay in the subarachnoid space for years if not removed at the time of the procedure.

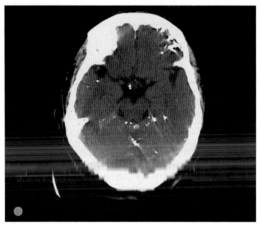

D1. Axial CT scan demonstrates multiple hyper-dense areas in the subarachnoid space.

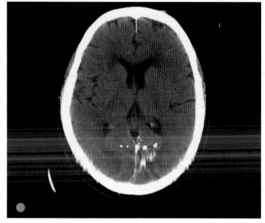

D2. Axial CT scan demonstrates multiple hyper-dense areas in the subarachnoid space.

MENINGITIS (BACTERIAL, FUNGAL, VIRAL)

Meningitis is an inflammation of the leptomeninges and subarachnoid space. It can be caused by a number of factors, including bacterial, fungal, and viruses. CT will initially demonstrate no abnormality of the subarachnoid spaces. Leptomeningeal enhancement may be seen in the subacute stage. The primary mechanism of this enhancement is breakdown of the blood–brain barrier without angiogenesis.

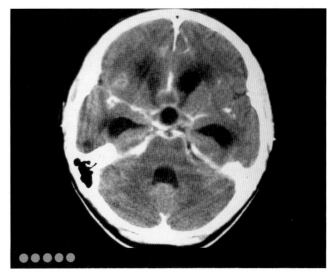

A. Axial CT with contrast shows enhancement along the suprasellar cistern, sylvian cistern, and interhemispheric fissure in a patient with bacterial meningitis. Dilatation of the anterior third and lateral ventricles is seen.

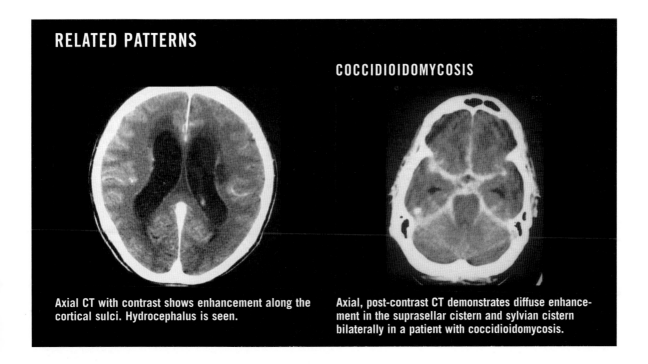

RELATED PATTERNS

COCCIDIOIDOMYCOSIS

Axial CT with contrast shows enhancement along the cortical sulci. Hydrocephalus is seen.

Axial, post-contrast CT demonstrates diffuse enhancement in the suprasellar cistern and sylvian cistern bilaterally in a patient with coccidioidomycosis.

DIFFERENTIAL DIAGNOSIS

At a Glance:

* *Granulomatous Disease*

* *Leptomeningeal Spread of Tumor* (not pictured)

GRANULOMATOUS DISEASE

Wegener's granulomatosis is a rare, multisystem disorder of unknown etiology. It is characterized by necrotizing granulomatous disease and/or vasculitis histopathologically. Most commonly this involves the upper and lower respiratory tract, with pulmonary involvement occurring at some stage of the disease in almost all patients. However, many other organ systems can also be affected including the kidneys, orbits and central nervous system. In the central nervous system, disease process may involve the pachymeninges and leptomeninges. Involvement may be focal or diffuse.

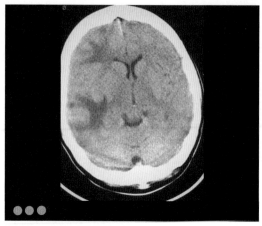

B1. Axial CT shows vasogenic edema in the right frontal and temporal lobes adjacent to sylvian fissure.

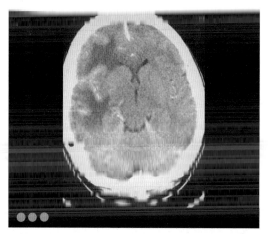

B2. Axial, post-contrast CT scan shows leptomeningeal enhancement in the region of right sylvian fissure in a patient with Wegener's granulomatosis.

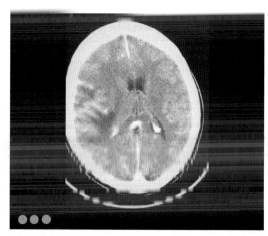

B3. Axial, post-contrast CT scan shows leptomeningeal enhancement in the region of right sylvian fissure in a patient with Wegener's granulomatosis.

MENINGEAL METASTATIC DISEASE

Non-contrast CT in patients with meningeal carcinomatosis may be normal initially. Subtle effacement of the sulci, high density within the sulci, or along the pachymeninges, may be seen as well as hydrocephalus. Thick, nodular pachymeningeal enhancement is usually seen on the post-contrast CT studies.

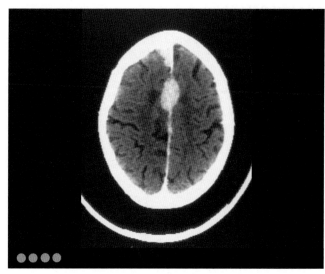

A. Axial, post-contrast CT in a patient with breast carcinoma reveals an ovoid area of enhancing mass along the falx extending to both sides of the falx, with another focus of enhancement on the right side anteriorly along the falx.

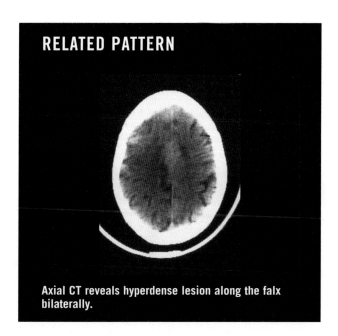

RELATED PATTERN

Axial CT reveals hyperdense lesion along the falx bilaterally.

DIFFERENTIAL DIAGNOSIS

At a Glance:

• *Granulomatous Disease*

• *Lymphoma* (not pictured)

GRANULOMATOUS DISEASE

Wegener's granulomatosis is a rare, multisystem disorder of unknown etiology. It is characterized by necrotizing granulomatous disease and/or vasculitis histopathologically. Many organ systems can be affected including the lungs, kidneys, orbits and central nervous system. In the central nervous system, disease process may involve the pachymeninges and leptomeninges. Involvement may be focal or diffuse.

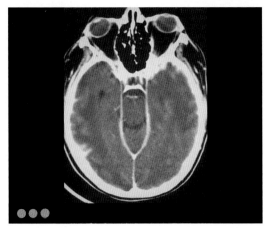

B1. Axial, post-contrast CT shows thick enhancement along the tentorium in a patient with Wegener's granulomatosis. Leptomeningeal enhancement is also seen in the right temporal region.

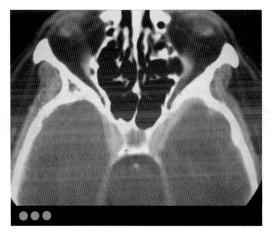

B2. Axial, post-contrast CT scan shows pachymeningeal enhancement along the left temporal fossa. Some leptomeningeal enhancement is seen in the right temporal region.

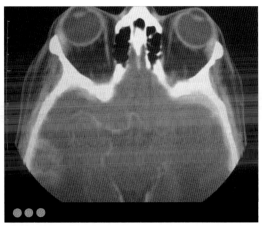

B3. Axial, post-contrast CT scan shows pachymeningeal enhancement along the left temporal fossa. Some leptomeningeal enhancement is seen in the right temporal region.

EPIDURAL HEMATOMA

An EDH is a biconvex collection of blood, which lies beneath the calvarium, external to the periosteal dura. It rarely extends beyond the suture margin due to the firm attachment of periosteal dura to the suture margin. An EDH most frequently occurs over the convexity from a lacerated meningeal or periosteal artery at the fractured bone edges. An EDH may also occur from the venous bleeding due to a dural sinus injury. An EDH is almost always the result of a coup injury at the site of impact. Conversely, a SDH is often the result of a contrecoup injury away from the impact site. An EDH may cross the midline by displacing the interhemispheric fissure and falx away from the inner table of the skull. An EDH may stop at the suture site due to the firm attachment of dura at suture.

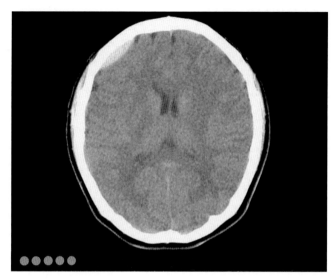

A. Axial CT reveals an extracerebral, lentiform blood collection in the right frontal region.

RELATED PATTERNS

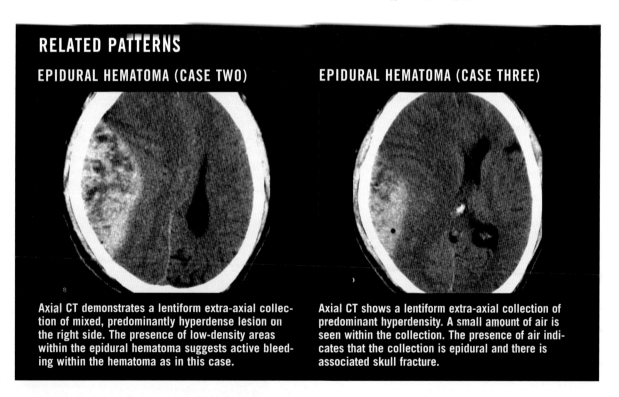

EPIDURAL HEMATOMA (CASE TWO)

Axial CT demonstrates a lentiform extra-axial collection of mixed, predominantly hyperdense lesion on the right side. The presence of low-density areas within the epidural hematoma suggests active bleeding within the hematoma as in this case.

EPIDURAL HEMATOMA (CASE THREE)

Axial CT shows a lentiform extra-axial collection of predominant hyperdensity. A small amount of air is seen within the collection. The presence of air indicates that the collection is epidural and there is associated skull fracture.

DIFFERENTIAL DIAGNOSIS

At a Glance:

- *Arachnoid Cyst*
- *Subdural Empyema*
- *Epidural Empyema*
- *Isodense Subdural Hematoma*
- *Mixed Subdural Hematoma*
- *Subdural Hematoma*

ARACHNOID CYST

Arachnoid cysts are benign cysts that occur in the central nervous system in relation to the arachnoid membrane. Communication with the subarachnoid space may or may not be present. They usually contain clear, colorless fluid similar to cerebrospinal fluid. Most are developmental in origin. A small number of arachnoid cysts are acquired and may be due to neoplasms, hemorrhage, or previous surgery. They constitute approximately 1% of intracranial mass lesions with the majority seen in the middle cranial fossa. Cysts in the middle cranial fossa are found more frequently in males than in females.

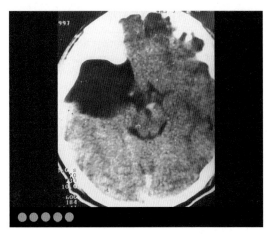

B. Axial CT shows a low attenuation lesion at the anterior right temporal fossa without mass effect.

SUBDURAL EMPYEMA

Subdural empyema is an intracranial focal collection of purulent material located between the dura mater and the arachnoid membrane. About 95% of subdural empyemas are located within the cranium and only 5% involve the spine. The most frequent location is the frontal fossa. Subdural empyema causes extrinsic compression of the brain by an inflammatory mass and inflammation of the brain and meninges. It has a tendency to spread quickly in the subdural space and the disease is life-threatening. In infants and young children, subdural empyema most often occurs as a complication of meningitis. In older children and adults, it usually occurs as a complication of paranasal sinusitis, otitis media, or mastoiditis.

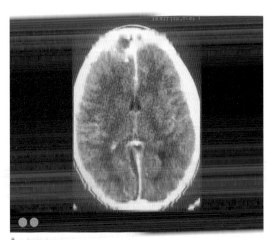

C. Axial, post-contrast CT shows an epidural empyema in the frontal region and a subdural empyema posteriorly along the falx on the right side.

EPIDURAL EMPYEMA

Cerebral epidural empyema is defined as a suppurative infection of the epidural space, which is the space between the dura mater and the inner table of the skull. In approximately 10% of cases, epidural abscess is associated with subdural abscess. The dura is tightly adherent to the skull, resulting in sharp demarcation and slow progression of the empyema. Intracranial epidural empyema can result from spread of infection to the epidural space from the paranasal sinuses, middle ear, orbit, or mastoids or as a complication of surgery. Cranial epidural empyema may rarely occur as a result of metastatic hematogenous seeding. Complications of epidural empyema include osteomyelitis, dural sinus thrombosis, subdural empyema, purulent leptomeningitis, and brain abscess.

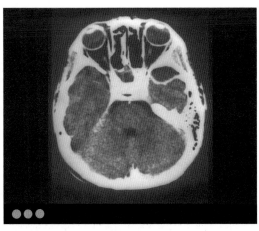

D. Axial, post-contrast CT reveals a lentiform fluid collection with marginal enhancement at left anterior temporal fossa.

ISODENSE SUBDURAL HEMATOMA

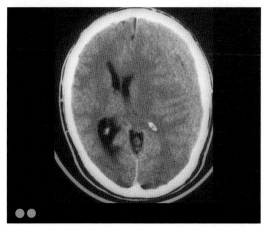

E1. Axial CT shows a crescent, isodense collection on the left. Note the displacement of the gray and white matter to the right, causing "buckling" of the white matter.

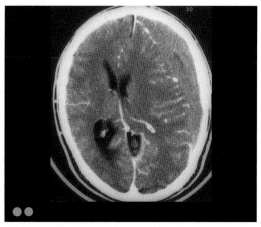

E2. Axial, post-contrast CT demonstrates a crescent collection outlined by the displaced, enhancing cortical veins.

MIXED SUBDURAL HEMATOMA

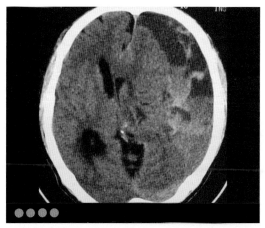

F. Axial CT demonstrates a crescent collection of mixed hyper- and hypodensity on the left side, indicating the presence of chronic subdural hematoma with recurrent episodes of re-bleeding.

SUBDURAL HEMATOMA

Subdural hematoma is an accumulation of blood between the meningeal dura and arachnoid mater. A **SDH** may occur from the rupture of bridging cortical veins, the bending of vessels from deceleration, or by direct injury to pial veins, great veins, or pacchionian granulation. A **SDH** tends to extend along the meningeal dura and the underlying arachnoid, forming a crescentic hematoma with a long tail. A **SDH** may extend from the convexity to the interhemispheric fissure and the tentorial edge. A **SDH** is not confined by the sutureline, but it cannot cross the midline due to the dural folding in the midline.

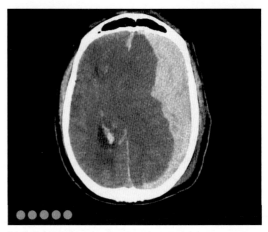

G. Axial CT shows a large, extracerebral, crescent blood collection on the left side.

DANDY–WALKER MALFORMATION

Dandy–Walker malformation consists of cystic dilatation of the fourth ventricle, vermian hypoplasia or agenesis, and large posterior fossa with high position of torcular. About 70–90% of patients have hydrocephalus, which often develops postnatally.

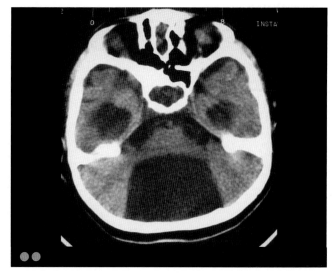

A. Axial CT shows a large cystic lesion in the retrocerebellar region. The fourth ventricle is not seen and is a part of this cystic lesion. There is agenesis of the vermia.

RELATED PATTERNS

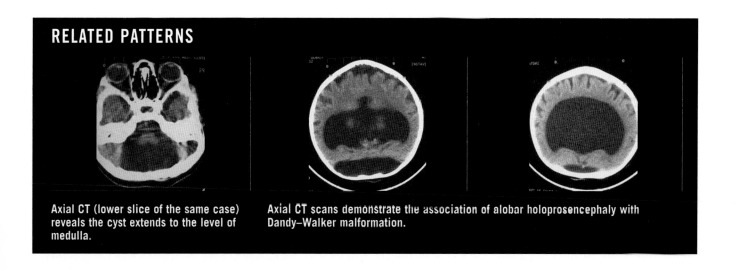

Axial CT (lower slice of the same case) reveals the cyst extends to the level of medulla.

Axial CT scans demonstrate the association of alobar holoprosencephaly with Dandy–Walker malformation.

DIFFERENTIAL DIAGNOSIS

At a Glance:

• *Arachnoid Cyst*

• *Giant Cisterna Magna*

ARACHNOID CYST

Posterior fossa **arachnoid cyst** is a retrocerebellar cyst that is not communicating with the subarachnoid space. The vermis, cerebellum, and fourth ventricle are normal but may be displaced by the cyst. The posterior fossa may be enlarged.

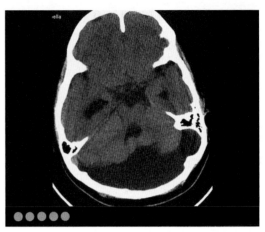

B. Axial CT shows a large retrocerebellar cyst. Note the vermis is seen between the cyst and fourth ventricle.

GIANT CISTERNA MAGNA

Giant cistern magna is a large retrocerebellar CSF collection. The fourth ventricle and cerebellar vermis are normal.

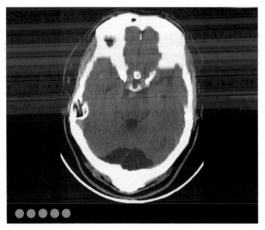

C1. Axial and sagittal reformatted CT images show a retrocerebellar cystic lesion, consistent with a giant cisterna magna.

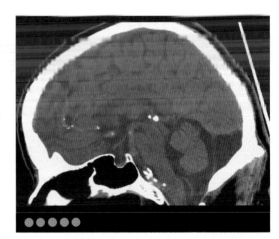

C2. Axial and sagittal reformatted CT images show a retrocerebellar cystic lesion, consistent with a giant cisterna magna.

Chapter 15

Extracerebral Masses

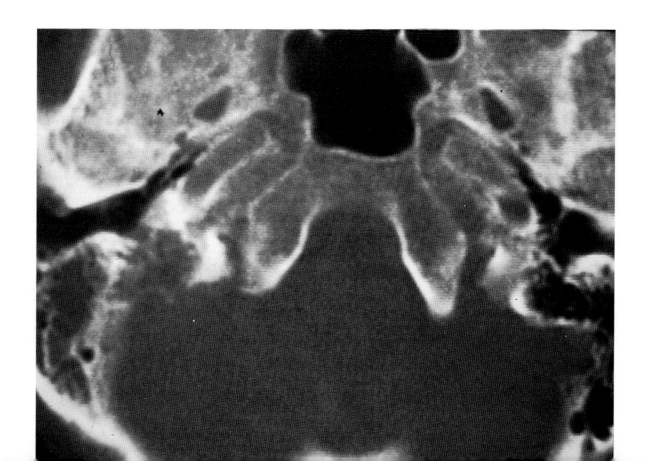

The right jugular foramen is larger than the left in 68%, equal in 12%, and smaller than the left in 20%, possibly due to the difference in the size of the sigmoid sinus and the jugular bulb. The jugular foramen is traditionally divided into a large posterolateral compartment (pars venosa) and a smaller anteromedial compartment (pars nervosa). The ninth cranial nerve goes through the pars nervosa, whereas the tenth and eleventh cranial nerves go through the pars venosa along with the jugular vein.

METASTASIS

Metastasis may show bone changes similar to glomus jugulare tumors but are usually much less vascular and do not show the "salt and pepper" appearance.

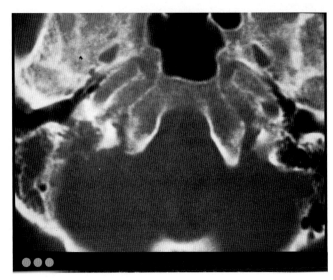

A. Axial CT shows mottled appearance of the right jugular foramen. Metastasis may show bone changes similar to glomus jugulare tumors on CT.

DIFFERENTIAL DIAGNOSIS

At a Glance:

- Glomus Jugulare
- High Jugular Bulb (Normal Variant)
- Meningiomas
- Schwannomas
- Cholesteatoma (not pictured)
- Chondrosarcoma (not pictured)
- Histiocytosis (not pictured)
- Lymphoma (not pictured)
- Plasmacytoma (not pictured)
- Thrombosis of Jugular Vein (not pictured)

GLOMUS JUGULARE

Glomus Jugulare tumors involve the jugular foramen and the skull base. Paraganglioma is the second most common tumor in the temporal bone after vestibular schwannoma. Paraganglioma consists of glomus jugulare, glomus tympanicum, and glomus vagale. These tumors are three times more common in females and are often multiple.

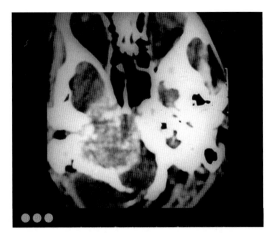

B. Axial, post-contrast CT shows a large enhancing mass in the region of right jugular foramen with marked bone erosion.

HIGH JUGULAR BULB (NORMAL VARIANT)

The jugular bulb is usually asymmetrical and the right jugular bulb often is larger than the left one. It is called a high jugular bulb, if it reaches above the level of lateral semicircular canal. When the bony septum that separates the jugular bulb from tympanic cavity is absent, it is called a dehiscent jugular bulb. Occasionally an outpouching of the jugular bulb is seen, it is called a jugular bulb diverticulum.

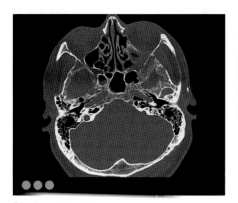

01. Axial CT demonstrates a round defect in the posterior aspect of the petrous bone on the right side.

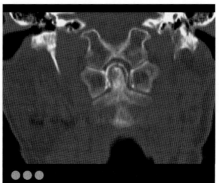

C2. Coronal and sagittal reformatted images show high position of the right jugular bulb.

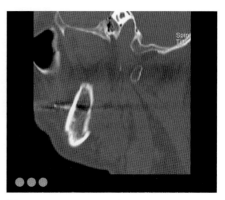

C3. Coronal and sagittal reformatted images show high position of the right jugular bulb.

MENINGIOMAS

Meningiomas arising from the jugular foramen are characterized by diffuse, centrifugal skull base infiltration. They extend laterally to involve the middle ear cavity, medially to involve jugular tubercle, hypoglossal canal, occipital condyle, and clivus. They extend inferiorly into the nasopharyngeal carotid space of the suprahyoid neck and superiorly into the dura of the cerebellopontine angle.

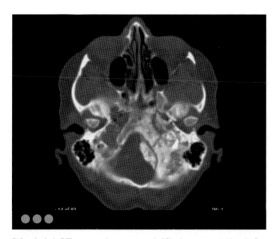

D1. Axial CT scan shows a calcified mass at the left jugular foramen with extension into the cerebellopontine angle cistern.

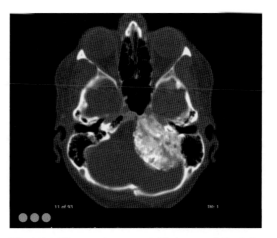

D2. Axial CT scan shows a calcified mass at the left jugular foramen with extension into the cerebellopontine angle cistern.

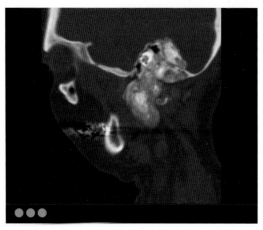

D3. Sagittal CT scan demonstrates a calcified mass through the jugular foramen extending upward to the cerebellopontine angle and downward to the nasopharyngeal carotid space.

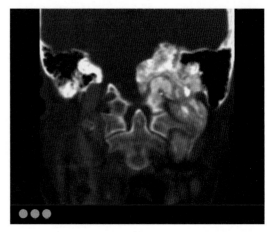

D4. Coronal CT scan demonstrates a calcified mass through the jugular foramen extending upward to the cerebellopontine angle and downward to the nasopharyngeal carotid space.

SCHWANNOMAS

Schwannoma of the cranial nerve IX, X, XI when arising from jugular foramen, cause sharp, smooth, rounded enlargement of the foramen on CT. They enhance homogeneously or contain cystic components on CT.

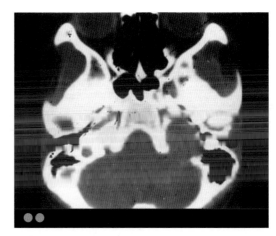

E. Axial CT shows marked enlargement of the left jugular foramen due to a ninth nerve schwannoma.

Clivus consists of a portion of the sphenoid bone and occipital bone in the base of the skull. The spheno-occipital synchondrosis can remain open in early childhood and fuses around the age of 15.

CHORDOMA

Chordomas represent less than 1% of all intracranial neoplasms and 2–4% of all primary bone tumors. Clivus is the second most common site of involvement only second to sacrococcygeal region. Chordomas arise from the remnants of primitive notochord, which extends from Rathke's pouch to the clivus, continuing caudally to the vertebral bodies. On CT, bone destruction involving the clivus associated with a soft tissue mass is seen. Calcification is seen in 50% of the cases and is better seen on CT. There are two types of chordomas histologically: typical and chondroid. The chondroid subtype is more commonly seen in the skull base, constituting up to one-third of cases in that region.

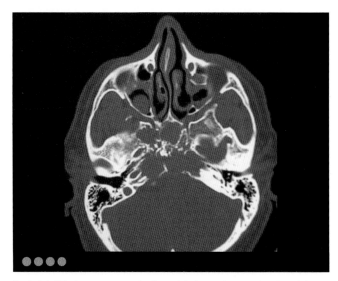

A. Axial CT shows a mass lesion with bony destruction involving the clivus and skull base.

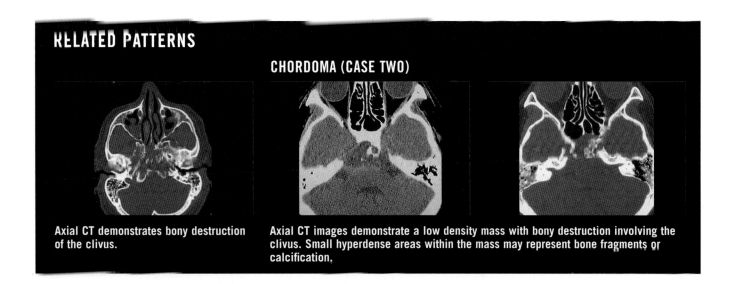

RELATED PATTERNS

CHORDOMA (CASE TWO)

Axial CT demonstrates bony destruction of the clivus.

Axial CT images demonstrate a low density mass with bony destruction involving the clivus. Small hyperdense areas within the mass may represent bone fragments or calcification.

DIFFERENTIAL DIAGNOSIS

At a Glance:

- *Adenoid Cystic Carcinoma*
- *Chondrosarcoma*
- *Giant Cell Tumor*
- *Lymphoma*
- *Meningioma*

- *Metastasis*
- *Nasopharyngeal Carcinoma*
- *Cholesteatoma (Atypical Location)* (not pictured)
- *Pituitary Adenoma (Invading the Clivus)* (not pictured)
- *Plasmacytoma* (not pictured)
- *Sphenoid Sinus Neoplasm* (not pictured)

ADENOID CYSTIC CARCINOMA

Adenoid cystic carcinoma represents less than 10% of all salivary gland neoplasms, but is about 40% of all malignancies of major and minor salivary glands. The characteristics of this tumor include slow growth, multiple recurrences, prolonged clinical course, and late metastasis. Adenoid cystic carcinoma occurs most frequently in the 5th decade of life. There is no sex predilection. It is the most common malignancy in the submandibular gland and the minor salivary glands. **Adenoid cystic carcinoma** has the tendency for perineural invasion, which is seen in about 80% of all patients.

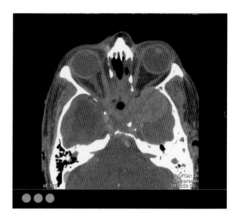

B. Axial, post-contrast CT shows mass at the ethmoid sinus, sphenoid sinus, left temporal fossa, left orbital apex with invasion of the clivus.

CHONDROSARCOMA

Chondrosarcoma consists of 20% of primary bone tumors, and 10% of chondrosarcoma occur in the bones of the face and skull base. They occur predominantly between the age of 20 and 50. There is a slight male preference of

all. They usually arise from different locations associated with sutures. CT shows a mass lesion slightly off midline with bone destruction, and sometimes with calcification. Contrast enhancement of the mass is inhomogeneous.

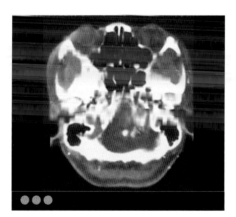

C1. Axial CT with soft tissue and bone window demonstrates a left cerebellopontine angle enhancing mass with calcification and erosion of the clivus and left petrous bone.

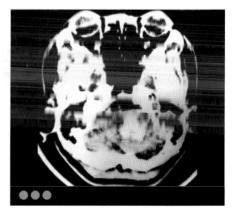

C2. Axial CT with soft tissue and bone window demonstrates a left cerebellopontine angle enhancing mass with calcification and erosion of the clivus and left petrous bone.

GIANT CELL TUMOR

Giant cell tumors of the clivus are rare. Giant cell tumors usually involve the epiphysis of long bones. Less than 1%

of giant cell tumors involve the skull. When skull is involved, they tend to preferentially occur in the sphenoid or temporal bones.

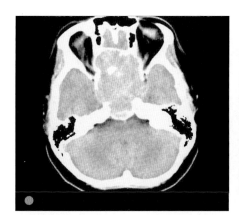

D1. Axial, post contrast CT shows an enhancing mass with bony destruction involving the clivus as well as the cribriform plate. There is extension of the mass into both temporal fossa and pre-pontine cistern.

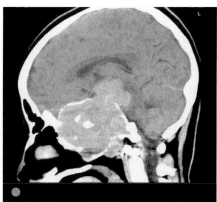

D2. Sagittal, post-contrast CT with bone window image reveals a large mass in the sphenoid and ethmoid sinuses with bony destruction of the clivus and cribriform plate. Intracranial extension of the mass is seen with marked compression of the brainstem.

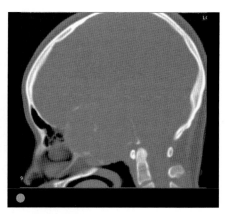

D3. Sagittal, post-contrast CT with bone window image reveals a large mass in the sphenoid and ethmoid sinuses with bony destruction of the clivus and cribriform plate. Intracranial extension of the mass is seen with marked compression of the brainstem.

LYMPHOMA

Lymphoma of the skull base and clivus are included in extra-cerebral lymphomas and are uncommon. As cranial base surgery becomes more common, it is important to be aware of lymphoma as a possible differential diagnosis of clival lesions.

Lymphoma involving the clivus may or may not demonstrate bone destruction.

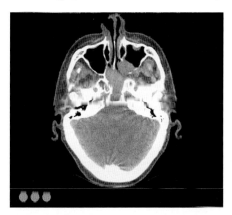

E1. Axial CT shows a soft tissue mass involving the sphenoid sinus and maxillary sinus with bony destruction of the clivus seen.

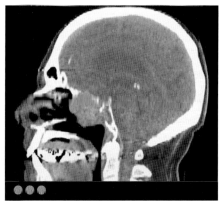

E2. Sagittal CT shows a soft tissue mass in the sphenoid sinus with bony destruction of the clivus and cribriform plate.

MENINGIOMA

Meningiomas are more commonly seen in middle aged women. While the majority of meningiomas are sporadic, they are also seen in the setting of previous cranial irradiation and in patients with neurofibromatosis type 2 (Chromosome 22). In addition meningiomas have estrogen sensitivity and may grow in size during pregnancy. Clival meningiomas arise from the clivus or petroclival junction medial to the trigeminal nerve. They may grow out along the petrous pyramid or into the cavernous sinus and middle cranial fossa. Large meningiomas may encase the basilar artery or its branches.

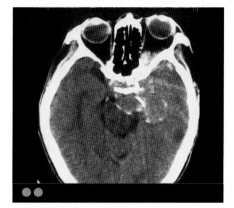

F. Axial CT shows a mass posterior to the dorsum sella and left parasellar region with calcification.

METASTASIS

Metastatic disease to the clivus is not uncommon. Bone destruction is seen on CT scans.

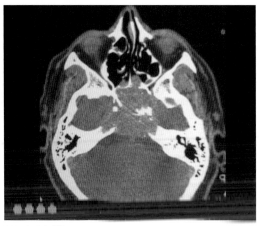

G1. Axial CT with soft tissue and bone window images shows bony destruction involving the clivus with a soft tissue mass extending into the prepontine cistern, displacing the brainstem posteriorly. Residual bony fragments are seen.

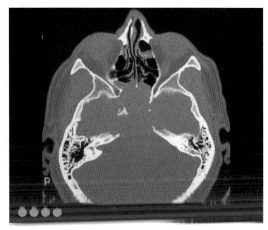

G2. Axial CT with soft tissue and bone window images shows bony destruction involving the clivus with a soft tissue mass extending into the prepontine cistern, displacing the brainstem posteriorly. Residual bony fragments are seen.

NASOPHARYNGEAL CARCINOMA

Posterior extension of **nasopharyngeal carcinoma** to involve the clivus and invade the dura with intracranial extension is not uncommon. Frequently, a recurrent **nasopharyngeal** carcinoma may present as a lesion involving the skull base and clivus with intracranial extension, whereas the primary site at nasopharynx may be normal following previous treatment.

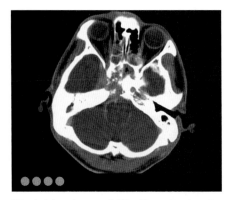

H1. Axial and coronal CT with contrast and bone window images show an enhancing mass involving the clivus with bone destruction. The mass is also seen in the sphenoid sinus and right cavernous sinus.

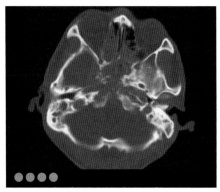

H2. Axial and coronal CT with contrast and bone window images show an enhancing mass involving the clivus with bone destruction. The mass is also seen in the sphenoid sinus and right cavernous sinus.

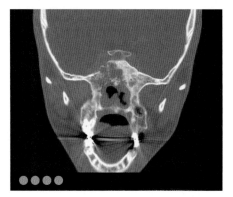

H3. Axial and coronal CT with contrast and bone window images show an enhancing mass involving the clivus with bone destruction. The mass is also seen in the sphenoid sinus and right cavernous sinus.

MENINGIOMA

There is a close relationship between the location of arachnoid granulation and prevalent site of origin of meningioma. They are frequently seen in the parasagittal region, along the convexity, sphenoid, and in the parasellar region. CT scan shows a hyperdense to isodense mass with well-defined margin. Tumor calcification and adjacent bony hyperostosis may be seen.

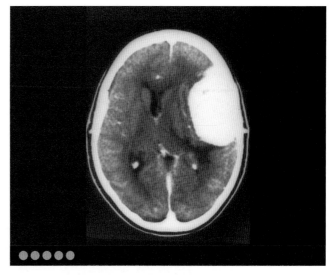

A. Axial post-contrast CT shows a large enhancing mass in the left frontal extradural space with a broad-based attachment to the dura.

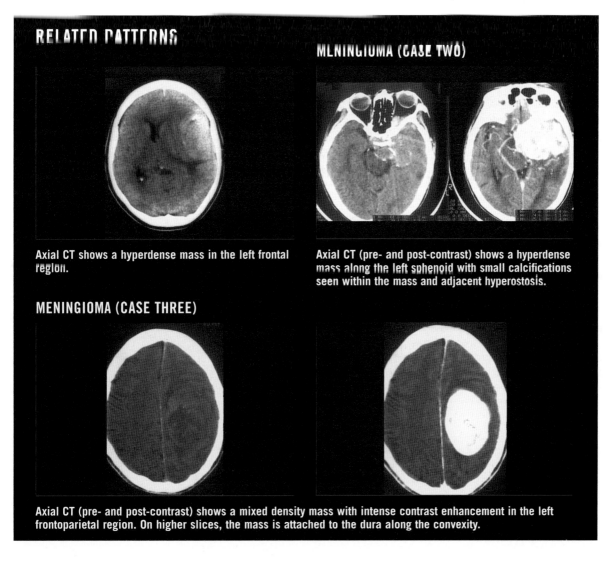

RELATED PATTERNS

Axial CT shows a hyperdense mass in the left frontal region.

MENINGIOMA (CASE TWO)

Axial CT (pre- and post-contrast) shows a hyperdense mass along the left sphenoid with small calcifications seen within the mass and adjacent hyperostosis.

MENINGIOMA (CASE THREE)

Axial CT (pre- and post-contrast) shows a mixed density mass with intense contrast enhancement in the left frontoparietal region. On higher slices, the mass is attached to the dura along the convexity.

DIFFERENTIAL DIAGNOSIS

At a Glance:

- *Hemangiopericytoma*
- *Lymphoma*

- *Metastatic Disease* (not pictured)
- *Plasmacytoma* (not pictured)
- *Sarcoidosis* (not pictured)

HEMANGIOPERICYTOMA

Hemangiopericytoma of the meninges is an aggressive, highly vascular neoplasm. It arises from vascular pericytes and is therefore a distinct entity. On imaging studies, it is a heterogeneous mass with cystic, necrotic areas, and prominent vascular channels. Bony erosion or destruction of the adjacent skull is frequently seen.

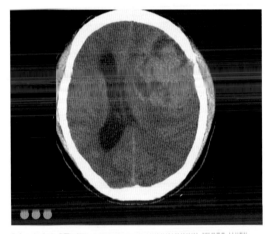

D1. Axial CT demonstrates a hyperdense mass with areas of central necrosis and adjacent bone erosion involving the skull.

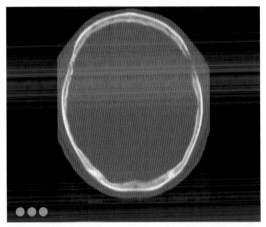

B2 Axial CT demonstrates a hyperdense mass with areas of central necrosis and adjacent bone erosion involving the skull.

LYMPHOMA

Primary non-Hodgkin's lymphomas of the extra-axial location with or without involvement of the skull are rare entities. They may present with a subcutaneous scalp lump clinically. Computed tomography scan shows an intracranial extra axial mass mimicking a meningioma. An associated calvarial lesion with soft tissue scalp swelling may also be seen. The classical CT appearances of lymphoma are of an isodense to hyperdense lesion with contrast enhancement.

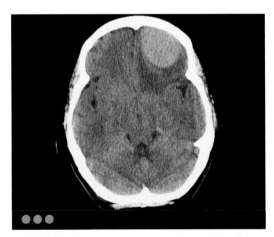

C. Axial CT demonstrates a hyperdense mass with surrounding edema in the left frontal region.

CHONDROSARCOMA

Approximately 10% of chondrosarcoma occur in the bones of the face and skull base. They occur predominantly between 20 and 50 years with a slight male preference of 2:1. They usually arise from different locations associated with sutures.

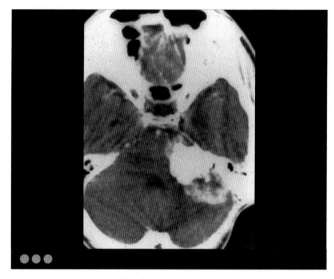

A. Axial, post-contrast CT shows an enhancing mass at the left CPA with calcification.

RELATED PATTERNS
CHONDROSARCOMA (CASE TWO)

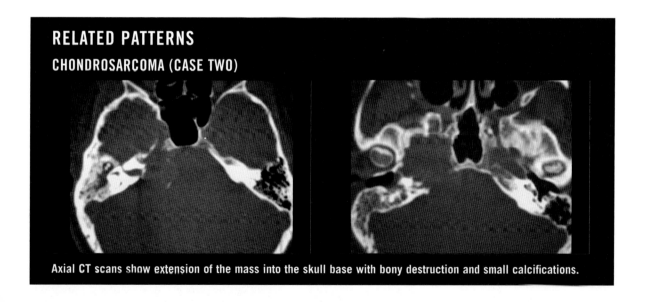

Axial CT scans show extension of the mass into the skull base with bony destruction and small calcifications.

DIFFERENTIAL DIAGNOSIS

At a Glance:

- *Cholesterol Granuloma*
- *Endolymphatic Sac Tumor*
- *Giant Cell Tumor*
- *Hemangiopericytoma*
- *Meningioma*
- *Vestibular Schwannoma*
- *Glomus Tumor* (not pictured)
- *Metastasis* (not pictured)

CHOLESTEROL GRANULOMA

Cholesterol granuloma is a histological term used to describe a tissue response to a foreign body such as cholesterol crystals. Following bleeding into the petrous bone or apex, hemoglobin is degraded and this causes formation and accumulation of cholesterol crystals. It may arise from any portion of the pneumatized temporal bone but most frequently involves the petrous apex.

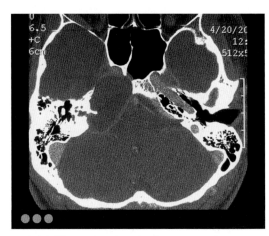

B. Axial CT reveals a low-density mass at the petrous apex associated with bone erosion. A thin rim of bone is seen surrounding the low-density mass.

ENDOLYMPHATIC SAC TUMOR

Endolymphatic sac tumor (ELST) has been known in the past by such synonyms as "Aggressive Papillary Middle Ear Tumor", "Heffner Tumor" and "Low-grade Adenocarcinoma of the Middle Ear." It is a rare neoplasm, affecting both sexes equally. Clinical symptoms include hearing loss and vestibular dysfunctions, facial nerve palsy. On CT, a multilocular mass lesion is seen with lytic changes involving the petrous temporal bone. Although these tumors are rarely seen in the general population, they are frequently found in patients with Von Hippel Lindau disease. Von Hippel-

Lindau disease is the only syndrome that has been identified to be associated with bilateral ELSTs. Endolymphatic sac tumors are usually located near vestibular aqueduct, centered between sigmoid sinus and the internal auditory canal. Involvement of the internal auditory canal, jugular bulb, and mastoid are common, as is erosion of the bone toward the vestibule of the labyrinth. Osseous margins have a geographic or "moth-eaten" appearance. Intratumoral bone appears reticular or spiculated with a thin peripheral rim of calcification. Involvement of the facial nerve and middle or posterior cranial fossa dura is also common.

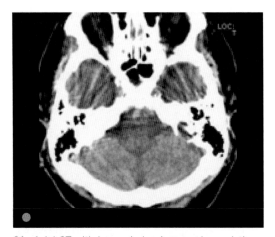

C1. Axial CT with bone window images show a lytic lesions at the left cerebellopontine angle involving the petrous temporal bone. A thin rim of peripheral calcification is seen.

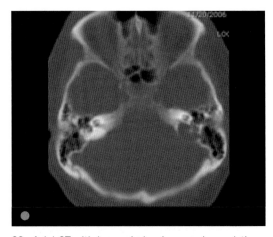

C2. Axial CT with bone window images show a lytic lesions at the left cerebellopontine angle involving the petrous temporal bone. A thin rim of peripheral calcification is seen.

GIANT CELL TUMOR

Giant cell tumor usually involve the long bones and rarely involve the cranium. In the skull, sphenoid bone is the commonest site, followed by temporal bone.

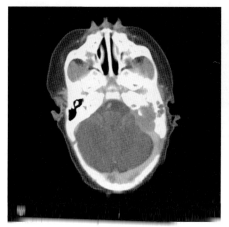 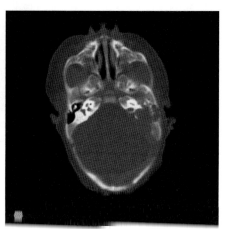

D1. Axial, post-contrast CT and bone window image demonstrates an enhancing mass with bone destruction involving the petrous temporal bone.

D2. Axial, post-contrast CT and bone window image demonstrates an enhancing mass with bone destruction involving the petrous temporal bone.

HEMANGIOPERICYTOMA

Hemangiopericytoma is a rare intracranial tumor that can mimic meningioma based on clinical presentation and imaging findings. Hemagniopericytomas are more likely to cause adjacent bone destruction than meningiomas. Hemangiopericytomas have been observed to occur in a number of intracranial compartments; however, involvement of the cerebellopontine angle is rare.

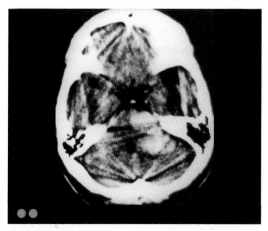 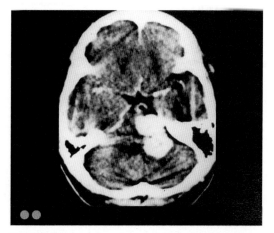

E1. Axial, pre- and post-contrast CT demonstrate a hyperdense mass in the left cerebellopontine angle cistern with intense contrast enhancement.

E2. Axial, pre- and post-contrast CT demonstrate a hyperdense mass in the left cerebellopontine angle cistern with intense contrast enhancement.

MENINGIOMA

Meningiomas in the cerebellopontine angle must be differentiated from schwannomas, which are seven times more common in this location. Meningioma tend to show isodensity on CT images and contrast enhancement is usually homogeneous. A dural tail is associated with meningioma. Schwannomas can involve the internal auditory canal, causing its enlargement. Meningiomas may extend into the internal auditory canal, but does not cause it to enlarge. Cystic changes are more common in schwannomas than meningiomas.

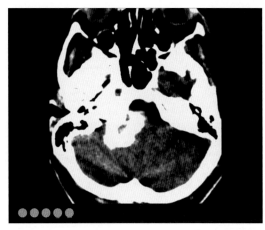

F. Axial, post-contrast CT demonstrates an enhancing mass at the right CPA. Meningioma usually has a broad-based attachment to the dura.

VESTIBULAR SCHWANNOMA

Schwannomas are typically round or ovoid lesions with a small portion extending into the internal auditory canal. Schwannomas tend to show hypodensity on CT images and contrast enhancement may be homogeneous or heterogeneous. Schwannomas can involve the internal auditory canal, causing its enlargement. Cystic changes are more common in schwannomas than meningiomas.

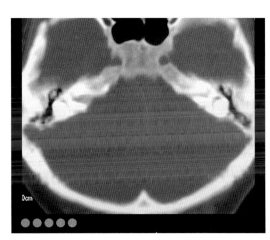

G. Axial CT with bone window shows widening of the right internal canal secondary to a vestibular schwannoma.

ESTHESIONEUROBLASTOMA

Esthesioneuroblastoma is a rare, malignant neoplasm arising from the olfactory epithelium located in the upper part of the nasal cavities. Molecular studies indicate basal progenitor cells of the olfactory epithelium as the origin of esthesioneuroblastoma. It represents 1–5% of malignant neoplasms of the nasal cavity. Clinical symptoms include epistaxis, nasal obstruction, and craniofacial pain.

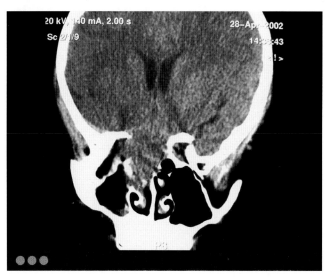

A. Coronal CT demonstrates a mass extending from ethmoid sinuses through the cribriform plate into the frontal fossa with bony destruction.

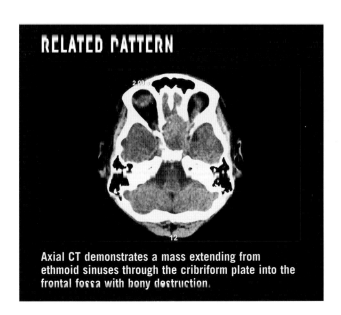

RELATED PATTERN

Axial CT demonstrates a mass extending from ethmoid sinuses through the cribriform plate into the frontal fossa with bony destruction.

DIFFERENTIAL DIAGNOSIS

At a Glance:

- *Juvenile Angiofibroma*
- *Lymphoma*
- *Sphenoid/Ethmoid Sinus Neoplasm (Adenoid Cystic Carcinoma)*
- *Chondrosarcoma* (not pictured)
- *Encephalocele* (not pictured)
- *Giant Cell Tumor* (not pictured)
- *Meningioma* (not pictured)
- *Metastasis* (not pictured)

JUVENILE ANGIOFIBROMA

Juvenile angiofibroma occurs adjacent to the sphenopalatine foramen in the nasal cavity. Large tumors are frequently bi-lobed or dumbbell-shaped, with one portion of the tumor filling the nasopharynx and the other portion extending to the pterygopalatine fossa. Lateral spread of the tumor is directed toward the pterygopalatine fossa, bowing the posterior wall of the maxillary sinus. Involvement of the cribriform plate is unusual.

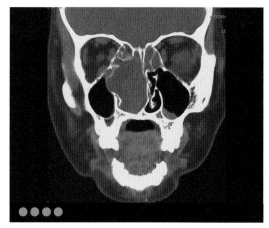

B1. Coronal and axial CT scans show a mass lesion involving the nasal cavity, ethmoid and sphenoid sinus in the region of cribriform plate.

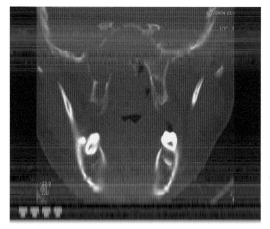

B2. Coronal and axial CT scans show a mass lesion involving the nasal cavity, ethmoid and sphenoid sinus in the region of cribriform plate.

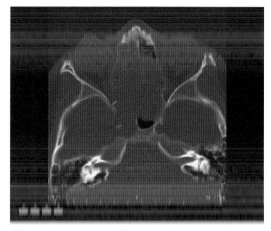

B3. Coronal and axial CT scans show a mass lesion involving the nasal cavity, ethmoid and sphenoid sinus in the region of cribriform plate.

LYMPHOMA

Lymphoid lesions of the head and neck mainly are seen in four areas: (1) Waldeyer's ring, (2) nasal and paranasal sinus, (3) oral cavity and (4) salivary glands. Each site is affected by lymphoid proliferation that is concordant with the biology of local lymphocytes. The nasal cavity and paranasal sinuses are the typical site of extranodal T-cell lymphoma, nasal type, a proliferation of cytotoxic, EBV infected cells. This lesion is sometimes difficult to distinguish from inflammatory, granulomatous processes, such as Wegener disease.

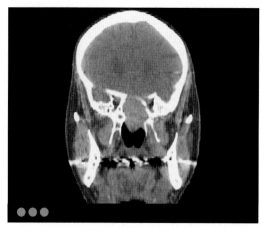

C. Coronal CT demonstrates a mass in the ethmoid and sphenoid sinus invading and destroying the cribriform plate.

SPHENOID/ETHMOID SINUS NEOPLASM (ADENOID CYSTIC CARCINOMA)

Although adenoid cystic carcinoma is a relatively common head and neck tumor, it is relatively rare in the ethmoid sinus. The tumor is slow growing, locally aggressive and associated with frequent recurrences. It is of particular interest due to its tendency to locally infiltrate neural structures and to spread perineurally. Intracranial involvement is reported as rare.

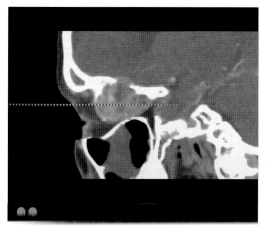

D1. Sagittal, post-contrast CT scan shows a mass lesion extending from the right ethmoid sinus into the right orbit with bone destruction of the orbital roof and cribriform plate.

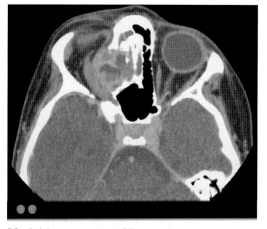

D2. Axial, post-contrast CT scan shows a mass lesion extending from the right ethmoid sinus into the right orbit with bone destruction of the orbital roof and cribriform plate.

LIPOMA

Lipomas are believed to result from the maldifferentiation of the meninx primitiva during the formation of the subarachnoid cistern and are associated with dysgenesis of the adjacent cerebral tissue in 55% of the cases. Their common locations include dorsal pericallosal, quadrigeminal cistern, superior vermian cistern, suprasellar cistern, cerebellopontine angle cistern, and sylvian fissure. On CT, they usually present a low-density mass of fat attenuation. Calcification is occasionally seen.

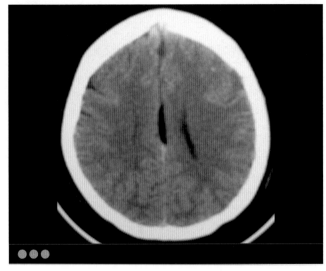

A. Axial CT demonstrates a low-density mass along the interhemispheric fissure, consistent with a lipoma. Its density is lower than the CSF in the adjacent lateral ventricle.

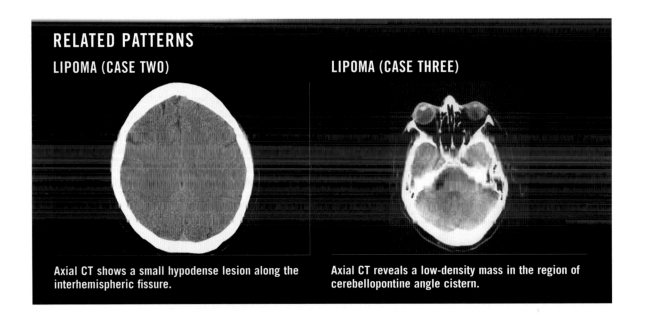

RELATED PATTERNS

LIPOMA (CASE TWO)

Axial CT shows a small hypodense lesion along the interhemispheric fissure.

LIPOMA (CASE THREE)

Axial CT reveals a low-density mass in the region of cerebellopontine angle cistern.

DIFFERENTIAL DIAGNOSIS

At a Glance:

- *Arachnoid Cyst*
- *CPA Epidermoid*
- *Frontal Dermoid*
- *Suprasellar Dermoid*

ARACHNOID CYST

Arachnoid cysts are extra-axial lesions that contain cerebrospinal fluid. They can grow slowly over time, causing remodeling of the adjacent skull. Arachnoid cysts arise from a splitting arachnoid membrane during its development. The most common location for arachnoid cysts is middle cranial fossa, followed by posterior fossa, suprasellar region, convexity, interhemispheric fissure in decreasing oeder.

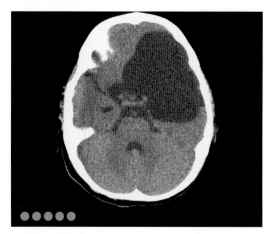

B. Axial CT shows a cystic lesion in the left fronto-temporal region.

CPA EPIDERMOID

Epidermoid cysts are benign congenital lesions of ectodermal origin. They consist of approximately 1% of all intracranial masses. Although these lesions are congenital, patients are usually not symptomatic until they are young or middle aged adults. On CT, they have a dirty CSF appearance.

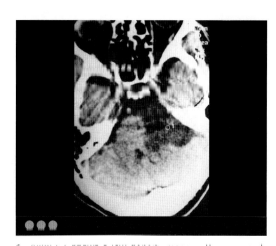

C. Axial CT shows a low-density mass in the region of left cerebellopontine angle cistern.

FRONTAL DERMOID

Intracranial **dermoids** are rare lesions and they are one-fifth as common as epidermoids. They are congenital tumors, but they only become symptomatic during the third decade of life due to their slow growth. Common locations include fourth ventricle, vermian, suprasellar, parasellar, subfrontal, and the facial region. **Dermoids** are composed of ectodermal elements and are lined with stratified squamous epithelium with skin appendage such as hair follicles, sebaceous and sweat glands.

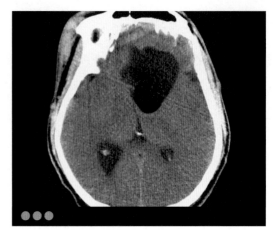

D. Axial CT shows a low-density mass in the left frontal region.

SUPRASELLAR DERMOID

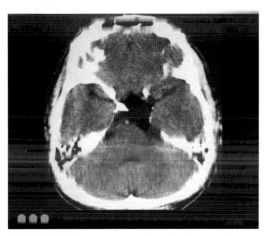

E1. Axial CT demonstrates a low-density mass in the suprasellar cistern with peripheral calcification on the left side. The low density is much lower than the CSF in the fourth ventricle.

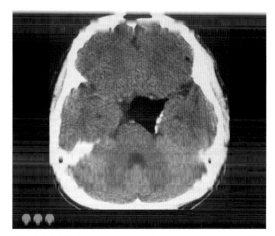

E2. Axial CT demonstrates a low-density mass in the suprasellar cistern with peripheral calcification on the left side. The low density is much lower than the CSF in the fourth ventricle.

Chapter 16

Intracerebral Masses

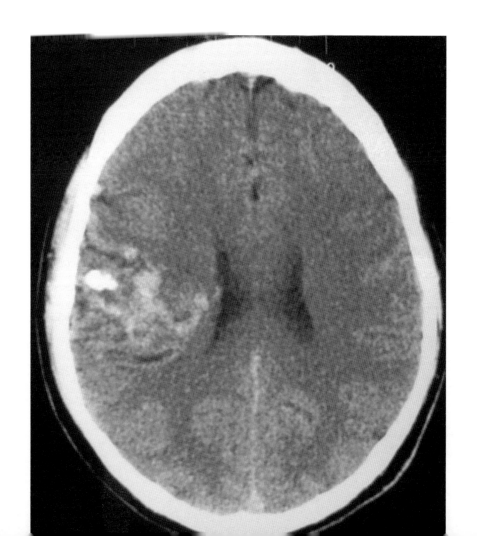

OLIGODENDROGLIOMA

There is a wide range of grades within the category of oligo-dendroglioma due to the tumor's heterogeneity of histopathology. Calcification is demonstrated in 50–90% of cases on CT. The tumor is a hypodense-to-isodense mass with foci of calcification or hemorrhage. About half of the tumor will show contrast enhancement and the other half will not enhance.

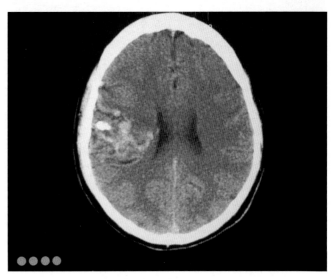

A. Axial CT demonstrates a right temporal, parietal, cortical based mass with curvilinear hyperdensity and calcification. There is minimal mass effect and no surrounding edema.

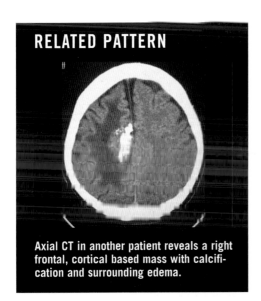

RELATED PATTERN

Axial CT in another patient reveals a right frontal, cortical based mass with calcification and surrounding edema.

DIFFERENTIAL DIAGNOSIS

At a Glance:

• *Ganglioglioma*

• *Low Grade Astrocytoma*

• *Dysembryoplastic Neuroepithelial Tumor (DNET)*

GANGLIOGLIOMA

Gangliogliomas are predominantly seen in children and young adults. They are the most common mixed glioneural tumors. Seizure is the most common clinical presentation.

Their common locations include temporal lobes, frontal lobes, anterior third ventricle, and cerebellum. They are typically hypodense or isodense on CT and appear cystic in up to 50% of the cases. Calcification and faint contrast enhancement may be seen.

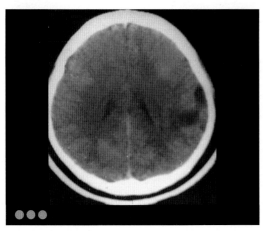

B1. Axial CT shows a cortical based mass of mixed density with solid and cystic components in the left frontal region.

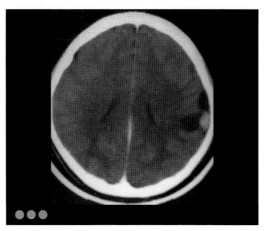

B2. Axial, post-contrast CT demonstrates a left frontal cortical based mass with an enhancing solid component and adjacent cystic components.

LOW-GRADE ASTROCYTOMA

Astrocytomas may show low density or isodensity on CT. Peritumoral edema is absent or minimal. Tumor calcification is detected in 20% of astrocytomas. The pattern of

contrast enhancement is quite variable with 40% of low-grade **astrocytomas** exhibiting some degree of contrast enhancement.

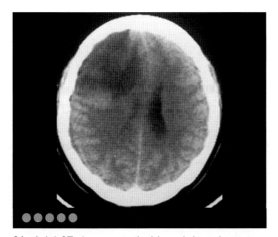

C1. Axial CT shows a cortical based, hypodense mass in the right frontal region.

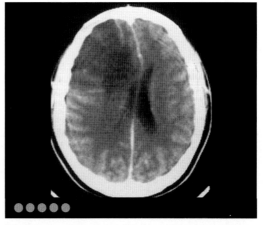

C2. Axial, post-contrast CT demonstrates no abnormal enhancement of the cortical based mass in the right frontal region.

605

DYSEMBRYOPLASTIC NEUROEPITHELIAL TUMOR (DNET)

DNET are most commonly seen in the temporal and frontal lobes. They are neuroepithelial tumors that present in patients with seizure in their second or third decade. They are superficially located and cortically based masses, often associated with underlying skull remodeling. The mass is hypodense on CT and grows very slowly. There is usually no surrounding edema. Focal cortical dysplasia can be associated with **DNET** in approximately 50% of the cases.

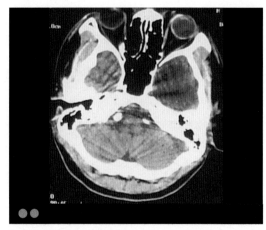

D. Axial CT shows a low-density mass in the left temporal lobe with slight expansion of the bony temporal fossa.

OLIGODENDROGLIOMA

These tumors typically involve the cerebral cortex and the subcortical white matter in the frontal and frontotemporal region. The tumor is hypodense to isodense with foci of calcification or hemorrhage. About half of the tumor will show contrast enhancement and the other half will not enhance. Cystic changes are frequently seen in oligodendroglioma. Peritumoral edema is mild or absent.

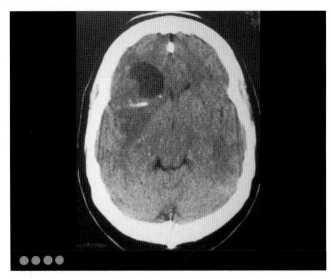

A. Axial CT demonstrates a cystic mass with adjacent calcifications in the right frontal lobe with mild surrounding edema.

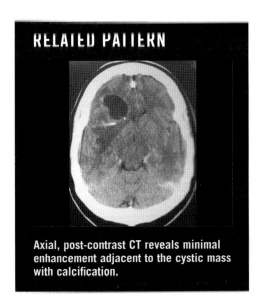

RELATED PATTERN

Axial, post-contrast CT reveals minimal enhancement adjacent to the cystic mass with calcification.

DIFFERENTIAL DIAGNOSIS

At a Glance:

- *Arachnoid Cyst*
- *Cysticercosis*
- *Echinococcus*
- *Ganglioglioma (Same Case as in Cortical Based Mass)*
- *Metastasis*
- *Pilocytic Astrocytoma*
- *Neuroepithelial cyst* (not pictured)

ARACHNOID CYST

Arachnoid cysts are benign cysts that occur in the central nervous system in relation to the arachnoid membrane. Arachnoid cysts usually contain clear, cerebrospinal fluid and do not communicate with the ventricular system. Most are developmental anomalies. A small number of arachnoid cysts may be acquired, such as those occurring in association with schwannomas or meningiomas, secondary to previous leptomeningitis, hemorrhage, or surgery. The majority of arachnoid cysts (50–60%) occur in the middle cranial fossa.

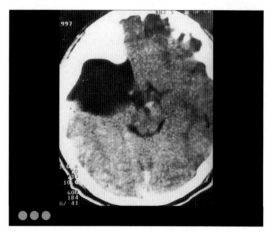

B. Axial CT shows a cystic lesion at the anterior aspect of the right temporal fossa without significant mass effect.

CYSTICERCOSIS

There are four stages of parenchymal cysticercosis cysts, namely, vesicular, colloidal vesicular, granular nodular and nodular calcified stages. In the vesicular stage, the cysts show very thin wall and clear fluid with a scolex. No contrast enhancement or edema is seen in this stage. In the colloidal vesicular stage, the cyst fluid becomes turbid and a ring-like enhancement is seen with surrounding edema. Scolex may not be seen due to cyst degeneration. In the nodular calcified stage, an enhancing nodule is seen with surrounding edema. In the nodular calcified stage, a calcific area is seen as a residua of the lesion.

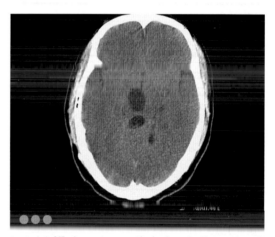

C. Axial CT shows two cystic lesions in the region of thalamus and midbrain due to cysticercosis.

ECHINOCOCCUS

Echinococcus is a parasitic disease. Echinococcus is the general term for three diseases caused by the larval stage of *Echinococcus* tapeworms. *Echinococcus granulosus* causes cystic echinococcus and is seen worldwide, in the rural areas. *Echinococcus multilocularis* causes alveolar disease and is seen only in the northern hemisphere. *Echinococcus vogeli* causes polycystic echinococcus and is seen in Central and South America.

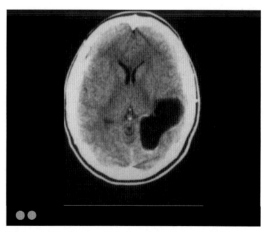

D. Axial CT shows a lobulated cystic mass with partial rim calcification in the left temporal, parieto-occipital region.

GANGLIOGLIOMA (SAME CASE AS IN CORTICAL BASED MASS)

Cystic appearance of **ganglioglioma** is seen in up to 50% of the cases.

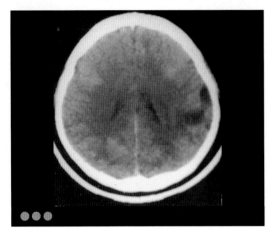

E1. Axial CT shows a cortical based mass of mixed density with solid and cystic components in the left frontal region.

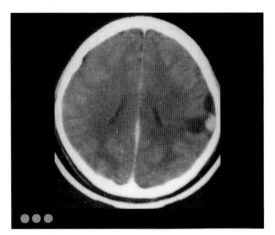

E2. Axial, post contrast CT demonstrates a left frontal cortical based mass with an enhancing solid component and apparent cystic component.

METASTASIS

Metastases are the most common masses in the supratentorial compartment in adults, consisting of 40% of intracranial neoplasms supratentorially. Approximately half of the metastatic lesions are solitary and the other half are multiple. Cystic metastases favor lung, breast, and gastrointestinal primary sites.

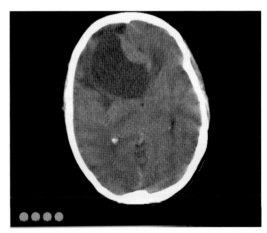

F. Axial CT shows a large cystic mass in the right frontal lobe with a solid component seen at its anterior medial aspect.

PILOCYTIC ASTROCYTOMA

Astrocytomas account for approximately 80% of intracranial gliomas and are the most common supratentorial tumor in all age groups. Astrocytomas are often divided into circumscribed or infiltrating tumors. Pilocytic astrocytomas and subependymal giant-cell astrocytomas are in the circumscribed group because they do not invade the surrounding structures. Pilocytic astrocytomas are usually located infratentorially and generally well circumscribed and often cystic. Supratentorial pilocytic astrocytomas are usually solid, cystic ones are unusual.

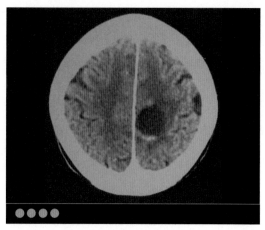

G. Axial, post-contrast CT shows a ring-like cystic lesion with partial rim enhancement.

OLIGODENDROGLIOMA

Calcification is demonstrated in 50–90% of **oligoden-drogliomas** on CT. The tumor is a hypodense-to-isodense mass with foci of calcification or hemorrhage.

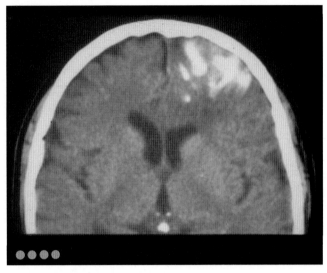

A. Axial CT shows a left frontal mass with calcification and minimal surrounding edema.

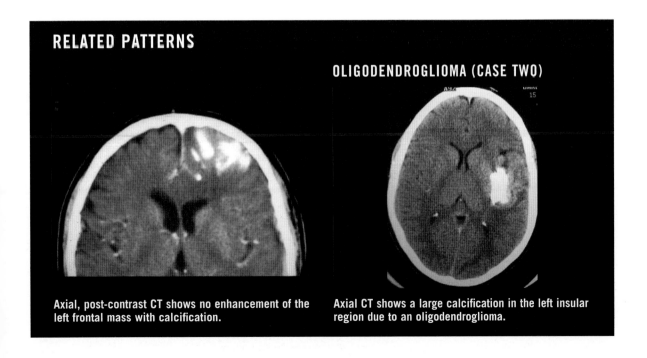

RELATED PATTERNS

OLIGODENDROGLIOMA (CASE TWO)

Axial, post-contrast CT shows no enhancement of the left frontal mass with calcification.

Axial CT shows a large calcification in the left insular region due to an oligodendroglioma.

ARTERIOVENOUS MALFORMATION

Arteriovenous malformations are the most common and most important congenital vascular anomaly. They are almost always solitary; a small number (2%) may be multiple. Approximately 80–90% of parenchymal **arteriovenous malformations** are supratentorial. They may occur anywhere in the brain, but a classic appearance is one in which the malformation has a wedge shape, with its base near the brain surface and its apex toward the ventricle. A non-contrast CT is useful in identifying calcification associated with AVM and acute hemorrhage.

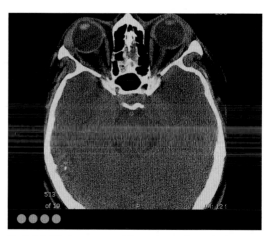

B. Axial CT shows a curvilinear hyperdense lesion with a small calcification in the right temporal region.

CALCIFIED ANEURYSM

A giant aneurysm (2.5 cm in diameter) can bleed just like any aneurysm. However, they tend to cause local mass effect and thrombus formation. Calcification is more common with giant aneurysms. A calcified giant aneurysm with thick wall or thrombus may not be treated easily with surgical clipping. Opening of the aneurysm and removing intra-aneurysmal clot may be necessary.

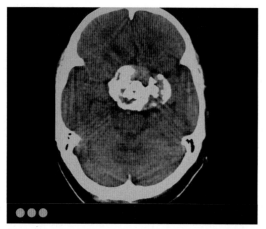

C1. Axial CT shows a large mass in the suprasellar region with calcification.

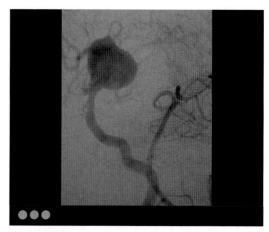

C2. A lateral veiw of the cerebral angiogram reveals a giant aneurysm in the supraclinoid internal carotid artery.

CAVERNOUS MALFORMATION

Cavernous angiomas are congenital vascular hamartomas composed of closely approximated endothelial-lined sinusoidal collections without significant amounts of interspersed neural tissue. Histopathologically, cavernous angiomas are characteristically lack of intervening neural tissue, whereas capillary telangiectasias exhibit significant amount of intervening neural tissue.

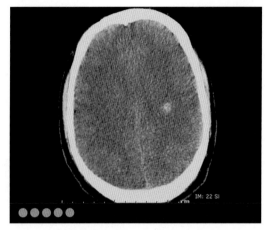

D. Axial CT demonstrates a round hyperdense lesion with specks of calcification.

DNET

DNETs are superficially located and cortically based masses, often associated with underlying skull remodeling. The mass is hypodense on CT and grows very slowly. There is usually no surrounding edema. Occasionally, calcification is seen within the mass.

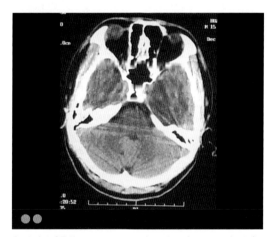

E. Axial CT demonstrates a low-density mass in left temporal lobe with specks of calcification.

EPENDYMOMA

Ependymomas constitute 2–6% of all gliomas. Only 40% of intracranial ependymomas occur in the supratentorial compartment. The reported incidence of parenchymal origin of the ependymomas varies from 55–85%.

EPENDYMOMA (CASE ONE)

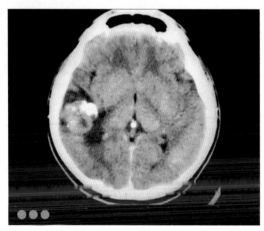

F1. Axial, pre- and post-contrast CT demonstrates a right temporal calcified mass with minimal contrast enhancement.

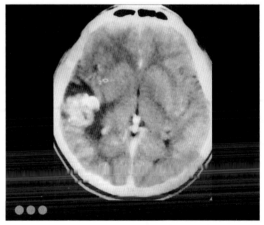

F2. Axial, pre- and post-contrast CT demonstrates a right temporal calcified mass with minimal contrast enhancement.

EPENDYMOMA (CASE TWO)

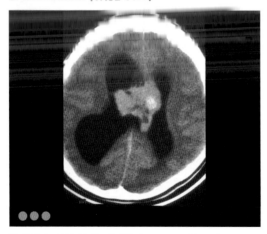

G. Axial, post-contrast CT shows an enhancing mass with calcification in the lateral ventricles, which are dilated.

GANGLIOCYTOMA

Ganglioglioma contains both glial and neuronal components and can undergo malignant degeneration (rarely). **Gangliocytoma** is composed entirely of neuronal components and is completely benign. Both occur primarily in children and young adults and affect the temporal lobes and cerebellum. One-third to one-half of gangliogliomas appear cystic; one-third have calcifications. **Gangliocytoma** is hyperdense on CT.

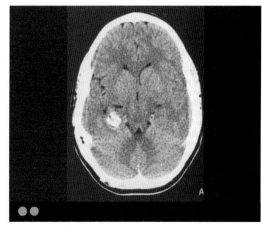

H. Axial CT shows a calcified mass in the region of right hippocampal formation.

GANGLIOGLIOMA

Gangliogliomas are typically hypodense or isodense on CT and appear cystic in up to 50% of the cases. Calcification is seen in 30% of the cases and faint contrast enhancement is seen in 50% of the cases.

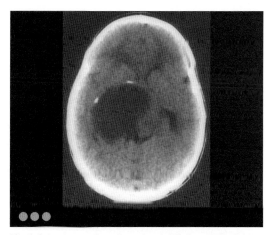

I1. Axial, pre- and post-contrast CT demonstrates a large low-density mass with small specks of calcification. Intense contrast enhancement is seen on the post-contrast image.

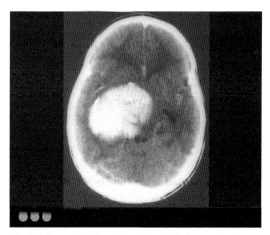

I2. Axial, pre- and post-contrast CT demonstrates a large low-density mass with small specks of calcification. Intense contrast enhancement is seen on the post-contrast image.

LOW-GRADE ASTROCYTOMA

Low-grade astrocytomas constitute about 25% of all cerebral gliomas. Peak incidence of low-grade astrocytoma is between the ages of 20 and 40 years and is generally 10 years below that for glioblastoma. **Astrocytomas** may show low density or isodensity on CT. Peritumoral edema is absent or minimal. Tumor calcification is detected in 20% of **astrocytomas.** In fact, the most common supratentorial tumor with calcification is **low-grade astrocytoma,** although oligodendroglioma has the highest frequency of calcification. The pattern of contrast enhancement is quite variable with 40% of **low-grade astrocytomas** exhibiting some degree of contrast enhancement.

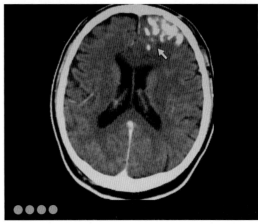

J. Axial CT shows a faintly enhancing mass with extensive calcification in the left frontal region.

MENINGIOANGIOMATOSIS

Meningioangiomatosis (MA) is a benign cerebral lesion characterized by leptomeningeal calcification and meningovascular proliferation. The commonest finding of **MA** on CT scan was a calcified, enhancing lesion with surrounding low density. **MA** usually appears in young patients and focal seizures and/or headaches are the most common presenting symptoms. **Meningioangiomatosis** may be associated with neurofibromatosis type I in 15% of the cases; the majority of MA is sporadic in nature.

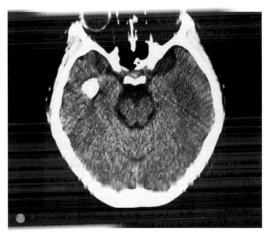

K. Axial CT shows a round calcific density in the right temporal lobe, due to meningioangiomatosis.

METASTATIC OSTEOSARCOMA

Metastatic osteosarcoma to the brain is rare. However, when an intracranial mass with calcification is seen, metastatic osteosarcoma should be included in the differential diagnosis.

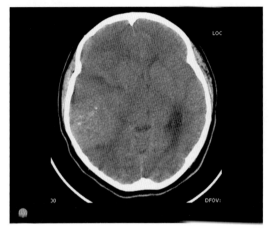

L1. Axial CT scans demonstrate a large, slightly heterogeneously hyperdense mass with faint calcification and a cystic component.

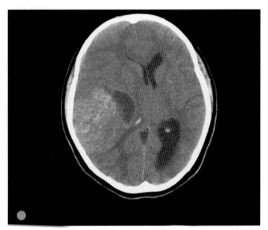

L2, Axial CT scans demonstrate a large, slightly heterogeneously hyperdense mass with faint calcification and a cystic component.

PILOCYTIC ASTROCYTOMA

Pilocytic astrocytomas in the supratentorial compartment tend to occur in the region of diencephalon, including the hypothalamus, visual pathway, optic chiasm, and basal ganglia. Cerebral location of the **pilocytic astrocytoma** is unusual. **Pilocytic astrocytomas** are cystic or multicystic, with a mural nodule in 55% of the cases and solid in 45% of the cases. Occasionally, calcification may be seen.

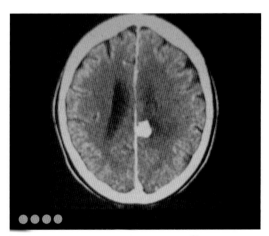

M. Axial CT shows a calcified mass with minimal surrounding edema in the left posterior frontal lobe.

617

METASTASIS

Since there is no blood–brain barrier involving metastatic disease, almost all the metastases show contrast enhancement, but the pattern may be solid, ring-like, irregular, homogeneous, or heterogeneous.

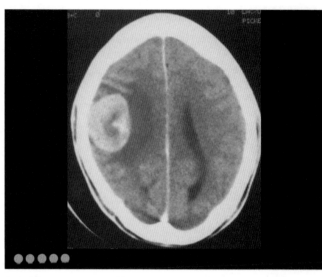

A. Axial, post-contrast CT shows a heterogeneously enhancing mass with a central low density and surrounding edema in the right frontal region. This is a case of metastatic melanoma.

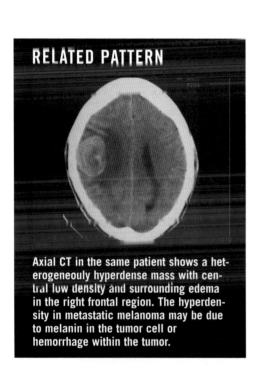

RELATED PATTERN

Axial CT in the same patient shows a heterogeneouly hyperdense mass with central low density and surrounding edema in the right frontal region. The hyperdensity in metastatic melanoma may be due to melanin in the tumor cell or hemorrhage within the tumor.

DIFFERENTIAL DIAGNOSIS

At a Glance:

- *Arteriovenous Malformation (AVM)*
- *Glioblastoma Multiforme*
- *Anaplastic Astrocytoma* (not pictured)
- *Ependymoma* (not pictured)

ARTERIOVENOUS MALFORMATION (AVM)

Arteriovenous malfromation consists of dilated feeding arteries, a nidus, and dilated draining veins. Associated aneurysms may be seen along the feeding arteries and draining veins. On CT, They are identified as curvilinear hyperdense areas intermixed with hypodense areas and calcification.

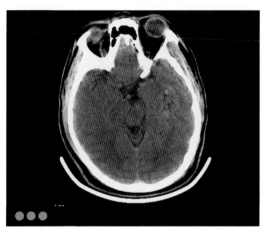

B1. Axial CT demonstrates a mass of heterogeneous density in the left temporal lobe. Heterogeneous contrast enhancement is usually seen (not shown here).

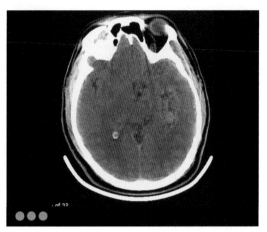

B2. Axial CT demonstrates a mass of heterogeneous density in the left temporal lobe. Heterogeneous contrast enhancement is usually seen (not shown here).

GLIOBLASTOMA MULTIFORME

GBMs tend to occur in elderly patients and clinical course is short, usually a few months. Secondary **GBMs** that arise from malignant dedifferentiation of AAs or low-grade astrocytomas tend to occur in younger age group and have a more retracted course over a few years. On CT, **GBMs** present as a necrotic mass with foci of hemorrhage. Patchy, irregular contrast enhancement is seen. Extensive surrounding edema is seen and tumor cells may be present in the areas of edema. Relative cerebral blood volume (rCBV) correlates with astrocytomas grade and vascularity on perfusion studies.

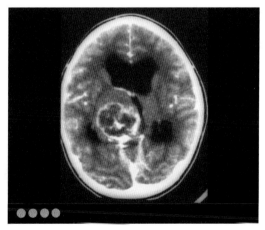

C. Axial, post-contrast CT demonstrates a multi-ring-like enhancing mass in the right thalamus with significant mass effect.

GBM (CASE TWO)

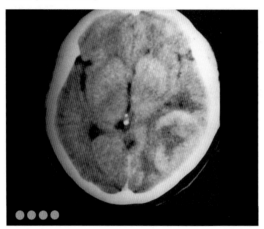

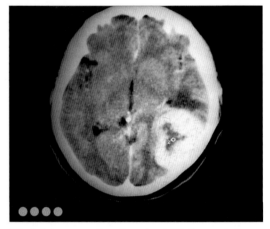

D1. Axial, pre- and post-contrast CT demonstrate a mixed density mass in the left temporal lobe with surrounding edema and heterogeneous contrast enhancment.

D2. Axial, pre- and post-contrast CT demonstrate a mixed density mass in the left temporal lobe with surrounding edema and heterogeneous contrast enhancment.

GBM (CASE THREE)

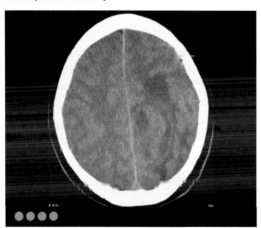

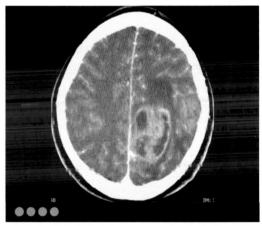

E1. Axial, pre- and post-contrast CT show a heterogeneous mass with irregular contrast enhancement and surrounding edema in the left frontoparietal, parasagittal region.

E2. Axial, pre- and post-contrast CT show a heterogeneous mass with irregular contrast enhancement and surrounding edema in the left frontoparietal, parasagittal region.

LYMPHOMA

About 10% of the patients with systemic lymphoma develop CNS involvement in clinical series, and secondary CNS lymphoma may be found in up to 26% of the cases in autopsy series. Primary CNS lymphomas are more common than secondary CNS lymphomas. Approximately 20–40% of lesions are multiple.

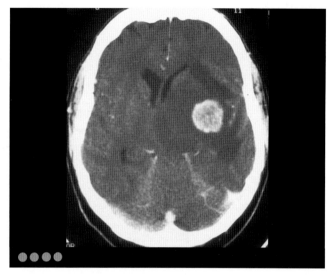

A. Axial, post-contrast CT image shows a large nodular enhancing mass in the left basal ganglia with surrounding edema.

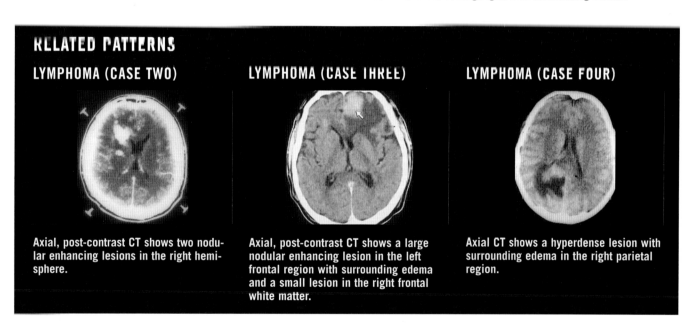

RELATED PATTERNS

LYMPHOMA (CASE TWO)

Axial, post-contrast CT shows two nodular enhancing lesions in the right hemisphere.

LYMPHOMA (CASE THREE)

Axial, post-contrast CT shows a large nodular enhancing lesion in the left frontal region with surrounding edema and a small lesion in the right frontal white matter.

LYMPHOMA (CASE FOUR)

Axial CT shows a hyperdense lesion with surrounding edema in the right parietal region.

DIFFERENTIAL DIAGNOSIS

At a Glance:

- *Aneurysm*
- *Cavernous Angioma*
- *Metastasis*
- *Vein of Galen Malformation*
- *Venous Malformation*

- *Cysticercosis* (not pictured)
- *Granuloma* (not pictured)
- *Histoplasmosis* (not pictured)
- *Multiple Sclerosis* (not pictured)
- *Sarcoidosis* (not pictured)
- *Toxoplasmosis* (not pictured)
- *Tuberculosis* (not pictured)

ANEURYSM

Intracranial aneurysms can be divided into developmental, infectious, traumatic and athrosclerotic types. Developmental aneurysms are most frequently seen at the bifurcation of major vessels whereas infectious and traumatic aneurysms tend to occur at the distal branches of the secondary vessels.

ANEURYSM (CASE ONE)

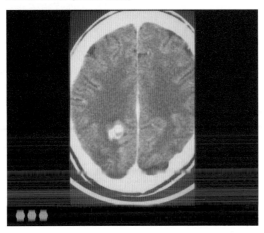

B1. Axial, post-contrast CT shows a nodular enhancing lesion in the left frontal region.

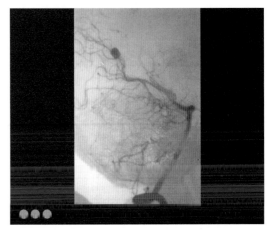

B2. Cerebral angiogram with vertebral injection demonstrates an aneurysm arising from a branch of posterior cerebral artery. This is a case of infectious aneurysm.

ANEURYSM (CASE TWO)

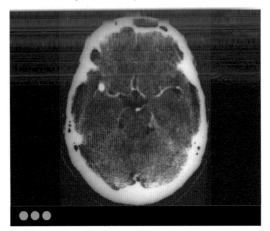

C1. Axial, post-contrast CT shows a nodular enhancing lesion in the region of right middle cerebral artery bifurcation.

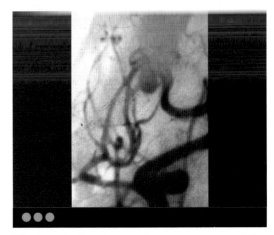

C2. A cerebral angiogram shows an aneurysm at the right middle cerebral artery bifurcation.

CAVERNOUS ANGIOMA

There are four types of vascular malformation, namely, arteriovenous malformation, cavernous angioma, capillary telangiectasia and developmental venous anomaly. Cavernous malformation are usually intra-axial in location, but they may be seen in extra-axial location, such as cavernous sinus.

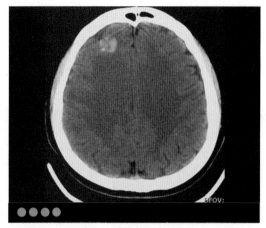

D. Axial CT shows a hyperdense lesion in the right frontal lobe.

METASTASIS

Intracranial metastatic disease is usually secondary to cancer of the lung and breast, followed by melanoma. About slightly less than half of the metastatic lesions are solitary and more than half are multiple. They may appear as nodular, or ring like enhancing lesions on contrast enhanced CT

METASTASIS (CASE ONE)

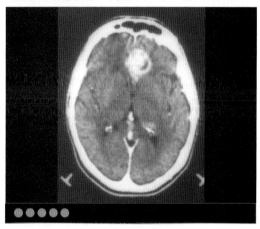

E. Axial post-contrast CT image shows an enhancing mass in the left frontal region.

METASTASIS (CASE TWO)

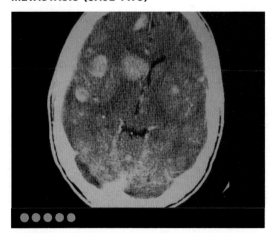

F1. Axial, post-contrast CT scan demonstrates multiple nodular enhancing lesions in both hemispheres in a patient with melanoma.

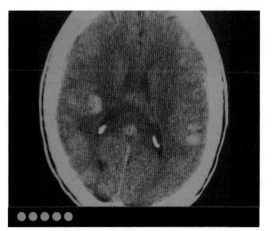

F2. Axial, post-contrast CT scan demonstrates multiple nodular enhancing lesions in both hemispheres in a patient with melanoma.

VEIN OF GALEN MALFORMATION

Vein of Galen Malformation is defined as an artriovenous fistula that drains into the vein of Galen, resulting in marked dilatation of the vein of Galen. The congenital malformation occurs during the 6–11 weeks of fetal gestational age. They are frequently seen in children and may cause high output cardiac failure due to rapid arteriovenous shunting in the newborns.

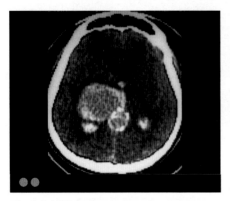

G1. Axial CT demonstrates a hyperdense, bilobular lesion with peripheral calcification in the region of vein of Galen

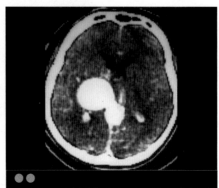

G2. Axial, post-contrast CT shows intense enhancement of the lesion.

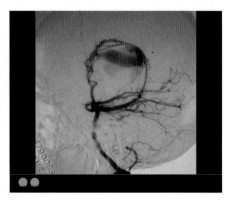

G3. A lateral view of vertebral angiogram reveals early filling in the vein of Galen malformation.

VENOUS MALFORMATION

Venous malformation is due to abnormal dilatation of the deep draining vein that drains the normal deep white matter. They may be associated with cavernous malformation and cavernous malformation is the usual source of hemorrhage.

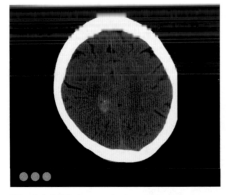

H1. Axial CT demonstrates a hyperdense lesion in the right centrum semiovale.

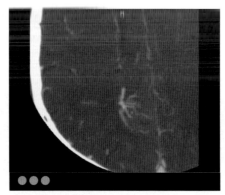

H2. CTA axial image reveals a developmental venous anomaly in the right frontal region.

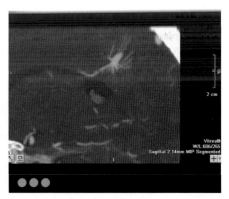

H3. CTA sagittal image reveals a developmental venous anomaly in the right frontal region.

ABSCESS

The most distinctive feature of abscess on imaging is the presence of a smooth, thin capsule with a moderate amount of cerebral edema. It is located at the corticomedullary junction and usually extends into the white matter. The abscess cavity has necrosis and liquefaction within its center. Contrast-enhanced CT scans show ring-like enhancement, which is usually thin and uniform in thickness. Occasionally, thick irregular ring enhancement may be seen—especially following partial treatment—and may mimic neoplasm.

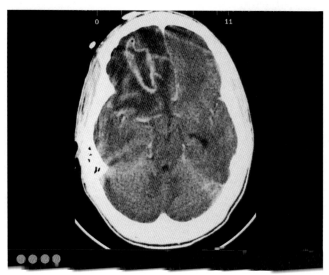

A, Axial post-contrast CT shows a ring-like enhancing lesion with surrounding edema in the right frontal region.

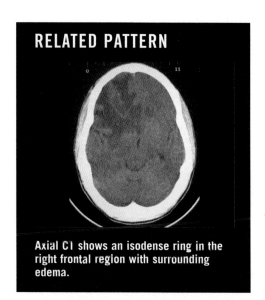

RELATED PATTERN

Axial CT shows an isodense ring in the right frontal region with surrounding edema.

DIFFERENTIAL DIAGNOSIS

At a Glance:

- *Metastasis*

- *Nocardia*

- *Toxoplasmosis*

- *Astrocytoma* (not pictured)

- *Cysticercosis* (not pictured)

- *Lymphoma* (not pictured)

- *Multiple Sclerosis* (not pictured)

- *Tuberculosis* (not pictured)

METASTASIS

The incidence of brain metastasis is rising with the increase in survival of cancer patients as a result of significant advances in cancer diagnosis and treatment. Approximately 40% of intracranial neoplasms are metastatic in nature. Multiple, large autopsy series suggest that, in order of decreasing frequency, lung, breast, melanoma, kidney and colon are the common primary sites. The most common location of brain metastasis is cerebrum (80–85%), followed by the cerebellum (10–15%), and the brain stem (3–5%). In more than half of the metastatic disease, lesions are multiple; solitary metastatic lesion is less common. Primary tumors that tend to produce multiple metastatic lesions include melanoma, lung and breast tumors. Intracranial metastases may be categorized by location as skull, dura, leptomeninges, and parenchymal brain metastases. Lesions of the brain and leptomeninges account for the majority (80%) of intracranial metastases.

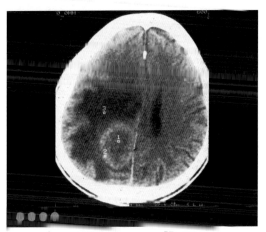

B1. Axial, pre-and post-contrast CT demonstrate a ring-like enhancing lesion with central low density and surrounding edema.

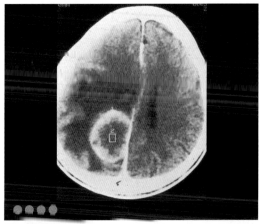

B2. Axial, pre-and post-contrast CT demonstrate a ring-like enhancing lesion with central low density and surrounding edema.

NOCARDIA

Nocardiosis is an uncommon bacterial disease that has traditionally been included in medical mycology. **Nocardia asteroides** is usually the causative organism. **Nocardia** is found in the soil worldwide. Nocardiosis occurs mostly in immunocompromised patients, patients with diabetes, and those with collagen-vascular disease or preexisting pulmonary disease. The organism is airborne, and the primary focus of infection is usually pulmonary. CNS involvement is usually secondary to hematogenous spread of pulmonary disease, and occurs in about 25% of patients. The most common manifestation is abscess formation, which may be multiple.

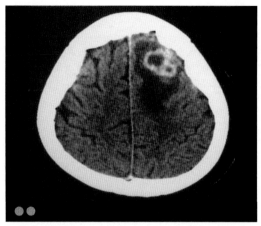

C. Axial, post-contrast CT demonstrates a ring-like enhancing lesion with an adjacent small ring in the left frontal region.

TOXOPLASMOSIS

Toxoplasma gondii infection of the CNS is seen in immunocompromised patients, including those with AIDS. The common locations are the basal ganglia and thalami. But they can be seen at the gray–white matter junction. Typically, ring-like enhancement is seen, but nodular enhancement or no enhancements are uncommon.

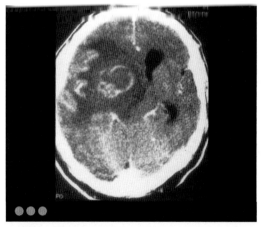

D. Axial, post-contrast CT shows a ring-like enhancing lesion in the region of right basal ganglia. Note the associated hydrocephalus caused by obstruction at the foramen of Monro by the mass.

LYMPHOMA

Primary CNS lymphomas are more common than secondary CNS lymphoma. Approximately 20 to 40% of lesions are multiple. When a butterfly lesion is seen involving the corpus callosum, lymphoma should be considered in the differential diagnsois.

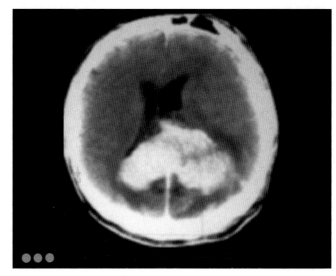

A. Axial, post-contrast CT shows a butterfly shaped enhancing mass crossing the corpus callosum,

DIFFERENTIAL DIAGNOSIS

At a Glance:

* *Lipoma of the Corpus Callosum*
* *GBM*
* *Agenesis of Corpus Callosum (not pictured)*
* *Metastasis* (not pictured)

LIPOMA OF THE CORPUS CALLOSUM

Intracranial lipomas are rare congenital lesions, being less than 0.1% of intracranial masses. Lipomas in the intracranial compartment originate from abnormal differentiation of mesenchymal tissue of meninx primitiva. Most of cases are pericallosal lesions, often associated with other defects of differentiation of the midline structures. They are usually asymptomatic. Lipomas of the corpus callosum are frequently associated with hypogenesis/agenesis of corpus callosum, which is seen in 90% of anterior lipomas and in 30% of posterior lipomas.

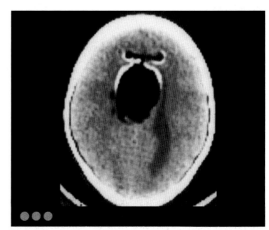

B. Axial CT demonstrates a low-density mass in the region of the corpus callosum with peripheral calcification.

GBM

Glioblastoma multiforme (GBM) is the most common and most malignant of all the gliomas. Of the estimated 17,000 primary brain tumors diagnosed in the United States each year, approximately 60% are gliomas. Gliomas comprise a heterogeneous group of neoplasms that differ in location, in age and sex distribution, in growth potential, in extent of invasiveness, in morphological features, in tendency for progression, and in response to treatments. Glioblastoma is composed of a heterogenous mixture of poorly differentiated neoplastic astrocytes. They primarily affect older adults, and children are rarely affected. They are usually located in the cerebral hemispheres although brainstem involvement may be seen in children.

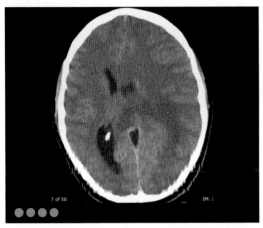

C1. Axial CT shows a mixed density mass in the left parietal region extending into the splenium of the corpus callosum.

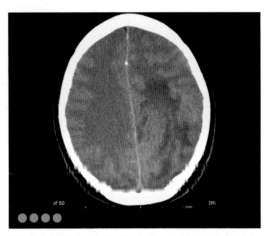

C2. Axial CT shows a mixed density mass in the left parietal region extending into the splenium of the corpus callosum.

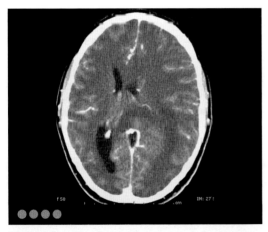

C3. Axial, post-contrast CT demonstrates a heterogeneously enhancing mass in the left parietal lobe with extension into the corpus callosum.

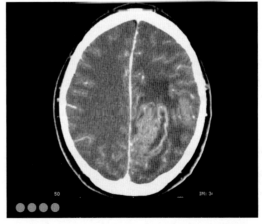

C4. Axial, post-contrast CT demonstrates a heterogeneously enhancing mass in the left parietal lobe with extension into the corpus callosum.

CYSTICERCOSIS

Parenchymal cysticercosis cysts can be in vesicular, colloidal vesicular, granular nodular, and nodular calcified stages in their natural evolution. In the nodular calcified stage, the cysts appear as focal calcifications.

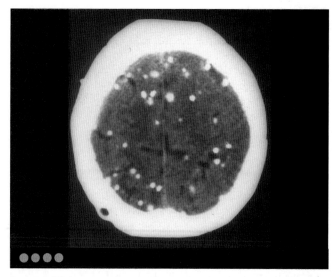

A. Axial CT demonstrates multiple small calcific densities, consistent with calcified granulomas.

DIFFERENTIAL DIAGNOSIS

At a Glance:

- *Tuberous Sclerosis*
- *Torch Infection*
- *Toxoplasmosis*
- *Tuberculosis* (not pictured)
- *Hyperparathyroidism* (not pictured)

TUBEROUS SCLEROSIS

Tuberous sclerosis is a multi-systemic disease. Intracranial lesions are classified into four major categories as follows: (1) Cortical tubers (hamartomas). (2) White-matter abnormalities. (3) Subependymal nodules (hamartomas). Periventricular subependymal nodules usually are present at birth and they have a tendency to become calcified with increasing age. (4) Subependymal giant cell astrocytomas, which are usually seen at the foramen of Monro in young adults.

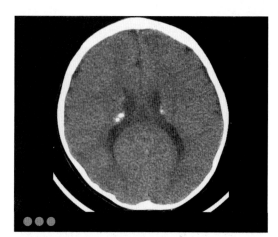

B. Axial CT demonstrates multiple calcific densities in the subependymal region.

TORCH INFECTION

Infections acquired in utero or during birth are a significant cause of fetal and neonatal mortality and an important factor to childhood morbidity. The original concept of the TORCH perinatal infections consist of five infections with similar clinical presentations. TORCH include Toxoplasmosis, Other (syphilis), Rubella, Cytomegalovirus and Herpes simplex virus. On CT, multiple intracranial calcifications may be seen, especially in the periventricular region.

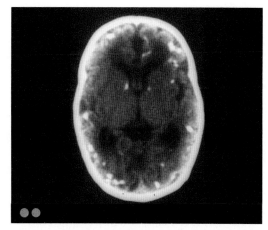

C. Axial CT reveals multiple intracranial calcifications in a child with prenatal infection of toxoplasmosis.

TOXOPLASMOSIS

Toxoplasmosis is caused by infestation with the parasite *Toxoplasma gondii*, a protozoan. The adult form usually occurs in immunocompromised patients or in patients with AIDS. Toxoplasmosis may appear as meningoencephalitis or as granulomas. In patients with AIDS, *Toxoplasma encephalitis* is the most common opportunistic infection. The granulomas may be situated at the corticomedullary junction or in the periventricular areas. Calcification may be seen in old, healed lesions.

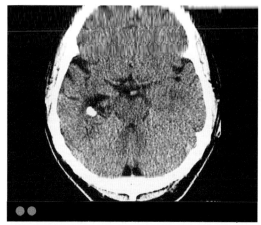

D. Axial CT demonstrate intracranial calcification in the right temporal lobe due to healed lesion of toxoplasmosis. Additional calcifications are seen on other images

16-9 Cystic Masses with an Enhancing Mural Nodule

When a cystic mass with an enhancing mural nodule is seen in the posterior fossa, the differential diagnosis is limited. In children or young adults, it is probably a juvenile pilocytic astrocytoma. In older patients above the age of 50, it should be considered as a metastatic lesion until proved otherwise. In patients between the ages of 30 and 40, it is probably a hemangioblastoma, although metastatic lesion is also a possibility.

PILOCYTIC ASTROCYTOMA

Cerebellar juvenile pilocytic astrocytomas are classified as WHO grade 1 astrocytoma. The majority of cerebellar astrocytomas are of the pilocytic variety (85%) and they occur within the first decade of life. On CT, they usually present as a cystic lesions with a mural nodule. The mural nodule enhances avidly on contrast enhanced images.

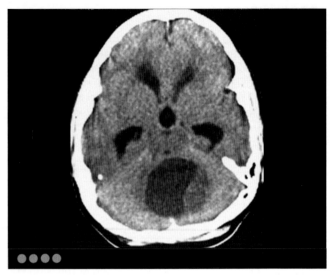

A. Axial CT shows a large cystic mass with a mural nodule in the posterior fossa. There is evidence of obstructive hydrocephalus.

DIFFERENTIAL DIAGNOSIS

At a Glance:

• *Hemangioblastoma* (not pictured)

• *Metastasis* (not pictured)

METASTATIC DISEASE

Metastases are usually well defined, and sharply marginated. Metastatic lesions may be associated with extensive edema or minimal edema, especially those cortical metastases. Almost all the metastases show contrast enhancement due to the lack of blood brain barrier, but the pattern may be nodular, ring-like, irregular, homogeneous or heterogeneous.

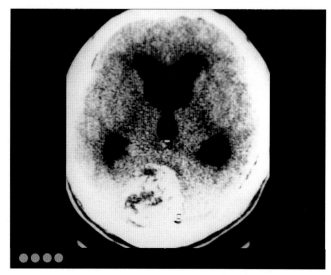

A. Axial, post-contrast CT shows a heterogeneously enhancing mass in the right cerebellum with obstructive hydrocephalus.

DIFFERENTIAL DIAGNOSIS

At a Glance:

- *Anaplastic Astrocytoma* (not pictured)
- *Ependymoma* (not pictured)
- *Glioblastoma Multiforme* (not pictured)

PNET

Some 25% of all pediatric intracranial tumors are medulloblastomas (**PNET**). The peak incidence is in the first decade. Males are two to four times more commonly affected than females. The medulloblastoma originates from poorly differentiated germinative cells of the roof of the fourth ventricle that migrate superiorly and laterally to the external granular layer of the cerebellar hemisphere. The medulloblastoma can occur anywhere along the path of migration. In children, they are usually midline lesions and in young adults, they are more likely to be laterally located in the cerebellar hemisphere. They are usually hyperdense masses on CT and show variable degree of contrast enhancement. Calcification and small cystic changes may be seen. Subarachnoid seeding of medulloblastoma occurs in up to 30% of the cases.

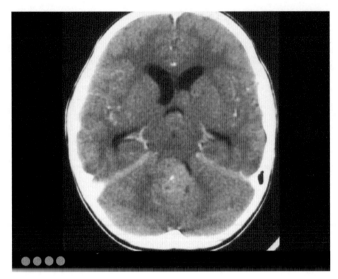

A. Axial, post-contrast CT shows a midline posterior fossa slightly enhancing mass with a speck of calcification and small cystic areas. Note the presence of nodular seeding in the third and left lateral ventricle with hydrocephalus.

RELATED PATTERNS

PNET (CASE TWO)

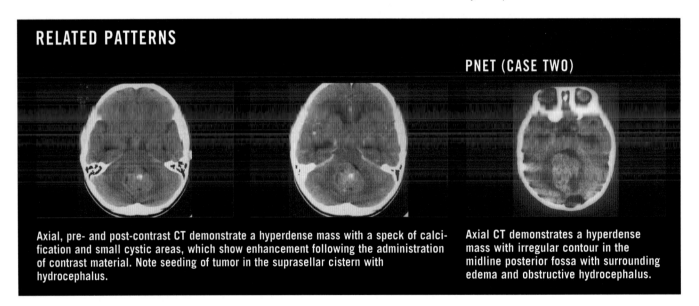

Axial, pre- and post-contrast CT demonstrate a hyperdense mass with a speck of calcification and small cystic areas, which show enhancement following the administration of contrast material. Note seeding of tumor in the suprasellar cistern with hydrocephalus.

Axial CT demonstrates a hyperdense mass with irregular contour in the midline posterior fossa with surrounding edema and obstructive hydrocephalus.

DIFFERENTIAL DIAGNOSIS

At a Glance:

- *Hemangioblastoma*
- *Astrocytoma* (not pictured)
- *Metastasis* (not pictured)
- *Sarcoidosis* (not pictured)

HEMANGIOBLASTOMA

Hemangioblastoma represents approximately 8–12% of all posterior fossa primary neoplasms. The peak age of presentation is 30–40 years. They are most commonly seen in the cerebellum, but can be found in the medulla and spinal cord. Approximately 60% are cystic and 40% are solid masses. Solid masses are nodular in shape. The solid masses exhibit intense contrast enhancement on CT.

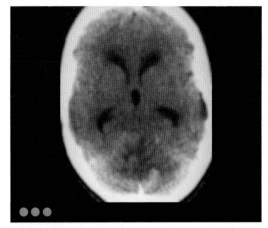

B1. Axial CT shows a slightly hyperdense mass in the left cerebellum.

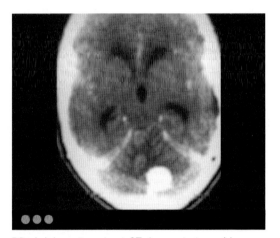

B2. Axial, post-contrast CT demonstrates avid enhancement of the mass.

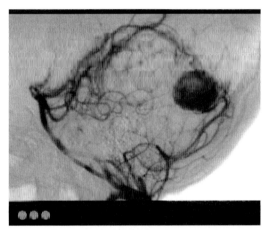

B3. A vertebral angiogram demonstrates a vascular mass with dense contrast stain.

METASTASIS

Metastases are usually well defined, and sharply marginated. Metastatic lesions may be associated with extensive edema or minimal edema, especially those cortical metastases. Almost all the metastases show contrast enhancement due to the lack of blood brain barrier, but the pattern may be nodular, ring-like, irregular, homogeneous or heterogeneous. When a single lesion is seen in the posterior fossa in a patient over 50 years of age, metastatic disease should be the first consideration.

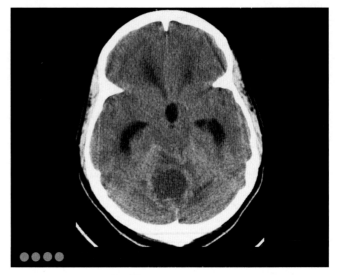

A. Axial CT shows a ring-like lesion in the middle of cerebellum with compression of the fourth ventricle and obstructive hydrocephalus (contrast-enhanced scan not shown)

DIFFERENTIAL DIAGNOSIS

At a Glance:

- *Abscess* (not pictured)
- *Astrocytoma* (not pictured)
- *Cysticercosis* (not pictured)
- *Multiple Sclerosis* (not pictured)
- *Tuberculosis* (not pictured)

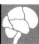

BRAINSTEM HEMORRHAGE

Brain stem hemorrhage may be due to various reasons including stroke and hemorrhage due to hypertension, vascular malformation, bleeding diathesis, anti-coagulant therapy, trauma, neoplasm and so on. Traumatic brainstem hemorrhage after blunt head injury is an uncommon event. The most frequent site of hemorrhage is the midline rostral brainstem.

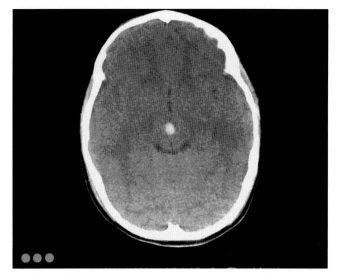

A. Axial CT shows a hyperdense area in the brainstem, consistent with hemorrhage due to trauma.

DIFFERENTIAL DIAGNOSIS

At a Glance:

- *Anaplastic Astrocytoma*
- *Glioblastoma Multiforme*
- *Metastasis*
- *Syphilis*
- *Brainstem Encephalitis* (not pictured)
- *Osmotic Myelinolysis* (not pictured)
- *Multiple Sclerosis* (not pictured)
- *Pilocytic Astrocytoma* (not pictured)

ANAPLASTIC ASTROCYTOMA

For patients with anaplastic astrocytomas, the tumor growth rate and interval between onset of symptoms and diagnosis is situated between low-grade astrocytomas and glioblastomas. Although highly variable, an interval of approximately 1.5–2 years between onset of symptoms and diagnosis is frequently reported. They can also occur as malignant dedifferentiation of a low grade tumor. Brain stem involvement is not common.

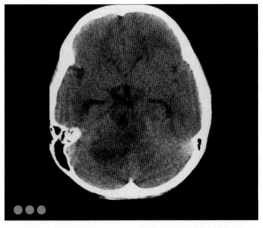

B1. Axial CT shows a low-density lesion in pons extending into the right brachium pontis.

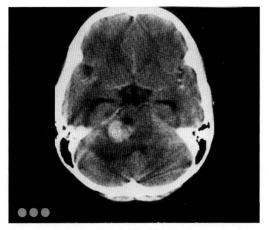

B2. Axial, post-contrast CT demonstrates some enhancement of the mass lesion.

GLIOBLASTOMA MULTIFORME

Glioblastoma multiforme exhibits tumor necrosis on microscopy, not seen on anaplastic astrocytoma. At least 2 genetic pathways have been documented in its development: de novo (primary) glioblastomas and secondary glioblastomas. De novo glioblastomas are more common. De novo GBM develops in patients in their sixties or seventies. In contrast, secondary GBM develops in younger patients and develops from a malignant transformation of a previously diagnosed lower grade tumor. Brain stem involvement is not common.

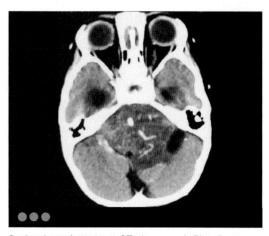

C. Axial, post-contrast CT shows an infiltrating, expansile mass involving the pons with patchy contrast enhancement.

METASTASIS

Almost all the metastases show contrast enhancement due to the lack of blood brain barrier, but the pattern may be nodular, ring-like, irregular, homogeneous or heterogeneous. Brainstem metastasis is rare.

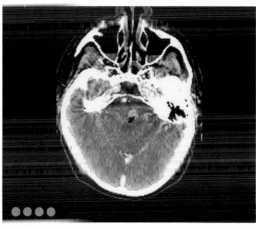

D. Axial, post-contrast CT demonstrates a nodular enhancing lesion in the brainstem.

SYPHILIS

Syphilis is a sexually transmitted disease caused by *Treponema pallidum*. Human beings are the only host. It is a disease of great chronicity. It is a systemic disease from the onset with florid presentations in every structure of the body. Syphilitic infection of the central nervous system is the most chronic, insidious meningeal inflammatory process. Neurosyphilis results from untreated syphilis. Brainstem involvement is seen with neurosyphilis.

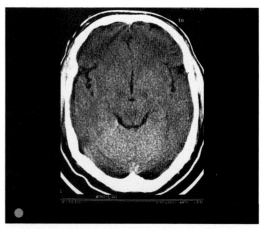

E. Axial CT shows a hypodense lesion in the midbrain due to syphilis.

Chapter 17

Mass Lesions in the Region of the Ventricular System

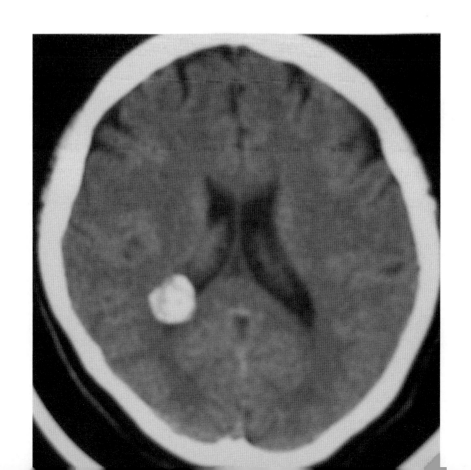

MENINGIOMA

Meningiomas are the most common nonglial primary neoplasms of the central nervous system. Meningiomas tend to occur in females between the ages of 40 and 70 years. The most common location of an intraventricular meningioma is in the atrium of the lateral ventricle. CT scan shows hyperdense to isodense mass with well-defined margin. Tumor calcification is frequently seen.

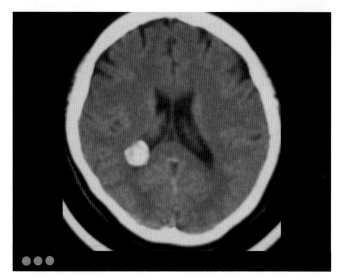

A. Axial CT demonstrates a hyperdense mass in the atrium of the right lateral ventricle, consistent with a calcified meningioma.

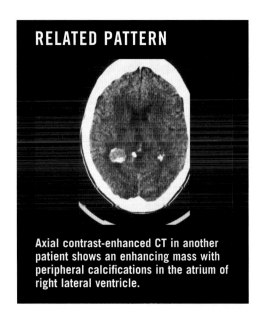

RELATED PATTERN

Axial contrast-enhanced CT in another patient shows an enhancing mass with peripheral calcifications in the atrium of right lateral ventricle.

DIFFERENTIAL DIAGNOSIS

At a Glance:

- *Central Neurocytoma*
- *Choroid Plexus Carcinoma*
- *Choroid Plexus Papilloma*
- *Ependymoma*
- *Metastasis*
- *PNET*
- *Subependymal Giant Cell Astrocytoma*
- *Cysticercosis* (not pictured)
- *Subependymoma* (not pictured)

CENTRAL NEUROCYTOMA

Central neurocytomas are seen in young adults and consist of 0.5% of primary brain tumors. They present as mass lesions in the body of lateral ventricle with cystic, necrotic change, and broad-based attachment of the superolateral ventricular wall. Tumor calcification is common. Homogeneous or heterogeneous mass with heterogeneous contrast enhancement is seen on CT.

CENTRAL NEUROCYTOMA (CASE ONE)

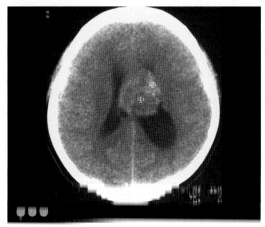

B. Axial, post-contrast CT shows an enhancing mass in the left lateral ventricle with calcification.

CENTRAL NEUROCYTOMA (CASE TWO)

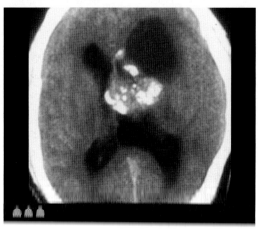

C. Axial, post-contrast CT shows an enhancing mass with calcification in the lateral ventricle.

CHOROID PLEXUS CARCINOMA (CPC)

The majority (80%) of **CPC** occurs in children, usually within the first 5 years of life and is equally distributed between male and female. Microscopic examination can differentiate **CPC** from papilloma; in that carcinoma is hypercellular, pleomorphic, with increased mitotic activity, cysts, necrosis, hemorrhage, microcalcifications, and brain invasion. **CPC** is a rapidly growing tumor that may seed the CSF pathways. Prognosis is poor with only 40% surviving at 5 years. It is very difficult to distinguish CPP from **CPC** with imaging studies as the two types of tumors have similar imaging characteristics. Generally speaking, **CPC** usually presents as a more heterogeneous lesion on imaging studies.

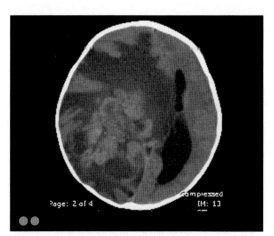

D1. Axial CT shows a large heterogeneous mass with cystic changes in the region of atrium of right lateral ventricle. A large amount of surrounding edema is seen.

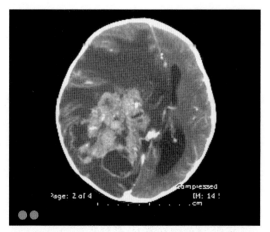

D2. Axial, post-contrast CT demonstrates a large heterogeneously enhancing mass in the region of the atrium of right lateral ventricle.

CHOROID PLEXUS PAPILLOMA

Choroid plexus papillomas consist of less than 1% of all intracranial neoplasms. They are among the most common brain tumors in children aged below 2 years. **Choroid** **plexus papillomas** are predominantly well-circumscribed, smooth, or lobulated masses that may display frondlike margins. They are of mixed density with intense contrast enhancement seen on CT. Calcification and hemorrhage are common.

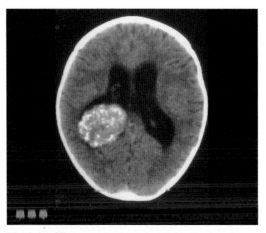

E1. Axial CT demonstrates a hyperdense mass in the atrium of the lateral ventricle with multiple punctate cacifications. There is associated hydrocephalus.

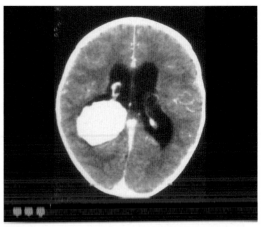

E2. Axial contrast-enhanced CT shows intense enhancement of this mass with lobulated margins.

EPENDYMOMA

Ependymomas constitute 2–6% of all gliomas. Only 40% of intracranial ependymomas occur in the supratentorial compartment. The reported incidence of parenchymal origin of the ependymomas varies from 55–85%. Parenchymal ependymomas are more commonly seen in the supratentorial compartment. **Ependymomas** are 4–6 times more common in children than in adults. CT shows a mass lesion that is hypodense to isodense to brain with dense punctate calcification, areas of necrosis or cystic changes. Hemorrhage may also be seen. Contrast enhancement is variable, from heterogeneous to homogeneous.

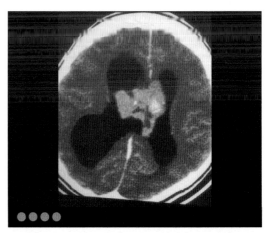

F. Axial contrast-enhanced CT shows an irregular enhancing mass with small cystic changes and calcifications in the lateral ventricle.

METASTASIS

Metastatic disease in the lateral ventricle usually occur in the glomus of the choroid plexus of the lateral ventricle and is due to hematogenous spread of the primary neoplasm. Since glomus of the choroid plexus is a highly vascular structure, its propensity for metastasis is expected.

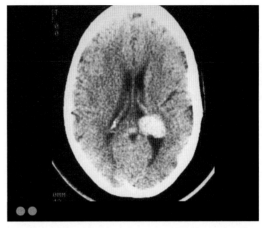

G. Axial, post-contrast CT demonstrates an enhancing mass in the atrium of the left lateral ventricle due to metastatic disease from renal cell carcinoma.

PNET

Primitive neuroectodermal tumors are usually seen in the posterior fossa in children. Supratentorial PNET is unusual, but also occur in children. Occasionally, they can be intraventricular in location.

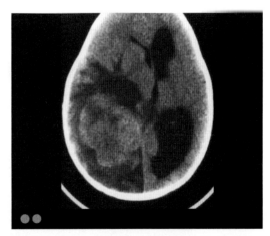

H. Axial CT demonstrates a heterogenous predominately hyperdense mass in the atrium and occipital horn of the right lateral ventricle. There is surrounding edema and hydrocephalus seen.

SUBEPENDYMAL GIANT CELL ASTROCYTOMA

Subependymal giant cell astrocytomas are found in 10–15% of the patients with tuberous sclerosis and are usually seen in patients below 20 years of age. They usually occur in the wall of the lateral ventricle near the foramen of Monro. On CT, they are a heterogeneous mass with hypodensity and isodensity. Calcification and cysts are commonly seen. Heterogeneous contrast enhancement is seen.

SUBEPENDYMAL GIANT CELL ASTROCYTOMA (CASE ONE)

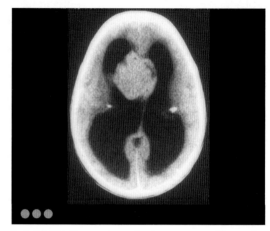

I. Axial CT shows a large isodense mass with small cystic area in the lateral ventricle adjacent to the septum pellucidum. Note the presence of hydrocephalus and subependymal calcifications.

SUBEPENDYMAL GIANT CELL ASTROCYTOMA (CASE TWO)

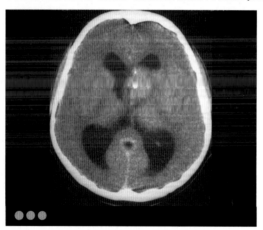

J1. Axial CT shows a hyperdense mass with calcification in the frontal horn of the left lateral ventricle adjacent to the septum pellucidum.

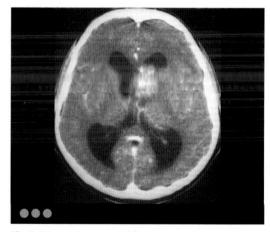

J2. Axial, post-contrast CT demonstrates an enhancing mass at the frontal horn of the left lateral ventricle.

644

MENINGIOMA

Intraventricular meningiomas are uncommon. They usually occur in the atrium of the lateral ventricle. Third ventricular meningiomas are rare. When an intraventricualr meningioma is seen in children, the possibility of neurofibromatosis type II should be entertained.

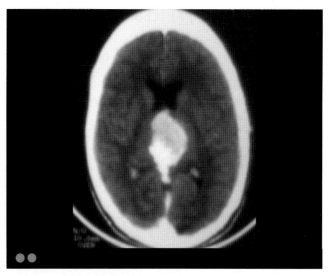

A. Axial contrast-enhanced CT demonstrates a homogeneously enhancing mass with a focal calcification in the third ventricle.

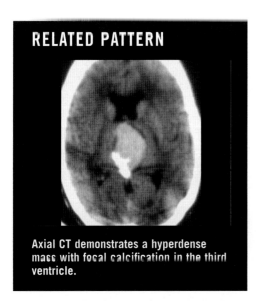

RELATED PATTERN

Axial CT demonstrates a hyperdense mass with focal calcification in the third ventricle.

DIFFERENTIAL DIAGNOSIS

At a Glance:

- *Choroid Plexus Papilloma*
- *Colloid Cyst*
- *Ependymoma*
- *Metastatic Adenocarcinoma*

- *Xanthogranuloma*
- *Central Neurocytoma* (not pictured)
- *Craniopharyngioma* (not pictured)
- *Cysticercosis* (not pictured)
- *Subependymoma* (not pictured)

CHOROID PLEXUS PAPILLOMA

Choroid plexus papillomas of the third ventricle are rare tumors seen in children. They tend to have smooth, or lobulated margins with frondlike appearance. They are usually hyperdense with calcification or hemorrhage on CT and intense contrast enhancement is seen.

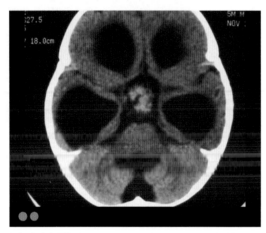

B1. Axial CT demonstrates a lobulated mass with contrast enhancement in the third ventricle.

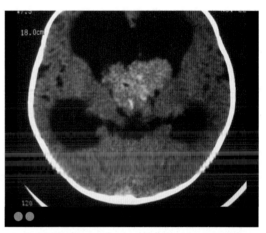

B2. Axial CT demonstrates a lobulated mass with contrast enhancement in the third ventricle.

COLLOID CYST

Colloid cysts are congenital in origin, but only 1.2% present before the age of 10. Most colloid cysts become symptomatic between the third and fifth decade. **Colloid cysts** occur most frequently in the anterior third ventricle, originating from the roof near the foramen of Monro. Less frequently, they may arise from and subsequently widen the septum pellucidum. These lesions are homogeneously hyperdense in two-thirds of the cases and isodense-to-hypodense in one-third of the cases.

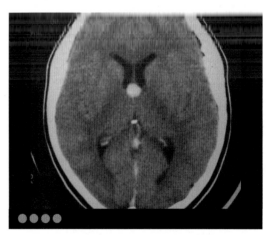

C. Axial contrast-enhanced CT demonstrates a hyperdense mass at the anterior third ventricle near the foramen of Monro (no definite contrast enhancement is seen as compared to pre-contrast study).

EPENDYMOMA

Ependymomas constitute 2–6% of all gliomas. Only 40% of intracranial ependymomas occur in the supratentorial compartment. The reported incidence of parenchymal origin of the ependymomas varies from 55–85% and supratentorial ependymomas are more likely to involve the parenchyma. Ependymomas are 4–6 times more common in children than in adults.

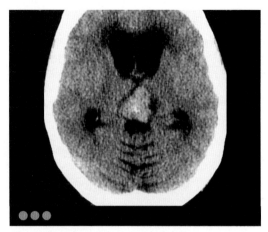

D. Axial CT shows a hyperdense mass with calcification in the third ventricle.

METASTATIC ADENOCARCINOMA (FROM COLON)

Intraventricular metastasis is more likely seen in the lateral ventricle, involving the ependyma and choroid plexus. Third or fourth ventricular involvement is rare. They are commonly seen in older patients in their 6th or 7th decade. Intraventricular metastases may be of variable density depending on their cell type on unenhanced CT. They usually show marked enhancement on contrast enhanced CT depending on their vascularity. Like metastasis elsewhere, calcification is unusual. In adults, metastases originate from carcinoma lung in more than half the cases, followed by breast and gastrointestinal malignancy, and renal cell carcinoma. However, in children, Wilm's tumor, retinoblastoma and neuroblastoma are the common primary sites to metastasize to brain.

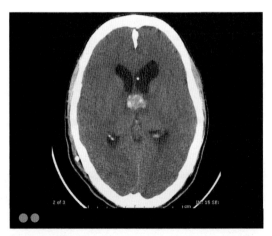

E1. Axial CT scan shows a hyperdense mass in the third ventricle. Note intraventricular blood in the occipital horn of the left lateral ventricle and hydrocephalus.

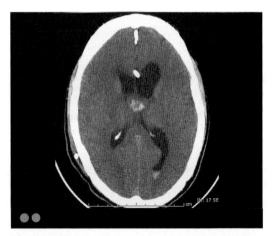

E2. Axial CT scan shows a hyperdense mass in the third ventricle. Note intraventricular blood in the occipital horn of the left lateral ventricle and hydrocephalus.

XANTHOGRANULOMA

Xanthogranulomas (XGs) are benign tumors typically composed of cholesterol clefts, macrophages, chronic inflammatory cellular reaction and hemosiderin deposits. Their incidence is approximately 1.6 to 7% of the cases in autopsy series. XG in the lateral ventricles are small lesions that do not obstruct the ventricle whereas those in the third ventricle are more likely to cause ventricular obstruction and be symptomatic. Lateral ventricular XGs are usually located in the glomus of choroid plexus. Third ventricular XGs can obstruct the foramen of Monro.

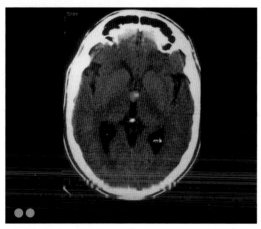

F1. Axial CT shows a hyperdense mass with calcification at the anterior third ventricle.

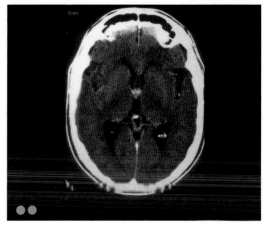

F2. Axial, post-contrast CT shows an enhancing lesion at the anterior third ventricle.

CHOROID PLEXUS PAPILLOMA

Distribution of choroid plexus papillomas varies between pediatric and adult patients. In children, most choroid plexus papillomas (80%) are located in the lateral ventricles whereas in adults, most choroid plexus papillomas are located in the fourth ventricle. Approximately 16% of choroid plexus papillomas are found in the fourth ventricle, and 4% are found in the third ventricle.

Choroid plexus papillomas are slightly hyperdense masses with lobulated margin. Calcification and hemorrhage may be seen within the mass. Intense contrast enhancement is seen following intravenous injection of contrast material.

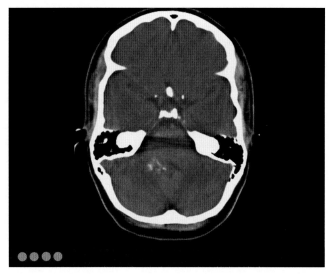

A. Axial CT demonstrates a heterogeneously hyperdense mass with punctate calcifications in the right lateral recess of the fourth ventricle.

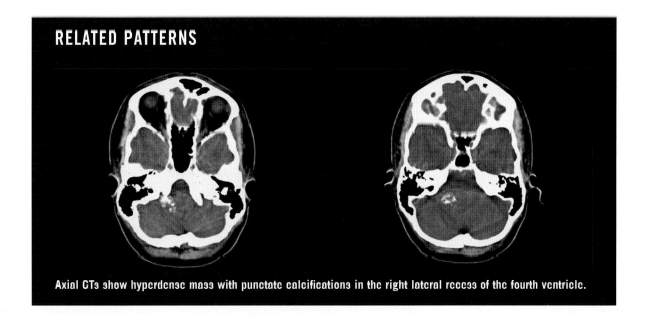

RELATED PATTERNS

Axial CTs show hyperdense mass with punctate calcifications in the right lateral recess of the fourth ventricle.

DIFFERENTIAL DIAGNOSIS

At a Glance:

- *Ependymoma*
- *Meningioma*
- *Cysticercosis* (not pictured)
- *Subependymoma* (not pictured)

EPENDYMOMA

Ependymomas constitute 2–6% of all gliomas. Approximately 60% of intracranial ependymomas occur in the infratentorial compartment. Infratentorial ependymomas usually arise from the fourth ventricle. Ependymomas are 4–6 times more common in children than in adults. CT shows a heterogeneous mass lesion with dense punctate calcification, areas of necrosis or cystic changes. Hemorrhage may also be seen. Contrast enhancement is variable, from heterogeneous to homogeneous.

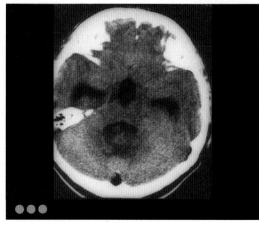

B. Axial CT shows a mixed hypo-, isointense mass in the region of fourth ventricle with obstructive hydrocephalus.

MENINGIOMA

Intraventricular meningiomas account for 2% to 5% of all meningiomas. They are found most frequently in the lateral ventricle (80%), followed by the third ventricle (15%), and the fourth ventricle (5%). Like meningiomas elsewhere, they are usually isodense on unenhanced CT. Calcification may be seen. Contrast enhancement is intense.

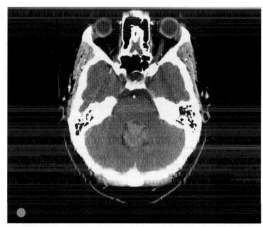

C. Axial, post-contrast CT demonstrates an enhancing mass in the fourth ventricle.

PINEOCYTOMA

Pineocytomas are seen in males and females equally. They can be seen in any age group, but are generally seen in older patients as compared to pineoblastomas. They are isodense-to-hyperdense on CT, and contrast enhancement is seen. Tumor calcification may be seen.

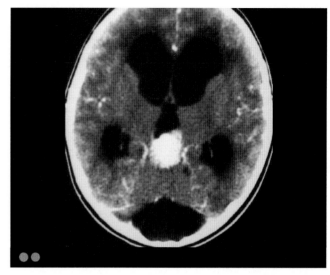

A. Axial contrast-enhanced CT shows an enhancing mass in the pineal region with obstructive hydrocephalus. Incidentally seen is the presence of an arachnoid cyst in the retrocerebellar region.

RELATED PATTERNS

PINEOCYTOMA (CASE TWO)

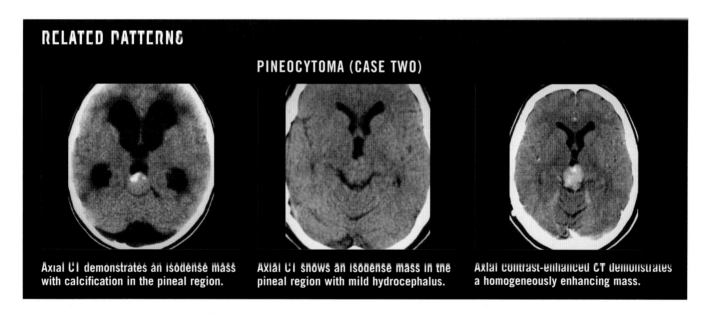

Axial CT demonstrates an isodense mass with calcification in the pineal region.

Axial CT shows an isodense mass in the pineal region with mild hydrocephalus.

Axial contrast-enhanced CT demonstrates a homogeneously enhancing mass.

DIFFERENTIAL DIAGNOSIS

At a Glance:

- *Germinoma*
- *Glioma*
- *Pineoblastoma*
- *Teratoma*
- *Germ Cell Tumors* (not pictured)

GERMINOMA

Germinomas are the most common pineal region neoplasm. They are seen in young males with a 9:1 male to female ratio. Occasionally a pineal region mass may be seen in association with a suprasellar mass. **Germinomas** are usually hyperdense on CT and homogeneous contrast enhancement is seen. Tumor calcification is not seen, although the tumor may engulf a calcified pineal gland.

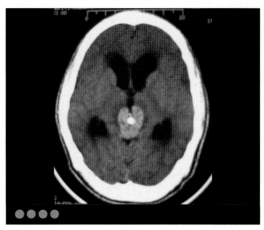

B. Axial contrast-enhanced CT shows an enhancing mass in the pineal region engulfing the calcification of pineal gland.

GLIOMA

Since the normal pineal gland contains fibrillary astrocytes, an astrocytoma may arise from the pineal gland. The majority of pineal region astrocytoma arises from the quadrigeminal plate or the thalamus.

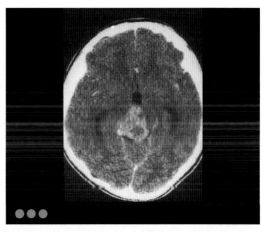

C. Axial contrast-enhanced CT shows a heterogeneously enhancing mass in the pineal region with obstructive hydrocephalus.

PINEOBLASTOMA

Pineoblastomas affect males and females equally and are predominantly seen in the first and second decade. They are about six times more common than pineocytomas. CT shows isodense-to-hyperdense mass with contrast enhancement. Calcification may be seen.

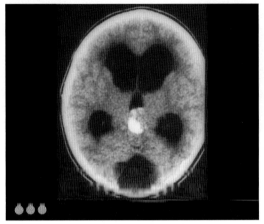

D1. Axial CT of a 12-year-old child shows an iso-dense mass with calcification in the pineal region with obstructive hydrocephalus.

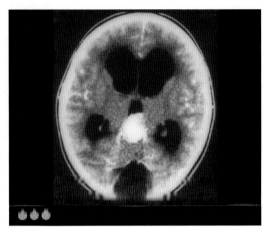

D2. Axial contrast-enhanced CT demonstrates intense contrast enhancement of the mass.

TERATOMA

The pineal region is the most common site of intracranial teratoma. Pineal **teratomas** are seen exclusively in young males. CT shows a well-demarcated mass with fat and calcification. Patchy contrast enhancement is seen.

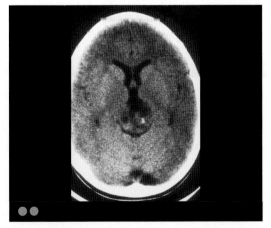

E1. Axial CT demonstrates a heterogeneous mass with calcification and fat (−58 HU) posteriorly.

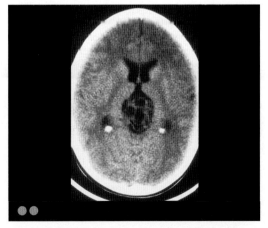

E2. Axial CT demonstrates a heterogeneous mass with calcification and fat (−58 HU) posteriorly.

SUBEPENDYMAL SEEDING OF NEOPLASM

Seeding of the neoplasms in the lateral ventricle involving the subependymal region can be due to a variety of malignant neoplasms, including PNET (medullobalstoma, pineoblastoma), GBM, malignant ependymoma, and so on. They are usually thick, nodular in appearance.

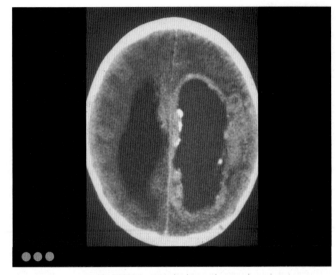

A. Axial post-contrast CT demonstrates subependymal enhancement in the left lateral ventricle and hydrocephalus in a patient with PNET in the posterior fossa.

RELATED PATTERNS

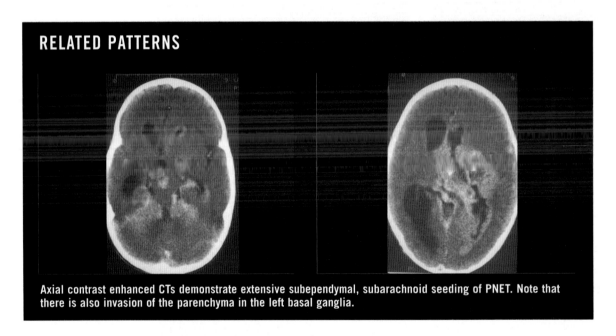

Axial contrast enhanced CTs demonstrate extensive subependymal, subarachnoid seeding of PNET. Note that there is also invasion of the parenchyma in the left basal ganglia.

DIFFERENTIAL DIAGNOSIS

At a Glance:

- *Lymphoma*
- *Ventriculitis (CMV)*
- *Sarcoid* (not pictured)
- *Tuberculosis* (not pictured)

LYMPHOMA

Primary lymphoma of the central nervous system (CNS) is usually a Non-Hodgkins B-cell type of lymphoma. They tend to occur in immunocompromised patients. Primary CNS lymphomas (70–90%) are more common than secondary CNS lymphomas. Approximately 10–30% of patients with systemic lymphoma develop CNS involvement. Secondary systemic and primary CNS lymphomas have similar imaging features on CT or MRI. Meningeal and ventricular involvement occurs more commonly in patients with secondary lymphoma. About half of the patients with lymphoma present with multiple tumor nodules.

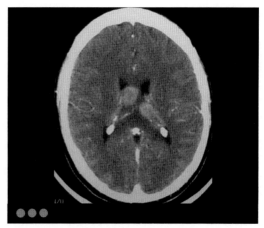

B1. Axial contrast-enhanced CT reveals enhancing masses in the lateral ventricles.

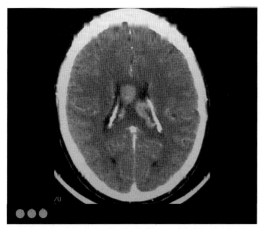

B2. Axial contrast-enhanced CT reveals enhancing masses in the lateral ventricles.

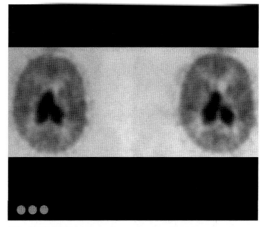

B3. FDG-PET image shows markedly increased uptake in the region of lateral ventricles.

655

VENTRICULITIS (CMV)

Ventriculitis may be due to bacterial, viral or fungal infection. They usually present as a smooth, uniform ependymal enhancement without nodularity. The imaging appearances of ventriculitis due to various etiologies are similar and cannot be differentiated one from another. MRI is more sensitive than CT in the detection of ventriculitis, especially with information from diffusion weighted sequence, FLAIR and contrast-enhanced FLAIR sequences.

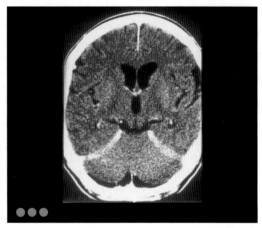

C. Axial, post-contrast CT demonstrates minimal periventricular enhancement and enhancement along the tentorium (MRI with contrast in this patient shows more obvious periventricular enhancement).

Chapter 18

Sellar and Parasellar Masses

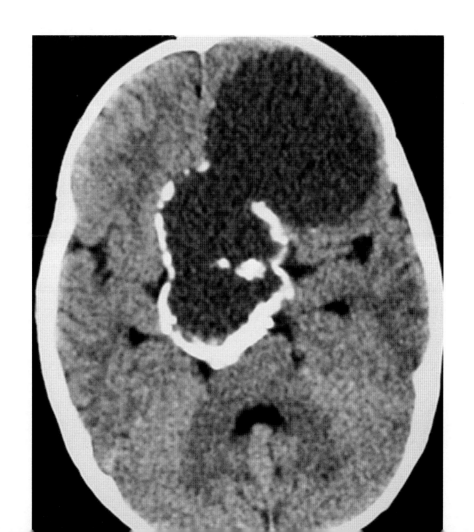

CRANIOPHARYNGIOMA

Craniopharyngiomas originate from the remnants of Rathke's pouch. They represent 3–5% of primary intracranial neoplasms. They have a bimodal age distribution; more than half occur in children and young adults. A second smaller peak occurs in the fifth and sixth decade. They are the most common neoplasm to calcify in children. Craniopharyngiomas are both intra- and suprasellar in about 70% of cases. They are suprasellar in only about 20% and intrasellar in 10% of cases. They are well-circumscribed, multi-lobulated masses with cystic and solid components. Calcification is present in 90% of the pediatric cases and 50% of the adult cases.

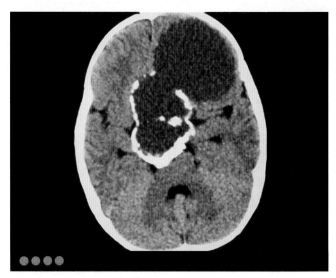

A. Axial CT shows a double ring-like lesion in the suprasellar and left frontal region with marginal calcification around and within the medial ring-like lesion.

RELATED PATTERNS

CRANIOPHARYNGIOMA (CASE TWO)

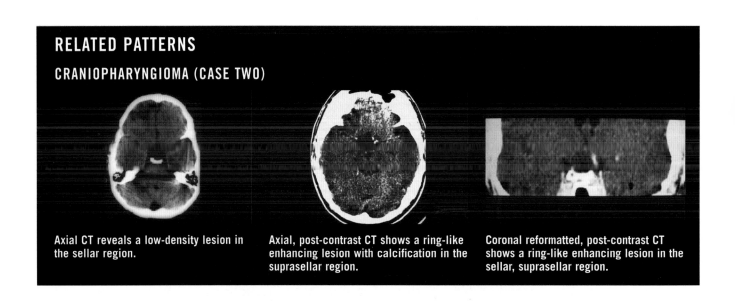

Axial CT reveals a low-density lesion in the sellar region.

Axial, post-contrast CT shows a ring-like enhancing lesion with calcification in the suprasellar region.

Coronal reformatted, post-contrast CT shows a ring-like enhancing lesion in the sellar, suprasellar region.

DIFFERENTIAL DIAGNOSIS

At a Glance:

- *Abscess*
- *Hypothalamic Gliomas*
- *Pituitary Apoplexy*
- *Rathke's Cleft Cyst*

- *Abscess* (not pictured)
- *Aneurysm* (not pictured)
- *Fungal Infection* (not pictured)
- *Pituitary Adenoma* (not pictured)
- *Tuberculosis* (not pictured)

ABSCESS

Pituitary abscess is a rare disease and its clinical presentations are non-specific. Pituiatry abscess can occur denovo in an otherwise normal pituitary gland or less frequently in a pre-existing pathology. Its density on CT is variable, probably related to its protein content.

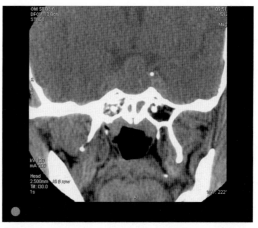

B. Coronal, non-contrast CT demonstrates a hyperdense mass in the sellar and suprasellar region.

HYPOTHALAMIC GLIOMAS

Hypothalamic gliomas occur more frequently during childhood and adolescence. In most of cases, it appears before the age of 15 and has a male to female ratio of 2:1. Optic pathway gliomas occur with a frequency of 15% among patients with Neurofibromatosis type I (von Recklinghausen disease). The tumors may be solid, gelatinous, or cystic.

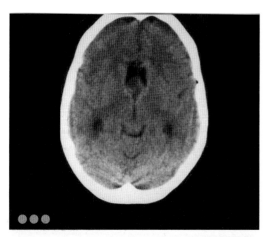

01. Axial CT shows a cystic lesion in the suprasellar region

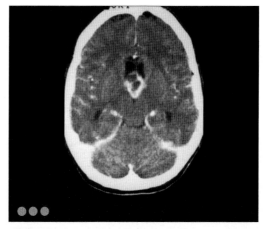

C2. Axial, post-contrast CT shows a multi-ring-like enhancing lesion in the suprasellar region.

PITUITARY APOPLEXY

Pituitary apoplexy is characterized by a sudden onset of headache, visual symptoms, altered mental status, and hormonal dysfunction due to acute hemorrhage or infarction of a pituitary gland. An existing pituitary adenoma is usually present. The male to female predominance is 2:1.

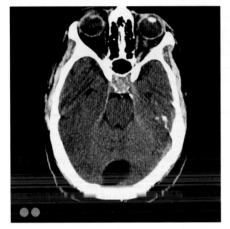 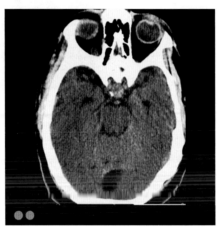 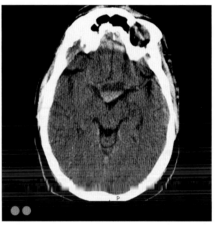

D1. Axial CT shows a hyperdense sellar mass, consistent with pituitary apoplexy.

D2. Axial CT shows a hyperdense sellar mass.

D3. Axial CT shows a fluid–blood level in the lesion.

RATHKE'S CLEFT CYST

Rathke's cleft cysts are lined by columnar or cuboidal epithelium. Cystic fluid within the **Rathke's cleft cysts** varies from serous to mucoid. Cyst with low protein content appears hypodense on CT. A cyst containing very high protein con-

centration appears hyperdense on CT. A mild rim of contrast enhancement is occasionally seen following the administration of contrast. Approximately 70% of the **Rathke's cleft cysts** are both intra- and suprasellar; 25% are intrasellar; and 5% are completely suprasellar.

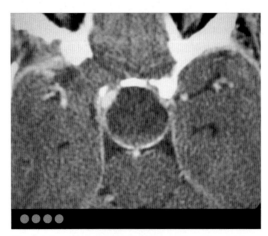 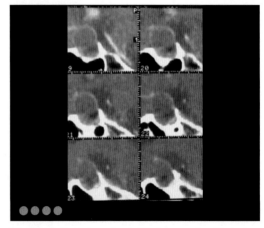

E1. Axial, post-contrast CT shows a ring-like enhancing lesion in the sellar and suprasellar region.

E2. Sagittal, post-contrast CT shows a ring-like enhancing lesion in the sellar and suprasellar region.

MENINGIOMA

Meningiomas arising from the tuberculum or diaphragma sellae may grow downward. Due to their proximity to the optic chiasm and the prechiasmatic portion of the optic nerves, compression of the chiasm or nerve is a common occurrence.

When they are in contact with the pituitary gland, it may be difficult to separate them. However, most of the time, a cleavage plane can be appreciated.

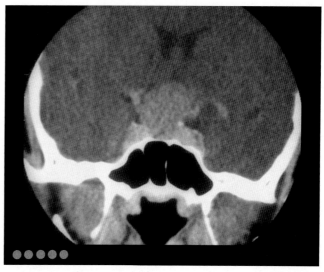

A. Coronal, post-contrast CT demonstrates a suprasellar enhancing mass.

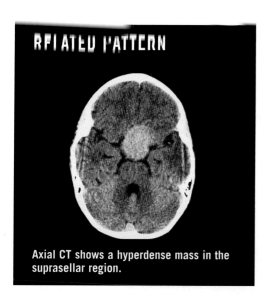

Axial CT shows a hyperdense mass in the suprasellar region.

DIFFERENTIAL DIAGNOSIS

At a Glance:

- *Aneurysm*
- *Germ Cell Tumor*
- *Craniopharyngioma* (not pictured)
- *Lymphocytic Adenohypophysitis* (not pictured)
- *Metastasis* (not pictured)
- *Pituitary Adenoma* (not pictured)
- *Sarcoid* (not pictured)

ANEURYSM

An **aneurysm** arising from the circle of Willis or cavernous internal carotid artery may project into the suprasellar cistern and/or sellar turcica. On CT, most **aneurysms** appear as a well-circumscribed, round, hyperdense mass in the sellar and suprasellar region with intense contrast enhancement. Although **aneurysms** are not solid unless they are thrombosed, they are included here to assure the awareness that they may mimic a solid mass.

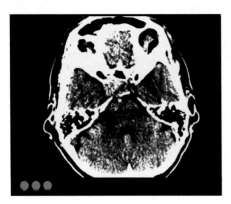

B1. Axial CT shows a hyperdense mass in the sellar and right parasellar region, mimicking a solid mass.

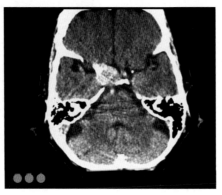

B2. Axial, post-contrast CT shows intense enhancement of the mass.

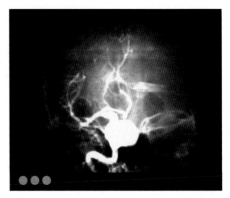

B3. Cerebral angiogram proved the mass lesion to be an aneurysm

GERM CELL TUMOR

Intracranial germ cell tumors are a heterogeneous group of tumors that can occur in all age groups. Germ cell tumors most frequently arise in the pineal region, followed by suprasellar region. Pineal region germ cell tumors are twice as common as suprasellar tumors. Between 5%–10% of germ cell tumors are found simultaneously in the suprasellar and pineal region at the time of initial diagnosis. Males are about twice more likely than females to develop germ cell tumors. In the pineal region, germinomas are predominantly seen in males whereas in the suprasellar region, germinomas are seen equally in males and females.

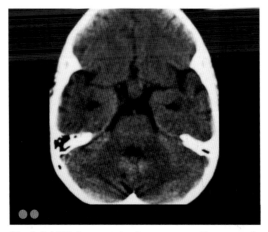

C1. Axial CT shows an isodense suprasellar mass.

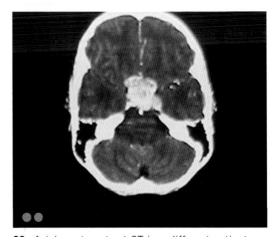

C2. Axial, post-contrast CT in a different patient shows an intensely enhancing suprasellar mass.

ANEURYSM

Curvilinear rim-like calcification is seen at the periphery of the aneurysm. Curvilinear calcification suggests an aneurysm but is a less specific finding because it can also occur in craniopharyngiomas and tumor of the clivus. Strong suspicion for aneurysm in the differential diagnosis of a suprasellar mass is important because the surgical approach for an aneurysm is different from that of a neoplasm. Serious consequence can occur if the neurosurgeon is not ready to deal with a bleeding aneurysm.

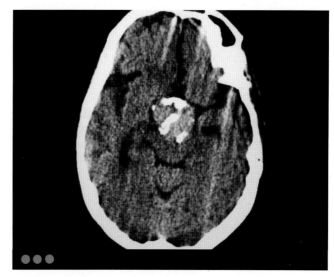

A. Axial CT shows a suprasellar mass with calcification.

RELATED PATTERN

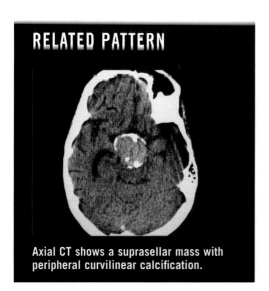

Axial CT shows a suprasellar mass with peripheral curvilinear calcification.

DIFFERENTIAL DIAGNOSIS

At a Glance:

- *Cavernous Angioma*
- *Craniopharyngioma*
- *Meningioma* (not pictured)

CAVERNOUS ANGIOMA

Cavernous angiomas can occur within the brain parenchyma, or less likely in the extra-axial location. Suprasellar cavernous angiomas are rare. They are usually heterogeneously hyperdense on CT. Calcification may be seen. Contrast enhancement may be seen. There is no surrounding edema or mass effect.

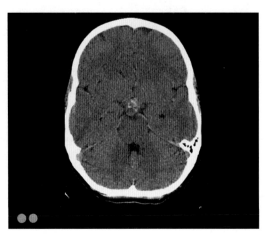

B1. Axial CT shows a suprasellar mass with calcification

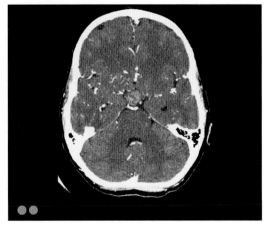

B2. Axial, post-contrast CT reveals an enhancing mass in the suprasellar region.

CRANIOPHARYNGIOMA

They have a bimodal age distribution; more than half occur in children and young adults. A second smaller peak occurs in the fifth and sixth decade. They are the most common neoplasm to calcify in children. Calcification is present in 90% of the pediatric cases and 60% of the adult cases.

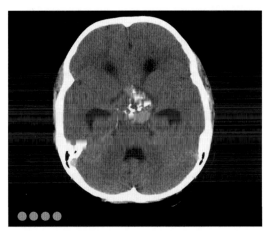

C. Axial CT reveals a suprasellar mass with multiple specks of calcification. Note that hydrocephalus with dilated ventricles is seen.

EPIDERMOID

Epidermoids are congenital masses, but their clinical presentation is usually in the third or fourth decade. They are predominantly located in basal cisterns and are usually lateral in location as opposed to the midline location of dermoids. Common locations include cerebellopontine angle, middle cranial fossa, suprasellar, and fourth ventricle. Epidermoids are composed of ectodermal elements and are lined with stratified squamous epithelium containing epithelial keratinaceous debris and cholesterol crystals.

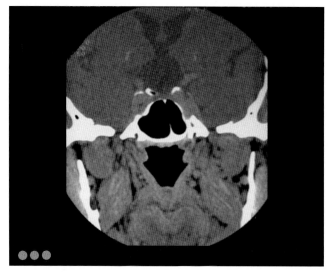

A. Coronal, post-contrast CT demonstrates a hypodense mass in the suprasellar cistern without enhancement.

DIFFERENTIAL DIAGNOSIS

At a Glance:

- *Dermoid*

- *Sphenoid Mucocele*

- *Arachnoid Cyst* (not pictured)

- *Cysticercosis* (not pictured)

- *Harmatoma of the Tuber Cinerium* (not pictured)

DERMOID

Dermoids are usually rounded, well-circumscribed, extremely hypodense lesions with a Hounsfield unit of -20 to -140, consistent with their lipid content. They are never associated with vasogenic edema and only rarely cause hydrocephalus. Peripheral capsular calcification is frequently seen. Contrast enhancement is rare but has been reported.

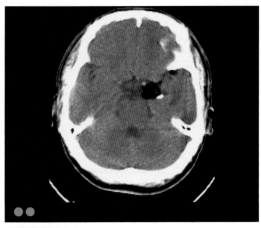

B. Axial CT shows a left parasellar, hypodense (fat density) mass with peripheral calcification.

SPHENOID MUCOCELE

Sphenoid sinus mucoceles are rare. They are usually due to previous trauma or chronic sinusitis. On CT, their appearance depends on their water content, high water content exhibits hypodensity. The wall of the involved sinus may be very thin because of constant and prolonged pressure of the mucocele. Sphenoid mucocele may extend superiorly to involve the sellar turcica and cause its erosion and enlargement.

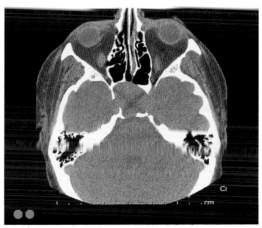

C. Axial CT demonstrates enlarged sella turcica in a patient with mucocele of the sphenoid sinus.

CAVERNOUS ANGIOMA

Parasellar cavernous hemangiomas may appear as hyperdense masses on CT and enhance avidly on post-contrast studies. They are difficult to remove surgically and tend to be adherent to the cavernous sinus and may also bleed profoundly.

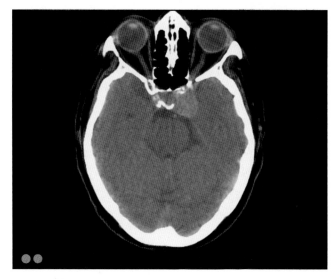

A. Axial CT shows a hyperdense mass in the region of left cavernous sinus with evidence of bony remodeling

RELATED PATTERNS

CAVERNOUS ANGIOMA (CASE TWO)

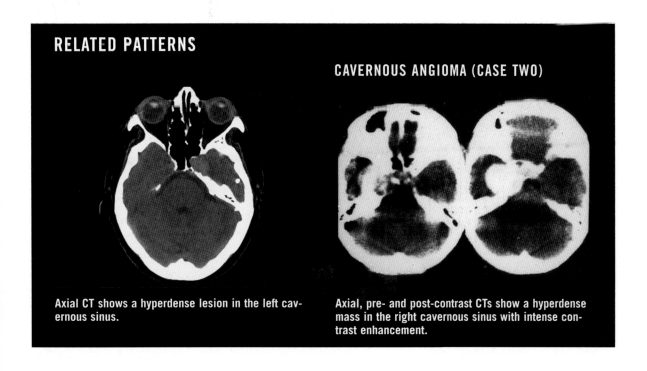

Axial CT shows a hyperdense lesion in the left cavernous sinus.

Axial, pre- and post-contrast CTs show a hyperdense mass in the right cavernous sinus with intense contrast enhancement.

DIFFERENTIAL DIAGNOSIS

At a Glance:

- *Aneurysm*
- *Carotid-Cavernous Fistula*
- *Dermoid*
- *Lymphoma*
- *Malignant Schwannoma*
- *Nasopharyngeal Carcinoma Invading Cavernous Sinus*

- *Sphenoid Sinus Tumor Invading Cavernous Sinus*
- *Teratoma*
- *Chondrosarcoma* (not pictured)
- *Fungal Infection* (not pictured)
- *Meningioma* (not pictured)
- *Other Granulomas (Including Tolosa-Hunt Syndrome)* (not pictured)
- *Sarcoid* (not pictured)
- *Tuberculosis* (not pictured)

ANEURYSM

An aneurysm arising from the circle of Willis or cavernous internal carotid artery may project into the cavernous sinus. On CT, most aneurysms appear as a well-circumscribed, round mass in the cavernous sinus region. The CT density of the aneurysm can be variable depending on the presence or absence of the blood clot within the aneurysm. A nonthrombosed aneurysm is readily detected on CT as a low density mass. Intense contrast enhancement is seen Following intravenous injection of contrast.

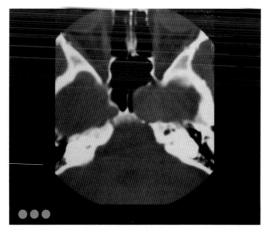

B1. Axial pre- and post-contrast CT scans demonstrate an intensely enhancing lesion in the region of left cavernous sinus with bone erosion.

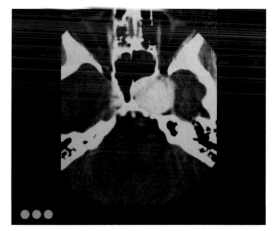

B2. Axial pre- and post-contrast CT scans demonstrate an intensely enhancing lesion in the region of left cavernous sinus with bone erosion.

CAROTID-CAVERNOUS FISTULA

Spontaneous or traumatic rupture of the wall of the intra-cavernous segment of the internal carotid artery or its dural branches results in sudden shunting of the arterial blood into the cavernous sinus. This can also occur due to rupture of an aneurysm located within the cavernous sinus. Tortuosity and dilatation of the superior ophthalmic vein is the hallmark on CT or MRI for the diagnosis of carotid-cavernous fistula. Focal bulging or expansion of the cavernous sinus is another sign of C-C fistula.

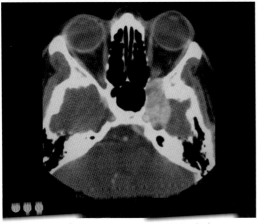

C1. Axial post contrast CT scan demonstrates dilatation of the left cavernous sinus and associated vein draining the fistula.

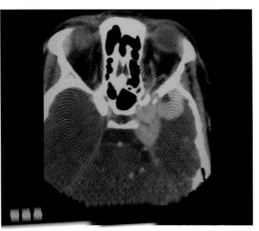

C2. Axial, post-contrast CT scan demonstrates dilatation of the left cavernous sinus and associated vein draining the fistula.

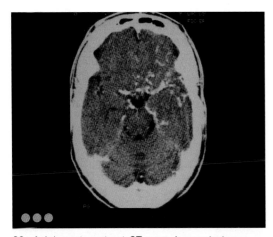

C3. Axial, post-contrast CT scan demonstrates dilated veins draining the c-c fistula.

DERMOID

Intracranial **dermoids** are rare lesions and are one-fifth as common as epidermoids. They are congenital tumors, but only become symptomatic during the third decade of life due to their slow growth. **Dermoids** are composed of ecto-

dermal elements and are lined with stratified squamous epithelium with skin appendage such as hair follicles, sebaceous, and sweat glands. On CT, they present as low-density masses with well-defined margin. The presence of an amorphous density (hair ball) and calcification may be seen.

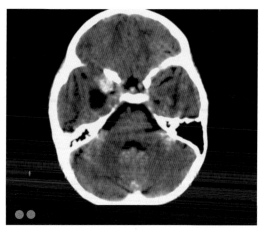

D1. Axial pre-contrast CT shows a right parasellar mixed density mass with contrast enhancement. The low-density area may be due to fat or fluid and Hounsfield unit can be used to distinguish the two, as fatty density is in the minus territory whereas fluid density is nearly zero.

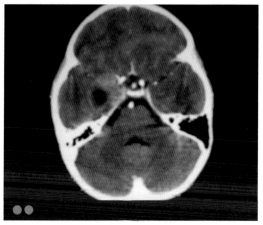

D2. Axial post-contrast CT shows a right parasellar mixed density mass with contrast enhancement. The low-density area may be due to fat or fluid and Hounsfield unit can be used to distinguish the two, as fatty density is in the minus territory whereas fluid density is nearly zero.

LYMPHOMA

Although primary CNS lymphomas involving the cavernous sinus is rare, they should be considered in the differential diagnosis of cavernous sinus lesions.

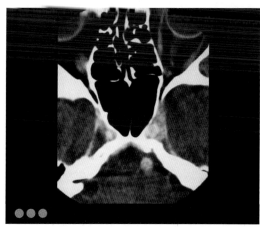

E. Axial, post-contrast CT shows an enhancing lesion in the left cavernous sinus due to lymphoma.

MALIGNANT SCHWANNOMA

Benign schwannoma of the trigeminal nerve comprises only 0.2–0.4% of all intracranial tumors and primarily arises in the gasserian ganglion. **Malignant schwannoma** of the trigeminal nerve is very rare.

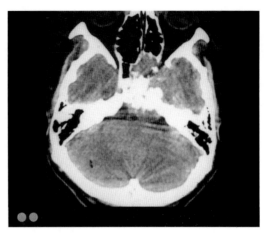

F. Axial CT shows a left parasellar mass extending into the posterior fossa and ethmoid sinus with bony destruction.

NASOPHARYNGEAL CARCINOMA INVADING CAVERNOUS SINUS

Nasopharyngeal carcinoma is a tumor arising from the epithelial cells that cover the surface of the nasopharynx. Although they are seen in any part of the world, they are prevalent in natives of southern China, Southeast Asia, and the Middle East/North Africa. The majority of tumors arise in the lateral walls of the nasopharynx, especially from the fossa of Rosenmuller and Eustachian tube cushions. These tumors can grow within the nasopharynx or can infiltrate in all directions locally. Skull base invasion is a common presentation (30%). Nasopharyngeal carcinoma can invade the cavernous sinus through the foraminal openings at the skull base, such as foramen lacerum or foramen ovale. It can also invade by direct erosion.

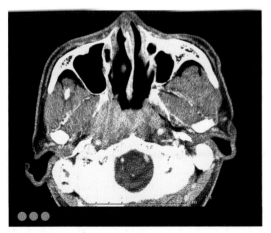

G1. Axial post-contrast CT demonstrates a right nasopharyngeal carcinoma with invasion of the right cavernous sinus.

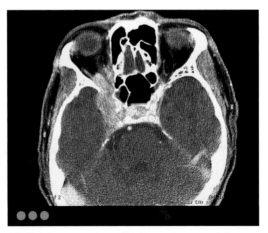

G2. Axial post-contrast CT demonstrates a right nasopharyngeal carcinoma with invasion of the right cavernous sinus.

SPHENOID SINUS TUMOR INVADING CAVERNOUS SINUS

Neoplasms of the sphenoid sinus can invade the cavernous sinus through direct erosion of the bony structure. Although it is uncommon, it should be considered in the differential diagnosis of cavernous sinus lesions.

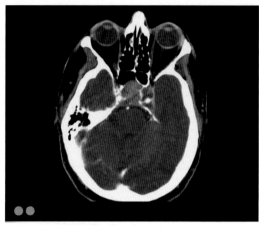

H. Axial, post-contrast CT shows an enhancing mass (small cell neuroendocrine tumor) in the sphenoid sinus invading the pituitary and left cavernous sinus.

TERATOMA

Teratomas represent approximately 0.5% of all intracranial tumors. These benign tumors contain tissue representative of all three germinal layers. Most **teratomas** are midline tumors located predominantly in the sellar and pineal regions. The presence of a teratoma in the cavernous sinus is very rare.

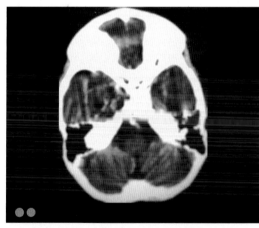

I. Axial, post-contrast CT shows a heterogeneous mass with patchy contrast enhancement.

Chapter 19

Vascular Lesions

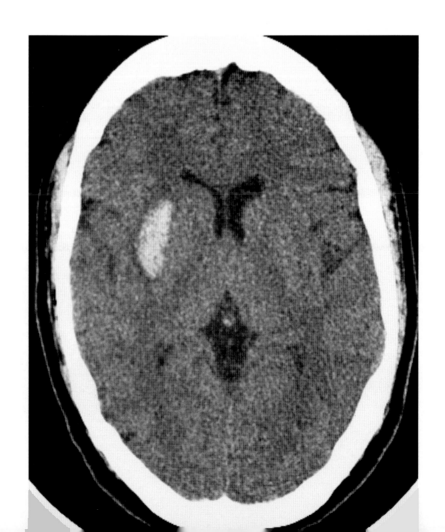

HYPERTENSIVE HEMORRHAGE

Hypertension is the most common cause of nontraumatic intracerebral hemorrhage in the brain. Intracerebral hemorrhage occurs when damaged arteries bleed directly into the brain parenchyma. The arteries in the brain damaged by exposure to chronic hypertension typically are the perforator arteries, such as lenticulostriate arteries, thalamoperforating arteries, which serve the basal ganglia and thalamus respectively. Other areas that also may be affected by hypertensive hemorrhage include the pons, centrum semiovale and the cerebellum. Hypertensive hemorrhages of the basal ganglia predominantly involve the putamen.

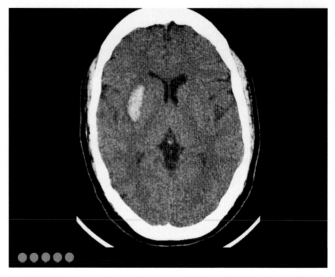

A. Axial CT shows a hyperdense area in the right basal ganglia, consistent with hypertensive hemorrhage.

DIFFERENTIAL DIAGNOSIS

At a Glance:

- Amyloid
- Aneurysm Rupture
- Arteriovenous Malformation
- Hemorrhagic Neoplasm (GBM)
- Hematoma Due to Trauma
- Moya-Moya Syndrome
- Pseudoaneurysm
- Venous Infarction Due to Sinus Thrombosis
- Cavernous Angioma (not pictured)
- Vasculitis (not pictured)

AMYLOID

Cerebral amyloid angiopathy is a disease due to the deposition of b-amyloid in the media and adventitia of small- and mid-sized vessels of the cerebral cortex and the leptomeninges. It is not associated with systemic amyloidosis. Cerebral amyloid angiopathy is one of the morphologic hallmarks of Alzheimer disease, but it is also often found in the brains of elderly healthy patients. Amyloid causes damage to the media and adventitia of cortical and leptomeningeal arteries, resulting in fibrinoid necrosis and microaneurysm formation, which could predispose the patient to intracerebral hemorrhage.

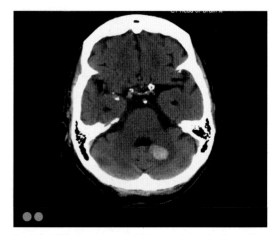

B. Axial CT shows an ovoid hemorrhage in the left cerebellum in a patient with amyloid.

ANEURYSM RUPTURE

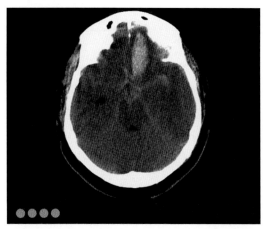

C1. Axial CT shows a hemorrhage in the left frontal lobe in addition to subarachnoid hemorrhage.

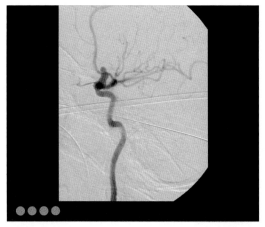

C2. Cerebral angiogram shows an aneurysm arising from the supraclinoid internal carotid artery at its junction with the ophthalmic artery.

ARTERIOVENOUS MALFORMATION

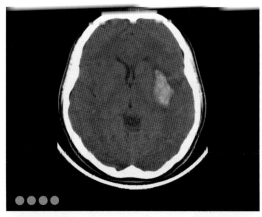

D1. Axial CT shows a hyperdense hemorrhage in the left basal ganglia due to a ruptured arteriovenous malformation.

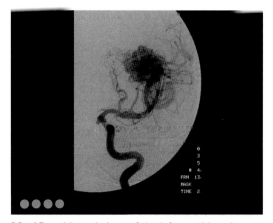

D2. AP and lateral views of the left carotid angiogram shows an arteriovenous malformation with dilated feeding arteries and early draining vein.

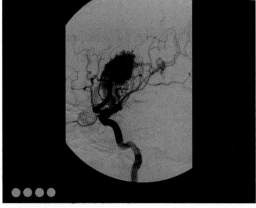

D3. AP and lateral views of the left carotid angiogram shows an arteriovenous malformation with dilated feeding arteries and early draining vein.

675

HEMORRHAGIC NEOPLASM (GBM)

The incidence of intracrebral hemorrhage due to neoplasm ranges from 1–14%. Primary iintracranial tumors that are frequently associated with hemorrhage include pituitary tumor, glioblastoma multiforme, ependymoma, choroid plexus papilloma, and meningioma. Secondary intracranial neoplasms that frequently bleed include melanoma, choriocarcinoma, renal cell carcinoma, thyroid cancer, breast and lung carcinoma.

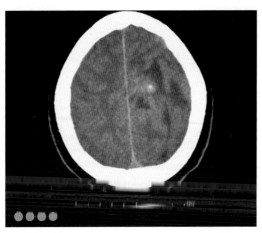

E1. Axial CT shows a heterogeneous mass with a small focus of hemorrhage in the left frontoparietal region.

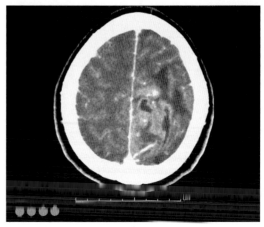

E2. Axial, post-contrast CT demonstrates heterogeneous enhancement of the mass in the left frontoparietal region.

HEMATOMA DUE TO TRAUMA

Trauma can cause intracerebral hemorrhage in addition to subdural hematoma, epidural hematoma, subarachnoid hemorrhage, and intraventricular hemorrhage. Delayed intracerebral hemorrhage can occur, and the duration of delay is usually within the first two weeks, especially the first 48 hours.

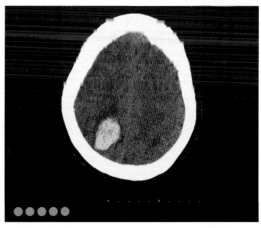

F. Axial CT shows a hyperdense hemorrhage in the right parietal region.

MOYA-MOYA SYNDROME

Moyamoya disease is a progressive occlusive disease of the intracranial vessels with particular involvement of the circle of Willis and the arteries that supply it. Moyamoya is a Japanese word meaning "puff of smoke". It describes the characteristic appearance of abnormal vascular collateral networks that develop due to stenosis of internal carotid arteries bilaterally. The characteristic pathological feature of moyamoya disease is intimal thickening in the walls of the terminal portions of the internal carotid arteries bilaterally. As a result, numerous small vascular channels are around the circle of Willis, giving a Moyamoya appearance.

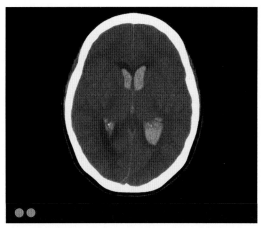

G1. Axial CT shows left periatrial intracerebral hemorrhage and extensive intraventricular hemorrhage.

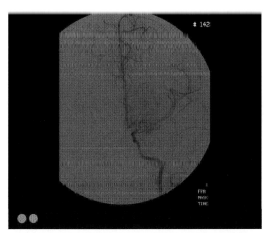

G2. AP view of bilateral carotid DSA demonstrates narrowing of the supraclinoid internal carotid arteries as well as proximal middle and anterior cerebral arteries. Collateral circulation from dilated lenticulostriate arteries presents as a puff of smoke type of appearance.

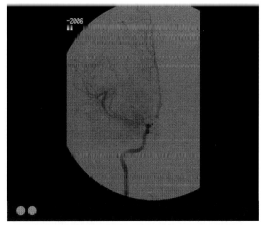

G3. AP view of bilateral carotid DSA demonstrates narrowing of the supraclinoid internal carotid arteries as well as proximal middle and anterior cerebral arteries. Collateral circulation from dilated lenticulostriate arteries presents as a puff of smoke type of appearance.

677

PSEUDOANEURYSM

Intracranial pseudoaneurysms are rare. They can be due to trauma, infection or tumor embolus. Traumatic aneurysms are usually seen at the peripheral cortical branches, where as infectious aneurysms can occur anywhere there is infection. Occasionally, a tumor emboli from atrial myxoma can cause a pseudoaneurysm.

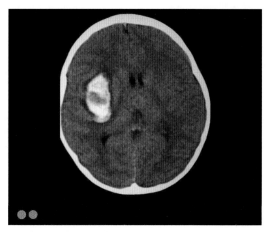

H1. Axial CT shows hemorrhage in the right basal ganglia.

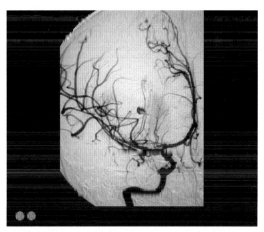

H2. AP and lateral views of the right internal carotid angiogram demonstrate a pseudoaneurysm arising from the lenticulostriate arteries.

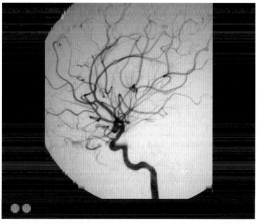

H3. AP and lateral views of the right internal carotid angiogram demonstrate a pseudoaneurysm arising from the lenticulostriate arteries.

VENOUS INFARCTION DUE TO SINUS THROMBOSIS

Hemorrhagic infarction is a complication of venous thrombosis. Venous thrombosis can occur in the sagittal sinus, transverse sinus, straight sinus and so on.

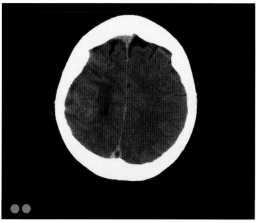

I. Axial CT shows an area of mixed hypo- and hyperdensity in the right frontal lobe due to a hemorrhagic venous infarction.

678

DENSE MCA

Early CT signs of cerebral infarction include:

1. "Dense MCA sign" is due to the presence of hyperdense clot in the middle cerebral artery on CT of the head without contrast.
2. "Insular ribbon sign" represents loss of gray-white differentiation at the insular cortex.
3. Effacement of cerebral sulci.

However, MRI with diffusion-weighted image is far more sensitive than CT for early detection of cerebral infarction. CT may not show acute infarct in the first 12–24 hours whereas MRI with diffusion imaging can demonstrate acute infarct as early as 30 minutes after the clinical onset.

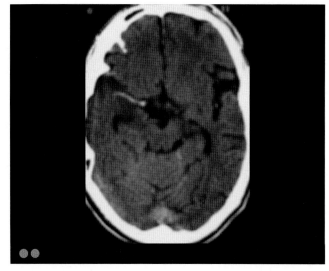

A. Axial CT demonstrates a dense right middle cerebral artery due to thrombus formation within the artery. Follow-up CT performed next day shows right middle cerebral artery territory infarct.

MCA TERRITORY INFARCT

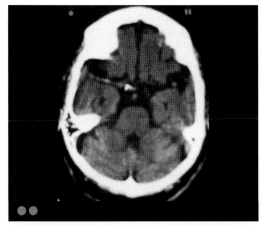

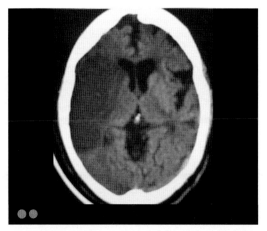

B1. Axial CT, obtained 24 hours following the initial CT, again shows a hyperdense right middle cerebral artery due to a thrombus in the right middle cerebral artery.

B2. Axial CT, obtained 24 hours following the initial CT, demonstrates an acute infarct in the right middle cerebral artery distribution.

Chapter 20

Lesions in the Cortical Gray Matter, White Matter, and Deep Gray Matter

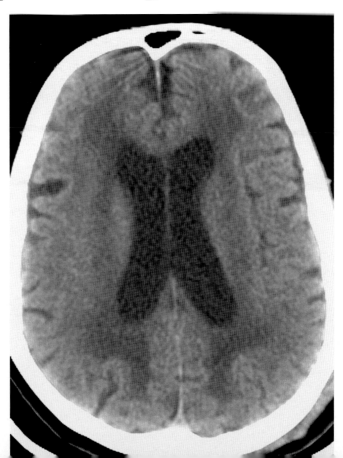

PERIVENTRICULAR WHITE MATTER ISCHEMIC CHANGES

Periventricular white matter low-density areas are seen in patients with chronic ischemic changes and are not necessarily symptomatic. They have been correlated with several factors including hypertension and silent stroke.

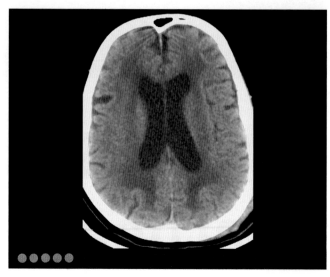

A. Axial CT shows periventricular hypodensity bilaterally due to chronic small vessel ischemic changes.

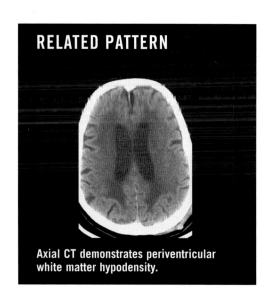

RELATED PATTERN

Axial CT demonstrates periventricular white matter hypodensity.

DIFFERENTIAL DIAGNOSIS

At a Glance:

- *Meningoencephalitis*
- *Multiple Sclerosis*
- *Posterior Reversible Encephalopathy Syndrome (PRES)*
- *Progressive Multifocal Leukoencephalopathy (PML)*
- *ADEM* (not pictured)
- *Vasculitis* (not pictured)

MENINGOENCEPHALITIS

CT findings are usually not useful in differentiating various types of viral meningoencephalitis. Low density edema in the white matter or high density hemorrhage may be detected by CT. CT can also be used to evaluate complications, such as hydrocephalus, hemorrhage or evidence of impending herniation.

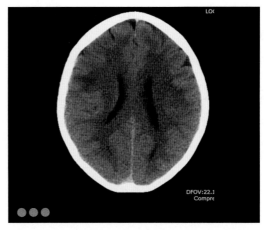

B. Axial CT shows ill-defined low-density areas in the periventricular white matter bilaterally in a patient with meningoencephalitis.

MULTIPLE SCLEROSIS

Multiple sclerosis is a demyelinating disease that is characterized by multiple inflammatory plaques of demyelination, involving the white matter of the central nervous system. Most common are among northern Europeans or people of northern European extraction. Females are affected more frequently than males with 3:2 ratios. CT scan shows hypodense to isodense lesions predominantly in the periventricular white matter with or without contrast enhancement. Large, mass-like plaques, or ring-like enhancing lesions can mimic neoplasm.

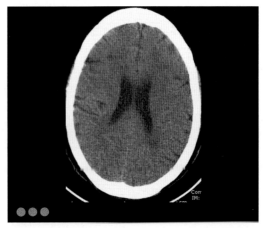

C. Axial CT shows low-density areas in the periventricular white matter in a patient with multiple sclerosis.

POSTERIOR REVERSIBLE ENCEPHALOPATHY SYNDROME (PRES)

As the name indicates, this is a reversible condition with abnormal hypodensity seen in the cortex and subcortical white matter in parietoccipital regions bilaterally on CT. Enhancement may or may not be seen. There are a diverse group of etiologies including preeclampsia-eclampsia, hypertension, cyclosporine, cisplatinum, SLE, cryoglobulinemia, and hemolytic uremic syndrome etc.

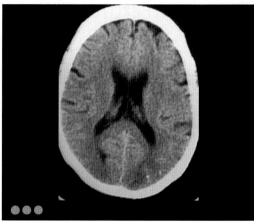

D. Axial CT demonstrates low density in parietooccipital region bilaterally involving the white matter as well as the gray matter.

PROGRESSIVE MULTIFOCAL LEUKOENCEPHALOPATHY (PML)

Progressive multifocal leukoencephalopathy (PML) is a fatal subacute progressive demyelinating disease seen in patients with impaired cell mediated immune response. The majority of PML cases involve patients who have AIDS. Other immunocompromised conditions, such as leukemia, lymphoma, collagen vascular disease, organ transplant etc, can be associated with PML. CT is not as sensitive for detecting white matter lesions as MRI. CT scans usually show several bilateral, asymmetric low density foci without significant mass effect. The lesions may involve the periventricular white matter, subcortical white matter with involvement of the subcortical U-fiber, or both. These lesions usually do not show contrast enhancement. Contrast enhancement is suggested to be an indicator of improved immune response.

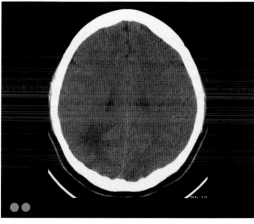

E. Axial CT shows low density in the parietal white matter bilaterally, worse on the right side in a patient with HIV infection.

CARBON MONOXIDE POISONING

Carbon monoxide toxicity is due to cellular hypoxia caused by interference of oxygen delivery. Carbon monoxide binds hemoglobin much more efficiently than oxygen, which results in functional anemia. CT scan may be normal or show bilateral basal ganglia low density. Cerebral edema may also be seen. CT findings may help to predict the outcome of patients as those with positive CT findings generally have neurologic sequelae.

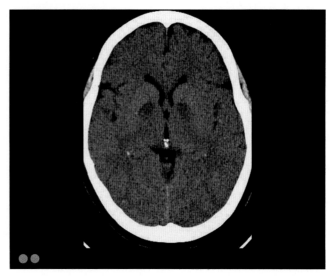

A. Axial CT demonstrates low density in the globus pallidi bilarerally.

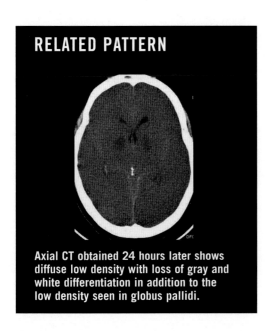

RELATED PATTERN

Axial CT obtained 24 hours later shows diffuse low density with loss of gray and white differentiation in addition to the low density seen in globus pallidi.

DIFFERENTIAL DIAGNOSIS

At a Glance:

- *Cryptococcus*
- *Vasculitis*
- *Huntington's Chorea*
- *Encephalitis* (not pictured)
- *Hypoglycemia* (not pictured)
- *Hypoxia* (not pictured)
- *Methanol* (not pictured)

- *Osmotic Myelinolysis* (not pictured)
- *Cockayne's Syndrome* (not pictured)
- *Creutzfelt-Jacob Disease* (not pictured)
- *Kearns-Sayre Syndrome* (not pictured)
- *Hallervorden-Spatz Disease* (not pictured)
- *Leigh's Disease* (not pictured)
- *Melas Syndrome* (not pictured)
- *Neurofibromatosis* (not pictured)
- *Pelizaeus-Merzbacher Disease* (not pictured)

CRYPTOCOCCUS

The majority of cryptococcal infections occur in patients with AIDS. Approximately 7–15% of patients with AIDS will eventually develop cryptococcal infection. Cryptococcal neoformans starts with pulmonary infection. The fungus disseminate from the lungs to other organs. Central nervous system infection has the most clinical manifestations. CT scans may show dilated perivascular spaces, cerebral edema, hydrocephalus, and atrophy.

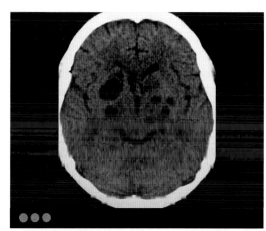

B. Axial CT shows multiple low-density areas in both basal ganglia due to dilated perivascular spaces in a patient with Cryptococcus infection.

VASCULITIS

Primary central nervous system vasculitis (PCNSV) is a rare form of vascular inflammatory disease. PCNSV diagnosis is established based on positive CNS tissue histopathology. Cerebral angiography may be negative in some cases although intracranial vascular stenosis can be demonstrated in some of the cases. Although no specific pattern for this entity exists on CT imaging, multiple infarcts of various ages in more than one vascular territory should raise the suspicion. CT angiography is now widely used and may replace conventional angiography as the primary imaging modality. The most frequent clinical presentations include hemiparesis, cerebral ischemia, headache and altered cognition.

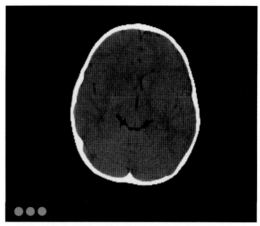

C. Axial CT shows low-density areas involving basal ganglia bilaterally, more on the right side.

HUNTINGTON'S CHOREA

Huntington disease (HD) is an adult-onset, autosomal dominant inherited disorder. It is associated with neuronal loss in the basal ganglia, especially the corpus striatum and deep layer of cerebral cortex. CT scans shows atrophy predominantly of the caudate nucleus and putamen, followed by the globus pallidus, thalamus, subthalamic nucleus, substantia nigra, and cerebellum.

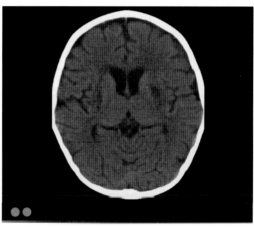

D. Axial CT reveals low-density area in both basal ganglia in a patient with Huntington's chorea.

FAHR'S DISEASE

Fahr's disease is a rare degenerative neurological disorder characterized by the presence of abnormal calcium deposits in the basal ganglia and associated cell loss in certain areas of the brain, particularly basal ganglia. Associated symptoms include progressive deterioration of cognitive abilities (dementia) and loss of acquired motor skills. Microcephaly, spasticity, seizure, and progressive neurologic deterioration is seen. The disease is often familial but may occasionally be sporadic.

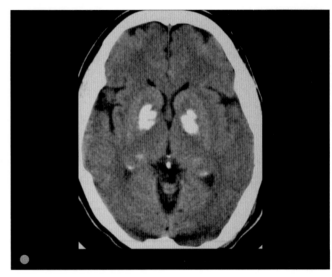

A. Axial CT reveals bilateral basal ganglia calcification along with calcification in the dentate nucleus in a patient with Fahr's disease.

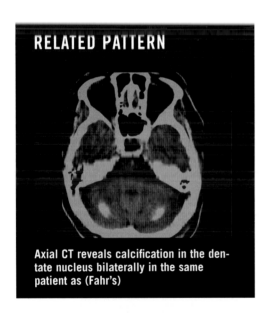

RELATED PATTERN

Axial CT reveals calcification in the dentate nucleus bilaterally in the same patient as (Fahr's)

DIFFERENTIAL DIAGNOSIS

At a Glance:

- *Physiologic Calcification*
- *Down's Syndrome*
- *Hyperparathyroidism*
- *Hypoparathyroidism*
- *Mineralizing Microangiopathy* (not pictured)
- *Toxoplasmosis* (not pictured)

- *AIDS* (not pictured)
- *Cockayne's Syndrome* (not pictured)
- *Hypoxic-Ischemic Encephalopathy* (not pictured)
- *Lead Intoxication* (not pictured)
- *Neurofibromatosis Type I* (not pictured)
- *Primary Hypothyroidism* (not pictured)
- *Pseudohypoparathyroidism* (not pictured)

PHYSIOLOGIC CALCIFICATION

The majority of the cases of basal ganglia **calcification** is idiopathic and of no clinical significance.

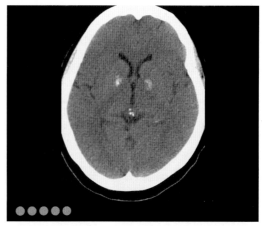

B. Axial CT shows idiopathic basal ganglia calcification in a 64-year-old male.

DOWN'S SYNDROME

Down syndrome is a congenital disorder due to trisomy 21. Down syndrome was named after John Langdon Haydon Down. The occurrence of Down syndrome increases with

maternal age especially in mothers aged 35 years or older. On CT scan, brachycephalic microcephaly, hypoplastic facial bones, widening of the pre dental space and basal ganglia calcification are seen.

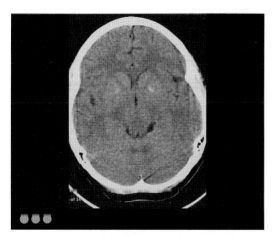

C1. Axial CT shows calcification in a 15-year-old patient with Down's syndrome.

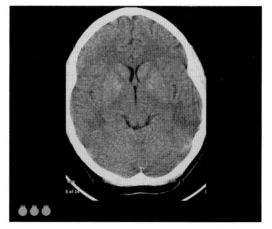

C2. Axial CT shows calcification in a 15-year-old patient with Down's syndrome.

HYPERPARATHYROIDISM

Primary hyperparathyroidism is caused by genetic mutation. Secondary hyperparathyroidism predominantly is due to chronic renal disease. Chronic hypocalcemia secondary hyperparathyroidism can also be the results of pseudohy-

poparathyroidism, vitamin D deficiency, and intestinal malabsorption syndromes. Hypertrophy of one or more of the four parathyroid glands is seen. CT scan of the head may show salt-and-pepper appearance of the skull, and intracranial calcification, especially in the region of basal ganglia.

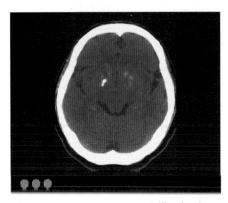

D1. Axial CT demonstrates calcification in both basal ganglia and in the periventricular white matter.

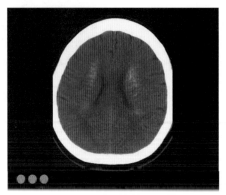

D2. Axial CT demonstrates calcification in both basal ganglia and in the periventricular white matter.

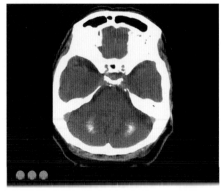

D3. Axial CT shows calcification involving both dentate nuclei.

HYPOPARATHYROIDISM

Primary hypoparathyroidism is a condition of inadequate parathyroid hormone (PTH) activity. In the situation of inadequate PTH activity, the ionized calcium concentration in the extracellular fluid is below the reference range. Primary hypoparathyroidism is a syndrome resulting from inadvertent surgical removal of parathyroid gland during surgery for thyroid gland or trauma. Secondary hypoparathyroidism is a physiologic condition in which PTH levels are low in response to a primary disease process that causes hypercalcemia. On CT, skull thickening, osteoporosis, poor dentition, Basal ganglia calcification may be seen.

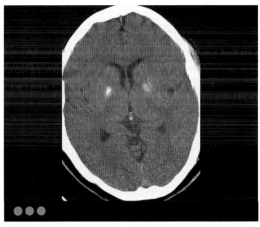

E. Axial CT demonstrates calcification in a 30-year-old patient with hypoparathyroidism.

690

CRANIOPHARYNGIOMA

Craniopharyngiomas can be histologically classified into three types: adamantinomatous, papillary, and mixed. The adamantinomatous type is predominantly seen in children (92–96%). Grossly, these tumors usually have both solid and cystic components. The fluid within the cysts has been historically described as "crankcase oil" because of its frequently dark and oily intraoperative appearance. The papillary type of craniopharyngiomas is more frequently seen in adults. They are well-circumscribed, pure, and solid masses. On CT, calcification is seen in 95% of the craniopharyngiomas in children and only 50% of the tumor in adults.

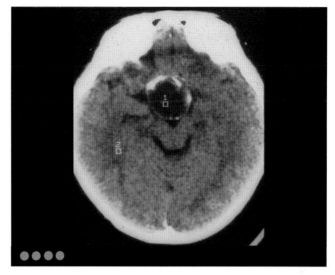

A. Axial CT reveals a curvilinear calcification in the suprasellar region. The differential diagnosis in this case is a suprasellar aneurysm.

DIFFERENTIAL DIAGNOSIS

At a Glance:

NEOPLASTIC

- Oligodendroglioma
- PNET
- Ganglioglioma
- Intraventricular Meningioma
- Meningioma
- Central Neurocytoma
- Pineoblastoma

INFECTIOUS

- Cysticercosis
- TORCH Syndrome
- Toxoplasmosis
- Tuberculoma (not pictured)

VASCULAR

- Aneurysm
- AVM Post-embolization
- Hemangioma

CONGENITAL

- Sturge Weber Syndrome (not pictured)
- Teratoma
- Tuberous Sclerosis

METABOLIC

- Hyperparathyroidism (not pictured)
- Parieto-occipital Calcification Due to Folate Deficiency in a Patient with Celiac Disease and Epilepsy

OLIGODENDROGLIOMA

Oligodendrogliomas constitute 5% of all cerebral gliomas. They are seen in young and middle aged adults. There is a male predominance of 2:1. These tumors typically involve the cerebral cortex and the subcortical white matter in the frontal and frontotemporal region. Calcification is demonstrated in 50–90% of oligodendrogliomas.

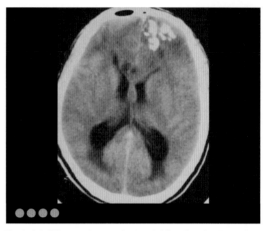

B. Axial CT reveals mottled calcification in the left frontal lobe with mass effect over the frontal horn of the left lateral ventricle. Abnormal low-density area is seen in the right frontal lobe. There is dilatation of the lateral ventricles seen. This is a case of high grade oligodendroglioma.

PNET

The term primitive neuroectodermal tumor or PNET is used to describe a group of tumors that exhibit similar cell types, but occur in different locations. Medulloblastoma, pineoblastoma, ependymoblastoma, retinoblastoma are all considered to be PNET. Medulloblastoma is the most common of all these tumors. PNETs generally occur in children. PNET of the brain can be divided grossly into infratentorial tumors (medulloblastoma) and supratentorial tumors (sPNET). The supratentorial tumors are much less common and are more likely to occur in young adults. Calcification may occur in PNET.

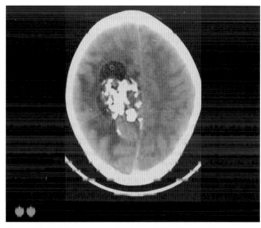

C. Axial CT shows mottled calcification with adjacent cystic areas and surrounding edema in the right frontal, parasagittal region. The pathological diagnosis is PNET.

GANGLIOGLIOMA

Gangliogliomas are predominantly seen in children and young adults. They are the most common mixed glioneural tumors. They can appear as cystic mass with a mural nodule in up to 50% of the cases. Calcification may be seen on CT.

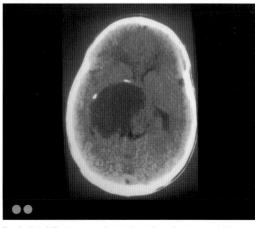

D. Axial CT shows a large low-density mass with small peripheral calcification.

INTRAVENTRICULAR MENINGIOMA

Intraventricular meningiomas are uncommon neoplasms. The incidence of lateral ventricular meningiomas is higher than those in the third or fourth ventricles. These tumors are usually asymptomatic in the early stage of the disease because ventricles of the brain provide space for tumor expansion, and until the cerebrospinal fluid pathways are mechanically occluded. The CT imaging features of intraventricular meningiomas are similar to dural based meningiomas. Tumor calcification may be seen. Avid contrast enhancement is usually seen following intravenous injection of contrast.

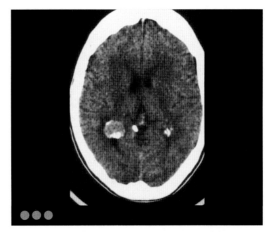

E. Axial CT reveals a mass lesion in the atrium of right lateral ventricle with calcification, consistent with intraventricular meningioma.

MENINGIOMA

Meningiomas are the most common nonglial primary neoplasm of the central nervous system. Extension of meningioma enhancement into adjacent dura may be seen in up to 60% of the cases. Tumor calcification is seen in 15% of the cases.

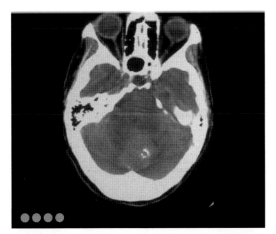

F1. Axial CT reveals a posterior fossa mass with calcification, consistent with a torcular meningioma.

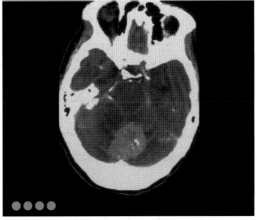

F2. Axial CT reveals a posterior fossa mass with calcification, consistent with a torcular meningioma.

CENTRAL NEUROCYTOMA

Central neurocytomas are seen in young adults and consist of 0.5% of primary brain tumors. They present as mass lesions in the body of lateral ventricle with cystic, necrotic change and broad-based attachment of the superolateral ventricular wall. Tumor calcification is common. Homogeneous or heterogeneous mass with heterogeneous contrast enhancement is seen on CT.

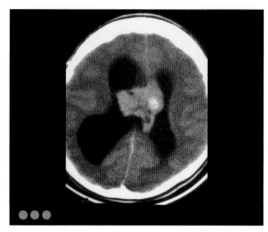

G. Axial CT shows an intraventricular mass in the lateral ventricle with focal calcification, consistent with a central neurocytoma.

PINEOBLASTOMA

Pineoblastomas affect male and female equally and are predominantly seen in the first and second decade of life. They are about six times more common than pineocytomas. Calcification may be seen in pineoblastoma. On CT, they show Slightly hypo- to iso-dense masses with calcification and contrast enhancement.

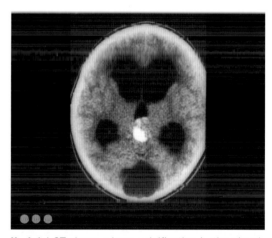

H. Axial CT shows a large calcification in the pineal region due to a pineoblastoma.

CYSTICERCOSIS

When cysticercosis cysts degenerate, they become calcified lesions with no edema or mass effect. Multiple intracranial calcification is frequently seen in patients with cysticercosis.

CYSTICERCOSIS (CASE ONE)

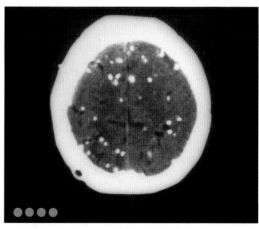

I. Axial CT shows multiple intraparenchymal calcifications due to healed lesions of cysticercosis.

CYSTICERCOSIS (CASE TWO)

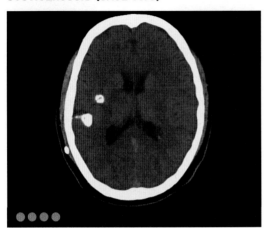

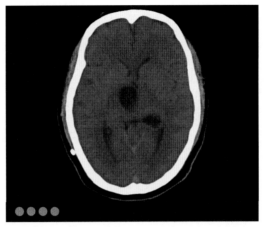

J1. Axial CT shows two relatively large calcifications in the right temporal region. Cysticercosis calcifications are usually small like those in case one. These large calcifications are occasionally seen.

J2. Axial CT shows a large cystic lesion in the right thalamus, consistent with a cysticercosis cyst.

TORCH SYNDROME

TORCH infection is usually caused by toxoplasmosis, other agents (syphilis), rubella, cytomegalovirus, and herpes simplex. **TORCH syndrome** refers to infection of pregnant women and a developing fetus or newborn by any of these infectious agents with similar clinical findings. CT scans frequently show intracranial calcification. Other congenital anomalies may also be demonstrated.

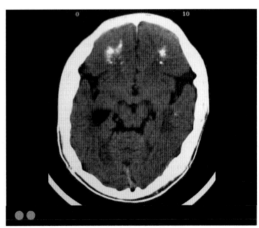

K. Axial CT shows bilateral frontal calcification in a patient with TORCH infection.

TOXOPLASMOSIS

Toxoplasmosis is a component of TORCH infection. TORCH syndrome refers to infection of pregnant women and a developing fetus or newborn by any of these infectious agents with similar clinical findings. CT scans frequently show intracranial calcification, sometimes in a periventricular distribution. Hydrocephalus may also be seen.

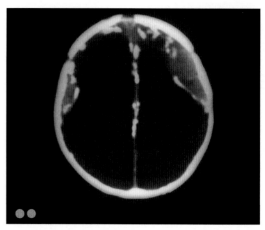

L. Axial CT shows marked hydrocephalus with periventricular calcification in a child with prenatal infection of toxoplasmosis. This is a case of TORCH syndrome.

ANEURY3M

Aneurysm wall may show calcification, especially those of giant aneurysms. Frequently, a fusiform aneurysm due to arteriorsclerosis can show calcification.

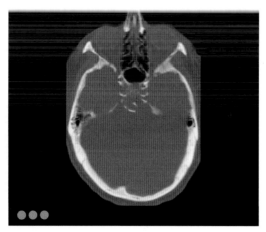

M1. Axial CT with soft tissue and bone window images show a calcified aneurysm of the basal artery.

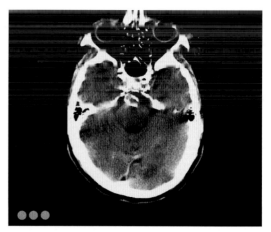

M2. Axial CT with soft tissue and bone window images show a calcified aneurysm of the basal artery.

AVM POST-EMBOLIZATION

Embolization material, such as glue or coil may mimic intracranial calcification on CT. AVM without any treatment may also show calcification.

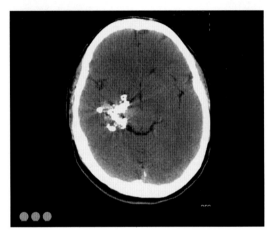

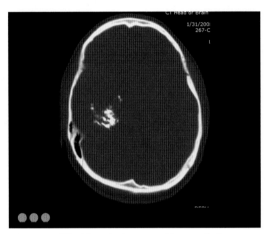

N1. Axial CT with soft tissue and bone window images shows irregular hyperdensity in the right temporal region in a patient post embolization for AVM. Hyperdense embolization material, such as glue, coil, may mimic calcification if appropriate window setting is not used to evaluate the hyperdensity.

N2. Axial CT with soft tissue and bone window images shows irregular hyperdensity in the right temporal region in a patient post embolization for AVM. Hyperdense embolization material, such as glue, coil, may mimic calcification if appropriate window setting is not used to evaluate the hyperdensity.

HEMANGIOMA

Intracranial hemangioma may show calcification within the mass.

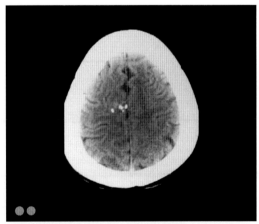

O. Axial CT demonstrates a hyperdense mass with calcification in the right frontal parasagittal region. The diagnosis is cavernous hemangioma.

TERATOMA

The pineal region is the most common site **of intracranial teratoma.** Pineal teratomas are seen exclusively in young males. CT shows heterogeneous signal intensity mass on. Focal fat can be seen as low density areas and calcification as high density areas.

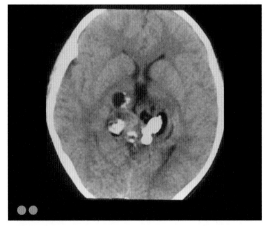

P. Axial CT shows a mass in the pineal region containing calcification, fat, and soft tissue. The diagnosis is pineal teratoma. Other calcified pineal masses include pineocytoma and pineoblastoma.

TUBEROUS SCLEROSIS

Tuberous sclerosis are usually seen in patients below 20 years of age. The tubers are actually harmatomas seen in the wall of the lateral ventricle and in the subcortical region. Calcification of the tubers in the subependymal region are frequently seen on CT.

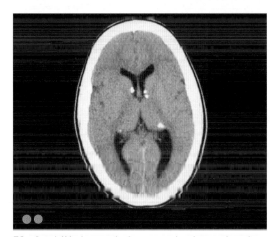

Q1. Axial CT demonstrates several subependymal calcifications around the lateral ventricle.

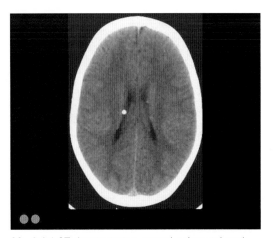

Q2. Axial CT demonstrates several subependymal calcifications around the lateral ventricle.

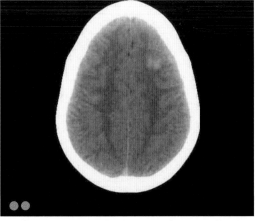

Q3. Axial CT shows hyperdense lesions in both the frontal lobes, consistent with subcortical tubers.

698

PARIETO-OCCIPITAL CALCIFICATION DUE TO FOLATE DEFICIENCY IN A PATIENT WITH CELIAC DISEASE AND EPILEPSY

The causes of intracranial parieto-occipital, cortical, or sub-cortical calcification in children are limited. Sturge–Weber syndrome and some atypical forms of other phakomatoses, intrathecal methotrexate and central nervous system irradiation, congenital folate malabsorption, and celiac disease. A definite association between epilepsy and celiac disease with folate deficiency has been recognized.

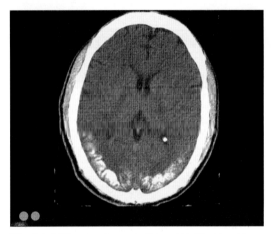

R1. Axial CT scan shows gyriform calcification in the parieto-occipital region bilaterally in a child with celiac disease.

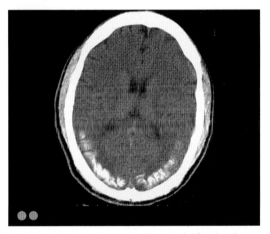

R2. Axial CT scan shows gyriform calcification in the parieto-occipital region bilaterally in a child with celiac disease.

HUNTINGTON'S DISEASE

Huntington's disease is a neurodegenerative disorder characterized by progressive choreoathetosis, psychological behavioral changes, and subcortical dementia. It is an autosomal dominant disease with a defective gene locus on chromosome 4. CT demonstrates diffuse cortical atrophy as well as atrophy of the caudate nucleus and, less frequently, of the putamen.

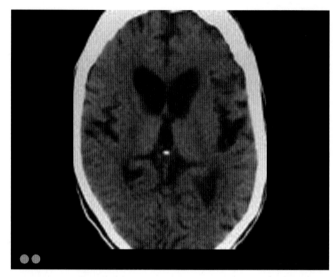

A. Axial CT demonstrates focal dilatation of the frontal horns of the lateral ventricles bilaterally secondary to atrophy of the head of the caudate nuclei.

DIFFERENTIAL DIAGNOSIS

At a Glance:

- *Caudate Infarct*

- *Alzheimer's Disease* (not pictured)

- *Multisystem Atrophy* (not pictured)

- *Parkinson's Disease with Dementia with Lewy Bodies* (not pictured)

CAUDATE INFARCT

Focal infarct of the caudate nucleus can result in focal dilatation of the frontal horn of the lateral ventricle. However, they are usually unilateral.

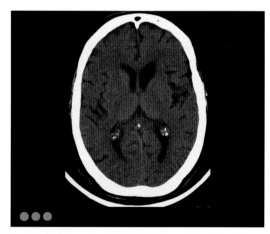

B. Axial CT reveals focal dilatation of the frontal horn of the left lateral ventricle due to an old infarct.

WERNICKE'S ENCEPHALOPATHY

Wernicke–Korsakoff syndrome is the most common deficiency syndrome related to chronic alcoholism. Wernicke's syndrome is the acute phase of the triad of oculomotor disturbance, cerebellar ataxia, and confusion. Korsakoff syndrome is a more chronic condition, which includes anterograde amnesia. Both syndromes are attributed to thiamine deficiency. CT shows hypodensity in thalamus bilaterally or in the midbrain.

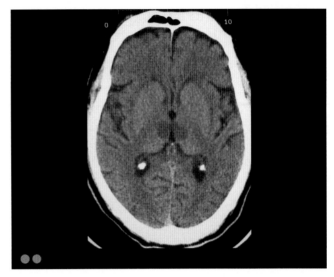

A. Axial CT demonstrates low-density areas in both thalami medially.

DIFFERENTIAL DIAGNOSIS

At a Glance:

• *Bilateral Thalamic Infarcts*

BILATERAL THALAMIC INFARCTS

A rare variation of the arterial blood supply in the thalamic and midbrain region is the artery of Percheron, which is a solitary arterial trunk that arises from the one of the proximal posterior cerebral arteries and supplies the paramedian thalami and rostral midbrain bilaterally. Occlusion of this artery can cause **bilateral thalamic infarction** as well as midbrain infarction.

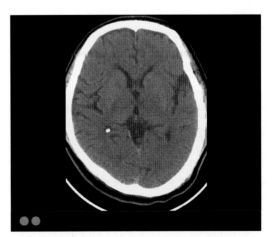

B. Axial CT shows low density in the medial aspect of thalamus bilaterally.

CEREBELLAR ATROPHY DUE TO SEIZURE MEDICATION (DILANTIN)

Chronic Phenytoin overdose has been implicated to cause cerebellar atrophy. Experimental studies have also shown loss of Purkinje cells and other evidence of cerebellar damage in animals given Phenytoin. However, some authors argue that seizure itself can cause hypoxic injury to the cerebellum with resultant atrophy.

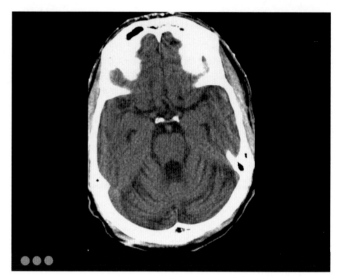

A. Axial CT demonstrates dilated fourth ventricle and prominent cerebellar sulci in a patient receiving seizure medication.

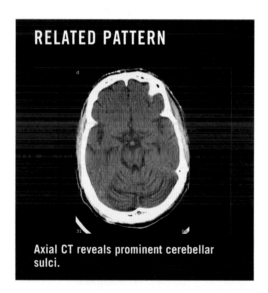

RELATED PATTERN

Axial CT reveals prominent cerebellar sulci.

DIFFERENTIAL DIAGNOSIS

At a Glance:

- *Olivopontocerebellar Degeneration*
- *Paraneoplastic Syndrome*
- *Alcoholism* (not pictured)
- *Hyperthyroidism* (not pictured)
- *Trauma* (not pictured)

OLIVOPONTOCEREBELLAR DEGENERATION

The olivocerebellopontine degenerations are progressive neurodegenerative disorders. Sporadic forms involve abnormalities of alpha-synuclein. Many specific genes have been implicated for the genetic forms. The pons is atrophic, especially in the area of the basis pontis. Volume loss of the cerebellum is seen, especially in the cerebellar white matter. Major neuronal loss occurs in the inferior olivary, arcuate, and pontine nuclei. The middle cerebellar peduncles show atrophy. The substantia nigra of the midbrain also shows evidence of tissue loss.

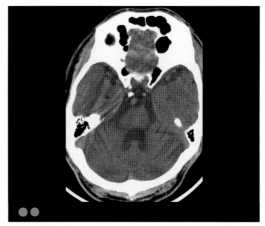

B. Axial CT shows dilated fourth ventricle and prominent cerebellar sulci.

PARANEOPLASTIC SYNDROME

Paraneoplastic cerebellar degenerations are disorders of the cerebellum, which are associated with certain neoplasms, particularly small cell lung carcinoma, ovarian cancer, uterine cancer, or breast cancer. These syndromes affect 1–3% of all cancer patients. They arise when tumors express proteins that are normally found only in neurons, and it is believed that the immune system, in its attempt to kill the tumor, also damages the cerebellum. Only about 1% of all persons thought to have a paraneoplastic syndrome turn out to have antibodies to neurons or Purkinje cells.

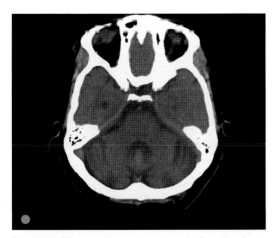

C1. Axial CT scan shows severe cerebellar atrophy in a patient with ovarian cancer.

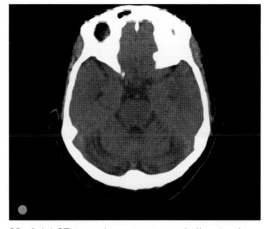

C2. Axial CT scan shows severe cerebellar atrophy in a patient with ovarian cancer.

SECTION II

SPINE

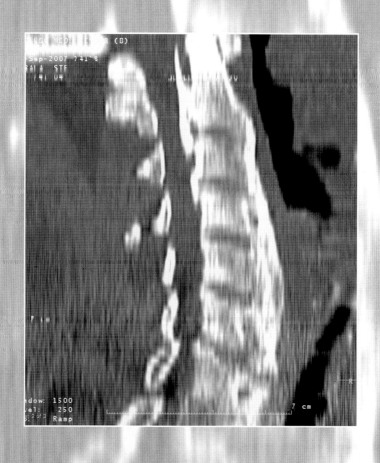

Chapter 21

Spinal Disease

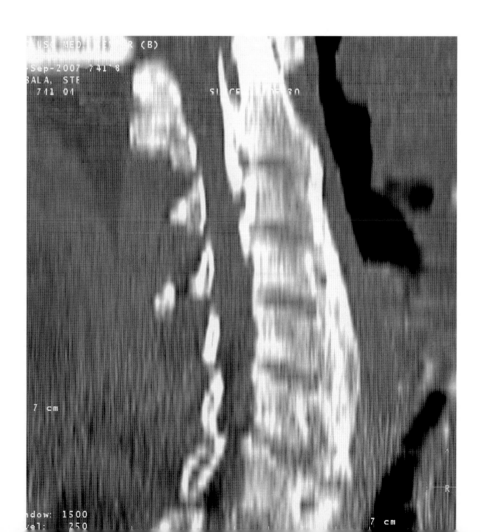

OSSIFICATION OF THE POSTERIOR LONGITUDINAL LIGAMENT

Ossification of the posterior longitudinal ligament (OPLL) is most prevalent in Asian population with most reports from Japanese literature and has a genetic linkage. Most individuals with this condition are asymptomatic and only a minority of them develop radiculopathy or myelopathy. Lesions of the posterior longitudinal ligament may include hypertrophy, calcification, and ossification. OPLL usually involves the cervical spine. Occasionally, it may be seen in the thoracic or lumbar region. OPLL is usually seen in the fifth to seventh decades with predominance in males. The ossified mass consists mainly of lamellar bone with areas of calcified cartilage in between. It expands in thickness and width beyond its anatomical boundaries and is firmly attached to the posterior margin of the vertebral bodies and annulus of the discs.

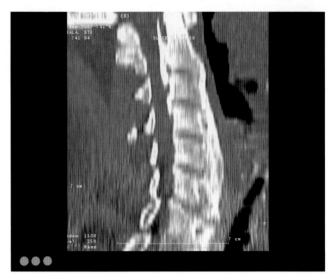

A. Sagittal reformatted CT image shows ossification of the posterior longitudinal ligament with spinal canal stenosis. In addition, there is ossification along the vertebral bodies anteriorly, consistent with diffuse idiopathic skeletal hyperostosis (DISH).

RELATED PATTERNS

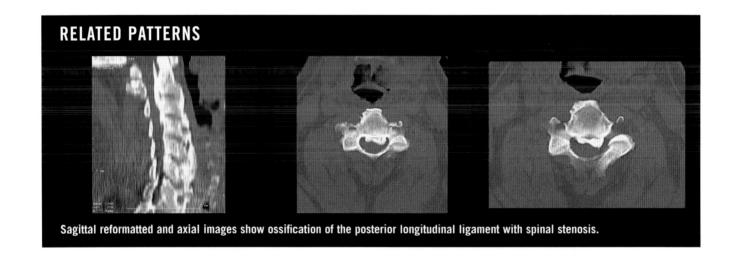

Sagittal reformatted and axial images show ossification of the posterior longitudinal ligament with spinal stenosis.

DIFFERENTIAL DIAGNOSIS

At a Glance:

- *Ossification of Ligament of Flavum*
- *Spondylosis*
- *Congenitally Short Pedicles* (not pictured)

OSSIFICATION OF LIGAMENT OF FLAVUM

Ossification of the ligamentum flavum (OLF) is the most common contributing factor in acquired thoracic spinal canal stenosis. It is known to occur frequently in the tho-racic spine and rarely in the cervical spine. The pathogenesis of ossification of the ligaments in OLF remains unclear. It has been reported that excessive exposure to fluoride can cause **ossification of the ligament of flavum.**

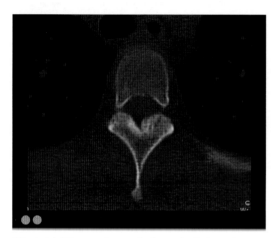

B1. Axial CT scan demonstrates spinal stenosis due to ossification/calcification of the ligament of flavum.

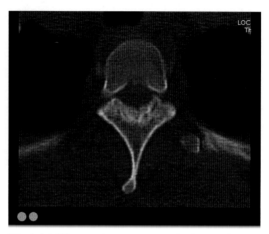

B2. Axial CT scan demonstrates spinal stenosis due to ossification/calcification of the ligament of flavum.

SPONDYLOSIS

Spondylosis is degenerative changes of the spine with aging. Degenerative or arthritic changes of the spine can involve the intervertebral discs, ligaments and facet joints surrounding the spinal canal. These changes include cartilaginous hypertrophy of the articulations surrounding the canal, intervertebral disc bulges or herniation, hypertrophy of the ligamentum flavum and bony osteophyte formation. CT scan shows osteophytes and endplate sclerosis, Schmorl's nodes, facet arthropathy and narrowing of the neural foramina.

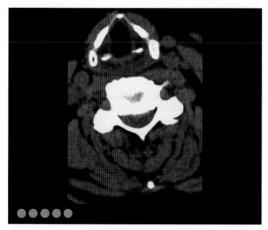

C1. Axial reformatted CT scan shows degenerative hypertrophic changes of the vertebral bodies with evidence of bony spinal canal stenosis.

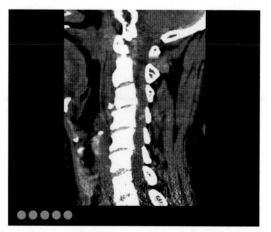

C2. Sagittal reformatted CT scan shows degenerative hypertrophic changes of the vertebral bodies with evidence of bony spinal canal stenosis.

709

SPONDYLOLISTHESIS SECONDARY TO SPONDYLOLYSIS

The spondylolytic (isthmic) type is due to the presence of defects in pars interarticularis and is the most common cause of spondylolisthesis. The defects separate the vertebra into two components. The portion of the vertebra posterior to the defects remain fixed, and the anterior portions are potentially allowed to slip forward relative to the posterior structures and the vertebral body below. Therefore, the bony spinal canal is widened at the level of spondylolisthesis.

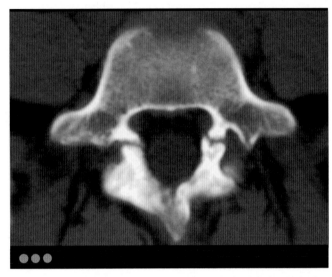

A. Axial CT reveals bilateral pars interarticularis defects. Note the spinal canal is widened.

RELATED PATTERNS

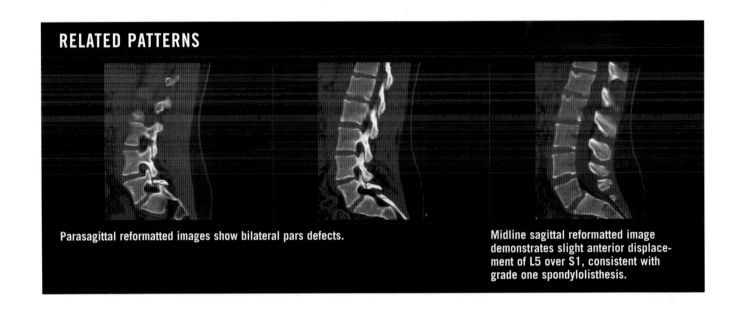

Parasagittal reformatted images show bilateral pars defects.

Midline sagittal reformatted image demonstrates slight anterior displacement of L5 over S1, consistent with grade one spondylolisthesis.

DIFFERENTIAL DIAGNOSIS

At a Glance:

- *Spondylolisthesis Due to Degenerative Changes of the Facet Joints*

SPONDYLOLISTHESIS DUE TO DEGENERATIVE CHANGES OF THE FACET JOINTS

In the degenerative type of spondylolisthesis, there is no pars interarticularis defect present. Long-standing intersegmental instability leads to degenerative spondylolisthesis. Arthritic changes develop in the facet joints. Eburnation and erosive changes occur, which may lead to abnormal vertical alignment of the articular surfaces allowing the inferior articular facet of the vertebral body above to slip forward in relation to the superior articular facet of the body below. Other factors include abnormalities of the ligaments and intervertebral disc. A constellation of these factors combined can cause spondylolisthesis. There is always associated spinal canal stenosis.

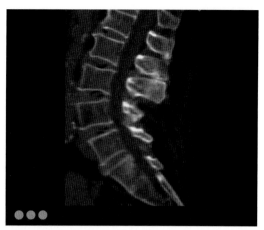

B1. Sagittal reformatted CT shows slight anterior displacement of L4 over L5.

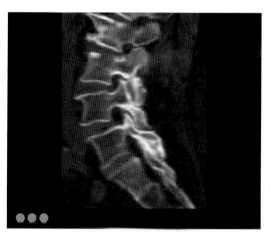

B2. Sagittal reformatted CT reveals slight anterior displacement of L4 over L5 and no evidence of pars defect.

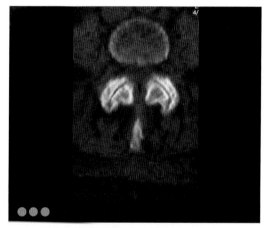

B3. Axial CT shows degenerative changes of the facet joints at L4-L5 level.

SPONDYLITIS

Early detection of infectious spondylitis is a challenge. CT scan is not as sensitive as MRI. It is a challenge to differentiate early infectious spondylitis from spondylosis. Correlation with clinical findings is essential.

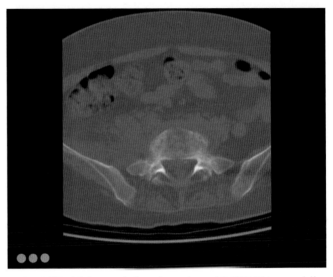

A. Axial CT with bone window shows irregular lytic changes of the S1 endplate.

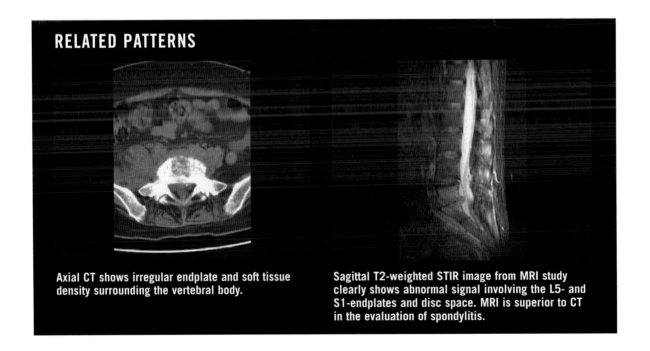

RELATED PATTERNS

Axial CT shows irregular endplate and soft tissue density surrounding the vertebral body.

Sagittal T2-weighted STIR image from MRI study clearly shows abnormal signal involving the L5- and S1-endplates and disc space. MRI is superior to CT in the evaluation of spondylitis.

DIFFERENTIAL DIAGNOSIS

At a Glance:

• *Tuberculosis*

• *Spondylosis* (not pictured)

TUBERCULOSIS

Differentiation of tuberculous spondylitis from pyogenic spondylitis can be a difficult task clinically and radiologically. Relative preservation of disc in patients with tuberculous spondylitis is thought to be due to the lack of proteolytic enzymes in the tuberculous mycobacterium. Tuberculous spondylitis tends to involve thoracic spine with resultant kyphotic deformity.

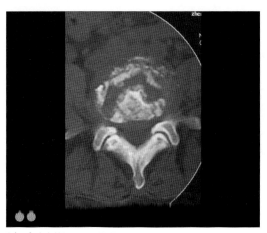

B1. Axial CT scan demonstrates irregular endplates with bone destruction and loss of disc space at L5-S1 level.

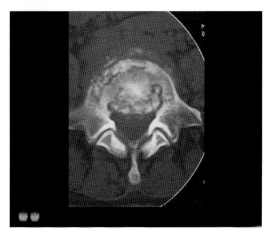

B2. Axial CT scan demonstrates irregular endplates with bone destruction and loss of disc space at L5-S1 level.

GIANT CELL TUMOR

Giant cell tumors are expansile, osteolytic lesions, but soft tissue mass without bony change can be seen. These tumors are often very vascular, containing osteoclast-like multinucleated giant cells. Most of the giant cell tumors of the spine occur in the sacrum.

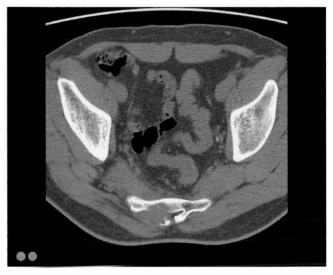

A. Axial CT shows a lytic lesion involving the sacrum on the right side with bone destruction.

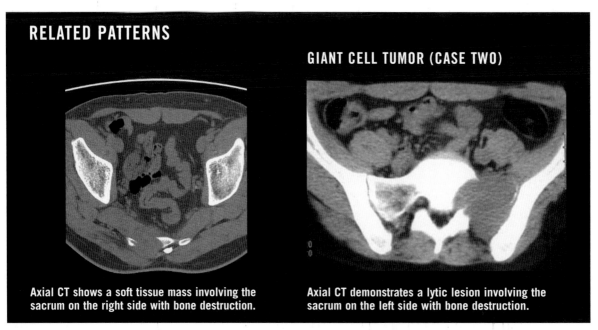

RELATED PATTERNS

GIANT CELL TUMOR (CASE TWO)

Axial CT shows a soft tissue mass involving the sacrum on the right side with bone destruction.

Axial CT demonstrates a lytic lesion involving the sacrum on the left side with bone destruction.

DIFFERENTIAL DIAGNOSIS

At a Glance:

- *Ankylosing Spondylitis*
- *Hemangioma*
- *Schwannoma*
- *Chordoma*
- *Ewing's Sarcoma*
- *Lymphoma*
- *Metastasis*

- *Aneurysm Bone Cyst* (not pictured)
- *Osteoblastoma* (not pictured)
- *Osteochondroma* (not pictured)
- *Radiation Osteonecrosis* (not pictured)
- *Multiple Myeloma* (not pictured)
- *Chondrosarcoma* (not pictured)
- *Osteosarcoma* (not pictured)
- *Angiosarcoma* (not pictured)

ANKYLOSING SPONDYLITIS

Ankylosing spondylitis is a chronic inflammatory disorder of unknown etiology with widespread musculoskeletal involvement. The most important features are sacroilitis as well as spondylitis. Abnormalities occur in joints and at the sites of attachment of ligaments and tendons to bone, with an overwhelming predilection for the axial skeleton. HLA-B27 antigen is found in a high percentage of patients with this disease. CT scans may be used to detect atlantoaxial joint instability, manubriosternal and costovertebral joint disease as well as sacroiliac joint disease.

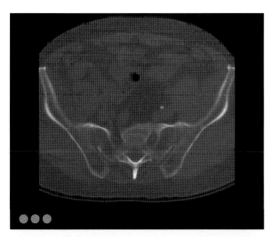

B1. Axial CT shows fusion of the S-I joints bilaterally.

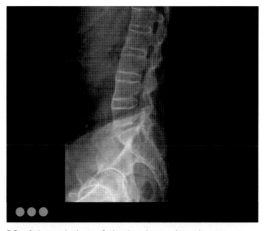

B2. A lateral view of the lumbar spine shows syndesmophytes involving all the lumbar vertebral bodies as well as fusion of the facet joints.

HEMANGIOMA

Hemangioma is the most common primary tumor of the spine, and it is frequently seen on the CT scan of the spine as an incidental finding. However, it is rarely seen in the sacrum.

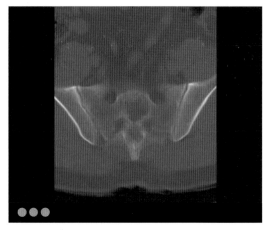

C. Axial CT demonstrates a lytic lesion with sclerotic margin involving the sacrum.

SCHWANNOMA

Schwannomas may arise from sacral nerve root sheath. They are usually seen as an intradural extramedullary mass and therefore are not true sacral neoplasms. They may be large and dumbbell shaped with extradural components that may erode and enlarge the sacral neural foramina.

SCHWANNOMA (CASE ONE)

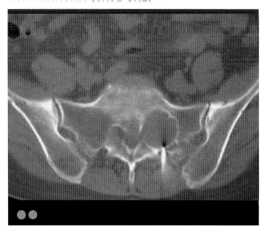

D1. Axial CT with bone and soft tissue window images shows erosion of the left S1 neural foramen with sclerotic margin.

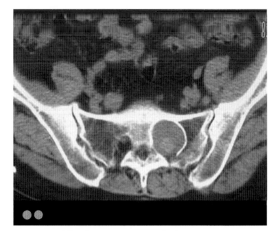

D2. Axial CT with bone and soft tissue window images shows erosion of the left S1 neural foramen with sclerotic margin.

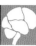

SCHWANNOMA (CASE TWO)

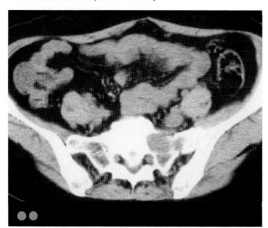

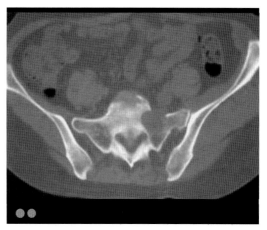

E1. Axial CT with soft tissue and bone window shows a mass with bone erosion involving the left side of sacrum.

E2. Axial CT with soft tissue and bone window shows a mass with bone erosion involving the left side of sacrum.

MALIGNANT SCHWANNOMA (CASE THREE)

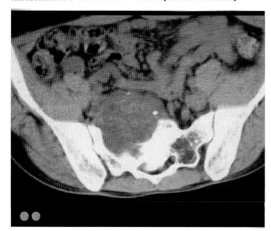

F. Axial CT shows bony destruction involving the right side of the sacrum with a large soft tissue mass. This is a case of malignant schwannoma.

CHORDOMA

Chordoma is a relatively rare tumor, representing only 2–4% of all primary malignant bone neoplasms. **Chordoma** is the most common primary malignant tumor of the spine (20–34%). The age range for chordoma is 30–60 years. The male to female ratio is 2–3:1. Tumoral calcification is frequently seen on CT.

CHORDOMA (CASE ONE)

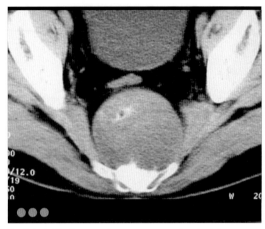

G. Axial CT shows a large pre-sacral soft tissue mass with evidence of bone destruction.

CHORDOMA (CASE TWO)

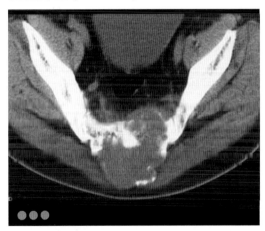

H1. Axial CT with soft tissue and bone window images demonstrates a large, lytic mass involving the sacrum.

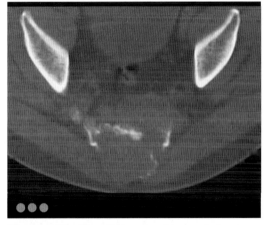

H2. Axial CT with soft tissue and bone window images demonstrates a large, lytic mass involving the sacrum.

EWING'S SARCOMA

Ewing's sarcoma tend to occur in patients younger than 30 years of age; pain is the most common presenting symptom. The sacrum and vertebral column, innominate bone, and bones of the lower extremity are the skeletal sites affected most frequently. Ewing's sarcoma is an aggressive tumor. CT findings include poorly defined osteolysis, erosion of the cortex, periostitis and soft tissue mass. In the spinal column, CT findings include bone destruction, pathological fractures and soft tissue mass.

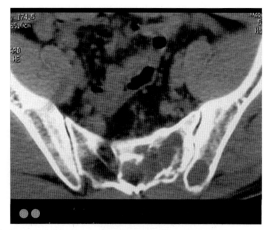

I. Axial CT shows a lytic lesion involving the left side of the sacrum extending into the sacral foramen. Another lytic lesion is seen involving the left ilium.

LYMPHOMA

Primary lymphoma of bone is a rare lesion but is the third most common primary malignant neoplasm of the sacrum. It may appear as either an aggressive lesion causing distinct bone destruction or as a permeative lesion, with a large associated soft tissue mass.

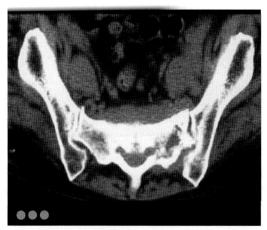

J1. Axial CT images with soft tissue and bone window show a flat, pre-sacral mass with lytic and sclerotic changes involving the sacrum.

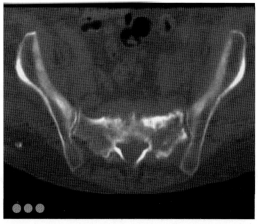

J2. Axial CT images with soft tissue and bone window show a flat, pre-sacral mass with lytic and sclerotic changes involving the sacrum.

METASTASIS

The spine including sacrum is a common site for metastatic disease. The more common primary tumors to metastasize to the spine are lung and breast carcinoma, followed by prostatic carcinoma. Any malignancy has the potential to metastasize to bone, and thus sacrum. Bony involvement results in epidural and paraspinal masses, which could cause nerve root compression.

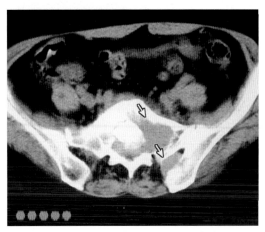

K1. Axial CT with soft tissue and bone window images shows lytic lesion involving the left side of the sacrum (arrows).

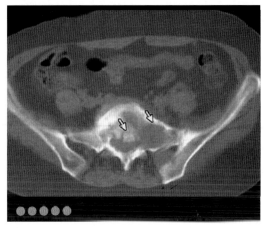

K2. Axial CT with soft tissue and bone window images shows lytic lesion involving the left side of the sacrum (arrows).

Chapter 22

Extradural Lesions

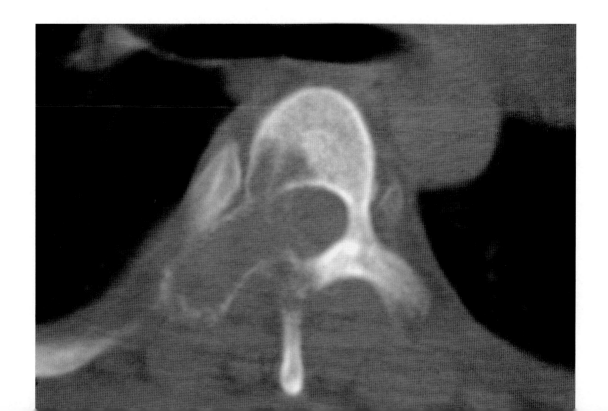

OSTEOBLASTOMA

The most common location for osteoblastoma is in the vertebral arch, mainly in the transverse and spinous processes. About 50% of the cases have vertebral body involvement. They are seen in young adults in the second and third decade. Patient usually complains of dull localized pain. An expansile lesion with multiple small calcifications and a sclerotic rim is seen.

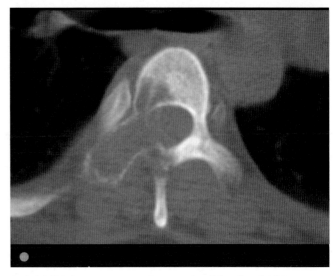

A. Axial CT shows an expansile mass involving the right transverse process, and part of the body and posterior elements with cortical thinning and bone erosion,

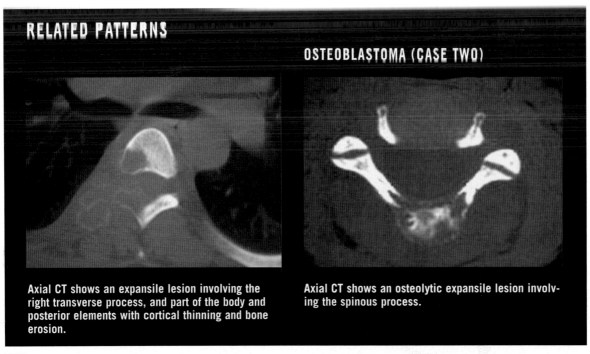

RELATED PATTERNS

OSTEOBLASTOMA (CASE TWO)

Axial CT shows an expansile lesion involving the right transverse process, and part of the body and posterior elements with cortical thinning and bone erosion.

Axial CT shows an osteolytic expansile lesion involving the spinous process.

DIFFERENTIAL DIAGNOSIS

At a Glance:

- *Aneurysm Bone Cyst*
- *Chondrosarcoma*
- *Chordoma*
- *Ewing's Sarcoma*
- *Giant Cell Tumor*
- *Metastatic Disease*

- *Osteochondroma*
- *Schwannoma*
- *Hemangioma* (not pictured)
- *Lymphoma* (not pictured)
- *Neuroblastoma* (not pictured)
- *Osteiod Osteoma* (not pictured)
- *Osteogenic Sarcoma* (not pictured)

ANEURYSM BONE CYST

Aneurysmal bone cyst (ABC) is a benign bone lesion and commonly affects young adolescents. It usually grows rapidly with hypervascularity. The majority of the **ABC** is seen before the age of 30. In the spine, it is usually an osteolytic lesion with predilection for posterior elements. Extensive bone destruction with vertebral body collapse can occur. Extension of the lesion into the spinal canal, adjacent ribs, and paravertebral soft tissue is seen.

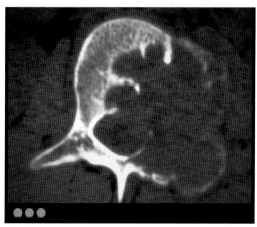

B. Axial CT shows a multi-lobulated, lytic lesion involving the vertebral body with erosion and expansion of the bony cortex.

CHONDROSARCOMA

They usually present as osteolytic, expansile lesions with amorphous calcification. Spine is only occasionally involved. Posterior elements may be involved. Chondrosarcoma may develop in a preexisting cartilaginous lesion or in association with Paget's disease, or previous radiation.

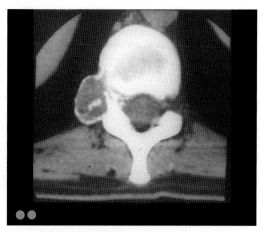

C. Axial CT demonstrates an expansile mass with ill-defined margin arising from the right side of the body and pedicle with internal calcification.

CHORDOMA

Chordomas are slow growing, locally invasive malignant tumors derived from remnants of the notochord. Sacrococcygeal involvement is seen in 50% of the cases and vertebral involvement is seen in 15% of the cases. They usually present with bone destruction with a soft tissue mass. Intervertebral disc may or may not be involved. Amorphous calcification and residual bone are better seen on CT.

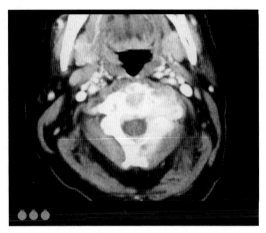

D1. Axial CT shows a destructive lesion involving the left transverse process and lamina of C2 vertebral body.

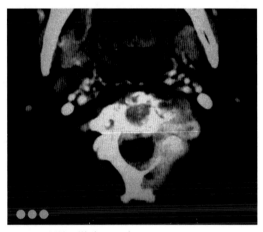

D2. Axial CT with bone window image shows a destructive lesion involving the left transverse process and lamina of C2 vertebral body.

EWING'S SARCOMA

Ewing's sarcoma presents as an ill defined, permeative destruction of the vertebral bodies associated with paraspinal mass. Collapse of the vertebral body may be seen. Primary Ewing's sarcoma of the spine is extremely rare; most spinal **Ewing's sarcoma** is metastatic in nature.

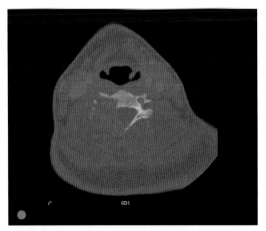

E1. Axial CT scan shows a soft tissue mass with bone destruction involving the right side of the vertebral body and posterior elements.

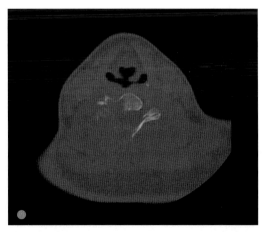

E2. Axial CT scan shows a soft tissue mass with bone destruction involving the right side of the vertebral body and posterior elements.

GIANT CELL TUMOR

Approximately half of the spinal **giant cell tumors** occur in the sacrum. Spinal **giant cell tumors** tend to occur earlier than those at other sites and have a peak incidence in the second and third decades. There is a 2:1 female predominance. Involvement of the spine occurs at the vertebral body and neural arch. A paravertebral mass may be seen. Imaging findings of **giant cell tumor** show an expansile lesion involving posterior elements and may appear to be aggressive. They can mimic aneurysm bone cyst. Dramatic increase in lesion size during pregnancy may occasionally be seen.

GIANT CELL TUMOR (CASE ONE)

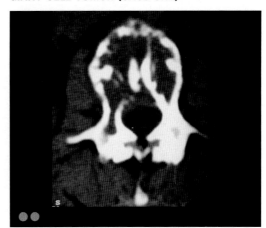

F. Axial CT with bone window shows lytic lesion involving the vertebral body with a small epidural component.

GIANT CELL TUMOR (CASE TWO)

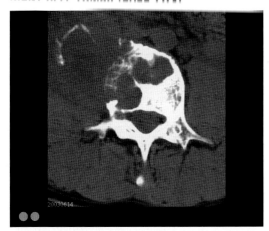

G1. Axial CT with bone window shows an expansile lytic lesion with soft tissue mass and displaced bony fragments.

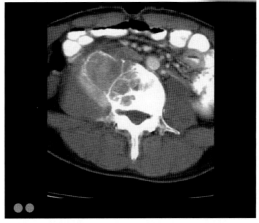

G2. Axial CT with bone window shows an expansile lytic lesion with soft tissue mass and displaced bony fragments.

METASTATIC DISEASE

Spinal **metastatic disease** most commonly involves the vertebral bodies, followed by pedicles and neural arch. They are most frequently seen in the thoracic spine, followed by lumbar spine. Most metastatic lesions are osteolytic. Osteoblastic lesions are seen in metastatic prostate carcinoma or breast carcinoma.

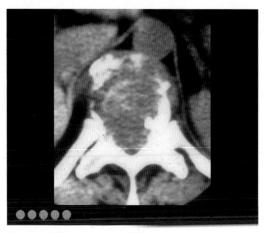

H1. Axial CT scan shows lytic lesions involving vertebral bodies with epidural mass

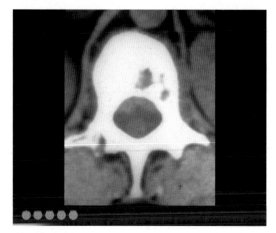

II2. Axial CT scan shows lytic lesions involving vertebral bodies with epidural mass.

OSTEOCHONDROMA

Osteochondroma is an overgrowth of cartilage and bone near the growth plate. This type of overgrowth can occur in any cartilaginous bone. It usually affects the long bones in the leg, the pelvis, or scapula. Osteochondroma rarely involves the spine, with a predilection for cervical or thoracic spine. It is seen between the ages of 10–30 years and affects males and females equally. Osteochondromas are usually located either on the posterior arch or on the anterolateral aspect of the vertebral body.

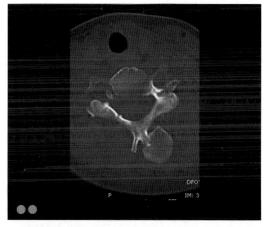

I. Axial CT shows focal bony growth from the spinous process.

SCHWANNOMA

Most schwannomas are intradural extramedullary in location. A combination of intradural and extradural components of the schwannomas may be seen. Occasionally, they can be purely extradural in location.

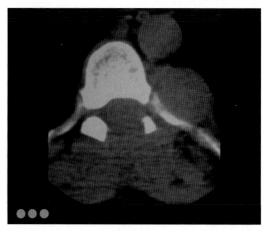

J. Axial CT shows a large left paraspinal mass. Note this patient had laminectomy and removal of the intradural component of the lesion previously.

BURST FRACTURE

Fractures in the lumbar spine can occur due to a number of reasons. In younger patients, fractures are usually due to car accidents, jumps or falls. In older patients, lumbar compression fractures can occur due to minor trauma, such as a fall. The most common underlying reason for fractures in older patients, especially women, is osteoporosis, followed by malignancy, infections, and renal disease. Burst fractures result from high-energy axial loading to the spine. They are usually seen in young patients with injuries caused by jumps or falls.

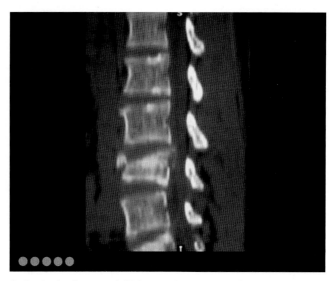

A. Sagittal reformatted CT image shows a burst fracture of L4 vertebral body.

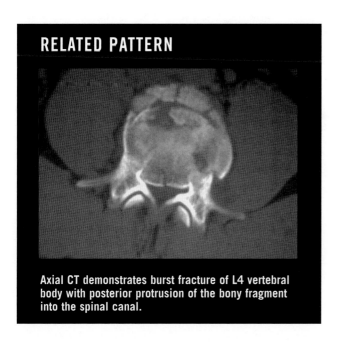

RELATED PATTERN

Axial CT demonstrates burst fracture of L4 vertebral body with posterior protrusion of the bony fragment into the spinal canal.

DIFFERENTIAL DIAGNOSIS

At a Glance:

- *Coccidiomycosis*
- *Echinoccocal Cyst*
- *Eosinophilic Granuloma*
- *Herniated Disc*
- *Lipoma*
- *Ossification of Posterior Longitudinal Ligament (OPLL)*

- *Renal Osteodystrophy*
- *Synovial Cyst*
- *Tarlov's Cyst*
- *Tumoral Calcinosis*
- *Epidural Cyst* (not pictured)
- *Epidural Abscess* (not pictured)
- *Epidural Hematoma* (not pictured)
- *Foreign Body* (not pictured)

COCCIDIOMYCOSIS

Coccidiomycosis is endemic in the Southwestern United States, especially in the San Joaquin Valley. Central nervous system involvement is usually the result of hematogenous spread of pulmonary lesions. There is a male predominance of 5 to 1. Meningeal involvement is the most common form. Lytic lesions involving the skull or spine are occasionally seen.

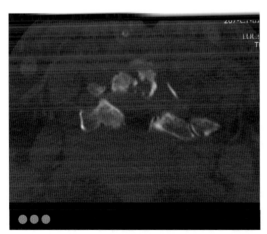

B1. Axial CT scan demonstrates lytic changes involving the cervical vertebral body with adjacent soft tissue mass seen on the left side. Note patient had previous laminectomy.

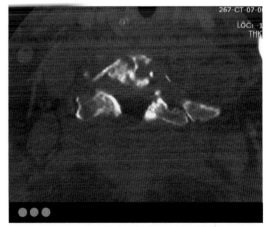

B2. Axial CT scan demonstrates lytic changes involving the cervical vertebral body with adjacent soft tissue mass seen on the left side. Note patient had previous laminectomy.

ECHINOCCOCAL CYST

Hydatid disease in humans is caused by the cystic (larval) stage of the tapeworm *Echinococcus granulosus*, which is endemic to the temperate climate. The disease is found worldwide, especially in the Middle East, Australia, and South America. In the United States, Echinococcus granulosus is seen in the western states including California, Arisona, New Mexico, and Utah. The most common sites of **echinococcus** infection are the liver, lungs, and brain in order of frequency. Bone involvement is uncommon, and spinal involvement is rare, with an incidence of less than 1%.

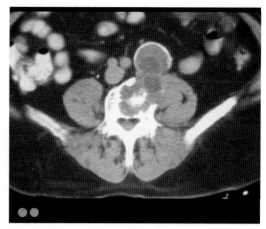

C. Axial CT demonstrates a lobulated cystic mass involving the vertebral body and anterior paraspinal tissue.

EOSINOPHILIC GRANULOMA

Eosinophilic granuloma is characterized by skeletal lesions, and it predominantly affects children, and young adults. Solitary lesions are more commonly seen than multiple lesions. Any bone may be involved including the skull, mandible, ribs, long bones of the upper extremity, pelvis, and spine. Vertebral body involvement may lead to flattening of the vertebral body, so called "vertebra plana".

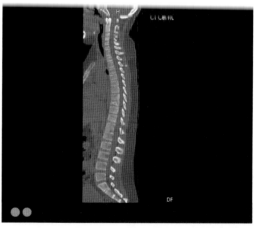

D. Sagittal reformatted CT shows loss of height of T9 vertebral body.

HERNIATED DISC

Lumbar disc herniation is the most common type of disc herniation. Thoracic disc herniation is the least common type. CT in the lumbar area demonstrates displacement of the anterior epidural and foraminal fat by herniated disc material, which may also obscure the nerve roots. Calcification of the herniated disc is more common in the thoracic spine. Little epidural fat is present in the cervical region, thus cervical herniations are not usually outlined by displaced fat but by subtle soft tissue encroachment upon the spinal canal.

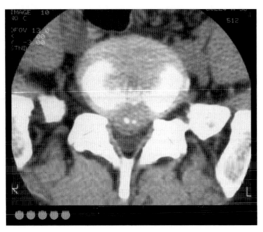

E1. Axial CT scan shows herniated disc centrally with compression of the thecal sac at L5-S1 level.

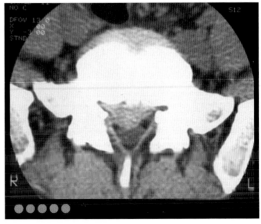

E2. Axial CT scan shows herniated disc centrally with compression of the thecal sac at L5-S1 level.

LIPOMA

Lipomas are believed to result from the maldifferentiation of the meninx primitiva during the formation at the subarachnoid cistern and are associated with dysgenesis of the adjacent neural tissue in 55% of the cases. The location for filum fibrolipomas is obvious; however, they may involve the conus superiorly and the epidural space inferiorly. On CT, they usually present a low-density mass of fat attenuation. Calcification is occasionally seen.

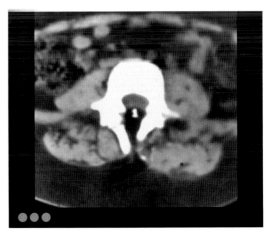

F. Axial CT shows a hypodense lesion with focal calcification at the posterior aspect of the spinal canal with spina bifida occulta.

OSSIFICATION OF POSTERIOR LONGITUDINAL LIGAMENT (OPLL)

Ossification of the posterior longitudinal ligament (OPLL) is commonly seen in the Asian people, and is well reported in Japanese literature. It appears to have a strong genetic predisposition. **Ossification of the posterior longitudinal lig-** ament represents a continuum, beginning with hypertrophy of the posterior longitudinal ligament followed by progressive coalescence of centers of chondrification and ossification. The majority (70%) of the cases involve the cervical spine, usually C2-C4, followed by 15% each for thoracic spine, usually T1-T4 and lumbar spine, usually L1-L3.

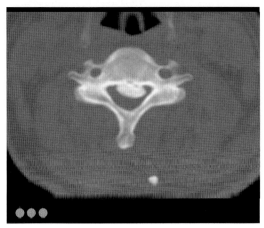

G1. Axial CT scan demonstrates ossification of the posterior longitudinal ligament extending from C3 through C5.

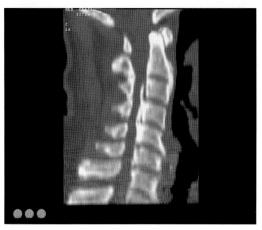

G2. Sagittal CT scan demonstrates ossification of the posterior longitudinal ligament extending from C3 through C5.

RENAL OSTEODYSTROPHY

Renal osteodystrophy is a global term used to describe all pathologic features of bony changes in patients with renal insufficiency. Osteomalacia is a part of the spectrum of osseous abnormalities that can be observed in patients with chronic renal failure. Renal osteodystrophy represents a constellation of findings including secondary hyperparathyroidism, rickets, osteomalacia, and osteoporosis. Features of rickets and osteomalacia are seen in children, whereas features of osteomalacia and secondary hyperparathyroidism are seen in adults. Imaging findings of renal osteodystrophy reflects a wide spectrum of these above mentioned disorders.

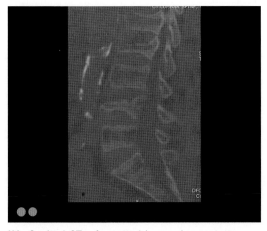

H1. Sagittal CT reformatted image demonstrates diffuse osteopenia with compression fractures of L2 and L4 vertebral bodies.

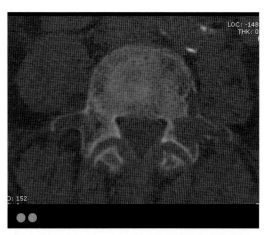

H2. Axial CT shows a a lucent lesion involving the left pedicle of L5, consistent with a Brown tumor.

731

SYNOVIAL CYST

Synovial cysts may be contiguous with the synovium or they may be juxtaarticular without synovial attachment. Some 75% occur at L4-L5 level, and most of the remain- der in L3-L4 and L5-S1 levels. Cysts are always seen adjacent to degenerative facet joints. The diagnosis of a **synovial cyst** can be made on CT by demonstrating an epidural cystic mass adjacent to degenerated facet joint.

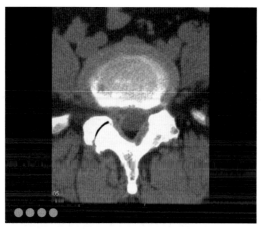

I1. Axial CT shows a soft tissue mass with low density centrally near the right facet joint.

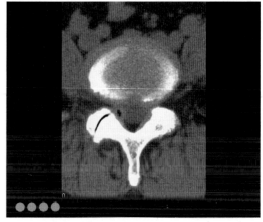

I2. Axial CT shows a soft tissue mass with gas centrally near the right facet joint. Note the gas in the right facet joint.

TARLOV'S CYST

Tarlov's cyst is an outpouching of the perineurial space on the extradural portion of the posterior sacral or coccygeal nerve roots at the junction of the root of the ganglion. Most cases are asymptomatic, but the cyst can impinge on the adjacent nerve roots causing low back pain or other neurological findings.

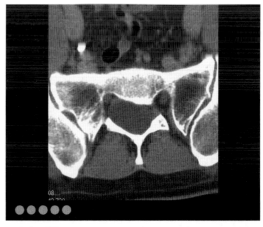

J. Axial CT demonstrates an expansile cystic lesion in the sacral canal with bony remodeling.

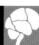

TUMORAL CALCINOSIS

Tumoral calcinosis is a rare disorder characterized by soft tissue calcification deposition, typically in a periarticular distribution most commonly seen in the regions of the hip, shoulder, and elbow. Spinal involvement is rare. The disorder was differentiated from dystrophic and metabolic calcifications in that patients had normal calcium levels and elevated phosphate levels. The disease has a familial predisposition and a higher incidence in the African American population. Tumoral calcinosis typically takes the form of calcium hydroxyapatite crystals surrounded by a foreign body giant cell reaction and histiocytes.

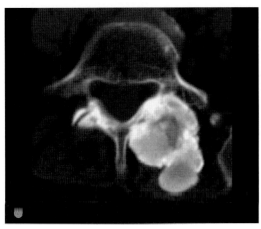

K1. Axial CT shows a large, calcified and lobulated bony mass in the region of left lamina and facet joint.

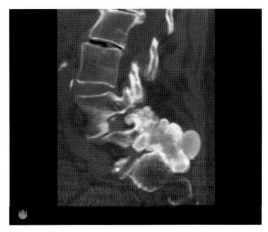

K2. Sagittal CT shows a large, calcified and lobulated bony mass in the region of left lamina and facet joint.

Chapter 23

Intradural Extramedullary Lesions

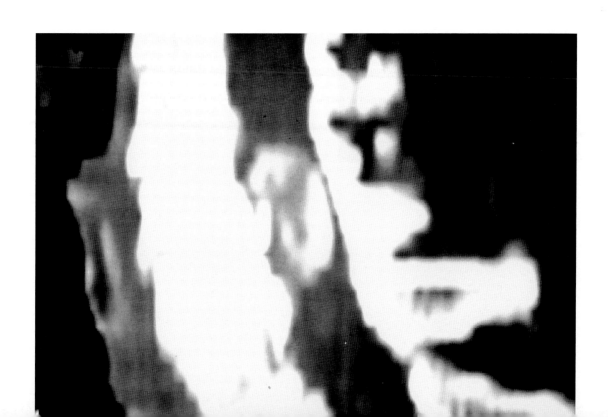

MENINGIOMA

Meningiomas comprise 25–45% of intraspinal tumors. Meningiomas typically present between the ages of 40 and 60 and demonstrate an up to 80% female preponderance. Approximately 80% of the spinal meningiomas occur in the thoracic region, 15% are cervical, 3% are lumbar, and 2% are located at the foramen magnum. Thoracic meningiomas tend to be located posterior or lateral to the cord. CT may show a hyperdense lesion due to psammomatous calcification. Homogeneous contrast enhancement is seen.

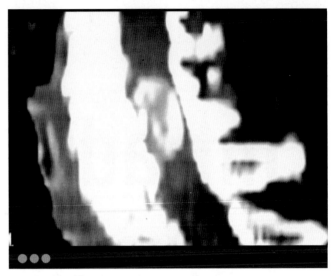

A. Sagittal reformatted CT shows a calcified intradural mass in the cervical region.

RELATED PATTERN

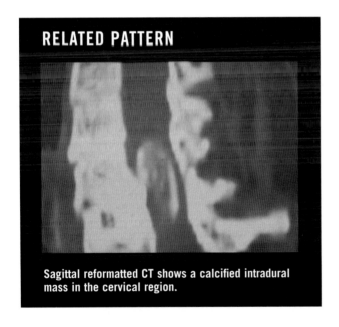

Sagittal reformatted CT shows a calcified intradural mass in the cervical region.

DIFFERENTIAL DIAGNOSIS

At a Glance:

- *Schwannoma*
- *Ependymoma (Rare)* (not pictured)
- *Metastatic Seeding* (not pictured)

SCHWANNOMA

Nerve sheath tumors consist of **schwannomas** and neurofibromas. Nerve sheath tumors have been reported to comprise 15–30% of primary spinal tumors. Nerve sheath tumors usually involve the dorsal nerve roots and may be located anywhere in the spine. The most common site is the thoracic spine (43%), followed by lumbar spine (34%). Approximately 70% are intradural, extramedullary, about 15% each are extradural and combined intradural/extradural, and less than 1% intramedullary in location. CT shows a soft tissue mass with associated focal bony changes. Homogeneous, intense contrast enhancement is seen.

SCHWANNOMA (CASE ONE)

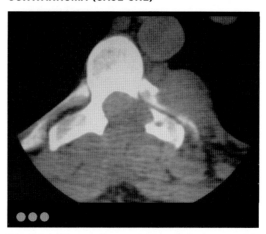

B1. Axial CT scan shows a left paraspinal mass with extension into the bony canal on the left side. Note status post laminectomy for this patient.

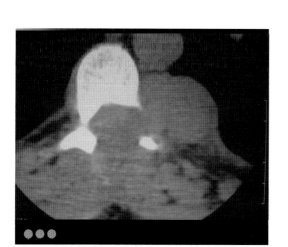

B2. Axial CT scan shows a left paraspinal mass with extension into the bony canal on the left side. Note status post laminectomy for this patient.

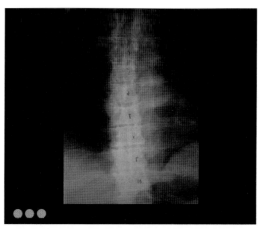

B3. A plain X-ray of the thoracic spine shows a left paraspinal mass at T6.

SCHWANNOMA (CASE TWO)

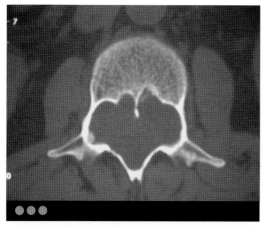

C. Axial CT shows lobulated expansion of the bony spinal canal due to a schwannoma.

737

SCHWANNOMA

Nerve sheath tumors usually involve the dorsal nerve roots and may be located anywhere in the spine. Sometimes, schwannomas can be cystic and exhibit ring-like contrast enhancement.

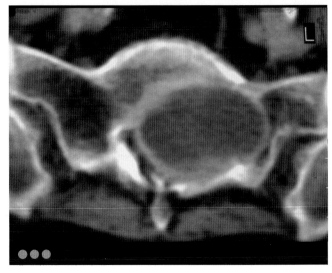

A. Axial, post contrast CT shows a cystic mass involving the sacrum on the left side.

DIFFERENTIAL DIAGNOSIS

At a Glance.

- *Epidermoid Cyst* (not pictured)

- *Metastasis* (not pictured)

- *Neuroenteric Cyst* (not pictured)

PART III

PLAIN RADIOGRAPHY

Chapter 24

Skull Defects and Lesions

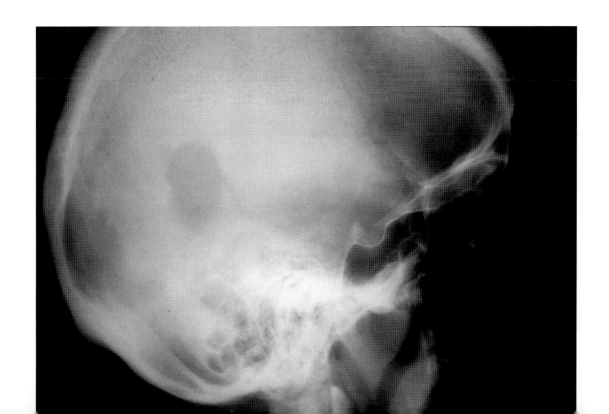

EOSINOPHILIC GRANULOMA (LANGERHAN'S CELL GRANULOMATOSIS)

Eosinophilic granuloma (EG) is a solitary, non-neoplastic proliferation of histiocytes. EG is a part of a spectrum of Langerhan's cell histiocytosis. It shows uneven destruction of the inner and outer table of the skull creating so-called "beveled edge" or "hole in a hole" appearance. "Button sequestrum" may be seen. The margin is usually not sclerotic.

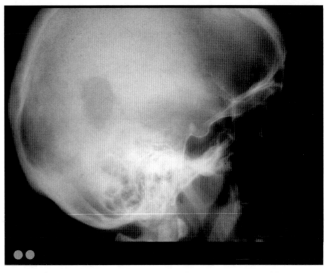

A. A lateral skull X-ray shows a lytic skull defect with irregular margin. Note there is no sclerosis around the defect.

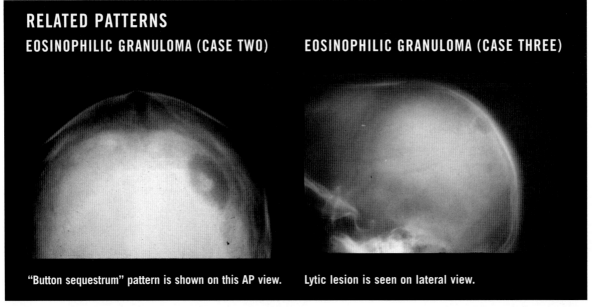

RELATED PATTERNS

EOSINOPHILIC GRANULOMA (CASE TWO)

EOSINOPHILIC GRANULOMA (CASE THREE)

"Button sequestrum" pattern is shown on this AP view.

Lytic lesion is seen on lateral view.

DIFFERENTIAL DIAGNOSIS

At a Glance:

- *Arachnoid Granulation (Normal Structure)*
- *Arachnoid Cyst*
- *Encephalocele*
- *Epidermoid*
- *Fibrous Dysplasia*
- *Hemangioma*
- *Leptomeningeal Cyst*
- *Meningioma*

- *Neurofibromatosis*
- *Paget's Disease*
- *Aneurysm Bone Cyst* (not pictured)
- *Metastatic Lesion* (not pictured)
- *Osteomyelitis* (not pictured)
- *Osteoblastoma* (not pictured)
- *Plasmacytoma* (not pictured)
- *Radiation Necrosis* (not pictured)
- *Venous Lake* (not pictured)

ARACHNOID GRANULATION (NORMAL STRUCTURE)

Arachnoid (pacchionian) **granulations** involve predominantly the inner table of the skull and are seen along the sagittal or transverse sinus. Well-defined cortical margin is seen. Occasionally they may be large enough to produce a deformity of the outer table of the skull.

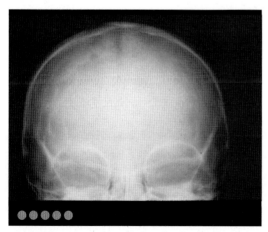

B1. AP and lateral views of the skull show remodeling of the inner table of the skull along the parasagittal region.

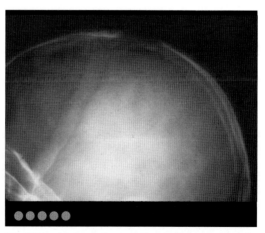

B2. AP and lateral views of the skull show remodeling of the inner table of the skull along the parasagittal region.

ARACHNOID CYST

Arachnoid cysts are cerebrospinal fluid collections covered by arachnoid cells and collagen that may develop between the surface of the brain and the calvarium or on the arachnoid membrane.

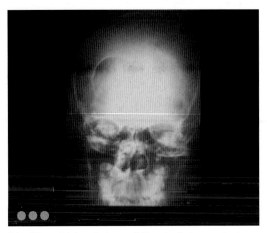

C1. AP and lateral views of the skull demonstrate a lytic skull defect caused by the remodeling of inner table of the skull by an arachnoid cyst.

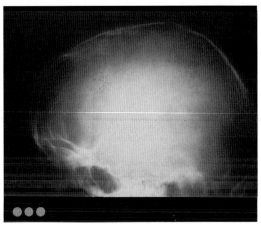

C2. AP and lateral views of the skull demonstrate a lytic skull defect caused by the remodeling of inner table of the skull by an arachnoid cyst.

ENCEPHALOCELE

An **encephalocele** is the result of failure of the surface ectoderm to separate from neuroectoderm. A skull and dural defect occurs, which allows the herniation of CSF, brain tissue, and meninges.

ENCEPHALOCELE (CASE ONE)

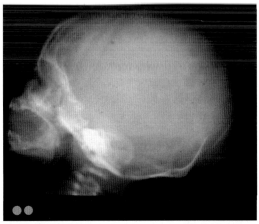

D. Lateral skull X-ray demonstrates the presence of an occipital encephalocele with a skull defect in the occipital bone.

ENCEPHALOCELE (CASE TWO)

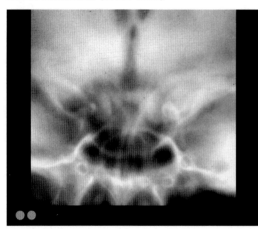

E1. AP and lateral tomograms demonstrate the remodeling of cribriform plate due to an encephalocele.

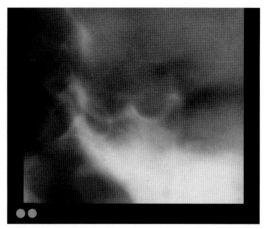

E2. AP and lateral tomograms demonstrate the remodeling of cribriform plate due to an encephalocele.

ENCEPHALOCELE (CASE THREE)

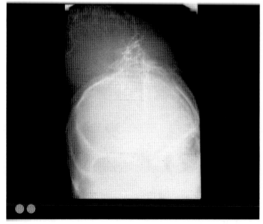

F. AP view of the skull shows a large frontal encephalocele with skull defect. The encephalocele is supplied by anterior cerebral arteries.

EPIDERMOID

Epidermoid exhibits purely lytic defect without calcification most commonly seen in temporal and occipital region. A sclerotic margin is seen. Only 10% of central nervous system **epidermoid** occurs in the diploic space.

EPIDERMOID (CASE ONE)

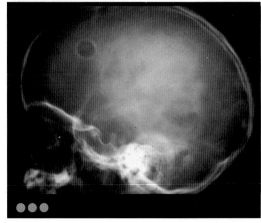

G. A lateral view of the skull demonstrates a round, radiolucent lesion with sclerotic margin. This solitary lytic lesion is an epidermoid.

EPIDERMOID (CASE TWO)

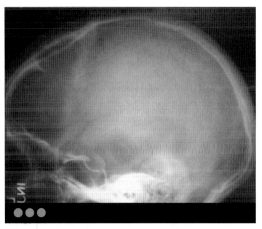

H1. Lateral and AP views of the skull demonstrate a lucent lesion with sclerotic margin.

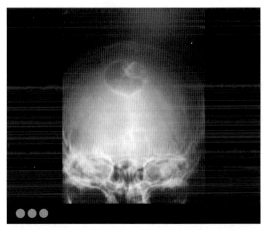

H2. Lateral and AP views of the skull demonstrate a lucent lesion with sclerotic margin.

FIBROUS DYSPLASIA

Fibrous dysplasia is a disease of unknown etiology in which the osteoblasts fail to mature and differentiate. The monostotic form (70–80%) is frequently asymptomatic and is discovered incidentally. Skull and facial bone involvement occurs in 20–30% of these patients. Skull abnormalities seen in fibrous dysplasia may be sclerotic or lytic. The lytic form usually involves the calvarium and consists of blister like expansion and thinning of the outer table, with a ground glass appearance centrally.

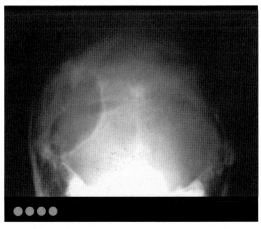

I. AP view of the skull shows a large skull defect with sclerotic margin.

HEMANGIOMA

Hemangiomas are lytic lesions with a "sunburst" or "soap bubble" appearance. Occasionally a sclerotic margin is seen. Hemangiomas arise from the diploic space and expand the outer table and are confined by the inner table.

HEMANGIOMA (CASE ONE)

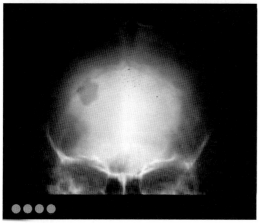

J1. AP view of the skull shows a lytic skull defect with lobulated margin.

HEMANGIOMA (CASE TWO)

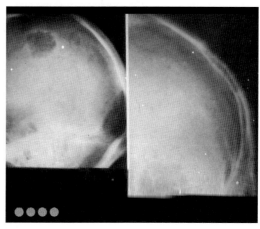

J2. AP and lateral views of the skull demonstrate a skull defect with honeycomb appearance.

HEMANGIOMA (CASE THREE)

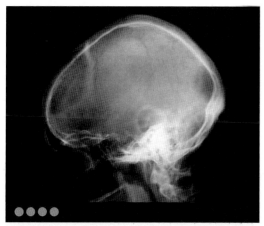

K1. Lateral and AP views of the skull reveal a defect with sclerotic margin and internal sunburst appearance.

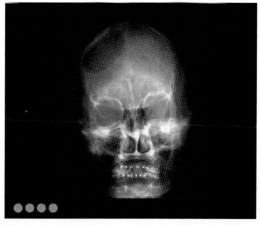

K2. Lateral and AP views of the skull reveal a defect with sclerotic margin and internal sunburst appearance.

LEPTOMENINGEAL CYST

Leptomeningeal cyst is a delayed complication of skull fracture with dural tear, usually occurring in a young child. The term "growing skull fracture" refers to interval enlargement of the skull defect on successive skull X-rays due to the erosion of the skull by herniated arachnoid with pulsating CSF.

LEPTOMENINGEAL CYST (CASE ONE)

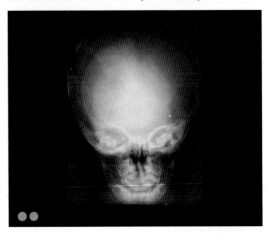

L1. AP and lateral views of the skull show a lytic skull defect with elongated margin.

LEPTOMENINGEAL CYST (CASE TWO)

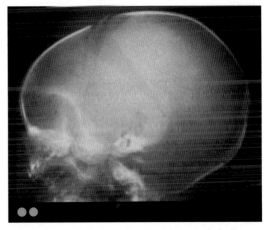

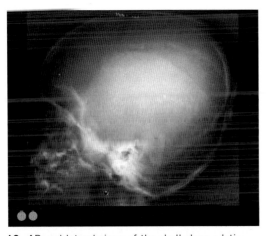

L2. AP and lateral views of the skull show a lytic skull defect with elongated margin

M. Lateral skull X-ray shows an elongated skull defect.

MENINGIOMA

Occasionally **meningioma** may show lytic changes. Meningiomas are usually associated with bony hyperostosis and calcification; bone destruction is unusual.

MENINGIOMA (CASE ONE)

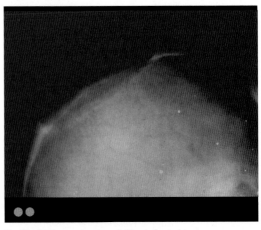

N. Skull X-ray shows a lytic defect due to meningioma.

MENINGIOMA (CASE TWO)

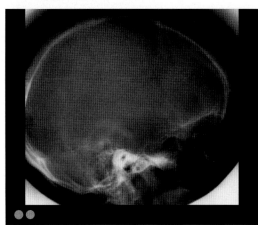

01. A lateral skull X-ray demonstrates focal mixed lytic and blastic changes of the skull in the frontal region.

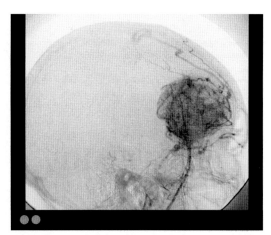

02. A lateral view of the cerebral angiogram shows a dense tumor vascular stain of a meningioma. The vascular stain in meningioma characteristically appears early and stays longer than other types of tumor stain.

NEUROFIBROMATOSIS

Skull defects associated with neurofibromatosis can occur along the sagittal suture (single) or lambdoid suture (uni- or bilateral). These are dysplastic changes of the skull secondary to **neurofibromatosis**.

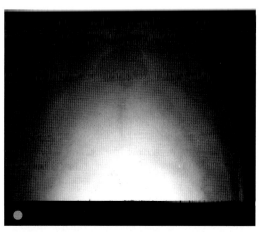

P. A skull defect is seen along the sagittal suture.

PAGET'S DISEASE

Skull involvement in **Paget's disease** is second in frequency only to involvement of the lumbar spine and pelvis. Three stages of **Paget's disease** are recognized. The osteolytic phase is most frequently seen in the skull, also known as osteoporosis circumscripta. It appears as a well-defined lytic lesion without a sclerotic margin. Suture line does not provide a barrier for growth of these lesions. The lytic phase is followed by evidence of osteogenesis. Areas of osteolysis and osteosclerosis merge imperceptibly with each other. The trabecular pattern is thickened and disorganized and the tables of the skull become thickened. The third stage of Paget's disease is the inactive or healing phase. The lesions become more sclerotic and thickening of the tables of the skull is more obvious.

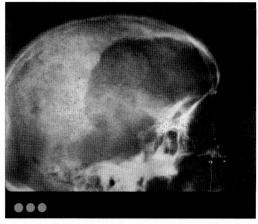

Q. A lateral view of the skull shows a large lytic defect due to Paget's disease.

METASTATIC LESIONS

Primary sites are usually breast, lung, prostate, kidney, thyroid, and melanoma. Diploic space is involved before the inner or outer table of the skull. Because of its rich blood supply, the calvarium is more commonly involved than the skull base.

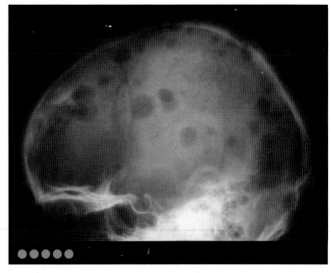

A. A lateral view of the skull shows multiple osteolytic defects, consistent with metastatic disease.

DIFFERENTIAL DIAGNOSIS

At a Glance:

- *Hyperparathyroidism*
- *Langerhan's Cell Histiocytosis*
- *Multiple Myeloma*
- *Parietal Foramina*
- *Arachnoid Granulation* (not pictured)
- *Osteomyelitis* (not pictured)
- *Radiation Necrosis* (not pictured)
- *Venous Lake* (not pictured)

HYPERPARATHYROIDISM

Among patients with primary **hyperparathyroidism**, calvarial changes occur in 10–20% of the cases. Pathologically, there is osteoclastic resorption in all tables of the skull, associated with reparative fibrosis and formation of immature bone. Mottled demineralization, followed by ground-glass appearance are the usual imaging findings.

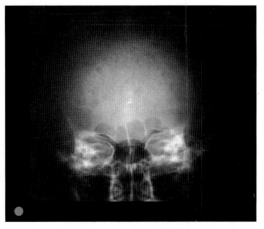

B1. AP and lateral views of the skull demonstrate multiple ill-defined lucent skull defects.

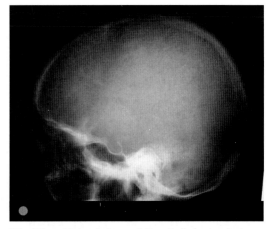

B2. AP and lateral views of the skull demonstrate multiple ill-defined lucent skull defects.

LANGERHAN'S CELL HISTIOCYTOSIS

Eosinophilic granuloma is characterized by skeletal lesions, and it predominantly affects children, and young adults. Solitary lesions are more commonly seen than multiple lesions. Any bone may be involved including the skull, mandible, ribs, long bones of the upper extremity, pelvis, and spine. Calvarial lesions have a classic "beveled edge" appearance.

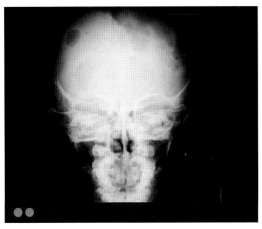

C1. AP and lateral views of the skull demonstrate multiple lytic skull defects.

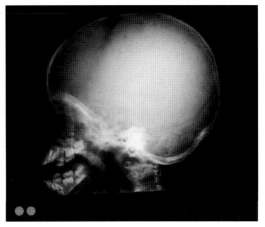

C2. AP and lateral views of the skull demonstrate multiple lytic skull defects.

MULTIPLE MYELOMA

Multiple myeloma manifests as an osteolytic process similar to metastatic disease. The skull is the third most frequently affected structure after the vertebral column and ribs. Mandibular involvement is seen in a third of the cases and may help to differentiate myeloma from metastatic disease.

MULTIPLE MYELOMA (CASE ONE)

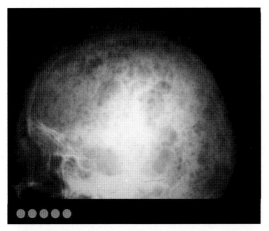

D. A lateral view of the skull demonstrates multiple, small and round defects with punched out appearance and without reactive sclerosis.

MULTIPLE MYELOMA (CASE TWO)

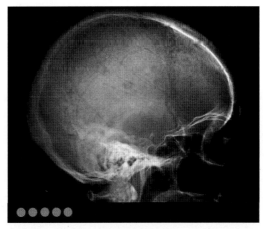

E. A lateral view of the skull shows multiple, scattered defects involving the skull.

751

PARIETAL FORAMINA (NORMAL STRUCTURE)

Parietal foramina are symmetrical normal structures seen on either side of the sagittal suture in posterior third of the parietal bone.

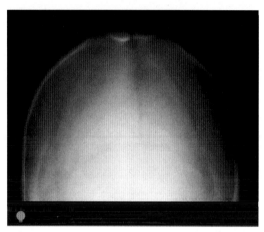

F1. AP and lateral views of the skull show symmetrical defects bilaterally.

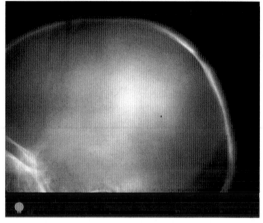

F2. AP and lateral views of the skull show symmetrical defects bilaterally.

OSTEOMA

Osteomas may involve either table, but more commonly the inner table of the skull. Osteomas appear as flat-based, well-marginated domes of dense bone. They do not involve the diploic space.

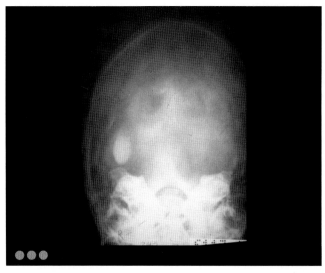

A. A Towne's projection X-ray shows a focal area of increased bony density with well-defined margin on the right side, consistent with an osteoma.

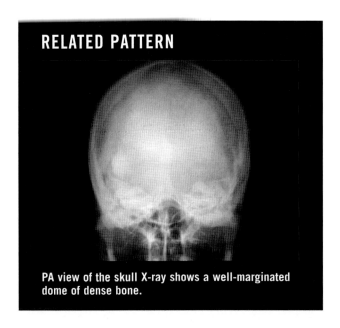

RELATED PATTERN

PA view of the skull X-ray shows a well-marginated dome of dense bone.

DIFFERENTIAL DIAGNOSIS

At a Glance:

- *Fibrous Dysplasia*
- *Hemangioma*
- *Hyperostosis Frontalis Interna*

- *Meningioma*
- *Chronic Osteomyelitis*
- *Metastasis* (not pictured)
- *Paget's Disease* (not pictured)

FIBROUS DYSPLASIA

Fibrous dysplasia is a skeletal developmental anomaly. The medullary bone is replaced by fibrous tissue. Malignant degeneration, although uncommon, may occur in fibrous dysplasia. On plain X-ray, it has a classic "ground glass" appearance.

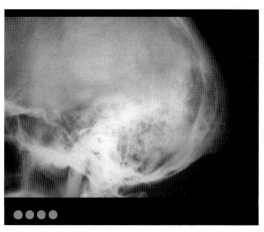

B. A lateral view of the skull shows focal thickening of the occipital bone due to fibrous dysplasia.

HEMANGIOMA

Hemangiomas arise from the diploic space and expand the outer table. There are four types of hemangioma, namely, capillary, cavernous, arteriovenous and venous types. Bone hemangiomas are predominantly of the capillary and cavernous types. Skull hemangiomas are usually of the cavernous variety.

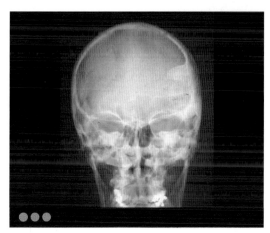

O. AP view of the skull shows a dense lesion with sclerotic margin and internal septa along the inner table of the calvarium on the left side.

HYPEROSTOSIS FRONTALIS INTERNA

Hyperostosis frontalis interna is an idiopathic benign condition with abnormal deposition of bone on the inner table of the frontal bone of the skull. It is usually seen in women.

It is important to recognize this entity and not to confuse it with pathological conditions. It may be a part of Morgagni's syndrome, which consists of hyperostosis frontalis interna, obesity, and virilism.

HYPEROSTOSIS FRONTALIS INTERNA (CASE ONE)

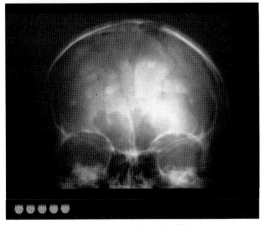

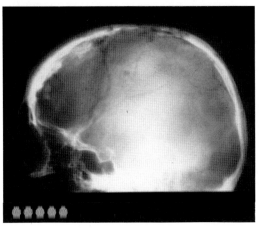

D1. AP and lateral views of the skull demonstrate multiple small foci of calvarial thickening involving the inner table in the frontal bone bilaterally.

D2. AP and lateral views of the skull demonstrate multiple small foci of calvarial thickening involving the inner table in the frontal bone bilaterally.

HYPEROSTOSIS FRONTALIS INTERNA (CASE TWO)

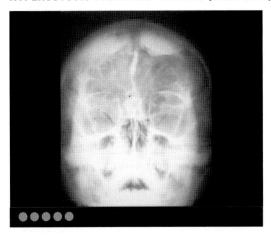

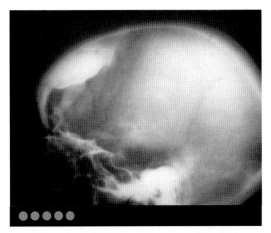

E1. AP and lateral views of the skull demonstrate focal skull thickening involving the inner table of the frontal bone bilaterally.

E2. AP and lateral views of the skull demonstrate focal skull thickening involving the inner table of the frontal bone bilaterally.

MENINGIOMA

The skull changes associated with **meningiomas** may be osteolytic (rare), osteoblastic, or mixed. Osteoblastic changes are more commonly seen.

MENINGIOMA (CASE ONE)

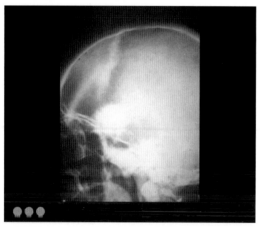

F. A lateral view of the skull shows focal increased bony density in the region of planum sphenoidale, consistent with a calcified meningioma.

MENINGIOMA (CASE TWO)

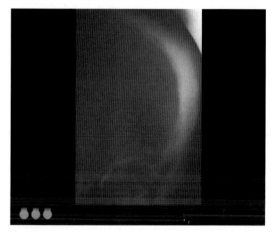

G. AP view of the skull shows focal thickening of the skull due to hyperostosis caused by meningioma.

MENINGIOMA (CASE THREE)

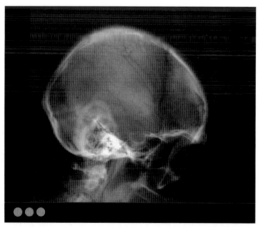

H. A lateral view of the skull reveals focal hyperostosis of the skull in the frontal region.

MENINGIOMA (CASE FOUR)

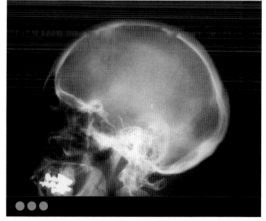

I. A lateral view of the skull demonstrates focal hyperostosis in the region of planum sphenoidale. It is sometimes called "blistering of the planum sphenoidale".

CHRONIC OSTEOMYELITIS

Osteomyelitis of the skull is a rare clinical entity. It usually occurs as a complication of previous trauma or sinusitis. Its complications can be life threatening and requires immediate treatment. However, the initial symptoms and signs are usually subtle and early diagnosis could be challenging. The incidence of calvarial osteomyelitis is about 1.5% of all osteomyelitis. Osteomyelitis usually present as lytic skull lesions. Chronic Osteomyelitis may show focal calvarial thickening on skull X-ray.

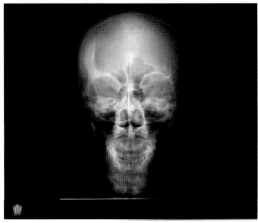

J1. AP and lateral views of the skull demonstrate focal calvarial thickening in the right frontal region due to osteomyelitis.

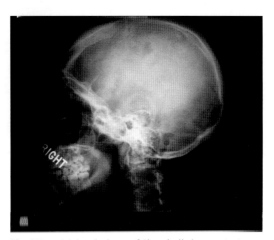

J2. AP and lateral views of the skull demonstrate focal calvarial thickening in the right frontal region due to osteomyelitis.

SHUNTED HYDROCEPHALUS

In children with hydrocephalus, skull thickening can develop following the placement of shunt to treat the hydrocephalus. With shunt placement, the cerebral volume will decrease and creating a space for skull to grow inward.

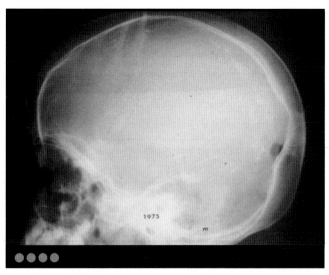

A. A lateral view of the skull shows diffuse thickening of the calvarium in a patient who had shunt placement for hydrocephalus. This condition occurs in children with long term shunt placement for hydrocephalus.

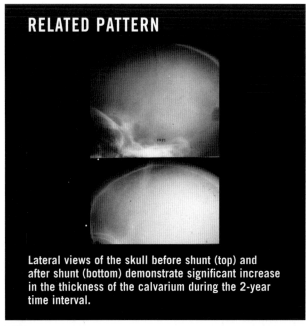

RELATED PATTERN

Lateral views of the skull before shunt (top) and after shunt (bottom) demonstrate significant increase in the thickness of the calvarium during the 2-year time interval.

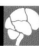

DIFFERENTIAL DIAGNOSIS

At a Glance:

- *Increased Intracranial Pressure*
- *Mucolipidosis*
- *Osteomyelitis*
- *Paget's Disease*
- *Acromegaly* (not pictured)

- *Anemias* (not pictured)
- *Fibrous Dysplasia* (not pictured)
- *Fluorosis* (not pictured)
- *Metastases* (not pictured)
- *Myelofibrosis* (not pictured)
- *Osteopetrosis* (not pictured)
- *Phenytoin* (not pictured)

INCREASED INTRACRANIAL PRESSURE

Increased intracranial pressure can cause calvarial thickening with increased digital marking, so called "silver beaten appearance".

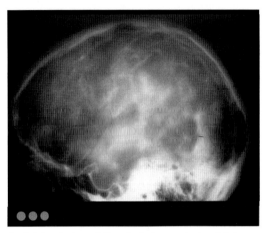

B. A lateral view of the skull demonstrates thickening of the skull with increased digital marking due to increased intracranial pressure.

MUCOLIPIDOSIS

Mucolipidosis are a group of rare, inherited metabolic disorders that affect the body's ability to carry out the routine turnover of various materials, such as carbohydrates or lipids within cells. Calvarial thickening, premature suture closure, shallow orbits, J-shaped sella are seen in mucolipidosis type III.

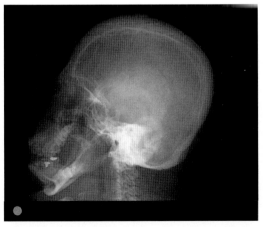

C1. Lateral and AP views of the skull reveal diffuse calvarial thickening in a patient with mucolipiodosis.

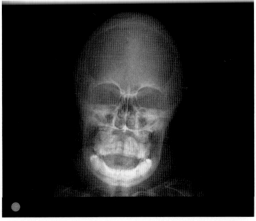

C2. Lateral and AP views of the skull reveal diffuse calvarial thickening in a patient with mucolipiodosis.

OSTEOMYELITIS

Osteomyelitis of the skull has a different appearance from that seen elsewhere. Periosteal reaction is extremely rare. Rapid and widespread involvement is the rule due to the extensive diploic venous network. Chronic **osteomyelitis** shows a mixed lytic and sclerotic pattern with the sclerotic process dominating. Underlying pathogen may be tuberculosis, syphilis, or fungus.

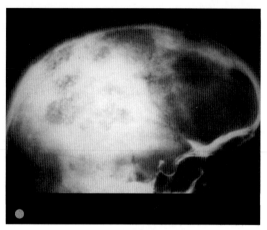

D. A lateral view of the skull shows patchy thickening of the skull due to chronic osteomyelitis.

PAGET'S DISEASE

The lytic phase of **Paget's disease** is followed by evidence of osteogenesis. Areas of osteolysis and osteosclerosis merge imperceptibly with each other. The trabecular pattern is thickened and disorganized and the tables of the skull become thickened. The third stage of **Paget's disease** is the inactive or healing phase. The lesions become more sclerotic and thickening of the tables of the skull is more obvious.

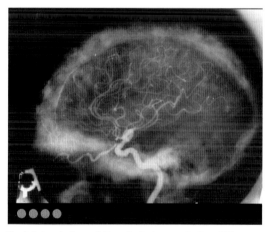

E. A lateral view of the skull demonstrates diffuse thickening of the calvarium with mixed density. Contrast is seen in the intracranial vessels.

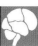

STURGE–WEBER SYNDROME

Sturge–Weber syndrome, also known as encephalotrigeminal angiomatosis, is a congenital vascular disorder of the brain, meninges, and the face in the trigeminal distribution, often involving the eye. The intracranial lesion is an ipsilateral leptomeningeal vascular malformation between the pia and arachnoid membranes. Abnormal cerebral venous drainage is the primary abnormality, with resultant venous hypertension leading to gradual cell death, progressive atrophy, and calcification of the cortex. A parietal, occipital location is most common. Angiomas may involve the choroid plexus and eye. Skull X-ray shows the typical "tram track" calcification and unilateral calvarial thickening.

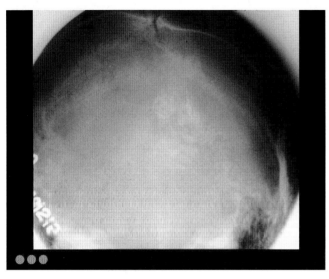

A1. AP and lateral views of the skull show calvarial thickening on the left side. The presence of tram-track type of calcification is also seen.

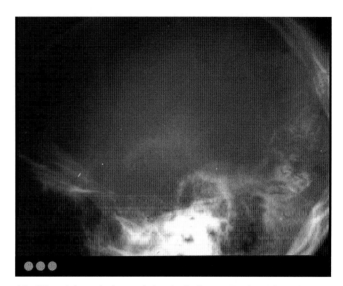

A2. AP and lateral views of the skull show calvarial thickening on the left side. The presence of tram-track type of calcification is also seen.

DIFFERENTIAL DIAGNOSIS

At a Glance:

• *Dyke-Davidoff-Mason Syndrome* (not pictured)

DOLICHOCEPHALY (SCAPHOCEPHALY)

Dolicocephaly is a type of craniosynostosis. It presents as an elongated, narrow skull secondary to total or partial premature closure of the sagittal suture. This creates a frontal bossing appearance due to the skull growth at the area of coronal sutures. It is also called scaphocephaly.

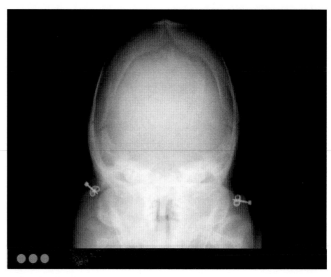

A. AP view of the skull shows an elongated, narrow skull secondary premature closure of the sagittal suture.

DIFFERENTIAL DIAGNOSIS

At a Glance:

- *Brachycephaly*
- *Plagiocephaly*
- *Trigonocephaly*

OTHER CRANIOSYNOSTOSIS

BRACHYCEPHALY

Bilateral coronal synostosis is more frequently seen in association with malformation syndromes. It is commonly associated with other sutural closure (50%).

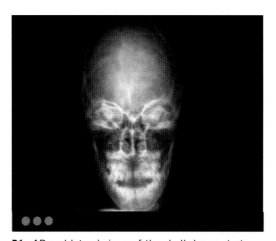

B1. AP and lateral views of the skull demonstrate shortening of the skull due to premature closure of the coronal suture.

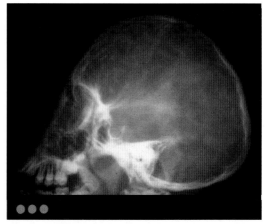

B2. AP and lateral views of the skull demonstrate shortening of the skull due to premature closure of the coronal suture.

PLAGIOCEPHALY

Premature closure of the coronal suture unilaterally causes unilateral flattening of the skull known as **plagiocephaly.**

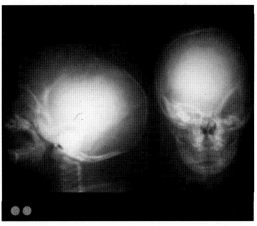

C. AP and lateral views of the skull show deformity of the skull with elevation of the left orbital rim.

TRIGONOCEPHALY

Premature closure of the metopic suture causes a keel shaped deformity of the anterior skull known as **trigono cephaly.** Secondary features include ethmoid hypoplasia, hypoterolism, and tilting of the orbits toward each other.

PITUITARY ADENOMA

Pituitary adenoma can cause the enlargement of the sellar turcica with erosion of the dorsum sella. Tilting of the floor of the sellar turcica may also be seen.

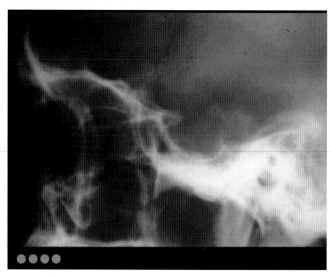

A. A lateral view of the sella turcica shows a ballooned sella turcica with expansion into the sphenoid sinus. The tip of dorsum and clinoids are displaced upward. No tumor calcification is seen. This enlargement of the sella turcica is due to a pituitary adenoma.

DIFFERENTIAL DIAGNOSIS

At a Glance:

- *Craniopharyngioma*
- *Hydrocephalus*
- *Increased Intracranial Pressure*
- *J Shaped Sella*
- *Aneurysm* (not pictured)
- *Empty Sella* (not pictured)

CRANIOPHARYNGIOMA

Craniopharyngioma can cause the enlargement of the sellar turcica if there is intrasellar extension of the tumor.

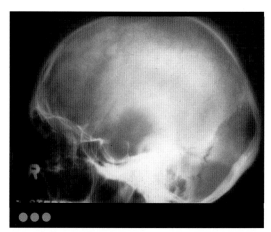

B. A lateral view of the skull shows enlarged sella turcica. Craniopharyngioma is frequently associated with suprasellar calcification.

HYDROCEPHALUS

Hydrocephalus can cause enlargement of the sellar trucica due to increased intracranial pressure. Sometimes, a dilated anterior third ventricle may herniate into the sellar turcica causing its enlargement.

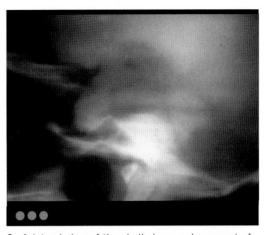

C. A lateral view of the skull shows enlargement of the sella turcica due to hydrocephalus. Note the contrast filled, dilated anterior third ventricle is seen extending into the sella turcica.

INCREASED INTRACRANIAL PRESSURE

Increased intracranial pressure can cause enlargement of the sellar turcica.

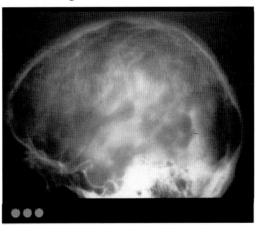

D. A lateral view of the skull shows enlarged sella turcica and increased digital markings of the skull due to increased intracranial pressure.

J-SHAPED SELLA

J-shaped sella can be due to Hurler's syndrome, hypothyroidism, optic glioma, neurofibromatosis, and arrested hydrocephalus. It may also be seen as a normal variant.

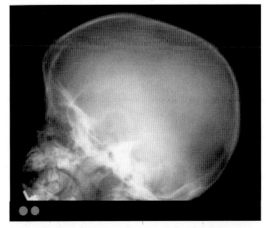

E. A lateral skull X-ray shows a J-shaped sella in a patient with Hurler's syndrome (mucopolysaccharidosis type I). Other diseases that can exhibit J-shaped sella include hypothyroidism, optic glioma, neurofibromatosis, mild arrested hydrocephalus, and a normal variant.

SUPRASELLAR CALCIFICATION

Craniopharyngioma is the most common cause of suprasellar calcification. Aneurysms may show curvilinear calcification. Adenoma with suprasellar extension rarely shows calcification.

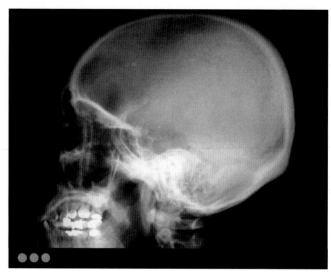

A. A lateral view of the skull demonstrates suprasellar calcification due to craniopharyngioma.

DIFFERENTIAL DIAGNOSIS

At a Glance:

- Oligodendroglioma
- Multiple Meningioma
- Dural Calcification
- Sturge–Weber Syndrome
- OMV Microcephaly
- Tuberculosis

- Pineal Region Calcification
- Tumor Calcification (not pictured)
- Vascular Calcification (not pictured)
- Aneurysm (not pictured)
- Arteriovenous Malformation (not pictured)
- Infectious Calcification (not pictured)
- Cysticercosis (not pictured)

OLIGODENDROGLIOMA

Calcification is seen in 30–40% of the cases of **oligodendroglioma** on plain X-ray and has a popcorn-like appearance.

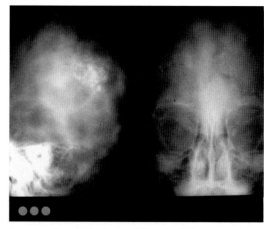

B. Lateral and AP views of the skull demonstrate calcification due to oligodendroglioma.

MULTIPLE MENINGIOMA

Calcification is seen in meningioma in about 15–20% of the cases. Multiple meningiomas can be sporadic, due to previous radiation or due to Neurofibromatosis type II.

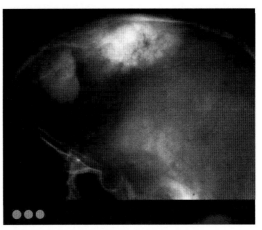

C. A lateral view of the skull shows multiple calcifications intracranially due to meningiomas.

DURAL CALCIFICATION

Calcification of the anterior portion of the falx is the most common **dural calcification**. Calcification of the dura of the superior sagittal sinuses is more common in females. Calcification of the tentorium is also commonly seen. Extensive **dural calcification** has been described in disorders of calcium homeostasis, pseudoxanthoma elasticum, and basal cell nevus syndrome.

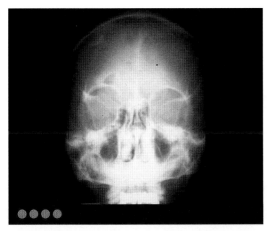

D1. AP and lateral views of the skull show dural calcification.

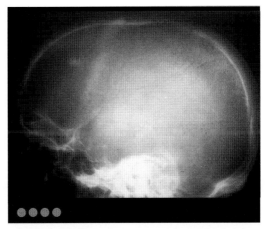

D2. AP and lateral views of the skull show dural calcification.

STURGE–WEBER SYNDROME

Sturge–Weber syndrome, also known as encephalotrigem-inal angiomatosis, is a congenital vascular disorder of the brain, meninges, and the face in the trigeminal distribution. Abnormal cerebral venous drainage is the primary abnormality, with resultant venous hypertension leading to gradual cell death, progressive atrophy, and calcification of the cortex. A parietal, occipital location is most common. Skull X-ray shows the typical "tram track" calcification and unilateral calvarial thickening.

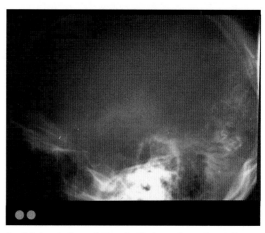

E. A lateral view of the skull shows tram-track type of calcification intracranially.

CMV MICROCEPHALY

Cytomegalovirus infection occurs in approximately 1% of all births. The symptoms and signs of the disease include microcephaly, impaired hearing, developmental anomalies, hepatosplenomegaly, seizures and chorioretinitis. The virus causes damage to the brain including polymicrogyria, gliosis of white matter, delayed mylination, intracranial calcifications, and Microcephaly.

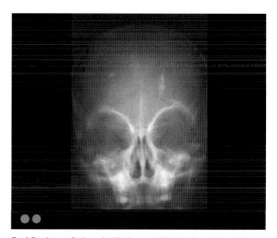

F. AP view of the skull shows bilateral periventricular calcification.

TUBERCULOSIS

Tuberculosis is a caseating granulomatous disease. Healed lesions of tuberculosis may show calcification.

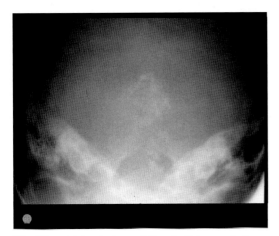

G1 AP and lateral views of the skull demonstrate the presence of amorphous calcification in the region of the fourth ventricle secondary to tuberculosis.

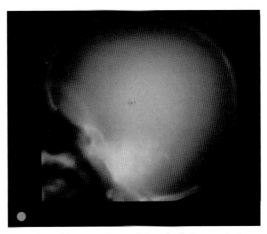

G2. AP and lateral views of the skull demonstrate the presence of amorphous calcification in the region of the fourth ventricle secondary to tuberculosis.

PINEAL REGION CALCIFICATION

Pineal calcification is seen on skull X-ray in 33–76% of the adults and is rare in children under the age of 6. The presence of **pineal calcification** in children less than 6 years should raise the suspicion of a pineal region neoplasm. Physiologic calcification is usually 3–5 mm in size. Calcification larger than 10 mm is probably associated with neoplasm.

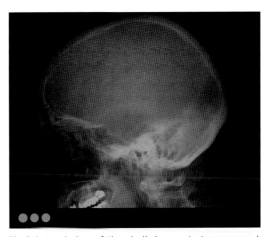

H. A Lateral view of the skull demonstrates a normal pineal calcification in an adult.

INDEX

777